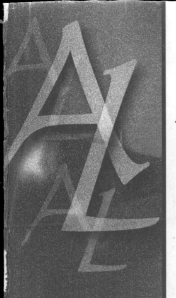

Applying the
ROPER·LOGAN·TIERNEY MODEL IN PRACTICE

Commissioning Editor: Ninette Premdas
Development Editor: Fiona Conn
Project Manager: Christine Johnston
Design Direction: Erik Bigland
Illustration Manager: Merlyn Harvey
Illustrator: Graeme Chambers

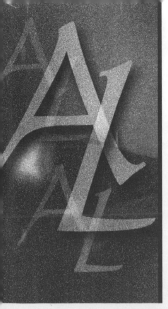

Applying the
ROPER • LOGAN • TIERNEY MODEL IN PRACTICE

Editor

Karen Holland BSc(Hons) MSc CertEd SRN
Professorial Fellow, School of Nursing, University of Salford, Salford, UK

Associate Editors

Jane Jenkins BA MSc SRN RNT
Senior Lecturer, School of Nursing, University of Salford, Salford, UK

Jackie Solomon MA PGDip SRN
Honorary Lecturer, School of Nursing, University of Salford, Salford, UK

Sue Whittam BA(Hons) MA RGN RCNT RNT
Head of Organisational Development and Learning, Bolton Hospitals NHS Trust, Bolton, UK

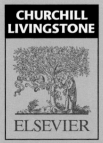

EDINBURGH LONDON NEW YORK OXFORD PHILADELPHIA ST LOUIS SYDNEY TORONTO 2008

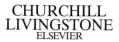

CHURCHILL
LIVINGSTONE
ELSEVIER

© 2003, 2008, Elsevier Limited. All rights reserved.

First edition 2003
Second edition 2008

ISBN: 9780443104053

British Library Cataloguing in Publication Data
A catalogue record for this book is available from the British Library

Library of Congress Cataloging in Publication Data
A catalog record for this book is available from the Library of Congress

Note

Knowledge and best practice in this field are constantly changing. As new research and experience broaden our knowledge, changes in practice, treatment and drug therapy may become necessary or appropriate. Readers are advised to check the most current information provided (i) on procedures featured or (ii) by the manufacturer of each product to be administered, to verify the recommended dose or formula, the method and duration of administration, and contraindications. It is the responsibility of the practitioner, relying on their own experience and knowledge of the patient, to make diagnoses, to determine dosages and the best treatment for each individual patient, and to take all appropriate safety precautions. To the fullest extent of the law, neither the Publisher nor the Authors assumes any liability for any injury and/or damage to persons or property arising out or related to any use of the material contained in this book.
The Publisher

The publisher's policy is to use paper manufactured from sustainable forests

Printed in China

Contents

Contributors

Karen Holland BSc(Hons) MSc CertEd SRN
Professorial Fellow, School of Nursing, University of Salford, Salford, UK

Helen Iggulden BA(Hons) MSc PGCE RGN
Lecturer, School of Nursing, University of Salford, Salford, UK

Jane Jenkins BA MSc SRN RNT
Senior Lecturer, School of Nursing, University of Salford, Salford, UK

Debbie Roberts PhD BSc(Hons) PGCert (Learning and Teaching) RGN
Lecturer in Nursing, School of Nursing, University of Salford, Salford, UK

Julia Ryan BA(Hons) MA RNT RN
Senior Lecturer, School of Nursing, University of Salford, Salford, UK

Jackie Solomon MA PGDip SRN
Honorary Lecturer, School of Nursing, University of Salford, Salford, UK

Susan Walker BSc(Hons) MA PGCE RGN
Lecturer in Nursing and Clinical Skills, School of Nursing, University of Salford, Salford, UK

Sue Whittam BA(Hons) MA RGN RCNT RNT
Head of Organisational Development and Learning, Bolton Hospitals NHS Trust, Bolton, UK

Acknowledgements

The task of writing this second edition would not have been possible without some help from each other as well as colleagues. We would particularly like to thank the non-editorial contributors again who have given us the benefit of their expertise and have delivered well-written and accessible information.

We wish to thank all those who have reviewed the book, in particular the students, both formally and informally for their helpful comments which have contributed to this revised second edition. We especially wish to thank Jean Williams, the Head Librarian at the Post Graduate Medical Education Centre in the Bolton Hospitals NHS Trust, for her support with searching the evidence.

All of us wish to thank our families for putting up again with angst and elation, and also for ensuring that we were fed and suitably hydrated!

We especially wish to thank Fiona Conn and Michèle le Roux, Development Editors at Elsevier, Christine Johnston, Project Manager, and Ninette Premdas, Commissioning Editor, for their support, constructive criticism and reassurance throughout the project. Thank you also to Jef Boys for his excellent editing and patience.

Finally we wish to thank again Nancy Roper, Winifred Logan and Alison Tierney for the model for nursing on which this book is based. Their perseverance over time during its development and the promotion of its use in practice, and its standing value as a framework for care delivery, are commendable. It is, in our experience, an invaluable resource for nurses in practice and as a tool for helping student nurses link theory and practice. This book would not be possible without what has become known as the Roper–Logan–Tierney model for nursing. It was with great sadness that we learnt of the death of Nancy Roper in 2004. She will be remembered not only for the development of the Roper–Logan–Tierney model of nursing but as a person who made a significant contribution to the nursing profession.

Preface

The Roper–Logan–Tierney model for nursing has been widely used in practice areas in the UK, and as a consequence has been used within many UK schools of nursing to teach students how to link the theory and practice of nursing (Roper et al 2000).

This book has been written to enable students and their teachers (in higher education and clinical practice) to explore the different dimensions of the model through a variety of case studies and exercises. The case studies can be viewed as 'triggers' for student problem-solving skills in using the model, not just as a checklist for assessment, but as an approach to patient care. They will also enable students to identify and understand how the model can help them in caring for patients and clients in a variety of practice settings. The chapters focus mainly on caring for adults and older people, although the influence of childhood on adult health and illness is explored in the different chapters in keeping with the elements of the model itself.

We do not offer a critique of the model, an issue which Roper et al (2000, p. 158) visit in their monograph. Rather we offer an exploration of how we believe the model can be used to guide practice in caring for patients, and to enhance student learning about a variety of patient-care situations. Like Roper et al (2000), we believe that its use in so many clinical practice contexts has established it as a valued framework for care delivery.

It is intended that the book will show, through each chapter and its associated case studies, exercises and information, how the Roper–Logan–Tierney model for nursing (Roper et al 1996) can be used as a model for:

- understanding how we live in society
- nursing practice
- care planning
- teaching and learning.

This is not intended to be a 'recipe book' for caring for patients, but to offer students the opportunity to evaluate their own learning and understanding of different aspects of daily living, and to integrate the knowledge and skills into their practice as student nurses. Their mentors, as qualified practitioners, will also benefit through having a book that will enable them to 'unpack' the aspects making up the whole of their care practice, so that the students can clearly see the 'parts' that make up this whole.

In developing the case studies we have drawn both from our own experiences of clinical practice and from those of our students and colleagues. It is not an easy task to develop case studies that do not stereotype people and groups in society, but for the purpose of teaching and learning it is often unavoidable in order to illustrate different care contexts. We have made every attempt to avoid this, however, as well as trying not to sensationalise care situations. We welcome comments on these issues from readers.

This book offers pathways of decision-making supported by an evidence base. Each chapter will explore the model of nursing through focusing on each Activity of Living (AL) in turn, but demonstrating the interconnectedness of each one. We demonstrate that the model makes nurses aware of the importance of such integrated knowledge to a holistic approach to care.

The chapters themselves follow a similar pattern but allow for the individual nature of each activity. Each has a number of case studies through which that activity is explored, as well as a wide range of exercises, some of which encourage reflection on practice and others that will stimulate further learning and exploration by the reader. The book also encourages skills in literature searching and in using the internet as an information resource. Each chapter offers a list of useful websites related to the Activity of Living, as well as a list of further reading to enhance learning. Although the book is mainly focused on the health care system and nursing practice of England/UK, we have, whenever possible, integrated knowledge and exercises that enable readers in other countries to use it as a valued resource for learning.

Chapter structure

Each chapter is divided into two parts: the model of living and the model for nursing. Combined, they make up the Roper–Logan–Tierney model for nursing.

In Section 1 the authors illustrate how the model can be used to learn about the issues affecting lifespan and age, the factors affecting health and how the dependence/independence continuum can be affected by both health and illness. The use of the twelve ALs to illustrate the model's usefulness means that the book can be used as a single resource, through demonstrating the interconnectedness of such factors as physiological and psychological bases for care.

In Section 2 we use this knowledge, to strengthen this interlinking and to describe and explore the nursing care of individuals with health problems that mainly affect one particular Activity of Living. We also show how these impact on the other ALs. All chapters offer evidence to support rationale for practice and the underpinning knowledge base for care.

A brief summary of chapter contents

Chapter 1 An introduction to the Roper–Logan–Tierney model for nursing

This chapter is an introduction to the model for nursing and the basic principles underlying it. It also explores the use of the nursing process, which is then used in different ways in each chapter. The main focus is assessment of the patient using the model, which is used to plan, set goals (patient's and nurse's) and implement and evaluate the care given.

Chapter 2 Nursing and the context of care

As nursing takes place in a social and political context, as well as a historical one, it is necessary to offer an introductory background into some of the issues affecting care delivery. This chapter focuses on issues such as the nature of nursing and health care, nursing practice, and international, professional and educational developments.

Chapter 3 Maintaining a safe environment

This chapter focuses on the AL 'maintaining a safe environment', and illustrates use of the model by focusing on such factors as the effects of stress and pollution on health and the importance of observations to maintain patient safety in the nursing care of patients undergoing surgical intervention.

Chapter 4 Communicating

This chapter highlights the importance of the AL 'communicating', not simply as an activity we all undertake in various ways, but also its relevance to how we undertake all the other ALs. There is a particular focus on neurological problems such as those caused by a cerebrovascular accident or stroke. The importance of understanding the communication needs of different cultural groups is also explored.

Chapter 5 Breathing

This chapter helps us to understand the impact on breathing of such factors as smoking and asthma, in particular the interrelationship between breathing and the cardiovascular system. Both are illustrated through the use of a case study, which shows the impact of smoking and asthma on an individual's breathing and lifestyle.

Chapter 6 Eating and drinking

This chapter focuses on how what we eat and drink influences our lifestyles and health, and vice versa. Issues such as poor nutritional status of patients in acute care and the effect of illness on eating and drinking are explored in the case studies and exercises.

Chapter 7 Eliminating

Getting rid of waste products from our bodies is a necessary part of ensuring a balanced metabolism. Issues such as incontinence of urine are dealt with sensitively, as are the effects of various bowel problems. The main case study highlights the problems and care associated with recurrent urinary tract infections and enlarged prostate gland.

Chapter 8 Personal cleansing and dressing

The importance of how we dress and how we ensure personal cleanliness is linked to our society and culture, as well as our age and gender. It is influenced by many factors, explored in the chapter, as well as health problems, which can cause difficulties in maintaining our normal personal cleansing and dressing behaviours. The impact of such potentially debilitating skin problems as psoriasis, and the effects of lack of mobility on being able to care for oneself, are explored in the case studies.

Chapter 9 Controlling body temperature

Ensuring a normal core body temperature is imperative for survival, and caring for people where this is compromised is an essential part of a nurse's work. This chapter illustrates potential imbalances through a case study, where a child's body temperature is raised, as well as the impact of such problems as heat stroke and hypothermia.

Chapter 10 Mobilising

This chapter focuses on the AL of mobilising and those factors that either help or hinder this. For some people being mobile means using a wheelchair and for others being able to walk using two legs. The main case study highlights the problems that arise when an 84-year-old lady living on her own has a fall, and the section on biological factors offers an understanding of the physiology of movement and joints to underpin the care offered to this lady.

Chapter 11 Working and playing

Being able to work and play is an essential part of maintaining the health and wellbeing of the individual. Being unable to do one or both of these can cause a variety of health and social problems. Examples in this chapter include a woman who becomes disabled due to a chronic back problem and a man who suffers from a myocardial infarction (heart attack) and is no longer able to be as physically active as he was. Again we see the importance of the model as a framework for assessing the potential factors influencing the care-planning cycle.

Chapter 12 Expressing sexuality

Expressing our sexuality occurs in different ways in different cultures and societies, and our sexual behaviour very often mirrors our social and cultural background. This chapter describes the physiological differences between men and women, and how their bodies function. The case studies focus on exploring how the model can help define sensitive nursing care for patients with health problems that have a direct impact both on the way in which they express their sexuality and on their sexual behaviour. Cultural issues related to expressing sexuality are also explored sensitively.

Chapter 13 Sleeping

Adequate sleep is essential for health and well-being. Being deprived of sleep can cause a variety of health problems and vice versa. This chapter explores a range of situations where sleep is compromised and the main case study focuses on the health problem of rheumatoid arthritis. Changes in sleep patterns and levels of consciousness are also explored, and how these are monitored, e.g. the Glasgow Coma Scale.

Chapter 14 Dying

The inclusion of dying as the final act of living (Roper et al 1996) illustrates the importance for nurses of understanding the way in which we manage this potentially distressing event in both our patients' and their families' and friends' lives. This chapter includes the sociocultural aspects of death and associated practices in relation to the dead and the dying, and the main case study focuses on the needs of a dying man, his partner and the nurses caring for him. It is an example of how the model can be used to highlight the different types of knowledge and care skills required to care for a dying person.

The appendices include a sample care plan document, an example of a care plan documentation audit tool and a tool for using as a guide to assessing patients in each of the Activities of Living.

Writing this revised book has, like its predecessor, been a challenge, particularly in terms of the responsibility of demonstrating how a model for nursing, which has become part of nursing culture, can be applied in practice. Despite this, we have gained from the experience, learning more about the Roper–Logan–Tierney model for nursing and its potential for both practice and education, and learning about the evidence base for care and the different ways of helping student nurses and their teachers gain access to this evidence. Since the first edition there have been many changes in both nursing and health care generally, not just in the UK but internationally. These changes are reflected throughout the revised chapters. We have also taken into account reviews of the first book and the results of student focus groups. It is clear from sales of the book that it fulfils a need, from both a student and a practitioner point of view. We are also delighted that the first edition has been translated in 2006 into the Japanese language.

Karen Holland
Jane Jenkins
Jackie Solomon
Sue Whittam
2008

References

Roper N, Logan WW, Tierney AJ 1996 The elements of nursing: a model for nursing based on a model of living, 4th edn. Churchill Livingstone, Edinburgh

Roper N, Logan WW, Tierney AJ 2000 The Roper–Logan–Tierney model for nursing based on activities of living. Churchill Livingstone, Edinburgh

A MODEL FOR PRACTICE

CONTENTS

An introduction to the Roper–Logan–Tierney model for nursing, based on Activities of Living

Karen Holland

INTRODUCTION

The Roper–Logan–Tierney model for nursing was initially created as an education tool for 'beginning nursing students and their teachers' (Roper et al 2000, p. 1). Since then it has been used extensively within the United Kingdom and other countries throughout the world as a framework for nursing care and practice and teaching and learning.

To enable both students and qualified practitioners to apply the model in practice and for nurse educators to use the model as an educational tool, there is a need to revisit some of basic underlying principles of the model.

This chapter will therefore focus on the following:

- an overview of the Roper–Logan–Tierney model for nursing
- the model of living
- Activities of Living
- lifespan
- dependence/independence continuum
- factors influencing the Activities of Living
- the model for nursing
- individualising nursing care and the nursing process.

AN OVERVIEW OF THE ROPER–LOGAN–TIERNEY MODEL FOR NURSING

The first model for nursing based on a model of living arose out of research undertaken by Nancy Roper in 1970. She sought to identify the core of nursing activities across any field of nursing practice, which could then be supported by knowledge, skills and attitudes required to work in the individual specialist fields, e.g. psychiatry, gynaecology, surgery, community or midwifery. As a result of this early work Roper, Logan and Tierney published *The Elements of Nursing* in 1980, identifying the individual aspects of the model as a whole and how nursing could use it as a framework for the care of patients in a wide variety of situations.

The model is divided into two parts: the model of living and the model for nursing.

THE MODEL OF LIVING

There are five components (concepts) in the model (see Fig. 1.1), namely:

- Activities of Living (ALs)
- lifespan
- dependence/independence
- factors influencing the ALs
- individuality in living.

ACTIVITIES OF LIVING (ALs)

Living is a complex process which we undertake using a number of activities that ensure our survival. Twelve such activities have been identified which are seen as the core of the model of living. These are:

- maintaining a safe environment
- communicating
- breathing
- eating and drinking
- eliminating
- personal cleansing and dressing
- controlling body temperature
- mobilising
- working and playing
- expressing sexuality
- sleeping
- dying.

Although each of these activities will be examined separately throughout the text it is important to remember that we do not undertake one at the exclusion of others. For example, we cannot conceive of eating and drinking without elimination, or breathing. They are simply different dimensions of our lives and the impact of illness on one activity can have a major impact on another (see model for nursing and each AL chapter). In order to ensure that there is a common understanding of these ALs when reading and using this book each one will now be

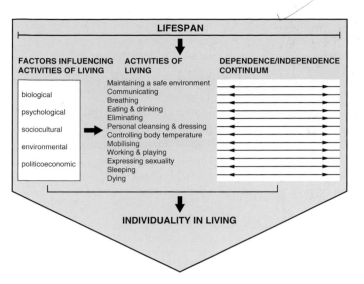

Fig. 1.1 The model of living (from Roper et al 1996, with permission).

described. More details in relation to these activities can be found at the beginning of every AL chapter.

Maintaining a safe environment

'In order to stay alive and carry out any of the other Activities of Living, it is imperative that actions are taken to maintain a safe environment' (Roper et al 1996, p. 21). These actions may include activities such as prevention of accidents in the home, driving carefully or washing hands after elimination.

Some of these activities, e.g. accident prevention, are not only the responsibility of the individual but of the society in which they live. They become shared responsibilities, which often need government legislation to ensure that they are carried out.

The environment in relation to the individual can also be thought of as having two elements, namely the external and the internal. For the purpose of this book the external is that which 'surrounds the body and provides the oxygen and nutrients required by all the body cells. Waste products of cellular activity are eventually excreted into the external environment. The skin provides a barrier between the dry external environment (the atmosphere) and the aqueous (water-based) environment of most body cells' (Waugh & Grant 2006, p. 4).

Ensuring that this external environment does not cause a threat to life through pollution, or destruction of the rainforests are two examples of maintaining a safe external environment. Examples of the impact of pollution from car exhausts on health can be seen in Table 1.1.

The internal safe environment is seen as:

> *the water-based medium in which the body cells exist. Cells are bathed in fluid called interstitial or tissue fluid. Oxygen and other substances they require must pass from the internal transport systems through the interstitial fluid to reach them. Similarly cellular waste products must move through the interstitial fluid to the transport systems to be excreted.* (Waugh & Grant 2006, p. 4)

This internal environment is maintained in a state of balance, i.e. homeostasis, which if threatened can pose a serious

Table 1.1 Potential harmful effects of automobile exhaust pollutants

Pollutant	Health effects	Environmental effects
Carbon monoxide (CO)	Lethal at high doses. At low doses can impair concentration and neuro-behavioural function. Increases the likelihood of exercise-related heart pain in people with coronary heart disease	Greenhouse gas contributing to global warming
Nitrogen oxides (NO_x)	May exacerbate asthma and possibly increase susceptibility to infections	Acid rain. Ground-level ozone precursor
Hydrocarbons (HC)	Low-molecular-weight compounds cause eye irritation, coughing and drowsiness. High-molecular-weight compounds can be mutagenic and carcinogenic	Ground-level ozone precursor
Benzene (C_6H_6)	Classified as a human carcinogen (Group 1) by the International Agency for Research on Cancer	
Ground-level ozone (O_3)	Irritates the eyes and air passages. Increases the sensitivity of the airways to allergy triggers in people with asthma. May increase susceptibility to infection	
Lead (Pb)	Impairs the normal intellectual development and learning ability of children	Ground-water pollution and particles in the air

Source: The European Fuel Oxygenates Association (www.efoa.org).

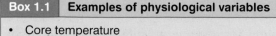

Box 1.1	**Examples of physiological variables**

- Core temperature
- Water and electrolyte concentrations
- pH (acidity or alkalinity) of body fluids
- Blood glucose levels
- Blood and tissue oxygen and carbon dioxide levels
- Blood pressure

From Waugh & Grant (2006), p. 6.

threat to the individual. Some of the factors which must be maintained within narrow limits can be seen in Box 1.1.

It is maintained 'by control systems that detect and respond to changes in the internal environment. A control system has three basic components: detector, control centre and effector' (Grant & Waugh 2006, p. 5). An example of a negative feedback mechanism which involves all three of these can be seen in Figure 1.2. A safe internal environment is therefore essential for survival (see Chapter 3).

Communicating

Roper et al (1996) see this activity in the following way:

> 66 *Human beings are essentially social beings and a major part of living involves communicating with other people in one way or another. Communicating not only involves the*

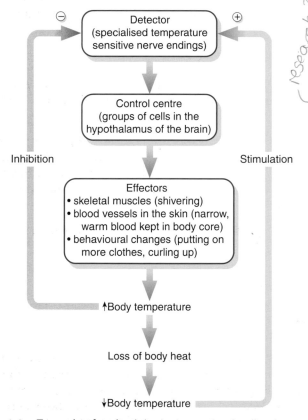

Fig. 1.2 Example of a physiological negative feedback mechanism: control of body mechanism (from Waugh & Grant 2006, with permission).

use of verbal language as in talking and writing, but also the non-verbal transmission of information by facial expression and body gesture. 99 (Roper et al 1996, p. 21)

The way in which we communicate will vary from culture to culture, especially in relation to nonverbal communication. Touching between men and women in public for example is not allowed in many cultures, e.g. Asian. To be able to communicate requires an individual to use their senses, such as sight, hearing and touch, so that when they lose the ability to use these, e.g. become deaf or blind, they need to acquire other means of communicating (see Chapter 4).

Breathing

Breathing is an activity that is essential for life itself and all other activities are therefore dependent on us being able to breathe. Breathing ensures that oxygen is taken into the body and carbon dioxide (a waste product of cell metabolism) is removed. This process helps maintain the body's homeostasis. Breathing is an effortless activity, and it is only when something happens to alter this that we become aware of it; for example, the effect of running a race or climbing a mountain (see Chapter 5).

Eating and drinking

Eating and drinking, as with breathing, are essential to maintain the body's homeostasis, and we need to eat the right food and drink the right fluids that ensure the correct balance. Eating and drinking are dependent on being able to afford to buy food and drink, and it should be remembered that there are many people who cannot afford to do so. People are dying from starvation in many countries, and (even in hospitals) research has shown that patients are suffering from starvation as a result of inadequate observation of their inpatient diets. Eating and drinking are also very social activities, and what we eat and drink is very much influenced by the culture in which we live (see Chapter 6).

Eliminating

In this book elimination is both urinary and faecal, yet remembering that elimination also occurs through breathing (external respiration). The metabolic waste products of the body are removed via the process of elimination, i.e. urinary elimination gets rid of urine from the body (kidney function) and faecal elimination gets rid of faeces (intestine function). Eliminating, like eating and drinking, is influenced by sociocultural factors. Many cultures have rituals and behaviours that govern these activities, and eliminating is a very private activity, unlike eating and drinking which are very social ones (see Chapter 7).

Personal cleansing and dressing

Roper et al (1996) chose to call this activity personal cleansing rather than washing, and have included the activities of perineal hygiene, care of the hair, nails, teeth and mouth, as well as handwashing, bodywashing and bathing. As with many other ALs it is influenced by sociocultural factors. Dressing, i.e. clothing, is influenced by culture and also by circumstances such as climate or being in hospital. Age and gender will also influence how we dress or manage our personal cleansing activities (see Chapter 8).

Controlling body temperature

Human beings are able to maintain their internal body temperature at a constant level due to a heat regulation system, but extremes in external temperatures can cause this to endanger normal living. Severe cold and heat can cause hypothermia or heatstroke, which if untreated can cause trauma or death.

In normal circumstances we are able to control our environment, e.g. central heating in winter, or take steps to manage it when required, e.g. wearing thermal underwear if working or holidaying in freezing conditions (see Chapter 9).

Mobilising

Roper et al (1996) see the AL of mobilising as including:

> 66 *The movement produced by groups of large muscles, enabling people to stand, sit, walk and run as well as groups of smaller muscles producing movements such as those involved in manual dexterity or in facial expressions, hand gesticulations and mannerisms: all of which are part of non-verbal communication.* 99 (Roper et al 1996, p. 22)

Movement is essential for many other ALs, such as working and playing or eliminating, and the effects of not being able to move, as can happen following trauma (e.g. spinal injury) or inflammatory disease (e.g. rheumatoid arthritis), can have a major impact on individual lifestyles and social activities (see Chapter 10).

Working and playing

Working for most people offers a way of obtaining income (money) to support how they live. Work can also be unpaid, as with housework or on a voluntary basis. For many women, housework and paid work are essential to maintain family life, but the social pressures on them undertaking both at the same time brings with it additional tensions. Unemployment can cause both health and social problems and both a lack of time and lack of money can prevent individuals from making time for 'play' activities. These can be varied, from visiting the theatre and cinema to exercising in a health and fitness club. Physical and mental health is affected by work and play (see Chapter 11).

Expressing sexuality

Expressing sexuality encompasses more than sex and sexual activity. It relates also to how we see ourselves and our bodies in relation to each other and how we behave in society. Being a man or woman will influence how we express ourselves, which may not always be in keeping with what is considered 'normal' for the majority. For example being a gay man or lesbian woman in a society that does not allow such relationships to be publicly acknowledged can be very traumatic for individuals who love one another and who wish to express this to others (see Chapter 12).

Sleeping

Sleep enables the body to relax from the 'stresses of everyday living' and it is also during sleep that 'growth and repair of cells takes place' (Roper et al 1996, p. 22). It is therefore essential that individuals have enough sleep to ensure this takes place, although this does differ from person to person. Being deprived of sleep can have a marked effect on the individual and their health (see Chapter 13).

Dying

It is the process of dying that is included here, not death 'which marks the end of life', and many people have to live with the fact that they face eventual death but not as an immediate event. This is not the same as the eventuality of death for all living things but having to live on a day-to-day basis knowing that there is no choice about prolonging life. For example, many individuals with cancer may have a short reprieve due to drug treatment, but will have to manage their daily lives with the knowledge that it is only temporary. Their family, friends and partners will also be affected by this knowledge. It is important to mention, however, that not everyone who has, or has had, cancer will necessarily die from its effects (see Chapter 14).

Exercise
1. Consider these Activities of Living and assess your own beliefs and/or practices in relation to each one.
2. How does this help you to understand the needs of others in relation to these activities? Discuss with a colleague.

LIFESPAN

The lifespan is a continuum (see Fig. 1.1) indicating movement of an individual from birth to death. Roper et al (1996, p. 23) state that:

> 66 *As a person moves along the lifespan there is a continuous change and every aspect of living is influenced by the biological, psychological, socio-cultural, environmental and politico-economic circumstances encountered throughout life.* 99

The lifespan is therefore inextricably linked to age. Roper et al (1996) have identified five stages of life:

- infancy
- childhood
- adolescence
- adulthood
- old age.

Each of us will live through these stages in different ways and not always successfully. Infancy may be a period of great vulnerability; babies born prematurely, for example, are especially vulnerable to infectious diseases, and those born in countries where there are no facilities to manage their health status may well not survive. Lack of food will add to their vulnerability (World Health Organization (WHO) 2002a). Some babies are born with health problems that will require long-term care and support, necessitating numerous visits and stays in hospital, e.g. sickle cell anaemia. These problems can very often lead to other needs at other stages of the lifespan.

Childhood experiences will depend on the culture to which we belong as well as the environment in which we live. This is especially seen in how children are reared by their parents and others. Knowledge and understanding of child-rearing practice is essential to understanding adult behaviour, especially during illness. For example, Andrews (2000, p. 139) highlights the differences between cultures, such as Anglo-American, where 'children are socialised from a very early age to learn to control their feelings and emotions, especially in public places' and those where such expression is not repressed and is socially acceptable, e.g. Italian or Indian.

Adolescence is a Western society concept, dominated by the stages of puberty. In certain cultures the end of childhood and onset of puberty is marked by special rituals which ensure that there is a clear transition from childhood to adulthood. Once puberty is reached, girls are very often married and become mothers themselves (La Fontaine 1985). Some adolescents experience psychological and emotional problems, some of which can require professional help and counselling. The outcome of these problems may well extend into adulthood.

Adulthood in Western society is identified by age rather than physiological body changes. Roper et al (1996, p. 39) state that 'early adulthood is considered to be a stage of relative stability, with both physical fitness and intellectual ability at their peak' but that 'with advancing age into the middle years of life, ill-health becomes more common'. They also state that 'there are two dominant areas of concern for all adults, namely work and family life'. The outcome of having neither can have a marked effect on an individual's life.

Old age is no longer seen as the end of one's active life, in either work or the home. A report on nursing older people (Department of Health (DoH) 2001a, p. 9) states that:

> 66 *People are living longer. The Office of Public Censuses and Surveys (1991) estimates that the average life span is increasing by 2 years per decade. Old age used to be defined as over 65, but now a large and growing proportion of the population is over 75, and the number of people over 85 has doubled since 1981. The population of older people is extremely heterogeneous and there is a great deal of debate in the academic literature about whether an increase in longevity means an extension of healthy active life or an extension of morbidity. The majority of those reaching old age are still in good health (Victor 1991) and it is clearly wrong to stereotype older people as infirm.* 99

Many of these issues will be discussed at relevant points throughout the book.

One can see from the above that the lifespan is linked closely with dependence and independence, in both health and illness.

Exercise

1. Consider the above statement and what it could mean for future health care provision.
2. Consider the lifespan as it applies to your own family. How many life groups are there?
3. Are you able to determine how your culture/society is influencing each age group?
4. Discuss your findings with a colleague from another culture/society and compare them in relation to each stage of the lifespan.
5. Consider how understanding the needs of different age groups will help you in your role as a nurse.

DEPENDENCE/INDEPENDENCE CONTINUUM

Roper et al (1996) state that:

> 66 *This component of the model is closely related to the lifespan and to the ALs. It is included to acknowledge that there are stages of the lifespan when a person cannot yet (or for various reasons can no longer) perform certain ALs independently. Each person could be said to have a dependence/independence continuum for each AL.* 99
> (Roper et al 1996, p. 23)

This relationship can be seen in Figure 1.1. Newborn and young babies can be seen to be very dependent on adults, as can those who may have sustained serious trauma resulting in being in a coma. Individuals may be dependent on equipment for their survival, e.g. artificial ventilation, or may be dependent on wheelchairs for their mobility. All of us are dependent on others in some way, e.g. transport or having somewhere to live, and the effect of lack of transport or housing can be seen to have a detrimental effect on the health and wellbeing of individuals. Without some kind of transport for example elderly people may become isolated in their communities. The devastating effects of lack of somewhere to live or shelter can be seen at the scenes of earthquakes or other natural or man-made disasters.

Dependence/independence status in each AL therefore is clearly linked to the factors which influence them.

FACTORS INFLUENCING THE ACTIVITIES OF LIVING

Although Roper et al (1996) indicate that there are numerous factors that could influence our daily lives, they decided that five main groups were sufficient to avoid over-complicating the model. These groups are:

- biological
- psychological
- sociocultural
- environmental
- politicoeconomic.

Biological

66 *For the purpose of this model of living, the term biological relates to the human body's anatomical and physical performance. This is partly determined by the individual's genetic inheritance and although the influence of heredity is usually more obvious in facial appearance and physique, it also affects each person's physical performance. The individual's physical endowment is inextricably linked with other factors – psychological, socio-cultural, environmental and politico-economic.* 99
(Roper et al 1996, p. 25)

This link can be seen when considering the lifespan. For example, if there is a hereditary link to height, e.g. being short, then as the child grows and is measured against the normal percentile for his/her age this factor can be taken into account in the overall assessment of the child's development. However, should that child also be deprived of food or physical care then this could exacerbate the problems of a short height and normal development. The biological factors associated with an ageing body also cause problems and may restrict the person's independence. For example it may cause us to become 'physically slower and weaker' but that should be no obstacle to 'maintaining regular physical activity' (Herbert 2006, p. 77).

Psychological

Intellectual development begins in infancy as a result of stimuli via the sense organs. Later in childhood and adolescence this continues through 'formal education and the pursuit of personal interest and leisure' (Roper et al 1996, p. 25). In adulthood work and a career are important. Ageing, however, causes 'intellectual functioning to become gradually less efficient and may cause problems with Activities of Living, for example, there may be difficulty with communication because the senses are less acute' (Roper et al 1996, p. 26). There is evidence 'that older people maintain their cognitive abilities into old age – demonstrated by the activities of members of the House of Lords, clergy and judicial system' (Ponto 2006, p. 44). Also many people are undertaking Open University courses on retirement. Emotional development is also closely linked to intellectual development and the lifespan – 'the need for love and belonging is crucial in young children; and from a stable and close relationship in infancy the child can grow with self-confidence and a feeling of worth' (Roper et al 1996, p. 26). One can see how an unhappy childhood and lack of emotional development could influence the way in which adults behave in relationships and when ill or needing care.

Sociocultural

The society and culture in which we live will also influence the intellectual and emotional development of an individual. What is considered the norm in one culture may be considered otherwise in another. Religion can have a major influence on lifestyle as can social class expectations and Roper et al (1996, p. 27) believe that 'where there is religious unity in a society, the culture and religion are almost inseparable'. It is, however, important not only to recognise the difference between culture and religion, but also how they are closely linked. Religion is a system of belief (a faith) whilst culture encompasses this and more. Leininger (1978, p. 491) for example defines it as:

66 *Culture is the learned and transmitted knowledge about a particular culture with its values, beliefs, rules of behaviour and lifestyle practices that guides a designated group in their thinking and actions in patterned ways.* 99

Both culture and religion have an impact on individual lifestyle.

Exercise
1. Consider how your culture influences your dependence on or independence from others.
2. How is social class or stratification illustrated in your culture?
3. Consider how religion influences your role and status in society.

Environmental

In Roper et al's (1996) model, environment factors include atmospheric components, clothing, household environment, vegetation and buildings. They separate atmosphere into three components, namely:

- organic and inorganic particles
- light rays
- sound waves.

These are described in Box 1.2.

Politicoeconomic

Roper et al (2000, p. 71) state that:

66 *For the purpose of this model of living the term politico-economic factors subsumes aspects of living which have a legal connection; frequently political and/or economic pressure and action is reflected in legislation.* 99

They focus in particular on the state, the law and the economy. They conclude that 'in the modern world, every citizen is the subject of a state' and that 'the citizen is legally bound to obey orders of the state and to a large extent, the individual's ALs are influenced by its norms. These norms are the laws and the state has the power to enforce the law on all who live within its frontiers' (Roper et al 2000, p. 72). The state has a significant influence and its power is considerable. Although in some countries individuals and groups can register their outrage at certain issues without harm, in many others to do so could place the individual and in many cases their families, in danger of their lives. The effects of such power can be seen in the number of refugees

| Box 1.2 | Atmospheric components |

Organic and inorganic particles

The atmosphere is in contact with exposed skin and outer garments on which it deposits inorganic matter such as particles, which are the products of combustion. Such particles can also be inhaled thereby relating it to the AL of breathing. In addition the atmosphere contains organic matter in the form of pollen, pathogenic microorganisms and vectors such as flies and lice. These can affect several ALs.

Light rays

Light rays are transmitted via the atmosphere; these can be from the sun providing daylight; from an electrically operated apparatus which provides light when natural lighting is inadequate or absent; from technological apparatus such as batteries and from burning candles. Light rays not only stimulate the sense of sight in normal eyes but also provide the ambience for such varied ALs as communicating, for example, for hearing impaired people to maximise the visual input into a conversation. Some of the sun's rays – ultraviolet – may burn the exposed skin or, after long exposure, may even cause cancer and may require people to take preventative action by applying screening lotion or wearing clothes which cover the skin – a relationship to the AL of personal cleansing and dressing.

Sound waves

Sound waves are also transmitted by the atmosphere and in various ways can influence different ALs. For example, those produced by speech are an essential part of communicating for most people. Those produced by professional vocalists could be said to relate to the AL of working while, for the majority of people, singing would involve the AL of playing. Sound waves may of course contribute to an emergency warning such as a fire alarm, which would certainly influence the ALs of mobilising and maintaining a safe environment.

From Roper et al (1996), p. 28.

Exercise

1. Identify how the state (Government) works in your individual society.
2. How is health and welfare managed?
3. Consider the effects of being a refugee and find out how many refugees, if any, the Government has accepted to stay in your country.

across the world. It is therefore important that this aspect of world politics is understood, as many nurses will come into contact with displaced people requiring health care.

To be able to use the model for nursing in different countries requires its application to be context specific – a task which can only be touched upon in a book such as this. It is a point of interest that our book has been translated into Japanese, indicating that the model is of value in helping Japanese student nurses understand the principles of applying it within the Japanese health care system (Kawashima 2006).

The world is becoming increasingly interdependent and this, according to Roper et al (2000, p. 74) 'appears to be leading the United Nations Organisation (UN) into a controversial sphere: the right to humanitarian intervention.'

They believe that the 'UN lacks the money and trained personnel to enforce humanitarian operations everywhere they might be needed in the world, but the issue is creating international controversy and sometimes, acrimony'. The impact is also felt by health care services worldwide as the UN responds to major humanitarian disasters and ethnic conflict (see www.unhcr.org for examples).

It can be seen from this overview of the five factors that they are inextricably linked and this needs to be considered when using the model as a framework for nursing care. This will be explored in each AL chapter.

INDIVIDUALITY IN LIVING

The fifth component is that of 'individuality in living' and stresses that each individual will experience and carry out the ALs differently. 'Each person's individuality in carrying out the ALs is, in part, determined by stage on the lifespan, and degree of dependence/independence, and is further fashioned by the influence of various biological, psychological, socio-cultural, environmental and politico-economic factors' (Roper et al 2000, p. 75). They consider that a 'person's individuality can manifest itself in many different ways' (see Box 1.3).

SUMMARY POINTS

1. The model of living has five components – Activities of Living, lifespan, dependence/ independence continuum, factors influencing the ALs and individuality in living.
2. The five factors influencing the ALs are: biological, psychological, sociocultural, and environmental and politicoeconomic.
3. The lifespan is divided into five stages: infancy, childhood, adolescence, adulthood and old age.

THE MODEL FOR NURSING

This section will focus on the model for nursing (see Fig. 1.3) which differs from the model of living in its fifth component – that of individualising nursing. Roper et al (2000, p. 77) state that:

Box 1.3	The Roper–Logan–Tierney model for nursing

- How a person carries out the AL.
- How often the person carries out the AL.
- Where the person carries out the AL.
- When the person carries out the AL.
- Why the person carries out the AL in a particular way.
- What the person knows about the AL.
- What the person believes about the AL.
- The attitude the person has to the AL.

From Roper et al (2000), p. 75.

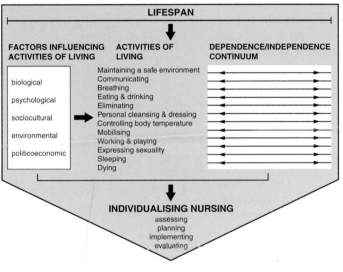

Fig. 1.3 The model for nursing (from Roper et al 1996, with permission).

66 *The objective in conceptualising living according to the first four concepts in the model of living is to identify each person's individuality in living, and this is the basis of our conceptualisation of nursing. The objective in conceptualising nursing according to the first four concepts in the model for nursing is to identify the individual's pattern of living (and actual or potential problems with any of the ALs) so that the nurse can individualise the nursing of that person taking account of that individual's lifestyle – and when appropriate taking account of family and/or significant others. Individualising nursing is accomplished by application to practice of the concept of the process of nursing comprising four phases.* 99 (Roper et al 2000, p. 78)

Assumptions on which the model is based

Nursing theorists who have developed model frameworks to explain and interpret the discipline of nursing make assumptions about how the world of nursing is viewed. They are indicative of the beliefs and values of the theorists. Roper et al (1996, p. 34) make the following assumptions in relation to their theory and model:

1. Living can be described as an amalgam of Activities of Living (ALs).
2. The way ALs are carried out by each person contributes to individuality in living.
3. The individual is valued at all stages of the lifespan.
4. Throughout the lifespan until adulthood, the individual tends to become increasingly independent in the ALs.
5. While independence in the ALs is valued, dependence should not diminish the dignity of the individual.
6. An individual's knowledge, attitudes and behaviour related to the ALs are influenced by a variety of factors which can be categorised broadly as biological, psychological, sociocultural, environmental and politicoeconomic factors.
7. The way in which an individual carries out the ALs can fluctuate within a range of normal for that person.
8. When the individual is 'ill' there may be problems (actual or potential) with the ALs.
9. During the lifespan, most individuals experience significant life events which can affect the way they carry out ALs, and may lead to problems, actual or potential.
10. The concept of potential problems incorporates the promotion and maintenance of health, and the prevention of disease; and identifies the role of the nurse as a health teacher, even in illness settings.
11. Within a health care context, nurses work in partnership with the client/patient who, except for special circumstances, is an autonomous, decision-making person.
12. Nurses are part of a multiprofessional health care team, who work in partnership for the benefit of the client/patient, and for the health of the community.
13. The specific function of nursing is to assist the individual to prevent, alleviate or solve, or cope positively with problems (actual or potential) related to the ALs.

Exercise
1. Consider these assumptions and compare them to other nursing models/theories.
2. How different are they in relation to these assumptions?

How these assumptions about living are linked to the assumptions about nursing will now be considered.

ACTIVITIES OF LIVING (ALs)

In Virginia Henderson's (1966) definition of nursing a link can be seen between the nurse and activities:

66 *The unique function of the nurse is to assist the individual, sick or well, in the performance of those activities contributing to health or its recovery (or to peaceful death) that he would perform unaided if he had the*

necessary strength, will or knowledge. And to do this in such a way as to help him gain independence as rapidly as possible. 99 (Henderson 1966, p. 15)

Henderson (1966) identified 14 activities where the nurse would help the patient by providing basic nursing care or provide conditions under which the patient could manage them unaided (see Box 1.4).

Roper et al (1996) developed these activities further and arrived 'after lengthy debate' to their decision of 12 ALs as described in their model (Roper et al 2000).

These ALs are:

- maintaining a safe environment
- communicating
- breathing
- eating and drinking
- eliminating
- personal cleansing and dressing
- controlling body temperature
- mobilising
- working and playing
- expressing sexuality
- sleeping
- dying.

It is important to note that these activities are interlinked in many different ways. For example, if an individual is having difficulties mobilising then this will also affect their need to eliminate, especially if the person is paralysed

and unable to walk to the toilet or feel that they need to empty their bladder or bowel.

Each of these ALs will be examined in depth in each of the AL chapters, along with the other concepts of the model as they affect that individual activity. The ALs are the main focus of the model. Nursing in relation to the model is seen by Roper et al (1996, p. 35) as (Box 1.5):

66 *helping people to prevent, alleviate or solve, or cope positively with problems (actual or potential) related to the ALs. Recognition of the fact that people's problems may be actual or potential means that nursing not only responds to existing problems but is also concerned with preventing problems, whenever possible.* 99

The focus in the next section of this chapter will be on the concept of 'individualising nursing'. Before beginning to examine this in more detail it is important to acknowledge, within a nursing context, how the ALs are influenced by:

- stage of the lifespan
- level of dependence/independence and methods of coping with dependence
- factors which have influenced/are influencing individual lifestyle, i.e. biological, psychological, sociocultural, environmental and politicoeconomic.

LIFESPAN

66 *In a nursing context, the lifespan serves as a reminder that nursing is concerned with people of all ages; that an individual may require nursing at any stage of the lifespan, from birth to death.* 99 (Roper et al 1996, p. 37)

Young babies and children admitted to hospital will also require different nursing skills to those for adults, and this is mirrored in the qualifications of nurses employed to nurse

Box 1.4	Activities for helping patients through basic nursing care

1. Breathe normally.
2. Eat and drink adequately.
3. Eliminate body wastes.
4. Move and maintain desirable postures.
5. Sleep and rest.
6. Select suitable clothes – dress and undress.
7. Maintain body temperature within normal range by adjusting clothing and modifying the environment.
8. Keep the body clean and well groomed and protect the integument.
9. Avoid dangers in the environment and avoid injuring others.
10. Communicate with others in expressing emotions, needs, fears or opinions.
11. Worship according to one's faith.
12. Work in such a way that there is a sense of accomplishment.
13. Play or participate in various forms of recreation.
14. Learn, discover or satisfy curiosity that leads to normal development and health and use of available health facilities.

From Henderson (1966), p. 16.

Box 1.5	Summary of the nursing function	
Prevent	→ **Potential problems** From becoming actual problems This may involve the person carrying out the preventative activities	
Alleviate or solve	→ **Actual problems** Appropriate activities may be carried out by the nurse The person may be able to continue the activities with the objective of preventing a recurrence of the actual problem	
Cope in a positive way	→ Any problems that cannot be solved	

From Roper et al (1996), p. 35.

children. Involvement of the family is also encouraged, to avoid the adverse effects of separation. Infant and childhood death, whilst it does occur in countries with a developed health care system, is not as visible as it is in those where natural and man-made disasters occur on a regular basis, e.g. Southern African countries (WHO 2002b), and where health care often has to take place in hazardous environmental conditions. The nursing of adolescents requires an understanding of their physical and emotional development, in particular when they may be faced with serious illness, such as insulin-dependent diabetes (diabetes mellitus), which requires a significant alteration to their previous lifestyle. The nursing needs of adults and older people will depend on the reason they encounter health professionals. Three illnesses that have become more common in middle age are heart disease, cancer and stroke – all of which are responsible for an increase in the death rate in late adulthood (Roper et al 1996). Nurses will also come across older people in the course of their work either in hospital or in the community given that more people are living longer. The National Service Framework (NSF) for older people indicated that:

66 *The number of people (in Britain) aged over 65 has doubled in the last 70 years and the number of people over 90 will double in next 25 years.* 99 (DoH 2001b)

Knowing how to care for older people and what happens during the process of ageing is therefore an essential part of the nurse's role if they are to ensure that the care they plan and deliver is to meet individual needs.

DEPENDENCE/INDEPENDENCE CONTINUUM

This continuum is an important component of the model for nurses. It reminds us that during our lifetime we can, depending on our health and life circumstances, move from the very dependent stage of infancy and childhood to the independent adult and older person stage. Ill health, however, could make us either partially or totally dependent in either one or more AL. The nurse will 'help people towards independence in the ALs and at other times help them to accept dependence' (Roper et al 1996, p. 42) This is indicated by arrows on the model framework (see Fig. 1.4), reminding us to assess the person's level of independence in each of the ALs and then 'judging in which direction, and by what amount they should be assisted to move along the dependence/independence continuum; what nursing assistance they need to achieve the goals set; and how progress in relation to these goals will be evaluated' (Roper et al 1996, p. 42).

FACTORS INFLUENCING THE ALs

To be able to use the model effectively requires the nurse to have knowledge of the five factors and how they

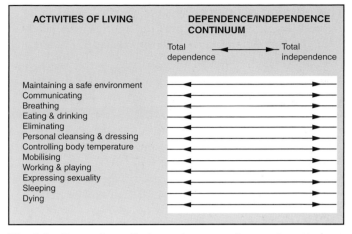

Fig. 1.4 Dependence/independence continuum (from Roper et al 1996, with permission).

influence the ALs. In the model for nursing sections in each AL chapter you will see how this knowledge is applied to patient care and how the factors are interrelated when assessing a patient's needs. Knowledge of the structure and function of the heart (biological factors), for example, will help the nurse explain what happens during a heart attack (myocardial infarction) as will knowledge of the effects of smoking or obesity on the heart when promoting healthy living. Understanding the possible psychological effects of having a heart attack (psychological factors) will also make it easier to explain to a patient's relatives how their family member is likely to respond to their illness. Likewise understanding the patient's beliefs about health and illness and their cultural and religious beliefs (sociocultural factors) will enable the nurse to offer the appropriate pain relief or manage personal cleansing and dressing needs. Where and how the patient lives (environmental factors) will be essential knowledge when considering their discharge home from hospital, as will knowledge of how the social services and the NHS work when discussing patient's rights with regard to treatment and care (politicoeconomic factors). As with the model of living the factors influencing the ALs interlink with the lifespan and the dependence/independence continuum to enable the nurse to adopt a holistic approach to nursing care.

INDIVIDUALISING NURSING CARE AND THE NURSING PROCESS

Each patient is unique, as is the nurse–patient relationship. The Roper et al (1996) model for nursing offers a framework for nurses to be able to ensure that this individuality is taken into account when undertaking nursing care. In order to ensure that all aspects of an individual's life are integrated into an effective plan of care, Roper et al (1996) use a problem-solving approach and the nursing process in conjunction with their model for nursing.

The nursing process

The nursing process is a systematic approach to planning and delivering nursing care. Yura & Walsh (1978) identified four main stages of this process, namely:

- assessment
- planning
- implementation
- evaluation.

Uys & Habermann (2005, p. 3) enlarge on these phases:

- collecting information and assessing the patient
- planning the care and defining the relevant objectives for nursing care
- implementing actual interventions
- evaluating the results.

They also point out that in some areas further stages are added to these, one being 'making a diagnosis' and that all the stages 'guide the production of nursing care plans and documentation of care in all fields of nursing' (p. 3).

Slevin (2003) summarises the nursing process method as:

> ❝ ... *a logical, purposive, goal-orientated, systematic and planned approach to the resolution of problems within nursing contexts. It is to a large extent linear and sequential in its orientation, usually involving stages that follow a general progression from the assessment of a situation, through the identification of problems and tentative solutions, resulting in a plan of action that following implementation is evaluated. There is recognition of the interactivity of the elements and the cyclical and progressive nature of the method; evaluative information leads to further modification of the assessment, the problem and the plan as implementation proceeds. The method is nevertheless characterized by adherence to a systematic logic that extends from the assessment through to the evaluation of outcomes.* ❞
> (Slevin 2003, p. 458)

The nursing process stages are similar to many other 'problem-solving' approaches, in particular the stages of research process, where gathering data and analysing them are fundamental to a successful outcome. It is however only 'partially implemented in practice in most countries, although it is now 40 years since its introduction' (Uys & Habermann 2005, p. 4). Research for this varies from country to country. Uys & Habermann (2005) offer many explanations for the variance and conclude that, despite dissatisfaction with the concept, no new system has yet replaced it. So what is this systematic approach?

Assessment

Roper et al (2000, p. 124) point out that, although 'the word assessment has generally been adopted for the first phase of the process of nursing', their view is that the word 'assessing' should be encouraged as it implies a more cyclical activity rather a 'once only' one. They use the word to include:

- collecting information about or from a person
- reviewing the collected information
- identifying the person's problems with ALs
- identifying priorities among problems.

The following questions may be asked regarding assessment:

- For whom is this information to be gained?
- What information is to be gained?
- How is this information to be gained?
- When is assessment undertaken?

The main data (information) come from the patient whenever possible (primary source) and any other data, e.g. from relatives, are a secondary source. It may not be possible, however, to obtain first-hand information from the patient, e.g. if they were unconscious, and 'second-hand' information thus becomes very important in helping the nurse and others to plan the care necessary.

Sources of data are:

- the patient
- family
- significant others
- health care professionals
- patient records/nursing notes.

Obtaining information on assessment

Data can be collected in a number of ways, but whatever data are obtained it is essential that the nurse ensures that they are kept confidential in accordance with their professional code of conduct and that any recorded data are protected (Department of Health 2000).

As with the research process, observation and interview are two key methods of obtaining information. Observation of a patient, however, must be systematic in order to ensure that nothing is missed. It is here that a framework, such as the Roper–Logan–Tierney model for nursing, is an essential tool. Other means of obtaining data are: physical examination of the patient, informal discussion with patient and significant others/family, and medical records. Objective data are essentially those which can be observed and measured, whereas subjective data are how the patient defines or reports their own experience, symptoms and feelings.

Exercise

Imagine that you have tonsillitis.

1. What objective data (symptoms) would we be able to identify?
2. What subjective data (symptoms) may you describe?

For 1. you may have considered symptoms such as having a high temperature and red swollen tonsils, and for 2. having a sore throat and feeling very weak and 'dizzy'. We can clearly see the first but it is only the patient who is experiencing the second.

Type of information obtained at assessment

Roper et al (2000, p. 127) point out that biographical and health data are vital to ensuring effective assessment of nursing needs. This will include 'name, sex, age, usual place of residence and the person or people to contact when the client requires the assistance of a friend or family member, or when the client's health status is giving cause for concern'. Individual surnames and names are very important information and ensuring that individuals are recognised by the correct name is vital to avoid potential harm, for example when administering medication. Addressing the patient by their correct name is also important in different cultures, where naming systems often require the surname to be placed before the first name. It is important to note that titles such as Mr or Mrs may not always be appropriate. Similar or identical surnames can also cause identification errors; hence it is essential that all names be recorded appropriately. How patients wish to be addressed needs to be determined. Nurses cannot assume that everyone wishes to be known by their first name nor that a request for formal address implies a lack of friendliness on the part of the patient (Holland & Hogg 2001).

The age of the patient is important as it indicates their position within the stages of the lifespan. Where someone lives can indicate the kind of community in which the patient lives, for example a small rural village or a flat in the middle of a large city. If they have no home, this can indicate that support services might be contacted in order to ensure care after discharge from hospital. Some health authorities in the UK employ community nurses to assess homeless patients' needs in the community and deliver care in a 'peripatetic' way, i.e. moving about from place to place to meet the patients. Wright & Tompkins (2005), in a WHO/ Europe report, consider that access to primary health care to be a prerequisite for effective treatment of health problems among homeless people (p. 4). Of course it is not only those who are homeless that require the support of social services and other agencies.

The type of house/living accommodation the patient lives in will also be important if they are to be discharged home into the community from hospital, and may require a visit by the occupational therapist who will assess the suitability of the home for safety and accessibility for the patient. Some people may live in more temporary accommodation or travel about in caravans, e.g. nomadic people in some parts of the world, or gypsy travellers.

Making sure to record the name of a contact person and significant other is essential. Next of kin is required for legal purposes (Roper et al 2000) and for contact in case of emergency. It is also important to know of significant others, such as friends or neighbours, who are the patient's support network. Again such information will be useful for planning discharge home from hospital.

The occupation of a patient is useful, in that again it helps build up a picture of the person now requiring health care and will ensure a more holistic approach. If, for example, a young patient has had to have both legs amputated, it helps in the counselling process to know that he was previously a very active person, e.g. a sports teacher. This may affect his recovery, knowing that he is no longer able to do this work as he did previously.

Information about cultural and religious beliefs and practices is essential to providing holistic care. As part of daily living these will need to be accommodated into the plan of care, and will also have a significant effect on the assessment of their needs in all the ALs. For example, if a patient is a Jehovah's Witness, the nurse will need to be aware of the religious beliefs with regard to blood transfusion, and if a patient is a Muslim, that for many Muslims daily prayer is very important and helping the patient to undertake this in the hospital routine will be part of the care planned (Holland & Hogg 2001).

Any recent life events or crises that nurses need to be aware of can also help in the provision of holistic care, such as a recent bereavement that may have taken place in hospital. This could cause the patient to worry that they may not come out of hospital alive either. There is a need to be aware of the current health problems and how they have affected the patient's life, including how they have changed their daily Activities of Living. If they are being cared for in the home, how has their illness affected what activities they could previously manage safely, such as getting out of bed during the night to go to the bathroom which may be on a different floor. Planning for discharge home if they are in hospital should begin when they are admitted, taking account of this biographical and health data and the main assessment of needs in the Activities of Living (see Box 1.6 for an example of discharge planning after surgery).

When assessment is undertaken

Beretta (2003) considers that assessment is undertaken on the following occasions:

- An assessment is usually carried out when the nurse first meets a patient or client, which may be on admission to hospital, on a visit to a clinic, or in the patient's or client's own home.
- Assessment may be carried out on a daily basis, to check the relevance of the care plan and to identify whether there is improvement or deterioration in the patient or client. This may mean the care plan has to be updated to accommodate new information gathered.
- Assessment is usually carried out before a patient or client is discharged home from hospital, to identify whether there is a need to continue care when the person is home. This may be a joint assessment involving other members of the multi-professional team, such as the physiotherapist, occupational therapist, social worker or the patient's GP (Beretta 2003, p. 123).

Obtaining information from the patient and others, however, is not enough to ensure successful care planning

Box 1.6	Practice application – preparation for discharge after surgery

Successful discharge planning should begin as soon as individuals enter the health care system. An early application of patients' perceptions of their problems, the support systems available to them and their coping abilities are pivotal to identifying the resource requirements for discharge. Regardless of whether patients are undergoing a minor procedure in a day-care setting or the most complex of operations, early planning can significantly and positively influence successful recovery.

Inappropriate discharge has been highlighted as a major reason for patient readmission. Poor and noncompliance with health information and medication are strongly linked to the quality of the discharge process.

Key educational aspects of a discharge plan

- General effects of surgery and/or anaesthesia (e.g. driving etc. may be restricted; need for rest, sleep etc.)
- Procedure specific advice (e.g. wearing anti-embolic stockings)
- Specific exercise activity (e.g. pelvic floor strengthening, walking and leg exercise)
- Dietary and nutritional advice (e.g. fruit, vegetable and fluid consumption to prevent constipation)
- Medication (e.g. dosage, side-effects and special instruction verbally and in written form), such as for pain relief
- Postoperative complication potential (e.g. advice on the recognition of bleeding, infection, persistent pain, limb swelling etc. and understanding of when to seek help is confirmed)
- Nurse and self-administered treatment (e.g. information on dressing changes, care of operation site, and suture clip/staple removal)
- Continuing and follow-up care (e.g. contact details and documentation for community nurse, outpatient and follow-up appointments)

From Brooker (2005), p. 159.

and goal setting. The information needs to be relevant and interpreted accurately. Also all information does not need to be obtained immediately, as more often than not patients are in an anxious state on admission to hospital or making first contact with health professionals. It is also inappropriate in emergency situations. For example, a patient admitted with a heart attack (myocardial infarction) is not going to be able to answer questions as to their lifestyle or social needs until they are in a stable condition. Recording the information obtained must also be accurate and clear – in order that patient care can be planned with confidence and based on substantiated data. Assessment is also a time for establishing a meaningful nurse–patient relationship, although as seen in Case study 1.1 (p. 18) this may not be the most immediate

action possible if the patient's health problem is critical. Roper et al (2000, p. 135) state that:

> *the objective therefore in collecting information about the ALs is to discover:*
> - *previous routines*
> - *what the person can do independently*
> - *what the person cannot do independently*
> - *previous coping behaviours*
> - *what problems the person has, both actual and potential, with relevant ALs.*

Identifying the person's problems is in fact the final activity of the assessing phase of the nursing process. Roper et al (2000, p. 135) point out that:

> *The nurse's role is to enable the patient/client to prevent, alleviate or solve, or cope positively with problems (actual or potential) related to the ALs. In many cases, the presence of actual problems (such as pain, bleeding, anorexia, pyrexia, acute depression, learning disability) may be obvious to the person and often is obvious to the nurse. But it has to be remembered that there may be a 'nurse-perceived' problem of which the patient is not aware (raised blood pressure being an obvious example) or a 'patient-perceived' problem (such as a particular worry or obsessive behaviour or suicidal tendencies) of which the nurse is not immediately aware. Being alert to these possibilities will ensure that they are explored in the course of the assessment.*

Identifying potential problems is very much dependent on the nurse's own knowledge of ill health, the possible complications and the underpinning cause including the altered physiology. In addition it is also dependent on the nurse's ability and skills to be able to use this knowledge to make, what are very often, critical decisions. Assessment is the key stage of the nursing process and all other stages (including reassessment) are dependent on how accurate this is in identifying patient needs and problems. Let us consider the kind of data that we need to obtain in relation to the 12 ALs (further information can be found in each AL chapter). It is acknowledged that using the model in practice will depend very much on the cultural and social context in which nursing exists. In some countries, the model framework will need to be adapted to allow for cultural differences as well as similarities and questions asked during the assessment will need to be adapted accordingly. It is also important to remember, however, that this takes into account both the nurse and patient's culture in this process. In New Zealand, for example, the concept of cultural safety has given rise to a complete change in how patient care is delivered and we can see how a definition of this recognises the importance of both the nurse and the patient culture in the case situation:

> *The effective nursing practice of a person/family from another culture is determined by that person or*

family. Culture includes, but is not restricted to, age or generation; gender; sexual orientation; occupation and socioeconomic status; ethnic origin or migrant experience; religious or spiritual belief; and disability.

The nurse delivering the service will have undertaken a process of reflection on his or her own cultural identity and will recognise the impact that his or her personal culture has on his or her professional practice. Unsafe cultural practice comprises any action which diminishes, demeans or disempowers the cultural identity and well-being of an individual. 99 (Nursing Council of New Zealand 2005)

In 1996 the Nursing Council of New Zealand introduced guidelines for cultural safety (referring to safe and competent practice) education for nursing and midwifery students (reviewed in March 2005). Through this education student nurses and midwives will:

66 • *examine their realities and the attitudes they bring to each new person they encounter in their practice*
  • *evaluate the impact that historical, political and social processes have on the health of people*
  • *demonstrate flexibility in their relationships with people who are different from themselves.* 99
(Nursing Council of New Zealand 2005, p. 8)

Although the guidelines have been adopted to meet the specific cultural needs of people in New Zealand the principles of safe and competent practice in cultural care are of value to other similar multicultural communities worldwide.

Given this multicultural nature of many countries today, together with international travel, it must also be noted that an awareness of cultural differences when using language in communicating with patients is essential to an effective assessment of individual needs (see Chapter 4). In fact being able to communicate, either verbally, visually or through touch is an essential prerequisite for effective assessment of any patient or client. It is also important to consider the physical setting for the assessment, e.g. comfortable for the patient, and that the nurse has acquired the appropriate interviewing skills, e.g. listening and observing, to carry it out.

Assessment of patient's ability to maintain own safe environment Data here will be of two main kinds – namely physical observations and verbal information. It will be essential for care planning to identify if the patient/client has any difficulties (actual problems) with maintaining their own internal safe environment. For example, if they have been bleeding heavily (haemorrhage) they will probably be having difficulty in maintaining a balanced homeostasis and will require immediate fluid/blood replacement in order to survive. Assessment of blood pressure, pulse and respirations will be essential data for the nurse and the

doctor to be able to plan care/treatment for the patient. The primary responsibility here is to maintain life and prevent deterioration by focusing on the physiological status of the patient.

It is also important to find out if the patient has any difficulties with their vision or hearing, which could compromise their physical safety. Questions such as 'Can the patient walk?' or 'How far can he/she walk?' may also be asked, and if the patient has a disability such as paraplegia (paralysed from waist down). Knowing this will also be important for ensuring that their skin integrity is maintained and that care can be instigated to ensure pressure sores do not develop. As well as its importance for patient care, the information is also very relevant for nursing practice. Knowing, for example, the patient is unable to move by himself also means that the nurse can plan for her own safe environment by ensuring that moving the patient is undertaken safely and with the right technique and equipment. The patient's relatives may also offer information here, if the patient is unable to do so. For example, if a patient has had a stroke and their speech has been impaired, the information a relative can give may be crucial in determining the cause of their illness or their capability to manage their own safety (see Chapter 3).

Assessment of communication skills/needs Effective communication is an essential prerequisite for effective nurse–patient relationships (Robinson 2002). It is important, for example, to know whether a patient can hear what is being said, can understand the language in which a question is being asked and can actually answer by either speaking or sign language. We often assume also that people can actually read the written information given to them, and assessing this deficit is potentially a very sensitive issue. There are, however, ways of ensuring that direct questioning on this issue is avoided, through, for example, observing the patient reading diet sheets and asking if there is a need for explanation. These are cues to making an assessment. Is the patient able to hear what you are saying? We cannot assume that because he or she is not wearing a hearing aid that they are not deaf. Does the patient normally wear a hearing aid and if so in which ear? Knowing this will help the nurse by ensuring that when speaking to the patient, they speak on the hearing side or speak more slowly and clearly.

Not speaking English, for example, can be a major communication barrier for patients and nurses working in a predominantly English-speaking society (and the same in other countries where another language is predominantly spoken) – but one that can easily be rectified through careful assessment of patient needs. Interpreters can contribute much to the assessment process, as can relatives. However, in some cultures, translating by men on behalf of women, or children on behalf of their parents, can cause untold embarrassment for all concerned and is to be avoided whenever possible. Very often accurate information will not be given, thus preventing a full assessment of patient needs (Holland & Hogg 2001). Other cues in assessing communication needs could relate to how the patient/client maintains contact with the nurse undertaking the assessment. For example, do they appear reluctant to make eye contact? Do they seem withdrawn and not wanting to talk? These kinds of cues could indicate that the patient is worried about something or frightened to ask about their health problems. It could also be indicative of some kind of depression. All cues need to be assimilated and actual or potential problems then identified (see Chapter 4).

Assessing a patient's breathing needs   Observing a patient's breathing is the first stage in assessing needs, i.e. ensuring that the patient is able to breathe and that there is a clear airway. The way in which a person breathes may be indicative of a number of immediate and long-term health problems. For example, if a patient has been admitted with an asthma attack, ensuring that they breathe effectively will be the nurse's first concern. Asking the patient to recall life history and other information will have to wait until their breathing has become more controlled and manageable for them. In some instances observing and then supporting an asthmatic's breathing could prevent them from requiring artificial mechanical support and ventilation.

As well as recording respirations per minute, the depth and regularity of their breathing is also important. They may be experiencing pain on breathing, resulting in their taking very shallow breaths. Long-term health problems affecting their breathing may have led the patient to adopt different positions in which their breathing becomes manageable – they may prefer to sit up using pillows or in a chair rather than a bed. Questions such as 'Do they have a cough?', 'Is it productive or a very dry cough?', 'If they are producing sputum – what colour is it?', 'Do they smoke?' and 'How many and how long have they smoked?' can lead to a picture of the patient's current and past health, and enable the nurse, doctor and other health professionals to plan care that will include realistic and manageable goals (see Chapter 5).

Assessing eating and drinking needs   Ensuring adequate hydration and nutrition is essential if health is to be maintained. Research has identified that patients suffer from malnutrition in hospital and that older people in particular are affected by lack of attention by nurses to their need for food and fluids (DoH 2001a). Assessment of individual eating and drinking needs will obviously depend very much on the patient's health problem or medical diagnosis. For example, a patient admitted to hospital for investigations of loss of weight and vomiting will need careful assessment of previous eating and drinking habits which will be important cues as to the reason for their current illness and symptoms. They may, for example, be alcohol dependent or may have a health problem such as anorexia nervosa. Past history of their patterns of eating and drinking are an essential part of the nursing assessment.

Have they likes or dislikes when it comes to food and drink? Are they eating a special diet? Do they have religious or cultural food and drink preferences? All these are questions that need to be determined during the assessment phase.

Other issues to take account of in order to ensure adequate hydration and nutrition are linked to physical activities. For example, can the patient cut up his or her own food? Have they got use of both hands? Are they able to swallow effectively?

All of these cues can then be examined as a group in order to be able to arrive at possible reasons for the patient's current problems, i.e. a diagnosis. The doctor will decide on a medical diagnosis which is inextricably linked to the nursing one – i.e. planning care requires an understanding of the underlying cause of the patient's illness in order to make sure that any care planned after the assessment will not further harm the patient (see Chapter 6).

Assessing a patient's elimination needs   Knowing about a patient's elimination habits is important, even if they are not experiencing problems directly linked to it. It is an aspect of living that some patients will find embarrassing to discuss and therefore requires sensitivity and sensitive questioning. For example, they may experience incontinence of urine when coughing or sneezing or they may have difficulty passing urine. This could be important information when patients have to go for surgery, especially postoperatively. It is important to know how often patients have their bowels opened in a day, if they take laxatives, especially if they are prone to constipation as this may require specific dietary measures, e.g. more fibre and fruit. If a patient has noticed any change from the normal bowel or urine output, it is necessary to determine what these are, e.g. colour, consistency, unusual smells. Some patients may have a colostomy or ileostomy from previous surgery and similar questions are just as relevant to them (see Chapter 7).

Assessing personal cleansing and dressing needs   Observation of the patient can provide a great deal of information about a patient's personal cleansing and dressing needs. For example if the community nurse has to undertake the assessment in the home, she can see what facilities are available for the patients to wash, bathe and dress themselves. In any situation the condition of clothing can be observed, is it clean or dirty? Has the patient been washing himself or herself or do they have a smell? This can also be linked to incontinence problems, especially in older people. Do they have skin problems such as psoriasis or eczema, which need additional care? Many patients will be embarrassed if they are no longer able to wash themselves and will need a great deal of reassurance that everything will be undertaken to ensure their privacy and dignity. In the community, day care services are available where people can be assisted with bathing on a daily or weekly basis.

If patients are not able to care for themselves they will be at a high risk of skin breakdown and pressure sores developing. Assessing their risk factor, by using a scoring system (Waterlow score for example) is an essential part of assessing personal cleansing and dressing needs (see Chapter 8).

Assessment of controlling body temperature needs

Assessing whether a patient has a normal or abnormal body temperature will entail both observation and measurement. Excessive perspiration or shivering, for example, could indicate a pyrexia (raised temperature), while the skin being very cold to the touch and white in appearance could indicate hypothermia (low temperature). Taking a patient's temperature using a thermometer of some kind, e.g. tympanic thermometer, will help to confirm this. Temperature is also affected by many factors that will indicate the treatment to be pursued (see Chapter 9). For example, a raised temperature 7 days postoperatively could indicate a wound infection, which would require antibiotics.

Assessment of mobility needs

It will be immediately apparent if a patient admitted to hospital, for example, arrives in a wheelchair, that their mobility is either temporarily or permanently affected. Determining which will require very sensitive questioning of the patient or anyone accompanying them. Determining how dependent the patient is for help to move about will be essential if the care planned is to be effective and avoid the potential problems associated with immobility (see Chapter 10). Questions include: 'Does the patient need mechanical aids to move about?', 'How restricted is their movement?', 'Is this restricted to one part of the body only?' and 'Does this vary in different situations or times of the day?' Knowing that someone has rheumatoid arthritis or has suffered a stroke, for example, will immediately alert the assessor that the patient could be in need of both physical aids and human assistance. A less apparent problem may be that mobility is impaired due to fear of falling, rendering the patient dependent on the nurse for a whole range of daily activities such as going to the toilet. Again sensitive questioning and nursing management of the situation is essential.

Assessment of working and playing needs

Knowing about an individual's employment is essential when planning effective care, especially if their illness prevents them from returning to that work. It may be that the individual is unemployed, and that this may affect their feeling of self-worth. An awareness of their normal leisure activities or hobbies may also be valuable, for example, in planning their discharge home from hospital. It may be necessary to communicate with other health and social care professions, such as the psychologist or social worker, to ensure that resources are available to enable them to manage not being at work due to their illness. Their work or leisure activity may have also contributed to their illness in some way. For example, they may have suffered a serious injury in the pursuit of rock climbing or been under stress due to working long hours (see Chapter 11).

Assessment of expressing sexuality needs

A discussion, rather than direct questioning, relating to expressing sexuality may be more appropriate and will need to be very sensitive and may not always be necessary for all patients. It is of obvious importance when patients are experiencing health problems related to sexual function, such as prostate or uterine cancer or termination of pregnancy. It is important to ensure, however, even when such questions are necessary during the assessment that these are asked sensitively and appropriately. For some men and women their cultural or religious beliefs may prevent them from giving appropriate responses, especially if interpreters or members of their own families are asked to translate (Holland & Hogg 2001, Robinson 2002). There are many health problems that affect sexual feelings and function, and the nurse needs to be aware of these in relation to the patients they care for (see Chapter 12).

Assessment of sleep needs

Sleep is essential for healthy living and recovery from illness. How much sleep individuals need will vary, but adults 'on average spend about one quarter to one third of their lives sleeping' (Roper et al 2000, p. 47). It is important to assess therefore the usual sleep patterns of the patient and whether they take any medication or other activities, e.g. a hot drink, to promote sleep. Asking whether they wake often in the night, for example, to go to the toilet is also important, especially if they are admitted to hospital where the environment is alien to them. Have they observed any change in their normal sleeping patterns? Do they need to sleep in the afternoon? These questions are very relevant when being admitted to a very busy surgical ward for example. Open visiting also means that the patient's day in hospital is now governed, not by patient needs necessarily but by convenience to their visitors. Restricted visiting times enabled patients who needed to rest and sleep the opportunity to do so without interruptions, and some ward areas still maintain this tradition. It is acknowledged, however, that open visiting is an opportunity for families to be involved in care. In Japan, for example, visiting a person who is sick in hospital is of cultural significance. It is a means of 'sustaining the identity of the patient as a social persona' and difficult to manage where there is restricted visiting to ensure adequate rest for the patient (Ohnuki-Tierney 1984) (see Chapter 13).

Assessment of needs in relation to death and dying

> ❝ *Dying is the final act of living. To die suddenly from natural causes in old age, and without loss of dignity, is what most people would regard as a 'good death'. However death is often preceded by a period of survival in a state of terminal illness, the duration of which may be prolonged, and perhaps accompanied by pain and distresses.* ❞ (Roper et al 2000, p. 51)

Assessing individual needs at such a time will require sensitivity and observation of both patients and their families, particularly concerning any cultural or religious needs they may have. Assessing the needs of relatives or significant others may take priority in the case of a sudden death of a patient following admission to hospital for example, as will assessing the needs of the family to start the bereavement process (see Chapter 14).

It is essential when considering the assessment of patients' needs that there is no unnecessary duplication of information by different health and social care professions. Being asked the same or similar questions by a number of people could be both distressing and unnecessary. The introduction of the single assessment process as outlined in the National Service Framework for Older People (DoH 2001b) is an excellent example of how this can be avoided. This process:

> 66 *recognises that many older people have health and social care needs, and that agencies need to work together so that assessment and subsequent care planning are person-centred, effective and co-ordinated. In particular, implementation will ensure that:*
>
> - *The scale and depth of assessment is kept in proportion to older people's needs*
> - *Agencies do not duplicate each other's assessments and*
> - *Professionals contribute to assessments in the most effective way.* 99 (DoH 2002)

SUMMARY POINTS

1. Each patient and their circumstances are individual and these need to be accommodated as much as possible into an individualised assessment.
2. There is no priority given in the assessment process to one specific Activity of Living, although the patient's illness will determine which activities are affected above others.
3. It is important to note that information about the patient is not only gained from the direct assessment itself. That is, information is also gained from other sources such as doctors' case notes and relatives.

Assessment framework in action Using a framework is essential to systematically gather information – in order to ensure accuracy and appropriateness of the data. It is also essential in order to be able to identify the actual or potential problems that the patient may experience. Consider the assessment stage in relation to the following patient (Case study 1.1).

Case study 1.1

Assessment of patient's actual and potential problems

Mr Davies, a 50-year-old man, has been involved in a road traffic accident. He has been admitted to the ward with a head injury and is unconscious.

We can see immediately that obtaining information from Mr Davies himself is not going to be possible as he is unconscious, and the serious nature of his illness requires information which must be prioritised in order to ensure his safety and wellbeing. We can assume that, as we know his name, secondary data from relatives and others will have been obtained or it may have been obtained from his wallet. Additional data such as information regarding his previous health, especially with regard to medication or illnesses that could contribute to his unconscious state, e.g. diabetes, will be essential. This first-stage assessment will have taken place in an accident and emergency unit or similar area.

On arrival to the ward it will be essential to continue to assess Mr Davies and identify his needs and problems. For example, the first question the nurse may ask is 'Can the patient maintain his own safe environment?' If yes, he does not have an actual problem or a need to have it maintained for him. If no, then he does have a problem and therefore goals, nursing actions and evaluation of the care need to take place.

Using the Roper et al (1996) model for nursing, what are Mr Davies's actual problems? (We can only assume some of

those in a hypothetical situation such as that described but this exercise will give you some indication of problem-solving using both the nursing process and a nursing model framework.)

His main (actual) problem will be that he is unable to maintain his own safe internal and external environment due to his unconscious state.

In order to meet this problem (problem is an unmet need) and to detect and prevent potential problems, some of the nursing actions (including continual gathering of certain types of data) and interventions will be as follows.

To maintain a safe internal environment (see Chapter 3):

- Position the patient (allowing for the head injury) to ensure a clear airway is maintained to prevent the potential problem of asphyxia.
- Observe pulse and blood pressure to detect the potential problem of raised intercranial pressure – indicated by a drop in pulse rate and a raised blood pressure.
- His temperature would be observed to detect the potential problem of damage to temperature control centre, indicated by high rise or severe drop in temperature.
- Observations need to be made of any head wound and any bleeding from the nose or ears which could indicate intercranial bleeding, and he is at risk of infection if he has an open head wound (potential problem). *(continued)*

Case study 1.1 *(continued)*

- Neurological observations would be undertaken – using, for example, the Glasgow Coma Scale for observations – to detect potential problems of intercranial changes and consciousness levels (as indicated by possible restlessness and changes in levels of consciousness).
- A safe external environment will be ensured by careful positioning of Mr Davies in the bed, ensuring that equipment for emergency care is within reach and in working order, e.g. oxygen, suction and emergency trolley with resuscitation equipment.

It is important when assessing a patient's needs/problems that priorities such as those above are determined. Other aspects of the model for nursing, such as lifespan, dependence/independence and factors influencing his health will become more important as his health improves. One influencing factor, however, will be important at this time, the sociocultural. It is important, given the seriousness of Mr Davies' condition, that his religious and spiritual needs are known. For example, he may be a Jehovah's Witness and have strong beliefs about treatment requiring blood transfusion, or he may be a Roman Catholic who attends mass regularly and would wish for a priest to visit him to offer prayers for his recovery.

Once we have ensured that his priority need is being met and his airway is clear and he is breathing normally, other actual problems can be assessed. For example:

- He will have an actual problem of immobility – due to his unconsciousness – and will therefore require his limbs to be moved and repositioned in order to ensure that the potential problem of breakdown in skin integrity (see Chapter 8) or deep vein thrombosis does not occur.
- He will have an actual problem of not being able to eliminate adequately or normally and he may be incontinent due to his unconsciousness or have urinary retention for the same reason (see Chapter 7).
- He will have an actual problem of not being able to eat or drink as he normally does. His nutrition and hydration needs will have to met by other means in order to ensure that the potential problem of dehydration and malnutrition does not occur (see Chapter 6).
- He will have an actual problem of not being able to meet his own personal cleansing and dressing needs (see Chapter 8).

Mr Davies will be constantly assessed and his care re-evaluated to an agreed care plan, and all members of the multidisciplinary team will make decisions about his care. His relatives/significant others will be included in his care whenever possible and he should be talked to at all times when care is carried out. Pemberton & Waterhouse (2006) inform us that research has shown that there is a possibility that patients can still hear conversations and voices even though they are unconscious (Podurgiel 1990).

It can be seen from this small case study the way in which a problem-solving approach to Mr Davies' care can be used, based on the data presented and also, most importantly, the knowledge of how to care for a patient with a head injury. In order to be able to ensure an accurate assessment of patient needs using the model for nursing (see Appendix 3) it is essential that nurses have knowledge of the anatomy and physiology and potential problems associated with the presenting illness (each chapter will explore this in detail).

Once the patient's needs have been assessed, using the Roper et al framework, all information/data acquired must be documented in the nursing care plan (see Appendix 2). These will vary in their structure according to individual organisations' own policies and developments.

Exercise

1. Using a care plan of your choice undertake an assessment of a patient/client.
2. Note the kind of skills you used in the assessment process and how these influenced the responses you received from the patient and their family.
3. Identify actual and potential problems that the patient has.

Planning

Care is planned according to the nature of the actual and potential problems identified, and is dependent on the nurse's knowledge of appropriate care to be given for that health problem and taking account of the individuality of the patient.

According to Roper et al (2000, p. 137) the objective of the plan is:

- to prevent identified potential problems with any of the ALs from becoming actual ones
- to solve identified actual problems
- where possible to alleviate those that cannot be solved
- to help the person cope positively with those problems that cannot be alleviated or solved
- to prevent recurrence of a treated problem
- to help the person to be as comfortable and pain-free as possible when death is inevitable.

To achieve the plan requires the nurse and the individual to set goals, both short term and long term for the actual and potential problems identified. Some of these will be goals for the nurse to achieve in relation to the patient. For example, if the patient has a raised blood pressure requiring medication, it is the nurse's task to ensure that the patient receives that at the appropriate times and in accordance with the doctor's prescription. On the other hand if the patient is very anxious about his blood pressure it could be their goal to try and reduce this anxiety by voicing their concerns and talking through any other activities they may have with the nurse. Roper et al (1996) point out these:

> *goals should be achievable within a person's individual circumstances, otherwise there is a danger of disheartenment. Whenever possible, goals should be stated in terms of outcomes which are able to be observed, measured or tested so that their subsequent evaluation can be accomplished. Whenever feasible, a time/date should be specified alongside a goal to indicate when evaluation should be undertaken.* (Roper et al 1996, p. 57)

Kemp & Richardson (1994, p. 38) state that 'One of the advantages of goal setting is that it can act as a stimulus for the patient – something that gives him a sense of purpose, something to work for'. They cite the following example to illustrate this:

> *Mr John Brown, a patient with bone metastasis, was at home receiving terminal care. He was being cared for by his wife Anne and the district nurse. He had become withdrawn and was apparently not interested in anything and said as much. He just wanted 'to get it over with'. Anne and the nurse discussed how they could help him. Anne said that he had been a keen gardener until recently. It was suggested to John that he plan a flower garden with Anne and supervise her carry out the work. This they did together. He sat in a chair whilst she dug the garden and planted the seeds. There is no doubt that these activities, which were achieved through a series of goal steps, enabled the patient to reach the goal, 'Planned and supervised the planting of a flower garden by March 1988'.* (Kemp & Richardson 1994, p. 38)

They concluded that 'by discussing a problem and identifying a person's strengths (in this case his love for his wife and his past interest) it was possible to motivate the patient and give him and his wife something to work for, which obviously helped them both' (Kemp & Richardson 1994, p. 39). Goals can be either immediate, e.g. resuscitating a patient following a myocardial infarction; short term, e.g. for a diabetic patient to learn how to self-medicate and give their own insulin injection; or long term, e.g. in the case of alcohol dependence, not drinking any alcohol at the end of 3 years.

Kemp & Richardson (1994) offer the following advice on writing goal statements (based on Mager 1975):

> *A goal may contain the following:*

- *Performance – the actual behaviour, communication or clinical features demonstrated by the patient, e.g. walks, recognises, writes, reports decreasing weight*
- *Condition – the environment or help required from a person and/or resources, e.g. with the aid of the Zimmer frame; supported by daughter; in the hall*
- *Criteria – the measurement of how well, how long, how far, how often, how much, e.g. walks with the*

Zimmer frame from the hall to the door twice a day; loss of weight – 1 kg in one week
- *Target – the predicted time by which the goal will be achieved and thus evaluated*
- *Review – a checking time may be necessary for some long term goals, when an evaluation statement should be written.* (Kemp & Richardson 1994, p. 39)

Setting and achieving goals will be dependent on the patient, his health problem and 'the resources available, together with the nurse's skills and experience in dealing with the particular problem' (Kemp & Richardson 1994, p. 41).

In addition to planning care and setting goals through verbal/nonverbal interaction between patient and nurse, it is customary to record or document the care planned, indeed all the stages of the nursing process are documented. This is essential for continuity of care and also as a legal document, which records evidence of care and treatment given by health care professionals (Walsh 2002).

Exercise

1. Consider the issues raised in Box 1.7. What are your experiences of documenting care?
2. Discuss with colleagues how you would ensure confidentiality in multidisciplinary documentation and your views on patient-held records.

Box 1.7	Documentation

All members of the health care team should share the patient's record. Increasingly, care teams are developing multidisciplinary documentation that places all the different professions' records in a single document. This greatly improves communication between different members of the health care team. If a patient has a chronic condition that is managed largely in the community but still requires occasional admissions either for acute exacerbations or respite care, the patient care record can be held by the patient. Some health staff find this a rather radical suggestion but it is increasingly gaining acceptance. If involving patients as partners in care is to be meaningful why not let them look at their own notes? It means staff know exactly what community care has been given before admission and vice versa on discharge. It becomes a means of providing information about the patient's condition and the health professionals' nursing care plans, and contributes to continuity of care. Accurate and comprehensive written documentation facilitates collaboration and cooperation among members of the various health care professions to ensure optimal use of resources on the patient's behalf. The record is a confidential document; it is available only to those participating in the care by permission of the patient and employer.

From Walsh (2002), p. 12.

Nursing care plans can either be handwritten or, as in some hospitals today, by inputting data into a computer (Walsh 2002). Some areas have standard nursing care plans, which although they appear to be contrary to the philosophy of nursing process and the Roper et al model for nursing, i.e. individualised care, can be used effectively. An example of their use would be in pre- and postoperative care where there are core nursing interventions to be undertaken in order to ensure a safe environment for all patients undergoing surgery. Nursing care plans vary in their format in different countries and different hospitals and community settings. The model for nursing used, as a framework for the nursing process and nursing care plans will also vary. However, most will reflect the stages of the nursing process, i.e. assessment, planning, implementation and evaluation.

Exercise

1. Find out what kind of care plan documentation is being used in the hospital or community where you work or are learning as a student nurse.
2. Identify what nursing model is being used as a framework for assessing, planning, implementing and evaluating care.
3. Discuss your findings with your colleagues and compare the use of these nursing care plans in practice.

Roper et al (2000, p. 140) summarise the planning phase of the nursing process by stating that:

> *It involves producing a nursing plan that contains the following information:*
>
> - *Stated goals or desired outcomes for each problem*
> - *A date on which the goals are expected to be achieved*
> - *The nursing interventions (and patient participation) to achieve the goals*
> - *The objective of the nursing plan is to provide the information on which systematic, individualised nursing can be based and implemented by any nurse.*

It is important to note here the need for any care planned to be based on best practice and best evidence in order to ensure quality care (Parsley & Corrigan 1999).

The development of integrated care pathways and resultant documentation may mean that the nursing care plan becomes an integral part of a multiprofessional document and care plan (Parsley & Corrigan 1999). According to Roper et al (2000, p. 143) documenting care can be seen to:

- be part of a monitoring programme related to the quality of nursing service
- provide factual information to managers when, because of staff shortages, items in the 'planned nursing' had to be omitted
- provide factual information to managers when a second best nursing intervention had to be planned because of lack of resources

- provide information that can be used in defence of patients' compliants in a legal context
- help nurses to describe nursing's contribution to the total health care programme, particularly important when submitting an application for adequate financial resources
- provide substantiation for adequate remuneration for nursing personnel
- contribute to a database for research in nursing.

Implementing

This is the third stage of the nursing process and is evidence of how the nurse intervenes to solve the actual or potential problems the patient/client may experience. The nurse plans and carries out the interventions by drawing upon a range of knowledge and skills and expertise in caring for patients in her own field of practice, as well as the expertise of nursing practice gained generally (see each AL chapter for examples of this 'expert practice' and intervention). An interesting example of how the Roper et al model for nursing was used to assess, plan and implement care in a very different environment to that of a Western hospital is seen in Heslop's (1991) care study of a sick Tibetan child (Tenzin) in a refugee settlement in Northern India. She used the model to work with the child's father (Sonam) to identify Tenzin's actual problems, discuss his management related to these problems and reassess them following implementation of the planned care. Despite the treatment and care, however, Tenzin eventually died from the diagnosed poliomyelitis but because of the collaborative approach between the nurse and the parent he was able to do so surrounded by his family at home.

Exercise

1. Using the assessment of a patient already undertaken (see exercise on p. 19) identify the interventions you plan to undertake to ensure that actual and potential problems are solved.
2. Using appropriate documentation record these interventions and identify who will be responsible for their action.
3. Discuss with your mentor or preceptor how you will involve the patient and others in the care to be implemented.

Evaluating Any care planned and implemented must have some outcome if it is to be worthwhile in terms of benefiting patients. Evaluating care also 'provides a basis for ongoing assessment and planning as the person's circumstances and problems change' (Roper et al 2000, p. 141). It is an opportunity for nurses to evaluate whether the care they have either managed or delivered themselves has been effective in meeting the goals that were set by them or by the patient. If the goals have been met then interventions will have been successful. If they have not then the nurse might ask the following (Roper et al 2000, p. 141):

1. Is it partially achieved and is more information needed before reconsidering whether or not to continue or adapt the intervention?
2. Is the problem unchanged or static and should the goal and the planned intervention be changed or stopped?
3. Is there worsening of the problem and should the goal and the planned nursing intervention be reviewed?
4. Was the goal incorrectly stated or inappropriate?
5. Does the goal require intervention(s) from other members of the health care team?

All four stages of the nursing process (including nursing diagnosis of actual or potential problems) are part of a cycle of care and should be responsive to change (see Fig. 1.5). In practice the documentation of patient care is recorded in nursing or patient care plans (paper or electronic). The Nursing and Midwifery Council (NMC) in the UK reinforces the professional and legal responsibilities that nurses have in ensuring the accuracy of care records and recommends the regular use of a care plan audit in order to protect patients and contribute to the body of practice evidence and quality of care, together with identifying future improvements (NMC 2007). An example of a simple audit tool can be found in Appendix 1.

Exercise

1. Using the nursing process and the Roper et al model for nursing as a framework undertake the total care of a patient. If you are a student ensure that this is supervised by a qualified nurse according to policy.
2. Analyse each stage of the nursing process undertaken and determine on what evidence the care was planned and delivered.
3. Summarise your learning needs following discussion with either your mentor or preceptor.

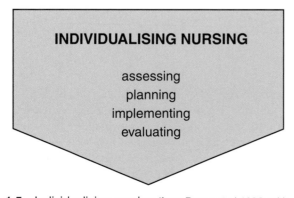

Fig. 1.5 Individualising nursing (from Roper et al 1996, with permission).

SUMMARY POINTS

1. The nursing process has four main stages, namely assessment (including nursing diagnosis of actual and potential problems) planning, implementing and evaluation.
2. Each stage is dependent on the effectiveness of the other in a cyclical process.
3. The Roper et al model for nursing is one framework that can be used to guide the nurse in the delivery of patient care and the design of the care plan documentation.

References

Andrews M 2000 Transcultural perspectives in the nursing care of children and adolescents. In: Andrews MM, Boyle JS (eds) Transcultural concepts in nursing care, 3rd edn. JB Lippincott, Philadelphia

Beretta R 2005 Assessment: the foundations of good practice. In: Hinchliffe S, Norman S, Schober J Nursing practice and health care, 4th edn. Arnold, London

Brooker C (ed) 2005 Mini encyclopaedia of nursing. Churchill Livingstone, Edinburgh

Data Protection Act 1998 Office of Public Sector Information, London

Department of Health 2001a Caring for older people: a nursing priority. DoH, London

Department of Health 2001b National service framework for older people. DoH, London

Department of Health 2002 The single assessment process – key implications for nurses. DoH, London (www.doh.gov.uk/scg/sap/nurses.html)

Herbert RA 2006 The biology of human ageing. In: Redfern SJ, Ross FM (eds) Nursing older people. Churchill Livingstone, Edinburgh, pp. 57–81

Henderson V 1966 The basic principles of nursing. International Council of Nurses, Geneva

Heslop P 1991 A preventable tragedy. Nursing Times 87(39): 36–39

Holland K, Hogg C 2001 Cultural awareness in nursing and health care. Arnold, London

Kawashima M (trans.) 2006 Applying the Roper-Logan-Tierney model in practice. Japanese translation, Elsevier, Tokyo

Kemp N, Richardson E 1994 The nursing process and quality care. Arnold, London

La Fontaine JS 1985 Initiation – ritual drama and secret knowledge across the world. Penguin Books, Harmondsworth, Middlesex

Leininger M 1978 Transcultural concepts, theories and practices. John Wiley, New York

Mager RF 1975 Preparing instructional objectives, 2nd edn. Fearnon Pitman, Belmont, CA

Nursing Council of New Zealand 2005 Guidelines for cultural safety, the Treaty of Witangi and Maori Health in nursing education and practice. Nursing Council of New Zealand, New Zealand

Nursing and Midwifery Council 2007 Record keeping guidance. NMC, London

Ohnuki-Tierney E 1984 Illness and culture in contemporary Japan. Cambridge University Press, Cambridge

Parsley K, Corrigan P 1999 Quality improvement in healthcare – putting evidence into practice, 2nd edn. Stanley Thornes, Cheltenham

Pemberton L, Waterhouse C 2006 The unconscious patient. In: Alexander MF, Fawcett JN, Runciman PJ (eds) Nursing practice, hospital and home (the adult). Churchill Livingstone, Edinburgh, pp 965–988

Podurgiel M 1990 The unconscious experience: a pilot study. Journal of Neuroscience Nursing 22(1): 52–53

Ponto MT 2006 The psychology of human ageing. In: Redfern SJ, Ross FM (eds) A textbook of gerontological nursing. Baillière Tindall, London

Robinson M 2002 Communication and health in a multi-ethnic society. The Policy Press, Bristol

Roper N, Logan W, Tierney A 1980, 1996 The elements of nursing, 1st edn, 4th edn. Churchill Livingstone, Edinburgh

Roper N, Logan W, Tierney A 2000 The Roper–Logan–Tierney model of nursing. Churchill Livingstone, Edinburgh

Slevin O 2003 Problem-solving frameworks: the nursing process approach. In: Basford L, Slevin O (eds) The theory and practice of nursing – an integrated approach to caring practice. Nelson Thornes, Cheltenham

Uys LR, Habermann M 2005 The nursing process: globalization of a nursing concept – an introduction. In: Habermann M, Uys LR The nursing process – a global concept. Churchill Livingstone (Elsevier), Edinburgh

Walsh M (ed) 2002 Watson's clinical nursing and related sciences, 6th edn. Baillière Tindall, London

Waugh A, Grant A 2006 Ross and Wilson anatomy and physiology in health and illness, 9th edn. Churchill Livingstone, Edinburgh

World Health Organization 2002a Child and adolescent health development. WHO, Geneva (www.who.int/child-adolescent-health)

World Health Organization 2002b Health conditions aggravate South Africa famine. WHO Press release, WHO 63, 5th August. WHO, Geneva (www.who.int/mediacentre/releases/who6)

Wright NMJ, Tompkins CNE 2005 How can health care systems effectively deal with the major health needs of homeless people? Health Evidence Network, World Health Organization Regional Office for Europe

Yura D, Walsh MB 1978 The nursing process: assessing, planning, implementing and evaluating. Appleton Century Crofts, New York

Further reading

Jamieson EM, McCall JM, Whyte LA 2002 Clinical nursing practices, 4th edn. Churchill Livingstone, Edinburgh

Robinson M 2002 Communication and health in a multi-ethnic society. The Policy Press, Bristol

Roper N, Logan W, Tierney A 1996 The Roper, Logan and Tierney model: A model in nursing practice. Chapter 12. In: Walker PH, Neuman B (eds) Blueprint for use of nursing models: Education, research, practice and administration. National League for Nursing, New York

Roper N, Logan W, Tierney A 2000 The Roper–Logan–Tierney model of nursing. Churchill Livingstone, Edinburgh

Useful websites

www.culturediversity.org (transcultural nursing concepts)
www.doh.gov.uk (Department of Health, UK)
www.icn.ch (International Council of Nurses)
en.wikipedia.org/wiki (Wikipedia (free encyclopedia) – definitions and examples of nursing process and other nursing terms)

Nursing and the context of care

Karen Holland

INTRODUCTION

Nursing takes place within a social and political context that is influenced by its history. Nurses need to be aware of the development of their profession in order to be able to understand the way in which factors outside their direct responsibility can have an influence on the care they give to patients and their families. This may be unique to each country in which that care is delivered. This care is also influenced by the way in which health care and nurse education is developed and managed.

Given the multicultural nature of societies throughout the world, and the way in which travel has made it easier for individuals from those countries to meet, it is important that some understanding of nursing practice in different countries is gained.

The essential requirement of nursing to be evidence based influences not only the way care is delivered but also the way in which students and qualified practitioners learn the skills of ensuring that the evidence is the best available.

To be able to use a model for nursing which has been developed over time to accommodate all manner of change, socially, politically and professionally, it is essential that the issues raised above be explored. The use of the model is dependent on understanding not only the factors influencing each Activity of Living (AL), but more importantly the nature of nursing as practised by nurses and the context in which that care takes place. This chapter is only an introduction to nursing and the context of care and you will be directed to further reading to enhance your understanding of the issues raised. This chapter will therefore focus on the following:

1. The nature of nursing and health care
   - the role and function of the nurse
   - knowledge for nursing practice
   - skills for nursing practice
   - health care.

2. Health care and nursing practice
   - NHS in the UK
   - new roles for nurses in patient care
   - evidence-based practice in nursing
   - multiprofessional collaboration
   - delivery of care.

3. International perspectives in nursing and health care.
4. Professional issues influencing nursing practice.
5. Nurse education – its development and current context.

THE NATURE OF NURSING AND HEALTH CARE

INTRODUCTION

Nursing as an occupation takes place in a number of health care settings and is a universally recognised profession. According to Savage (1993):

> 66 *The mission of nursing in society is to help individuals, families and groups to determine and achieve their physical, mental and social potential, and to do so within the challenging context of the environment in which they live and work. This requires nurses to develop and perform functions that promote and maintain health as well as prevent ill-health. Nursing also includes the planning and giving of care during illness and rehabilitation, and encompasses the physical, mental and social aspects of life as they affect health, illness, disability and dying.* 99 (Savage 1993, p. 15)

THE ROLE AND FUNCTION OF THE NURSE

The functions that a nurse has in society are seen to derive from this mission and should remain constant 'regardless of the place (home, workplace, school, university, prison, refugee camp, hospital, primary health care clinic or other site) or time in which nursing care is given, the health status of the individual or group to be served or the resources available' (Savage 1993, p. 16). These functions can be seen in Box 2.1.

Box 2.1	Summary of the functions of the nurse

1. Providing and managing nursing care

- Assessing the needs of the individual, family, group or community and identifying the resources required and available to meet them.
- Identifying the needs that can be met most appropriately and effectively by nursing care and those that should be referred to other professionals.
- Ranking the health needs that can best be met by nursing care in order of priority.
- Planning and providing the nursing care required.
- Involving the individual (and where appropriate, family and friends) in all aspects of care and encouraging community participation (if relevant and acceptable), self-care and self-determination in all matters related to health.
- Documenting what is done at each stage of the nursing process and using the information to evaluate the outcome of the nursing care given, in terms of the individual, family, group or community, the nurse involved and the system within which the nursing care was given.
- Applying accepted and appropriate cultural, ethical and professional standards.

2. Teaching patients or clients and health care personnel

- Assessing the individual's knowledge and skills relating to the maintenance and restoration of health.
- Preparing and providing the information needed at an appropriate level.
- Organising or participating in health education campaigns.
- Evaluating the outcome of such educational programmes.
- Helping nurses and other staff to acquire new knowledge and skills.
- Applying accepted and appropriate cultural, ethical and professional standards.

3. Acting as an effective member of a health care team

- Collaborating with individuals, families and communities and other health workers to plan.
- Acting as a leader of a nursing care team, which may include other nurses and auxiliary personnel as well as users of nursing services.
- Delegating nursing activities and tasks to other nursing personnel and supporting them in their work.
- Negotiating the user's participation in the implementation of his or her care plan.
- Collaborating with other people in multidisciplinary and multisectoral teams in planning, providing, developing, coordinating and evaluating health services.
- Collaborating with other health professionals in maintaining a safe and harmonious working environment that is conducive to team work.
- Being actively involved in policy making and programme planning, in setting priorities and in the development and allocation of resources.
- Participation in the preparation of reports to authorities and politicians at the local, regional or national level and, when appropriate, to the mass media.

4. Developing nursing practice through critical thinking and research

- Launching innovative ways of working to achieve better results.
- Identifying areas for research to increase knowledge or develop skills in nursing practice or education and participating in such studies as required.
- Applying accepted standards and appropriate cultural, ethical and professional standards to guide research in nursing.

From Savage (1993).

Another more well-known definition of the role and function of the nurse is that of Virginia Henderson (1966):

> The unique function of the nurse is to assist the individual, sick or well, in the performance of those activities contributing to health or its recovery (or to peaceful death) that he would perform unaided if he had the necessary strength, will or knowledge. And to do this in such a way as to help him gain independence as rapidly as possible. This aspect of her work, this part of her function, she initiates and controls, of this she is master. In addition she helps the patient to carry out the total program whether it be for the improvement of health or the recovery from illness or support in death. (Henderson 1966, p. 15)

Exercise

Consider these two descriptions of the functions and role of the nurse and discuss your responses with colleagues.

1. How does your own experience of nursing compare with Henderson's definition?
2. How many of Savage's functions of a nurse have you undertaken in your role as either a student or qualified nurse?
3. What do you consider to be the most rewarding functions of your role as either a student or qualified nurse?
4. How does the society/culture in which you live influence how you carry out these functions?
5. Do these definitions remain valid in today's nursing context?

In relation to Point 4 you may have considered the following issues:

- the status of nursing in different countries
- the health and illness beliefs of patients
- the health care system in which nursing exists.

For example, multiprofessional collaboration will be difficult to implement in a health care system which promotes a hierarchy of status, and where the medical team is considered to make all the decisions regarding patient care. Henderson's definition implies that nurses are only there to 'carry out the therapeutic plan as initiated by the physician', and this may still be the case in many countries. However, certainly in the United Kingdom this is no longer the situation, with new roles enabling nurses to have much more of a lead in decision-making regarding patients' treatment and care (Humphris & Masterson 2000). These issues are explored later in the chapter.

KNOWLEDGE FOR NURSING PRACTICE

As we can see from Savage's description (Box 2.1), undertaking the role of a nurse will require an extensive knowledge and skills base with which to practise in an accountable way and this is drawn from a number of other disciplines as well as from the art and science of nursing itself. Those which have had a significant impact on nursing care include:

- sociology
- biological science
- psychology
- ethics
- anthropology
- health promotion
- politics and social policy
- research
- management
- economics.

We can see the influence of these disciplines in Roper et al's model itself, in particular the factors influencing the Activities of Living, e.g. biological (biological sciences), psychological (psychology), sociocultural (sociology and anthropology), environmental (health promotion and social policy) and politicoeconomic (politics and economics). (Further details can be found in each AL chapter.) How has nursing used the source of knowledge from these disciplines? To be able to answer this question in its entirety is beyond the scope of this chapter. However, a brief explanation of each discipline and a link to nursing will be offered.

Sociology

Jones (1994) defined sociology as follows:

> *Sociology is the systematic study of human society. It provides us with evidence and explanations of how society works, of the actions of individuals and groups, of patterns of similarity and difference between people (within a single society and between societies), of the distribution of social resources and economic and political power. Sociology is concerned both with studying individuals (social actors or agents) operating in the social world and with trying to understand how the social world 'works' by investigating how social structures and relationships develop, persist and change.* (Jones 1994, p. 40)

Thinking of nursing, and the contexts in which it takes place, it can be seen that it offers a rich 'social world' for sociological investigation. Porter (1998, p. x), however, notes that sociologists 'have not paid great attention to the actual work that nurses do'. In 1991 he chose to study effects of the nursing process on the working lives of nurses in an intensive care unit (Porter 1991) and one of his findings was that despite nurses having 'considerable informal input into decisions' that the most important ones 'about care were made by physicians, nursing care plans being constructed in response to those decisions' (Porter 1998, p. 79). Are Porter's findings still valid?

With the development of new nursing roles such as nurse consultants it could be argued that this is no longer the case. Fairly & Closs (2006) in their evaluation of a nurse consultant's clinical activities and the search for patient outcomes in critical care illustrate this change with the following example of a nurse consultant's narrative:

> *A 39 year old male was admitted for abdominal pain and at the time I saw that he did not have a medical diagnosis ... (She then reads his notes and begins to talk to him.) After I questioned him further he said that he had not informed a member of medical or nursing staff that he took recreational drugs. The medical team were subsequently informed about this. As the patient had not been seen by a doctor that morning I carried out a physical examination, listened to heart and breath sounds and in view of his breathlessness, low oxygen saturation and deterioration in blood gases instructed that his oxygen be increased. I also noted that the patient had previously been receiving regular fruesemide prior to hospital admission and in view of his positive fluid balance, suggested that it be recommenced. I also suggested that the patient should have a 12 lead ECG in view of his heart rhythm. The ECG was performed and fruesemide recommenced. Arterial blood gases, oxygen saturation and respiratory status improved with increased oxygen concentrations.* (Fairley & Closs 2006, p. 1109)

We can see here that it was the nurse that made the initial decisions with regard to treatment and patient care.

Your answers may well be influenced by the way society as a whole and/or how the medical profession in your country views nurses and their role in patient care.

Biological science

Davey (1992, p. 42) stated that 'biology is the scientific study of the structure and function of living things and of the interactions of organisms with each other in the natural world and with their environment'. Roper et al (1996, p. 25), in the model for nursing, use the term as it relates to 'the human body's anatomical and physiological performance'. Knowledge of this is essential if nurses are to understand the nature of disease and patient symptoms, as well as help to promote healthy living. Examples of this interdependence are to be found in all AL chapters, e.g. in Chapter 5 it can be seen how a knowledge of gaseous exchange can help to understand the effects of smoking on breathing.

Psychology

Psychology considers the understanding of experience and behaviour of the individual especially relevant to nursing, considering that it involves caring for individuals. It includes understanding of emotional and intellectual development (Roper et al 1996). Knowledge of psychology would, for example, be important if you were to understand a child or adult's fear of hospitals, as would understanding how people behave when in stressful situations. Nursing is also an interpersonal activity (e.g. nurse–patient, nurse–nurse, nurse–doctor interactions) with communication (both verbal and nonverbal) being an essential aspect of care. We also communicate through different media, such as television, music, newspapers and books.

Ethics

Cooper (2001) states that 'ethics is the study of what is right or good'. She offers the following observations of its links to nursing:

> *Ethical nursing practice is based on general knowledge about ethical frameworks and principles, professional codes and guidelines, and particular knowledge of one's values and the values of the patient. Knowing about ethics however is not the same as developing ethical nursing practice. Moving from knowing about ethics to being an ethical nurse is similar to developing any other nursing skill. What is required is an intention to learn, self-reflection about values, as skilful teacher, dialogue with others and practice.* (Cooper 2001, p. 46)

The UK Nursing and Midwifery Council's Code of Professional Conduct (NMC 2004a) offers nurses an ethical framework in which to practise. Ethical principles guide nurses' actions and choices when faced with an ethical dilemma, for example not agreeing with the active resuscitation of a person who has told you they have no wish for this to happen. This may involve being an advocate for the patient, an advocate being 'one who supports or champions another, often because an individual, for whatever reason, is not in a position to speak adequately or effectively for him- or herself' (Wallace 2002, p. 10).

Anthropology

Anthropology can be defined as the 'study of human nature, human society and human history' (Schultz & Lavenda 1990, p. 4) and a central concept is culture.

Madeline Leininger, an American nurse and an anthropologist, has used this concept in the development of transcultural nursing which she states is a subfield of nursing, i.e. that it is:

> *the comparative study and analysis of different cultures and sub-cultures in the world with respect to their caring behaviour, nursing care, and health–illness values, beliefs and patterns of behaviours with the goal of generating scientific and humanistic knowledge in order to provide culture-specific and culture universal nursing care practices.* (Leininger 1978, p. 8)

Other nurses such as Holden & Littlewood (1991) and Savage (1995) have used anthropology to view nursing very differently. Savage, in her ethnographic study of nurse–patient interaction, for example, linked her finding of 'closeness' in nursing with kinship and family relationships. Littlewood (1991) discusses the way in which nursing is viewed as being 'polluting or dirty' work, a theme which is also developed in the work of Jocalyn Lawler (1991) on body care in nursing work.

Exercise
1. How does your culture influence your beliefs about health and illness?
2. Discuss with colleagues how different cultural beliefs can influence patient care.
3. Identify in clinical practice situations where your beliefs about health and illness have been different to your patients' and reflect on your actions.

Health promotion and education

Walsh (2002, p. 16) points out that 'given the difficulties surrounding the definition of health, there is little agreement about what constitutes health promotion and how it differs from health education'. He does offer, however, what he calls a very 'commonsense definition of health education', i.e. 'as teaching individuals about steps they can take to enhance their health (e.g. exercise) and avoid disease (e.g. use a condom during sex)'. If this is then linked to Tones's (1993) definition, i.e. 'Health promotion = health education × healthy public policy', then he concludes that 'in this view health education is seen as empowerment which, when combined with a health-orientated public policy, leads to the promotion of health' (Walsh 2002). Nurses have a major role in promoting health and wellbeing,

---

Exercise
1. Find out what are the main health education issues facing health and social services in your country.
2. Consider one of these in more detail and find out what is being undertaken with regard to health promotion, education and their outcomes.

---

as well as preventing disease, and Roper et al see this as being an essential factor in the model for nursing (Roper et al 2000, p. 102).

Politics and economics

Nursing exists in a political world, where the actions of government affect the way in which it is delivered, e.g. setting down legislation as to what competencies nurses need, and also affect individuals who require nursing care, e.g. investing in new hospitals or making patients pay for their medication prescriptions. Roper et al (2000) explain the role of the state in a modern world and point out that:

> *the State is the apex of the modern social pyramid and has supremacy over other forms of social groupings, so, in general terms, the State regulates human activities of living. For example, in relation to the AL of mobilizing, traffic regulations are enforced by the State. However the State is dependent on the economic system that underlies legal order; only limited social progress is possible when a State has a precarious economic base.* (Roper et al 2000, p. 72)

Health economics is not a subject, in the past, that has been promoted in the nursing curriculum. However, as Morris (1998, p. vii) points out, this is now becoming increasingly important for nurses 'as efficient and cost-effective use of resources is seen as necessary for the provision of a high-quality nursing service'.

Exercise
1. Identify the countries where the health service is not free at the point of need.
2. How is patient care determined in those countries?
3. What impact does having to pay for care have on nursing practice?

A useful website for information on health care systems and health policy in Europe and the United States of America is that of the European Observatory on Health Systems and Policies (www.euro.who.int/observatory).

Research

The ability to understand research and critically appraise evidence is essential to taking forward the current NHS agenda in the UK (Department of Health (DoH) 2000). Grant & Massey (1999, p. 117) state that 'the primary goal of nursing research is to develop a specialised, scientifically based body of knowledge unique to nursing' and in basic terms this research can either be quantitative (positivistic) or qualitative (interpretive); the former Grant & Massey (1999) define as 'research which examines specific phenomena' (e.g. testing hypotheses) and the latter 'research which explores human experiences as they are lived' (e.g. living with a chronic illness). Hamer & Collinson (1999) indicate that there are different forms of evidence arising from the above approaches and that it is essential that they are appraised, using set criteria, for their usefulness and quality (see p. 33).

Exercise

1. Find three nursing research articles (nursing care) which have described three different research approaches (methodologies).
2. Read the articles and discover how the findings of the research could help nurses deliver care.
3. Consider how you would go about changing practice based on their findings.

Management

Watkins (1997, p. 15) stated that 'nurse managers require knowledge derived from the study of leadership, organisations and management if they are to provide managerial leadership in addition to the theory necessary for professional leadership'. Understanding how to manage change, how organisations function and how to ensure that the care being delivered is of a high quality are only three elements of the management role of a nurse. Others include managing conflict, decision-making and effective communication. Management can occur at different levels of the organisation, from being responsible for managing individual patient care on a day-to-day basis to being responsible for directing a whole service such as a primary care trust. Changes taking place in health and social care in the UK, as in other countries, however, now require that leadership and management are teased apart, and leadership development has become a key component of the modernisation agenda with the launch of the NHS Modernisation Agency – National Nursing Leadership Project in April 2001 (DoH 2001). This project concluded in 2004. For further information see the NHS Leadership Centre website at www.modern.nhs.uk/leadership. You will also see that the NHS Modernisation Agency was superseded in 2005 by the NHS Institute for Innovation and Improvement (www.institute.nhs.uk), which seeks to:

- work closely with clinicians, NHS organisations, patients, the public, academia and industry in the UK and world-wide to identify best practice
- develop the NHS's capability for service transformation, technology and product innovation, leadership development and learning
- support the rapid adoption and spread of new ideas by providing guidance on practical change ideas and ways to facilitate local, safe implementation
- promote a culture of innovation and lifelong learning for all NHS staff (www.wise.nhs.uk).

The difference between managers and leaders can be seen in Box 2.2.

Box 2.2	Contrasting the roles of managers and leaders

Role of the manager	Role of the leader
Create stability	Be proactive
Take control	Have integrity, an ethical
Accomplish tasks	approach and sound
Possess authority	principles
Hold power from their position	Thrive on change, challenge the status quo
Plan, organise and control human and material resources	Inspire followers
	Have vision
	Be willing to take risks
Enforce policy and procedures	Value people
	Develop relationships
Maintain hierarchical rule	Communicate effectively
Put the organisation before people	Not hold power through position or authority
	Empower others

Adapted from Sofarelli & Brown (1998).

Exercise

1. Consider your normal 'working' day and map out the key areas of activity.
2. What knowledge did you use from any of the above disciplines to carry out nursing activities?
3. Discuss with colleagues or tutors how this knowledge was integrated into nursing practice and consider the value it had for patient care.

SKILLS FOR NURSING PRACTICE

In order to carry out nursing care and related activities, nurses require a number of skills, ranging from practical and technical to problem-solving and critical thinking. These could be seen as the key skills of nursing practice. The exact need for those skills has altered over time and nursing has had to respond accordingly. Let us examine what these skills are.

Exercise

Consider the extract from Lucy Seymer's book on the Nightingale Training School – 1860–1960 in Box 2.3.

1. What similarities can be seen between these expectations and those of your training and education?
2. What practical skills used by the probationers would still be appropriate in today's nursing practice?
3. Identify those duties that are no longer undertaken and consider what influenced their demise.

Box 2.3	Duties of a probationer under the 'Nightingale Fund'

You are required to be:
Sober, honest, truthful, trustworthy, punctual, quiet and orderly. Clean and neat.
You are required to become skilful:

1. in the dressing of blisters, burns, sores, wounds and in applying fomentations, poultices and minor dressings;
2. in the application of leeches, externally and internally;
3. in the administrations of enemas for men and women;
4. in the management of trusses, and appliances in uterine complaints;
5. in the best method of friction to the body and extremities;
6. in the management of helpless patients, i.e. moving, changing, personal cleanliness of feeding, keeping warm (or cool), preventing and dressing bed sores;
7. in bandaging, making bandages and rollers, lining splints;
8. in making the beds of patients, and removal of sheet whilst patient is in bed;
9. you are required to attend at operations;
10. to be competent to cook gruel, arrowroot, egg flip, puddings, drinks for the sick;
11. to understand ventilation, or keep the ward fresh by night as well as by day; you are to be careful that great cleanliness is observed in all utensils; those used for secretions as well as those required for cooking;
12. to make strict observations of the sick in the following particulars – the state of secretions, expectoration, pulse, skin, appetite; intelligence, as delirium or stupor; breathing, sleep, state of wounds, eruptions, formation of matter, effect of diet or of stimulants and of medicines;
13. and to learn the management of convalescents.

From Report of the Committee of the Council of the Nightingale Fund, for the year ending 24th June 1861. Seymer (1960), p. 151.

Many of these prescribed duties have been replaced because of the influence of medical advances and technology, e.g. most nurses no longer have to make bandages or use poultices. Some duties, however, are unchanged, albeit carried out with more advanced resources. Skills such as observation, taking the pulse, wound care and preventing pressure sores remain an essential part of nursing work. (These skills and others undertaken by the nurse will be evident throughout each AL chapter.) Other skills such as application of leeches were abandoned but are now being reintroduced into mainstream health care for a variety of conditions, one being in the treatment of osteoarthritis pain according to a small study being undertaken in Germany (Arthritis Research Campaign 2001).

HEALTH CARE

Proctor (2000, p. 58) notes that the term 'health care' is commonly used to describe the work of the health services, and the professions that carry out this care include medicine, nursing, physiotherapy, midwifery and occupational therapy (see Fig. 2.1 for other members of the team who assist the patient, their families and carers).

Wallace (2002, p. 69) points out that 'the health services require a range of health care professionals each with their own unique role, although partnership working is becoming more and more common as cross-boundary activity is increasing'. We can see the effect of this in the development of new roles in nursing in the UK (see p. 32). Integration between health and social care is also an influencing factor, in particular in the development of primary care trusts (PCTs) (DoH 1999b). The publication of the White Paper *Our Health, Our Care, Our Say* (DoH 2006a) sets out how this integration is to take place. For example (DoH 2006b, p. 20):

> *One of our main aims for the future is to make sure that health and social services will work together and share information to give 'joined-up' care to the people they work for. Services will share information about the people in their care so that health, housing, benefits and other needs are considered together. By 2008 anyone with long term health and social care needs should have an integrated Personal Health and Social Care Plan, if they want one. All Primary Care Trusts and local authorities should have joint health and social care managed networks and/or teams for people with complex needs. We will also be building modern NHS Community hospitals which will offer integrated health and social care services.*

The work of the health care professions has developed in response to the need of people and both have been influenced by the political and social context in which they exist. For example, most of the health care needs of people in countries such as Ethiopia or India are very different from the health care needs of those in the USA or the UK. Africa, for example, 'has been hardest hit by the HIV/AIDS pandemic', whilst in the UK and the USA the effects of living style (e.g. high-cholesterol foods, smoking and alcohol) can be seen in the number of people with coronary heart disease (World Health Organization (WHO) 2001a). These needs are also affected by other conditions outside the control of people, with climate and weather being the most dramatic influence. Consider the devastating effects of the famine in Southern Africa where 'health conditions are putting 12–14 million people at particular risk during the ongoing shortage of food' (WHO 2002).

Advances in medicine and a significant improvement in the quality of life for people in many countries of the world have also brought with them one of the most significant influences on the future of health care generally. This relates

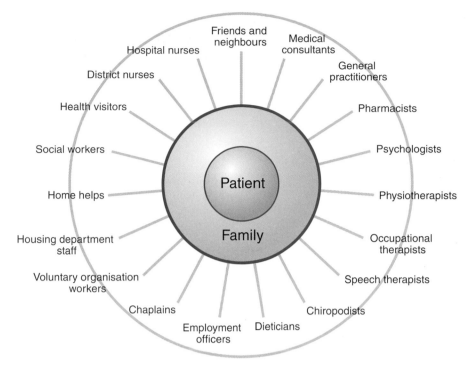

Fig. 2.1 Members of the team (from Roper et al 1996, with permission).

specifically to the rise in the number of older people in the world. A WHO (1997) press release reported that:

> 66 *By 2020 the world will have more than 1 billion people age 60 and over, and 710 million of these will live in developing countries. Today there are an estimated 540 million people in the world aged 60 and over, 330 million of whom live in developing countries.* 99

Ageing, however, does not mean ill-health. The WHO Global Movement for Active Ageing (WHO 2001c) suggests that 'if ageing is to be a positive experience, longer life must be accompanied by improvements of the quality of life of those who reach old age' and that it 'requires policies and strategies that value older people's contribution to their families, communities and economies and that enable them to maintain an optimal level of well being'. They suggest that 'Health is key to Active Ageing' and that 'maintaining good health throughout one's lifespan is essential to extend healthy life expectancy and maintain quality of life in old age' (WHO 2001c). Caring for the elderly person is a theme in many of the AL chapters, e.g. Chapter 10 (Mobilising) and Chapter 8 (Personal Cleansing and Dressing).

What significance therefore have all these issues for nursing practice? This will now be explored.

HEALTH CARE AND NURSING PRACTICE

Before the role of nursing in health care can be understood it is necessary to understand the health care system and its associated development in different countries. This section will initially focus on the health care system in the United Kingdom.

THE NATIONAL HEALTH SERVICE IN THE UK

The National Health Service (NHS) was set up as a result of a series of post-World War II developments, the National Health Service Act 1946 and the birth of the Welfare State (Baly 1995). It came into operation on 5 July 1948, and, apart from some charges to prescriptions and appliances, the majority of treatments were free of charge. Its introduction necessitated a significant change to nursing, and the resultant Nurses Act of 1949 saw a reconstituted General Nursing Council (GNC) and a new training scheme for nurses. The basic principles inherent in the setting up of the NHS remained until the new National Health Service and Community Care Act in 1990. This Act provided a framework for a closer working relationship between health and social care services, together with an increased consumer involvement in decision-making about service provision. This would have a direct effect on how nurses, for example, involved patients in their own care decisions – an important aspect when considering using a nursing model by which to assess, plan, implement and evaluate care. It also had an impact on where that care took place – in particular the shift to care in the community. There were, however, serious difficulties with the implementation of 'Government's new health market in the NHS' (Fatchett 1998, p. 29) but with the General Election of 1992 the election of the Conservative Government for another term of office ensured that the principles of the internal health market would be embedded in the UK health care system. 1997 saw the Labour Government being elected into office and it was faced with a major challenge to reform the NHS. The White Paper *The New NHS – Modern, Dependable* (DoH 1997) set out this reform, which sought to keep what worked from the previous system, whilst ensuring that care delivery was improved for everyone who made use of the NHS. Improving health and reducing inequalities were cornerstones to its implementation, as was the need for 'quality' and its monitoring. The publication of *A First Class Service – Quality in the New NHS* (DoH 1998) provided the evidence of how this was to be undertaken, e.g. the setting up of the National Institute for Health and Clinical Excellence (NICE), Clinical Governance and the Commission for Health Improvement. The impact of the NHS changes were to be significant to those who were employed to deliver the care as well as to the organisations in which they worked. Some of the most significant changes for nurses in the UK and the way in which they deliver care to the patient have been:

- the introduction of new roles for nurses
- implementation of evidence-based nursing practice
- multiprofessional collaboration.

These remain key issues. However, there have been further significant developments in the NHS in the UK since the first edition of this book. In particular are the recent changes to the way in which primary care and ambulance trusts in England are organised and managed. These include a reduction in their number: primary care trusts from 303 to 152 and ambulance trusts from 29 to 12 (DoH 2006a). The other major change includes the involvement of service users in the management of their own care and in nursing education (Warne & McAndrew 2005).

THE INTRODUCTION OF NEW ROLES FOR NURSES

Cameron (2000, p. 14) highlights two major initiatives that 'encouraged the development of new roles for nurses as well as for other health care professionals'. These were the waiting list initiatives and the reduction in junior doctors' hours.

For both the Conservative and Labour Governments the issue of long waiting lists has been problematic, and, despite steps to reduce it, some patients were still having to wait 2 years or more for admission to hospital (Cameron 2000). However, this trend has now changed, for a variety of reasons, with a reduction in waiting lists across the UK. In February 1999, for example, the Government announced a '£20 million boost to reduce waiting lists and waiting times' (DoH 1999a) by investing in new surgical equipment and facilities as part of modernising the NHS. In 2006 the following NHS waiting list figures were released, showing an improvement since 2000:

Inpatient waiting times

- The number of patients, for whom English commissioners are responsible, waiting over 26 weeks at the end of May 2006 was 58. Of these 58, 24 were English residents waiting in Welsh hospitals.
- The number of patients, for whom English commissioners are responsible, waiting over 13 weeks at the end of May 2006 was 198 600, an increase of 600 from April, but a fall of 59 200 from May 2005.

Outpatient waiting times

- The number of patients, for whom English commissioners are responsible, waiting over 13 weeks for first outpatient appointment at the end of May 2006 was 199. Of these 199, 115 were English residents waiting in Welsh hospitals.
- The number of patients, for whom English commissioners are responsible, waiting over 11 weeks at the end of May 2006, was 40 500, up 5100 from April 2006. (www.dh.gov.uk/publicationsandstatistics/pressreleases (DoH 2006b))

Long hours had been considered part of a junior doctor's working week but in 1991 the Government directed employers to begin to reduce them so that 'by the end of 1996 no junior doctor was supposed to be contracted to work more than 56 hours a week' (DoH 1991). To enable this to occur the Government allocated funding for the development of new clinical roles (Humphris & Masterson 2000). The reduction in junior doctors' hours meant that they would no longer be in a position to ensure continuity of care for patients, and there was a possibility of patients having to wait for assessment and treatments. Alongside this reduction in their hours was also a reduction in the number of doctors in employment. New roles for nurses were therefore encouraged and a plethora of specialist roles appeared. For example, night nurse practitioners, nurse-led services in preoperative assessment clinics and nurse endoscopists. The publication of the *Scope of Professional Nursing Practice* (UKCC 1992a) further enabled nurses, midwives and health visitors to expand their role beyond the boundaries of their professions, and Cameron (2000, p. 11) believes that:

> ❝ *Without doubt such professional developments helped demolish unhelpful barriers between health-care professions with the result that nurses could develop their roles into areas that previously were firmly within the domain of medicine.* ❞

Other roles which have developed have been the nurse consultant role (see p. 9) and more recently in the UK the advanced practitioner in such fields as critical care (DoH 2006c). This critical care practitioner role is described in the document as 'being based on the medical model of teaching, responsibility and care delivery and is designed to develop a high level, trained, accredited, recognised, transferable practitioner to address a service need in critical care' (DoH 2006c, p. vi). It is acknowledged 'that the role described crosses the professional boundaries of many functions within critical care, including medicine, nursing, technical, physiotherapy and clinical pharmacology'.

> **Exercise**
> 1. Read this document (available at www.dh.gov.uk) and consider its implications for the health care professions working within a critical care setting in the UK and non-UK settings.

It is important to reflect that in other countries nurses have been undertaking many roles and tasks that have been viewed as those of doctors in the UK. This is seen in the number of health initiatives reported by the WHO (2001b, p. 13), who also report that 'research conducted in North America and the United Kingdom on the nurse practitioner role supports positive results in patient outcomes, satisfaction and cost'.

> **Exercise**
> 1. What new roles would help you as a qualified nurse to assess, plan, implement and evaluate the care given to patients?
> 2. Discuss with colleagues what impact new roles have had on how you deliver care to patients.

To facilitate your discussion you may wish to read the book by Humphris & Masterson (2000).

IMPLEMENTATION OF EVIDENCE-BASED NURSING PRACTICE

The need to provide evidence that the care you deliver is both effective and appropriate has arisen because of the changes within the health service, in particular successive governments' drive for quality and improvement in care delivery. Evidence can be from different sources and have different levels and forms (Hamer & Collinson 1999; Craig & Smyth 2002). Examples of evidence are audit findings and research. The University of York, NHS Centre for Reviews and Dissemination has set out a hierarchy of evidence, with well-designed randomised controlled trials (RCTs) being number one. Hamer & Collinson (1999, p. 19) state that:

> 66 *All research evidence is susceptible to variation and not all research is equal: the domination of the positivist, natural science paradigm as embodied in the medical sciences has placed it in a stronger position.* 99

They identify the following research designs in their deliberations on the appropriateness of different forms of evidence: randomised controlled trials, case-controlled studies, cohort studies, surveys, qualitative studies and professional consensus.

> **Exercise**
> 1. Identify one area of nursing practice that you encounter in your workplace and determine what the underpinning evidence is.
> 2. Identify the research methodologies and methods that were used in the studies.
> 3. How do you ensure that the care planned and implemented is underpinned by an evidence base?

In response to the latter you may have considered keeping yourself up to date professionally, undertaking a course of study to be able to review the evidence and its quality, or even setting up a journal club where you and colleagues can discuss evidence available and how you plan to implement this in your area of work.

It is now an important part of the nurse's role to ensure that the care delivered is based on evidence from both nursing research and other sources (Hamer & Collinson 1999).

MULTIPROFESSIONAL COLLABORATION

Fatchett (1998) states that 'the promotion of the concept of collaboration has been and remains an important theme underpinning current health policy activity' and offers the following reasons for 'the apparent surge' in its popularity:

- a growth in the complexity of health and welfare services
- expansion of knowledge and subsequent increase in specialisation
- a perceived need for the rationalisation of resources
- a need for lessening the duplication of care
- the provision of a more effective, integrated and supportive service for both users and professionals. (Fatchett 1998, p. 135)

For nurses this means working in partnership not only with other health professionals but also with the users of health services (Ross et al 2005). Despite the various debates about professional boundaries (Gabe et al 1994) there has been a major shift towards creating an integrated and collaborative approach to care development and delivery (D'Amour & Oandasan 2005).

Examples of where this has been successful are in the development of pathways of care. Johnson (1997, p. 11) explains these as:

> " *Pathways of care amalgamate all the anticipated elements of care and treatment of all members of the multi-disciplinary team, for a patient or client of a particular case-type or grouping within an agreed time frame, for the achievement of agreed outcomes. Any deviation from the plan is documented as a 'variance'; the analysis of which provides information for the review of current practice.* "

Exercise

1. How could the Roper, Logan and Tierney model for nursing be used as a framework for documenting care as part of an integrated care pathway?
2. Find an example of an integrated care pathway (see *Journal of Integrated Care Pathways* at www.rsmpress.co.uk/jicp/html and www.lcp-marie-curie.org.uk) and compare it to the nursing care document found in Appendix 2. What are the key differences in the nursing sections of an integrated care pathway document?

You may have considered that the model would be invaluable as an assessment tool within an integrated care plan or you may decide to use it as a framework for ensuring that all aspects of an individual patient's life are considered. For example, if you were developing a pathway for caring for patients following a stroke the team would need to ensure that all the factors influencing the Activities of Living were included. To assess and plan the need for speech and language therapy would need a knowledge of the biological factors that have led to the stroke and also why speech is impaired.

It is important to remember that multiprofessional collaboration is not about dissolving professional boundaries but about understanding and recognising the value each profession has to play in the care and wellbeing of the patient (Howarth et al 2004, Holland et al 2006). This will then avoid the duplication of care practices and provide a more integrated and personalised service. Howarth et al (2004) recommended that:

- Role awareness should become an essential element of all programmes relating to preparing the workforce to deliver integrated health and social care.
- When developing new roles ensure that there has been organizational preparation for their introduction into the workforce.
- Shared learning initiatives between health and social care workforce students in practice should be encouraged to develop awareness and understanding of team roles.
- A variety of innovative learning opportunities need to be considered, including role shadowing, secondments to work with multiprofessional team and interprofessional education.

- Role awareness education for service users/carers should be considered essential to ensure effective communication and appropriate use of services. (Howarth et al 2004, p. 4)

D'Amour & Oandasan (2005) state that 'Interprofessional collaboration is a key factor in initiatives designed to increase the effectiveness of health services currently offered to the public' and believe that crucial to its success is understanding of the concept of collaboration. They conclude in their review of the literature that there were four key themes which underpinned this, namely sharing, partnership, interdependency and power (D'Amour & Oandasan 2005, p. 126).

Exercise

1. What is your experience of multiprofessional/interprofessional collaboration in the clinical environment?
2. How did working with other professions enhance the care delivered to patients?
3. How many different professions have you worked alongside in practice?
4. How aware were you of their professional roles?

DELIVERY OF CARE

Care is delivered in a number of different settings and in different ways. In many countries this setting can be divided into two main areas, namely hospital and community, with the latter encompassing a range of environments from care homes to health centres. In other countries care is delivered at the point of need and often in difficult and hazardous environments, e.g. refugee camps in war-torn countries.

In the UK there have been major changes to how care is delivered in the community, in particular through the developing integration of health and social care services, as well as the involvement of service users in their own care management. The setting up of the Primary Care Trusts is an example of how this collaboration and integration was being promoted (see Box 2.4). This change continues with the publication of the White Paper *Our Health, Our Care, Our Say* (DoH 2006a) which further promotes the integration of health and social care services.

Exercise

1. Consider the delivery of care in different countries.
2. How many of these promote the delivery of care through integration of health and social care services?
3. How are service users and their carers involved in the delivery of care?

Box 2.4	Devolution day for the NHS: Half a century of centralised healthcare is drawing to a close

Primary Care Trusts (PCTs) are free-standing, legally established, statutory NHS bodies that are accountable to their Health Authority. PCTs have the same overall functions as Primary Care Groups, thus allowing continuity with the strategic plans developed by them for their community. PCTs offer an unparalleled opportunity for local stakeholders – family doctors, nurses, midwives, health visitors, the professions allied to medicine, social services and the wider community they serve – to shape services to provide better health and better care.

PCTs will take responsibility for securing the provision of the fuller range of services for the local populations as Strategic Health Authorities step back from a hands-on commissioning role. They will take on responsibility for all family health services practitioners allowing a coherent view of the development of all the NHS services in the area. PCTs will have responsibility for the management, development and integration of all primary care services including medical, dental, pharmaceutical and optical.

Primary Care Trusts bring a range of benefits to patients, the community and professionals:

- better support to practices
- better support to individual clinicians
- better integrated services
- better access
- better action to improve public health
- bringing decision-making closer to patients and local communities.

From Department of Health (2002).

INTERNATIONAL PERSPECTIVES IN NURSING AND HEALTH CARE

In 2001 the World Health Organization (WHO 2001b) published its summary document *Strengthening Nursing and Midwifery*, which reported on the contribution that nursing and midwifery had made to health and development during the period 1996–2000. The importance of these professions can be seen from the introduction (p. 1):

> 66 *Despite differences in local contexts, nursing and midwifery services are an essential foundation and support for every health system. These services are found wherever health services are delivered, regardless of the service level, speciality area or service location.* 99

The report highlighted a number of challenges and strategic issues confronting nursing and midwifery services worldwide which need to be considered in the future as a result of their evidence. Some of these are:

- increasing case loads leading to stress and poor quality of services
- increased mobility of health workers – likely to aggravate 'provider' shortages in some areas, exacerbated by increased consumer awareness of and demand for nursing and midwifery services (p. 5)
- knowledge explosion and access to technology solutions
- epidemiological changes and service response – in particular the re-emergence of infectious diseases and increases in chronic health conditions, women's health issues and an ageing population
- poverty – nurses are not always recognised for what they can contribute to health care in different countries
- human rights and gender – women are still systematically discriminated against in many countries – both as providers and users of health care services.

Nurses and midwives are very often the prime carers in health care, with no easy access to medical services. The WHO cites a number of initiatives where nurses have made a difference to health care:

1. In Senegal and South Africa nurses are involved in facilitating community participation as well as in supervising and implementing programmes to combat HIV/AIDS.
2. In Thailand, nurses and midwives provide a variety of mental health services including education, prevention and management of stress, conflict resolution, group and family therapy and community-based and mobile mental health clinics.
3. In Bahrain, nurses run diabetic clinics and cardiac rehabilitation programmes (WHO 2001b, p. 12).

Exercise
1. Undertake a literature search to determine how nursing is developing in the various health care systems which exist in the world and determine if you can identify common themes emerging.

Some of the issues you may come across relate to the three universal themes that Salvage (1993) reports on, namely power, gender and medicalisation – which she states are all closely linked. **Power** is usually lacking even where there is a nursing voice at strategic level. **Gender** – women make up the majority of the nursing workforce and in many countries they 'suffer gender discrimination in both their personal and working lives'. **Medicalisation** – 'where medicine dominates every European health system to a greater or lesser extent' and nurses are seen as more or less assistants to the doctors. This can cause an undervaluing of nursing work and their caring role (Salvage 1993, p. 5).

Some of the issues you may have discussed in relation to these questions may have included those surrounding the professionalisation of nursing, in particular the relationship between doctors and nurses. Understanding what it is to be a profession and a professional is essential if you are to be part of a team delivering care to those who are the vulnerable in society due to illness or other causes such as disability.

PROFESSIONAL ISSUES AND NURSING PRACTICE

So what is a profession? One sociologist who studied the sociology of professions was Talcott Parsons, and from his work arose the 'trait theory' of what a profession is. Jones (1994) noted that these 'traits' were:

- theory of knowledge underlying and informing the practice of the profession
- code of ethics (accepted rules) regulating practice
- control of entry to the profession, through tests, training and so on, and through disciplinary powers
- professional authority over the layperson, based on specialist knowledge
- confidential nature of the patient–client relationship
- existence of a professional culture: that is, an agreed way of behaving, which may be designed to exclude/impress.

You may have considered that yes, nursing is a profession, based on the fact that there is a developing body of knowledge informing nursing practice, based on research and other forms of evidence; there is a code of ethics or rather a code of professional conduct; entry to the profession is also controlled through registration with a professional body such as the Nursing and Midwifery Council in the UK; nurses do have more detailed knowledge than the patient; and there is confidentiality between the nurse and the patient (albeit within a sphere of accountability and 'doing the patient no harm'). The existence of a professional culture can be seen in the way nurses behave and practise but this may not be as easy to demonstrate in terms of evidence as the other 'traits'. Being a professional would encompass adhering to a code of professional conduct and ensuring that whoever called themselves a nurse had the right to do so (professional regulation). Let us consider some of these 'traits' and how they influence the care that you give to patients and work with colleagues.

PROFESSIONAL REGULATION

In the UK, until 2002 the nursing profession was regulated by two professional bodies, namely the United Kingdom Central Council for Nursing, Midwifery and Health Visiting (UKCC) and the four National Boards in England, Scotland, Wales and Northern Ireland. The functions were different but they complemented one another. The UKCC set a code of professional conduct for registered nurses, midwives and health visitors to ensure that they maintained agreed standards of professional behaviour and practice (UKCC 1992b). This was revised in 2002 as part of the new Nursing and Midwifery Council (NMC) and came into effect in June 2002 (see Box 2.5).

For student nurses and midwives the NMC has guidance on clinical experience (NMC 2005) which encompasses some of the principles of the Code of Professional Conduct. For example in relation to accountability they state that:

> *as a pre-registration student you are not professionally accountable in the way that you will be after you come to register with the NMC. This means that you cannot be called to account for your actions and omissions by the NMC. So far as the NMC is concerned, it is the registered practitioners with whom you are working who are professionally responsible for the consequences of your actions and omissions. This is why you must always work under direct supervision. This does not mean however that you can never be called to account by your university or by the law for the consequences of your actions or omissions as a pre-registration student.* (NMC 2005)

Full details of the Code of Professional Conduct as well as other professional body documents can be found at www.nmc-uk.org.

Codes of professional conduct are also found in other countries where there is a recognised training and education programme for nurses. In Australia, for example, there is both a code of professional conduct and a code of ethics. The Australian Code of Professional Conduct (ANC 2003) has eight standards – each of which is further divided into

Box 2.5 **Code of Professional Conduct**

As a registered nurse or midwife, you are personally accountable for your practice. In caring for patients and clients, you must:

- respect the patient or client as an individual
- obtain consent before you give any treatment or care
- protect confidential information
- cooperate with others in the team
- maintain your professional knowledge and competence
- be trustworthy
- act to identify and minimise risk to patients and clients.

These are the shared values of all the United Kingdom health care regulatory bodies.

1.1 The purpose of the NMC Code of Professional Conduct is to:
- inform the professions of the standard of professional conduct required of them in the exercise of their professional accountability and practice
- inform the public, other professions and employers of the standard of professional conduct that they expect of a registered practitioner.

1.2 As a registered nurse, midwife or specialist community public health nurse you must:
- protect and support the health of individual patients and clients
- protect and support the health of the wider community
- act in such a way that justifies the trust and confidence the public have in you
- uphold and enhance the good reputation of the professions.

1.3 You are personally accountable for your practice. This means that you are answerable for your actions and omissions, regardless of advice and directions from another professional.

1.4 You have a duty of care to your patients and clients who are entitled to receive safe and competent care.

1.5 You must adhere to the laws of the country in which you are practising.

From NMC (2004b).

a series of explanatory statements (see www.anmc.org.au/publications for full details). One can see the similarities with the NMC Code of Conduct.

Code of Professional Conduct (Australian Nursing Council 2003)

A nurse must:

1. Practise in a safe and competent manner.
2. Practise in accordance with the agreed standards of the profession.
3. Not bring discredit upon the reputation of the nursing profession.
4. Practise in accordance with the laws relevant to the nurse's area of practice.
5. Respect the dignity, culture, values and beliefs of an individual and any significant other person.
5. Support the health, wellbeing and informed decision making of an individual.
6. Promote and preserve the trust that is inherent in the privileged relationship between a nurse and an individual and respect both the person and their property.
7. Treat personal information obtained in a professional capacity as confidential.
8. Refrain from engaging in exploitation, misinformation and misrepresentation in regard to health care products and nursing services.

The Australian Nursing Council (ANC 2002) have also developed a Code of Ethics for nurses, their rationale being that:

> ❝ *Nursing practice is undertaken in a variety of settings. Any particular setting will be affected to some degree by processes which are not within a nurse's control or influence. These include resource constraints, institutional policies, management decisions and the practice of other health care providers. Nurses also recognise the potential for conflict between one person's needs and those of another, or of a group or community. Such factors may affect the degree to which nurses are able to fulfil their moral obligations and/or the number and type of ethical dilemmas they may face.* ❞ (www.anmc.org.au/codeofethics)

This Code consists of six broad value statements (with explanatory statements to support them). The purpose of the Code is to:

- identify the fundamental moral commitments of the profession
- provide nurses with a basis for professional and self reflection on ethical conduct
- act as a guide to ethical practice
- indicate to the community the moral values which nurses can be expected to hold.

The six value statements are:

1. Nurses respect persons' individual needs, values, culture and vulnerability in the provision of nursing care.
2. Nurses accept the rights of persons to make informed choices in relation to their care.
3. Nurses promote and uphold the provision of quality nursing care for all people.
4. Nurses hold in confidence any information obtained in a professional capacity, use professional judgement where there is a need to share such information for the

therapeutic benefit and safety of a person and ensure that privacy is safeguarded.

5. Nurses fulfil the accountability and responsibility inherent in their roles.
6. Nurses value environmental ethics and a social, economic and ecologically sustainable environment that promotes health and wellbeing.

Exercise

1. Consider both the NMC and ANC Codes of Professional Conduct and Ethics and identify the similarities between them.
2. How can the Roper et al model for nursing help you to ensure that the Codes are adhered to? For example, ensuring that cultural needs are taken account of in the assessment process or ensuring that informed consent is obtained prior to surgery as part of ensuring and maintaining a safe environment.
3. Access the ANC website and read the full Code of Professional Conduct and Code of Ethics. Using the internet and other sources, search for other nursing codes of professional conduct in other countries and discuss them with colleagues.

This kind of regulation is termed 'self-regulation' but as Basford (2003, p. 88) outlines, this does not 'mean that a profession is totally autonomous and therefore totally self-regulating'. She states that all members of a profession are subject to 'the laws of the land' and that these include: criminal law, employment law, civil law and public law. An example of how a nurse came to break the law is seen in the case of Beverly Allit, convicted of murdering children in her care on a paediatric ward in the UK (Clothier et al 1994).

Patient care is therefore dependent on nursing practice that is based on a professional and ethical code. So how is it possible to ensure that those entering the profession are fit for taking on the title of nurse and will adhere to the code of professional conduct?

It is pertinent at this stage to look at the education and training of nurses, in particular the content of their 3-year programme which will ensure they are prepared for becoming a qualified nurse.

NURSING EDUCATION – ITS DEVELOPMENT AND CURRENT CONTEXT

In order to understand the present context, it is important to reflect on the past.

Nursing as a predominantly female occupation has been subjected to major changes since its origins in the late 1800s. The Nurses Registration Act 1919 ensured that the public were protected from untrained women who would no longer be able to call themselves 'nurse' without membership on the register. Since that time there have been numerous attempts to reform nursing and nurse education and training, with the result that in the UK in 1989, as a result of implementation of Project 2000 recommendations (UKCC 1987), all probationer nurses were recognised as students within the university (higher education) sector. In the USA, however, this had long been recognised as an essential prerequisite to ensuring professional status for nursing and the graduate nurse was well established within American health care.

Another major development taking place in the UK which is influencing the development of all the health and social care professions is interprofessional education (Barr 2002, Royle et al 1999, Miller et al 1999). To be able to deliver the current and future health and social care agenda requires a workforce that is interdependent as well as working interprofessionally (Audit Commission 2001). A major project has been undertaken in England. This is the 'Creating an Interprofessional Workforce' programme (www.cipw.org.uk).

NURSE EDUCATION IN THE UK

The current provision of education for pre-registration student nurses in the UK is at two levels: graduate and diplomat, with the majority qualifying with a Diploma plus their Registered Nurse (RN) qualification. Prior to 2000, student nurse Diploma-level education consisted of a 3-year programme, with an 18-month common foundation and an 18-month branch in one of four areas of practice, namely adult nursing, children's nursing, mental health nursing and learning disability nursing. At the end of that time students were expected to be able to meet the 13 competencies of Rule 18A (UKCC 1989 – Amendment of Nurses Act 1979). These can be seen in Box 2.6.

As a result of a number of research studies into the effectiveness and appropriateness of the Project 2000 course (Jowett & Walton 1994, Macleod Clark et al 1996) and also a UKCC commission into pre-registration education (UKCC 1999) Rule 18A was superseded by a new set of rules and competencies (Statutory Instrument 2000 No. 2554 – The Nurses, Midwives and Health Visitors (Training) Amendment Rules Approval Order 2000, www.hmso.gov.uk) and a new course was proposed which had a 1-year foundation and 2-year branch programme. The standards of proficiency for entry to the register (NMC 2004b) are more specific in what is expected of a student nurse after 1-year foundation and on qualifying (see Boxes 2.7 and 2.8).

It can be seen throughout the competency statements that the Code of Professional Conduct and ethical practice

| Box 2.6 | Statutory Instrument 1989 No.1456 |

Schedule 2 – The Nurses, Midwives and Health Visitors (Training) Amendment Rules 1989 – The Nurses, Midwives and Health Visitors Act 1979
Preparation for entry to Parts 12, 13, 14 and 15 of the register 18A

(1) The contents of the Common Foundation Programme and the Branch Programme shall be such as the Council may from time to time require.

(2) The Common Foundation Programme and Branch Programmes shall be designed to prepare the nursing student to assume the responsibilities and accountability that registration confers, and to prepare the nursing student to apply knowledge and skills to meet the nursing needs of individuals and of groups in health and in sickness in the area of practice of the Branch Programme and shall include enabling the student to achieve the following outcomes:

(a) The identification of the social and health implications of pregnancy and childbearing, physical and mental handicap, disease, disability, or ageing for the individual, her or his friends, family and community.

(b) The recognition of common factors which contribute to and those which adversely affect physical, mental and social wellbeing of patients and clients and take appropriate action.

(c) The use of relevant literature and research to inform the practice of nursing.

(d) The appreciation of the influence of social, political and cultural factors in relation to health care.

(e) An understanding of the requirements of legislation relevant to the practice of nursing.

(f) The use of appropriate communication skills to enable the development of helpful caring relationships with patients and clients and their families and friends, and to initiate and conduct therapeutic relationships with patients and clients.

(g) The identification of health-related learning needs of patients and clients, families and friends and to participate in health promotion.

(h) An understanding of the ethics of health care and of the nursing profession and the responsibilities which these impose on the nurse's professional practice.

(i) The identification of the needs of patients and clients to enable them to progress from varying degrees of dependence to maximum independence or to a peaceful death.

(j) The identification of physical, psychological, social and spiritual needs of the patient or client; an awareness of values and concepts of individual care; the ability to devise a plan of care, contribute to its implementation and evaluation; and the demonstration of the application of the principles of a problem-solving approach to the practice of nursing.

(k) The ability to function effectively in a team and participate in a multiprofessional approach to the care of patients and clients.

(l) The use of the appropriate channel of referral for matters not within her sphere of competence.

(m) The assignment of appropriate duties to others and the supervision, teaching and monitoring of assigned duties.

Available from Her Majesty's Stationery Office (www.hmso.gov.uk).

Exercise

1. Discuss with colleagues and tutors the possibility of having the same competencies for entry to the register in all nursing courses worldwide.
2. What would be the benefits and drawbacks of this view?
3. Compare the competency statements for your nursing registration with that prescribed by the NMC in the UK.

are essential to being able to become a registered nurse with the NMC in the United Kingdom. Other countries have similar competencies to be achieved but there are no universally agreed competencies which would enable nurses to move freely across international boundaries. It is beyond the scope of this book to consider the reasons for this; however, some of these could be attributed to the social, political,

cultural and economic climate of each country and the lack of consensus internationally about the role and function of the nurse.

NURSE EDUCATION WORLDWIDE

Nursing is a worldwide occupation and as such requires its education and training programmes to ensure that there are some commonalities between international boundaries. How nursing has developed in each country will depend, however, not only on its historical context, but most importantly on the social, political and economic needs prevalent at the time. Patient needs will also differ as a result of this. It can be seen how nursing has responded to change by the way in which its status as a profession has changed in different countries.

Box 2.7	Nursing outcomes – to be achieved for entry to branch (after 1 year)

Domain – Professional and Ethical Practice

- Discuss in an informed manner the implications of professional regulation for nursing practice.
- Demonstrate an awareness of the NMC Code of Professional Conduct; standards of conduct, performance and ethics
- Demonstrate an awareness of, and apply ethical principles to, nursing practice.
- Demonstrate an awareness of legislation relevant to nursing practice.
- Demonstrate the importance of promoting equity in patient and client care by contributing to nursing care in a fair and antidiscriminatory way.

Domain – Care Delivery

- Discuss methods of, barriers to and the boundaries of effective communication and interpersonal relationships.
- Demonstrate sensitivity when interacting with and providing information to patients and clients.
- Contribute to enhancing the health and social wellbeing of patients and clients by understanding how under the supervision of a registered practitioner:
  – contribute to the assessment of health needs
  – identify opportunities for health promotion
  – identify networks of health and social care services.
- Contribute to the development and documentation of nursing assessments by participating in comprehensive and systematic nursing assessment of the physical, psychological, social and spiritual needs of patients and clients.
- Contribute to the planning of nursing care, involving patients and clients and where possible their carers, demonstrating an understanding of helping patients and clients to make informed decisions.
- Contribute to the implementation of a programme of nursing care, designed and supervised by registered practitioners.

- Demonstrate evidence of a developing knowledge base which underpins safe nursing practice.
- Demonstrate a range of essential nursing skills, under the supervision of a registered nurse, to meet individual needs which include: maintaining dignity, privacy and confidentiality, effective communication and observation skills, including listening and taking physiological measurements; safety and health, including moving and handling and infection control; essential first aid and emergency procedures, administration of medicines; emotional, physical and personal care, including meeting the need for comfort, nutrition and personal hygiene.
- Contribute to the evaluation of the appropriateness of nursing care delivered.
- Recognise situations in which agreed plans for nursing care no longer appear appropriate and refer these to an accountable practitioner.

Domain – Care Management

- Contribute to the identification of actual and potential risks to patients, clients and their carers, to oneself and to others and participate in measures to promote and ensure health and safety.
- Demonstrate an understanding of the role of others by participating in interprofessional working practice.
- Demonstrate literacy, numeracy, and computer skills needed to record, enter, store, retrieve and organise data essential for care delivery.

Domain – Personal and Professional Development

- Demonstrate responsibility for one's own learning through the development of a portfolio of practice and recognise when further learning is required.
- Acknowledge the importance of seeking supervision to develop safe nursing practice.

From NMC (2004b).

In Brazil, for example, the introduction of undergraduate programmes for nurses 'elevated nursing to the status of a liberal profession, and the nursing faculty assumed major roles in nursing education' (Neves & Mauro 2000). However, it took 14 years of lobbying the government for approval to be given for a new curriculum which was established in 1994 but 'was already outdated, and is failing to attend the societal demands of the nursing profession' (Neves & Mauro 2000, p. 4). The way in which nursing responds to changes in society is illustrated in Primomo's (2000) description of the way in which Japanese nurses are trying to manage the increasing ageing population and also the changing societal values in relation to family structure and women's roles. She states that:

66 *By increasing efforts to move nursing education into the university setting and by focusing curriculum on community-based care, nurses should be better prepared to meet the needs of its ageing society and function in autonomous roles. As the profession continues its efforts to become involved in health policy at the national and local level it is anticipated that nurses will have even greater opportunities to improve health and health care for the Japanese population.* 99 (Primomo 2000, p. 15)

Box 2.8	Standards of proficiency for entry to register

Domain – Professional and Ethical Practice

- Manage oneself, one's practice and that of others, in accordance with the NMC's Code of Professional Conduct: standards for conduct, performance and ethics, recognising one's own abilities and limitations.
- Practice in accordance with an ethical and legal framework which ensures the primacy of patient and client interest and wellbeing and respects confidentiality.
- Practise in a fair and antidiscriminatory way, acknowledging the differences in beliefs and cultural practices of individuals and groups.

Domain – Care Delivery

- Engage in, develop and disengage from therapeutic relationships through the use of appropriate communication and interpersonal skills.
- Create and utilise opportunities to promote the health and wellbeing of patients, clients and groups.
- Undertake and document a comprehensive, systematic and accurate nursing assessment of the physical, psychological, social and spiritual needs of patients, clients and communities.
- Formulate and document a plan of nursing care, where possible in partnership with patients, clients, their carers and family and friends, within a framework of informed consent.
- Based on the best available evidence, apply knowledge and an appropriate repertoire of skills indicative of safe nursing practice.

- Provide a rationale for the nursing care delivered which takes account of social, spiritual, legal, political and economic influences.
- Evaluate and document the outcomes of nursing and other interventions.
- Demonstrate sound clinical judgement across a range of differing professional and care delivery contexts.

Domain – Care Management

- Contribute to public protection by creating and maintaining a safe environment of care through the use of quality assurance and risk management strategies.
- Demonstrate knowledge of effective interprofessional working practices which respect and utilise the contributions of members of the health and social care team.
- Delegate duties to others, as appropriate, ensuring that they are supervised and monitored.
- Demonstrate key skills.

Domain – Personal and Professional Development

- Demonstrate a commitment to the need for continuing professional development and personal supervision activities in order to enhance knowledge, skills, values and attitudes needed for safe and effective nursing practice.
- Enhance the professional development and safe practice of others through peer support, leadership, supervision and teaching.

From NMC (2004b).

The demand for nurses has, however, 'outpaced the supplies, due to the development of advanced medicine, increase in the number of hospital beds and the ageing of patients. Japan is now in a state of chronic nurse shortages in terms of both quality and quantity' (www.nurse.or.jp/na).

In addition to these issues there has been a drive for interprofessional education as in the UK. In Canada, for example, this has been directly linked to health care through the development and promotion of a model of 'collaborative patient-centred practice'. (See Health Canada website for full details of this model and other papers linked to interprofessional learning, education and practice: www.hc-sc.gc.ca.)

It can be seen from the examples cited that there is much in common between nursing in different countries and the importance of how society, politics and economics influence not only our understanding of patients needs but also to how nursing itself is developed, managed and delivered. The Roper et al model for nursing incorporates these dimensions in the model of living (see Chapter 1).

SUMMARY POINTS

1. Nursing exists in a social, political and economic context.
2. To use the model for nursing requires an understanding of the role of the nurse as it exists across international boundaries.
3. The education of nurses is essential to the delivery of effective patient care that meets the needs of individuals and their families as appropriate to that society's needs.

References

Arthritis Research Campaign 2001 Leeches – a treatment for knee osteoarthritis? (www.arc.uk/newsviews/press/aug20)
Audit Commission 2001 Hidden talents – education, training and developments for healthcare staff in the NHS. Audit Commission, London

Australian Nursing Council 2003 Code of professional conduct. (www.anmc.org.au/publications)

Australian Nursing Council 2002 Code of ethics. (www.anmc. org.au/codeofethics)

Baly M 1995 Nursing and social change, 3rd edn. Routledge, London

Barr H 2002 Interprofessional education – today, yesterday and tomorrow. LTSN for Health Sciences and Practice, London

Basford L 2003 Professionalisation. In: Basford L, Slevin O (eds) Theory and practice of nursing. Nelson Thornes, Cheltenham, pp 133–140

Cameron A 2000 New role developments in context. In: Humphris D, Masterson A (eds) Developing new clinical roles. Churchill Livingstone, Edinburgh, pp 7–24

Clothier C, MacDonald C, Shaw D 1994 Independent enquiry into deaths and injuries on the Children's Ward at Grantham and Kestoran General Hospital during the period February to April 1991 (Allitt Inquiry). HMSO, London

Cooper C 2001 The art of nursing – a practical introduction. WB Saunders Co, Philadelphia

Craig JV, Smyth RL 2002 The evidence based practice manual for nurses. Churchill Livingstone, Edinburgh

D'Amour D, Oandasan I 2005 Interprofessionality as the filed of interprofessional practice and interprofessional education: An emerging concept. Journal of Interprofessional Care 1: 8–20

Davey B 1992 Biological perspectives. In: Robinson K, Vaughan B (eds) Knowledge for nursing practice. Butterworth Heinemann, Oxford, pp 42–59

Department of Health 1991 Hours of work of doctors in training, the new deal. Executive letter 82. DoH, London

Department of Health 1997 The new NHS – modern, dependable. White paper, December. DoH, London (www. doh.gov.uk/nhsind.html)

Department of Health 1998 A first class service – quality in the new NHS. DoH, London

Department of Health 1999a Waiting times – modernisation fund investment, £20 million boost to reduce waiting lists and waiting times. Department of Health Press Release, 22nd February (www.doh.gov/nhsexec/modfund.html)

Department of Health 1999b Primary Care Trusts – establishing better services. DoH, London (www.doh.gov.uk/pricare/pcts. html)

Department of Health 2000 Towards a strategy for nursing research and development, p 10. DoH, London

Department of Health 2001 NHS national nursing leadership project. DoH, London (www.nursingleadership.co.uk)

Department of Health 2002 Devolution day for the NHS: half a century of centralised healthcare is drawing to a close. Milburn, Department of Health, Press Release 1st April (www.doh.gov. uk/pricare/pcts.html)

Department of Health 2006a White paper: Our health, our care, our say. DoH, London

Department of Health 2006b Brief guide: White paper: Our health, our care, our say. DoH, London

Department of Health 2006c The National Education and Competence Framework for Advanced Critical Care Practitioners – a discussion document. DoH, London

Fairly D, Close SJ 2006 Evaluation of a nurse consultant's clinical activities and the search for patient outcomes in critical care. Journal of Clinical Nursing 15:1106–1114

Fatchett A 1998 Nursing in the new NHS – modern, dependable? Baillière Tindall, London

Gabe J, Kelleher D, Williams G 1994 Challenging medicine. Routledge, London

Grant AB, Massey VH 1999 Nursing leadership, management and research. Springhouse Corporation, Springhouse, Pennsylvania, PA

Hamer S, Collinson G (eds) 1999 Achieving evidence based practice. Baillière Tindall/Royal College of Nursing, Edinburgh

Henderson V 1966 The nature of nursing. Collier-Macmillan, New York

Her Majesty's Stationery Office 1989 Statutory Instrument 1989 no. 1456, Schedule 2 – The Nurses, Midwives and Health Visitors (Training) Amendment Rules 1989 – The Nurses and Midwives and Health Visitors Act 1979. HMSO, London (www.hmso.gov.uk)

Holden P, Littlewood J 1991 Anthropology and nursing. Routledge, London

Holland K, Warne T, Lawrence K 2006 The project experience. Shaping the Future for Primary Care Education and Training Project: Finding the evidence for education and training to deliver integrated health and social care, Vol 9. University of Salford

Howarth M, Grant M, Holland K 2004 A systematic view of the literature. Shaping the Future for Primary Care Education and Training Project: Finding the evidence for education and training to deliver integrated health and social care, Vol 1. University of Salford

Humphris D, Masterson A 2000 Developing new clinical roles – a guide for health professionals. Churchill Livingstone, Edinburgh

Johnson S 1997 Pathways of care. Blackwell Science, Oxford

Jones LJ 1994 The social context of health and social work. Macmillan Press, Basingstoke

Jowett S, Walton I 1994 Challenges and change in nurse education – a study of the implementation of Project 2000. National Foundation for Educational Research in England and Wales, Slough

Lawler J 1991 Behind the screens – nursing, somology and the body. Churchill Livingstone, Edinburgh

Leininger M 1978 Transcultural concepts, theories and practices. John Wiley and Sons, New York

Littlewood J 1991 Care and ambiguity: towards a concept of nursing. In: Holden P, Littlewood J (eds) Anthropology and nursing. Routledge, London, pp 179–180

Macleod Clark J, Maben J, Jones K 1996 Project 2000: Perceptions of the philosophy and practice of nursing. English National Board, London

Miller C, Ross N, Freeman M 1999 Shared learning and clinical teamwork: new directions in education for multiprofessional practice. English National Board, London

Morris S 1998 Health economics for nurses – an introductory guide. Prentice Hall, Hemel Hempstead

Neves EP, Mauro MYC 2000 Nursing in Brazil: trajectory, conquests and challenges. Online Journal of Issues in Nursing 5(2):1–14 (www.nursingworld.org)

Nursing and Midwifery Council 2004a Code of professional conduct; standards for conduct, performance and ethics. NMC, London

Nursing and Midwifery Council 2004b Standards of proficiency for pre-registration nursing education. NMC, London

Nursing and Midwifery Council 2005 An NMC guide for students of nursing and midwifery. NMC, London

Porter S 1991 A participant observation study of power relations between nurses and doctors in a general hospital. Journal of Advanced Nursing 16(6):728–735

Porter S 1998 Social theory and nursing practice. Macmillan Press, Basingstoke

Primomo J 2000 Nursing around the world: Japan – preparing for the century of the elderly. Online Journal of Issues in Nursing 5(2):1–20 (www.nursingworld.org)

Proctor S 2000 Caring for health. Macmillan Press, Basingstoke

Roper N, Logan W, Tierney A 1996 The elements of nursing. Churchill Livingstone, Edinburgh

Roper N, Logan W, Tierney A 2000 The Roper–Logan–Tierney model of nursing. Churchill Livingstone, Edinburgh

Ross A, King N, Firth J 2005 Interprofesional relationships and collaborative working: encouraging reflective practice. Online Journal of Nursing Issues (www.nursingworld.org)

Royle J, Speller V, Moon A 1999 Exploring interprofessional education and training needs in public health. Wessex Institute for Health Research and Development, University of Southampton

Savage J (ed) 1993 Strengthening nursing and midwifery to support health for all. WHO Regional Publications, European Series, No. 48. World Health Organisation, Copenhagen

Savage J 1995 Nursing intimacy. Scutari Press, London

Schultz EA, Lavenda RH 1990 Cultural anthropology, 2nd edn. West Publishing, St Paul

Seymer L 1960 Florence Nightingale's nurses – The Nightingale Training School 1860–1960. Pitman Medical Publishing, London

Sofarelli D, Brown D 1998 The need for nursing leadership in uncertain times. Journal of Nursing Management 6:201–207

Tones K 1993 Theory of health promotion; implications for nursing. In: Wilson-Barnett J, Clark J (eds) Research in health promotion and nursing. Macmillan, London

UKCC 1987 United Kingdom Central Council for Nursing, Midwifery and Health Visiting, Project 2000: the final proposals (Project Paper 9). UKCC, London

UKCC 1989 Amendment of Nurses Act 1979. UKCC, London

UKCC 1992a Scope of professional practice. United Kingdom Central Council for Nursing, Midwifery and Health Visiting, London

UKCC 1992b Code of professional conduct. UKCC, London

UKCC 1999 Fitness for practice. The UKCC Commission for Nursing and Midwifery Education, UKCC, London

Wallace M 2002 A–Z guide to professional healthcare. Churchill Livingstone, Edinburgh

Walsh M (ed) 2002 Watson's clinical nursing and related sciences, 6th edn. Baillière Tindall, Edinburgh

Warne T, McAndrew S 2005 Using patient experience in nurse education. Palgrave Macmillan, Basingstoke

Watkins M 1997 Nursing knowledge in nursing practice. In: Perry A (ed) Nursing – a knowledge base for practice, 2nd edn. Arnold, London, pp 1–32

World Health Organization 1997 Global movement for healthy ageing. Press release WHO/69 26th September. WHO, Geneva (www.int/archives)

World Health Organization 2001a Life course perspectives on coronary heart disease, stroke and diabetes – key issues and implications for policy and research. Summary report of a meeting of experts, 2–4 May. WHO, Geneva

World Health Organization 2001b Strengthening nursing and midwifery – Progress and future directions – 1996–2000. World Health Organization, Geneva

World Health Organization 2001c The global movement for active ageing. World Health Organization, Geneva (www.int/hpr/globalmovement/index.html)

World Health Organization 2002 WHO and the humanitarian crisis in South Africa. doc.4/8/2002. World Health Organization, Geneva (www.who.int/disasters/emergency.cfm)

Further reading

Allen D 2001 The changing shape of nursing practice – the role of nurses in the hospital division of labour. Routledge, London

Baxter C (ed) 2001 Managing diversity and inequality. Baillière Tindall/Royal College of Nursing, Edinburgh

Bishop V, Scott I (eds) 2001 Challenges in clinical practice. Palgrave, Basingstoke

Chiarella M 2002 The legal and professional status of nursing. Churchill Livingstone, Edinburgh

Ewens A 2002 The nature and purpose of leadership. In: Howkins E, Thornton C (eds) Managing and leading innovation in health care. Baillière Tindall/Royal College of Nursing, London, pp 69–90

Hyde J, Cooper F (eds) 2001 Managing the business of health care. Baillière Tindall/Royal College of Nursing, Edinburgh

McCabe C, Timmins F 2006 Communication skills for nursing practice. Palgrave Macmillan, Basingstoke

Useful websites

www.chi.gov.uk (Commission for Health Improvement)

www.doh.gov.uk (UK Department of Health)

www.nursingboard.ie (Irish Nursing Board, An Bord Altranais)

www.nice.org.uk (National Institute for Health and Clinical Excellence)

www.nursingcouncil.org.nz (Nursing Council of New Zealand)

www.nursingworld.org (*Online Journal of Issues in Nursing* – a free peer-reviewed electronic journal – with links to other useful websites)

NURSING AND THE ACTIVITIES OF LIVING

CONTENTS

Maintaining a safe environment

Susan Whittam

INTRODUCTION

Keeping ourselves safe is thought to be a basic survival skill, which all individuals possess, yet there are times when we are either unaware or unable to control the ability to do this. Throughout the world there are many differences in the types of hazards and risks that people are exposed to and just as many differences in the way that people manage their own safety. The inclusion of this AL in the Roper et al (1996, 2000) model is to draw your attention to the importance of being able to recognise the threats that exist to human survival and wellbeing and identify the impact that this may have upon any individual at any given time in their lives. The model helps us to develop our understanding by essentially focusing upon three key areas of concern as follows:

- the human body's ability to protect itself and the biological mechanisms that it employs to carry this out
- the ability that individuals have to make choices and take action to keep safe and free from danger
- the identification and understanding of the dangers and hazards that exist in the surrounding environment (including the health care environment) and how they pose a threat to individual safety and wellbeing.

These three areas of concern will be discussed throughout this chapter within the framework of the model and will help to develop an understanding of the AL and enable nursing interventions to be as individualised and effective as possible. Like most things in life it is not until something goes wrong, do we seek to understand how our bodies or everyday life around us function. Often concern for our own health and safety only becomes heightened when we become ill, have an accident or hear about a tragedy or event that has had terrible human consequences.

By using the framework of the Roper et al (1996, 2000) model in the following way we can begin to examine and identify how complex and varied health and safety issues really are and also identify the interrelatedness that exists between the other ALs. This chapter will therefore focus on the following:

1. **The model of living**
   - maintaining a safe environment in health and illness across the lifespan
   - dependence and independence in the activity of maintaining a safe environment
   - factors influencing the activity of maintaining a safe environment.

2. **The model for nursing**
   - nursing care of individuals with health problems that are affecting their ability to undertake the activity of maintaining a safe environment
   - that the health care environment is in itself a hazardous place and that patient safety is of paramount importance.

THE MODEL OF LIVING

MAINTAINING A SAFE ENVIRONMENT IN HEALTH AND ILLNESS ACROSS THE LIFESPAN

This component of the model describes the importance that safety plays at various stages of the lifespan. Safety is viewed as being a basic human survival skill and the model helps us to identify how this is achieved or compromised in normal everyday life. When applying the model in practice you will need to acknowledge that as people move across the lifespan they will encounter continuous changes in the way in which they ensure their survival and wellbeing, take risks and avoid hazards. This requires consideration of both the *internal* and the *external* environment. Essentially the internal environment considers the biological and psychological factors that may threaten safety and the external environment relates to the impact that sociocultural, economic and the surrounding environment may have upon health, for example:

- *Internal:* Injuries and diseases causing physiological and psychological disturbances.
- *External:* Accidents influenced by physical, psychological, sociocultural, environmental or politicoeconomic changes or limitations.

By understanding the basic needs and activities of individuals or groups there is the opportunity for the practice of nursing to become more supportive and effective. The lifespan stages identified with the activity of maintaining a safe environment are as follows.

Childhood

Before birth, babies are totally dependent upon other human beings for their survival. In some cases there may be a known risk to the health and wellbeing of the unborn child, such as cystic fibrosis, heart defects and Down syndrome. Through the provision of good prenatal care and continuous improvements in knowledge and technology many physical and genetic disorders can be detected and treated prior to conception and birth (Kumar & O'Brien 2004, Williams 2006).

Under normal circumstances the health of the unborn child is dependent upon the health and wellbeing of the mother in order to ensure the best chance of survival at birth and during the early weeks of life. To increase knowledge about common genetic disorders and the help and advice available to parents complete the following exercise.

Exercise

Down syndrome, heart defects, sickle cell anaemia and cleft palate are four examples of genetic/birth disorders.

1. What techniques are used for detection of these?
2. What advice and support can parents expect to receive?

It is important to know that the provision and access to a range of support services will be influenced by a number of personal and social factors such as individual and social responsibility, personal finance, national wealth, geographical location, culture and social class. At any time advice and support needs to be handled very sensitively and in accordance with individual need. You may also discover that there are huge variations across the world in the provision of screening programmes, treatment and care. This will be further discussed in the sections related to sociocultural, environmental and politicoeconomic influences upon the AL of MSE.

During birth the safety of the mother and the baby is critical as they are both at risk from a number of hazards and complications, many of which can be detected through a collaborative multiprofessional approach to good pre- and antenatal care (Department of Health (DoH) 2004a, Campbell & Graham 2006, Walsh 2006). In the UK, support for a healthy pregnancy and safe childbirth is provided by midwives whose practice is statutorily regulated to ensure optimum safety to both mother and child. Whilst maternal deaths are rare in the UK the World Health Organization (WHO) has pledged to reduce the maternal mortality rate

by three-quarters by the year 2015, estimating that as many as 529 000 women die every year as a result of pregnancy or childbirth, 99% of which occur in developing world countries such as Africa, Asia, Latin America and the Caribbean (World Health Organization (WHO) 2006a).

The responsibility for the safety of babies and toddlers within the home primarily rests with the family. The Royal Society for the Prevention of Accidents publishes up-to-date information about a whole range of accidents and indicates that despite many years of safety campaigning, the home continues to be a most hazardous place (Department of Trade and Industry 2002, Royal Society for the Prevention of Accidents (RoSPA) 2004). The three most serious types of accident are:

- impact accidents (bumps, falls and collisions)
- heat accidents (burns and scalds)
- ingestion and foreign body accidents (poisoning, choking and suffocation are most common in children under 4 years of age).

Exercise

1. To find out more about home safety browse through the RoSPA website (www.rospa.co.uk). You will find there are a series of projects that can help you to undertake home safety assessments and up-to-date information about accident statistics.
2. Consider how you might use the information on the website to help patients and families improve safety within their own homes.

Despite medical advances every year 12 million children, predominantly in the developing world, die before reaching their fifth birthday from common treatable diseases such as acute respiratory infections, diarrhoeal diseases, malaria, measles and malnutrition (WHO 1999). Many countries are able to provide support for education, health and immunisation to reduce unnecessary health risks, but personal choices, beliefs, economic wealth, traditions and cultures all play a part in the extent to which the health safety of children and adolescents can be assured.

When children start nursery and school they begin to experience an early and gradual independence. They become more adventurous and daring and increasingly exposed to outdoor school and play activities. Accident statistics show that from 0 to 14 years children require careful supervision in order to prevent many common accidents associated with road traffic, falls, fire, poisoning and drowning. Despite the fact that fewer children are being killed, every year in the UK two million children attend accident and emergency departments, many of whom are disproportionately from disadvantaged families (Child Accident Prevention Trust 2006).

In the UK, schools play an important part in ensuring premises are safe and teaching children about accident prevention using the Injury Minimization Programme for Schools (IMPS) (Frederick & Barlow 2006). Teaching safety in the home is dependent upon the ability of family members and more difficult to legislate against, requiring families to understand where dangers may lie and take action to prevent accidents occurring. Many voluntary and charitable organisations provide information and run national campaigns to help reduce accident rates (See useful websites at the end of this chapter.)

Exercise

In order to discover how children learn about safety:

1. Reflect on your own childhood. How did you learn about dangers within and outside the home?
2. Find out what personal safety topics are taught to primary school age children. (Browse the Injury Minimization Programme for Schools website, www.impsweb.co.uk.)

Adolescence

Greater independence from parental control is known to coincide with greater risk-taking in this age group, resulting in an increase of accidents and deaths, with road and pedestrian injuries accounting for the largest number (National Institute for Health and Clinical Excellence (NICE) 2006). Increased risk-taking is influenced by a number of factors such as gender, culture, peer pressure and deprivation, in which drugs and alcohol play a significant role. In the UK a number of government departments are working together to prevent and reduce the accident rates by 2010 (Department of Transport 2000, 2004, Department of Health 2002a).

Exercise

1. Identify the risks that you faced as an adolescent. Are they the same as those facing adolescents today?
2. List the dangers that currently face adolescents. What information or agencies are concerned with reducing risks to health?

Risk patterns change over time, resulting in new risks emerging continually. Often parents, as well as adolescents, are ill-prepared for managing risks, and this exercise should help to develop an understanding of why health and safety education is an important aspect of public health (see Chapter 12 for issues related to sexual health risks and adolescents).

Adulthood

Independence and personal choice in adulthood expose individuals to a huge range of activities within the home,

at work and in the pursuit of leisure, each activity carrying with it some degree of risk to safety. Young adults will perhaps be encountering many new activities for the first time and may be unaware of the threats to their own or other people's safety. At work there will be a number of specific risks associated with the type of work that is undertaken for which a joint responsibility for safety between the individual and the employer is expected. Within this age group, however, it is the home that continues to pose the greatest threat to personal safety, causing accidents associated with falls, fires, faulty appliances, poisoning, gardening and home improvement activities. UK home accident figures show that almost 4000 people die and 2.7 million people each year seek treatment in accident and emergency departments; suffering from injuries to the head, arms and legs caused by slips, trips and falls from stairs, chairs and ladders (RoSPA 2002, 2005a).

Exercise

Explore how adults obtain information regarding safety.

1. Browse the RoSPA website for accident rate data which it produces for the Department for Trade and Industry.
2. Determine how you could use the information contained within the website to:
   - improve safety for yourself and your family
   - understand the implications of the data for the provision of health services
   - support the specific needs of patients that you encounter.

The task of ensuring public safety is enormous, particularly when individuals and groups have different perceptions about what constitutes a safety precaution. It is important to appreciate this when helping patients to adopt different lifestyles. Because of different attitudes and perceptions some issues receive more public attention than others.

Old age

Today many people are living longer and as a result it is becoming more difficult to determine what constitutes a normal ageing process. Generally speaking, ageing is observable by the onset of certain age-associated changes; however, this can affect individual people in different ways, giving rise to the question of whether health changes are as a result of old age or through the presence of disease. Nevertheless the physiological changes that are associated with ageing mean that elderly people become more prone to injury and ill health due to a deterioration in the functioning of body systems, resulting in some common disorders, such as arthrosis, heart and lung failure and dementia (Weinert & Timiras 2003).

Ultimately a deterioration in health leads to an increasing dependence upon others in order to maintain a personal level of safety.

Exercise

In order to increase your understanding of promoting safety in old age:

1. Find out what accidents elderly people are most likely to encounter.
2. Identify which of these occur (a) in the home, (b) outside the home.
3. List the most common disorders that affect older people.
4. Find out what agencies/services exist in your area to help elderly people avoid accidents.

In industrialised societies, through demographic and social changes, there is a greater need to provide public services to support the needs of older people. Often older people have to cope with living alone along with failing health and the increased risk of accidents, abuse and even attack. In order to meet the growing health and social care needs of older people, the UK has seen an increased demand for nursing and residential home care and pressure to improve the services. In response to the problem in 2001 the Government published a *National Service Framework for Older People* that includes specific targets related to reducing accidents and promoting health and safety (DoH 2001a, 2006a).

DEPENDENCY/INDEPENDENCY

The degree of independence associated with the AL of maintaining a safe environment both internally and externally is essentially linked to age. Dependency is at its greatest in infancy, is affected by ill health, injury and disability and is expected to gradually increase in old age. The speed at which individuals achieve independence is essentially a gradual process; however, dependency can occur gradually or suddenly. For example, an individual can be rendered unconscious instantaneously either by disease, injury or anaesthesia. However, it is apparent that a person can never achieve complete independence within the AL, as there will always be a degree of dependency upon either other people or the surrounding environment in order to ensure safety. There are many examples of how events and the behaviour of others can compromise safety, such as individuals with mental health problems, learning disabilities or physical disabilities, or those living where there is social unrest or risk of man-made or natural disasters. In relation to the body's internal environment independence is maintained through good health. There is, however, a

risk to the body's normal ability to function at any stage of the lifespan, by the presence of disease, trauma or any other abnormal state.

Exercise

How does society value independence and what are its attitudes towards dependence? Ask three different people what their attitudes are in relation to the following:

1. A middle-aged adventurer who climbs Mount Everest or sails around the world single-handed.
2. A young person who backpacks around the world or takes a holiday in a resort notorious for excessive alcohol- and drug-taking.
3. A person with mental health problems living, with difficulty, in the community.
4. An elderly person with no family support remaining living in his/her own home.

Discuss your views with colleagues.

Attitudes to the above will vary, dependent upon personal experiences and beliefs. This will be further explored in the following section.

FACTORS INFLUENCING THE AL OF MAINTAINING A SAFE ENVIRONMENT (MSE)

The AL of MSE is complex and multidimensional. This next section will help to develop an understanding of the complexity of the AL by discussing the importance that each of the factors plays in understanding the needs of patients. Each of the factors as described by the model will now be explored.

Biological factors

The function of keeping the body in a healthy state and correcting any disturbances relies upon several biological functions working effectively, which are chiefly controlled by the nervous system. The systems work in conjunction with one another to carry out a series of very complex cellular processes that are triggered by changes either within the body (internal) or around it (external). In order to accurately assess and observe both the health and altered states of patients, it is vital that you understand what the systems are and how they work. For ease it is useful to identify the systems in relation to the functions they serve internally and externally as follows:

- the internal environment which is concerned with homeostatic balance, stability, protection and repair (autonomic nervous system, immunity and tissue repair)
- the external environment and the body's ability to avoid danger, and cope with changes (the sensory system or somatic nervous system).

Internal environment and related systems

Homeostasis   To maintain the internal environment, the body relies upon an intricate and highly organised system of intercellular communication and control. The control process is known as homeostasis. In health the mechanisms are so efficient they are hardly noticeable, but in ill health states the mechanisms become disturbed and over time have difficulty in coping effectively. Dependent upon the underlying problem (pathophysiology) patients are often able (unless unconscious) to describe how unwell they feel. Together with patient accounts and a range of physiological observations it is possible to determine the root cause of the problem and the extent to which the homeostatic mechanisms are coping. When control breaks down, if not detected, the body will eventually reach a stage where homeostasis cannot be restored and normal cellular function will become seriously affected. This state is referred to as shock, and it is important to be aware that not only seriously ill or injured patients are at risk from it. Early detection of shock is vital, for if not supported by external means, death is likely to occur.

Homeostatic control   The overall process of homeostasis is controlled by the nervous system, and it is responsible for constantly detecting and reversing the effects of even the slightest changes in cellular activity (see Fig. 3.1). The role played by the nervous system is to initiate specific required responses in other parts of the body to achieve stability and balance. Communication with other parts of the body is achieved through the activation of nervous responses, chemical transmitter substances and hormones. Together the nervous (neural) and hormonal control systems complement each other to maintain homeostasis in many different ways. The responses occur at various speeds and are influenced by the nature in which the body needs to react and restabilise (see Montague et al 2005, Section 1).

Neural control   Neural control of homeostasis is governed by the autonomic nervous system by transmitting fast electrical messages along nerve fibres to the internal organs. The system is divided into two distinct parts, the sympathetic and the parasympathetic, each having specific effects upon internal organs in order to control homeostasis (see Fig. 3.2).

Hormonal control   Hormones are chemical substances secreted mainly by endocrine glands under the control of the hypothalamus. They each have a specific role to play in maintaining homeostasis and travel to their target via the bloodstream. The response is much slower than that of the nervous system but more widespread (see Kindlen 2003, ch. 11). Figures 3.3 and 3.4 show the position of the major endocrine sites and the hierarchy of control from the hypothalamus. Hormones are released in response to homeostatic changes and are controlled by high or low hormone levels (see Fig 3.5).

Protective and defence mechanisms   The human body provides a series of protective and defence mechanisms in many ways. The skeleton forms protective cavities for vital organs such as the brain, spinal cord, heart and lungs. The skin acts as a barrier to protect the body against potentially harmful microorganisms, as well as being capable of interacting with the external environment through sensory nerve receptors. Other associated skin structures such as hair, nails, lymph, sweat and sebaceous glands all contribute towards protecting the body's inner and outer surfaces (see Fig. 3.6).

There are many potentially harmful agents that have the capacity to breach the body's defence mechanisms. When this happens the body relies upon the immune system to activate lymphocytes and destroy the invading organism (see Alexander et al 2006, ch. 16). The development of the immune system is based upon a process of exposure, recognition and response to particular harmful organisms throughout the entire lifespan, hence the immune system is as individual as the person (see Fig. 3.7).

At birth the immune system is underdeveloped and newborn babies for the first few months of life have to rely upon the antibodies passed from the mother via the placenta. These are classed as natural ways to build up immunity; however, the process can be artificially assisted through programmes of vaccination and immunisation (see Fig. 3.8). Disorders of the immune system are usually classed as being congenital or acquired and cause either a deficiency or overactivity resulting in a greater susceptibility to infections. Excessive hypersensitivity to foreign organisms causes an inappropriate reaction known as anaphylactic shock. This causes an acute inflammatory reaction that can develop within minutes and can be life-threatening as seen in asthma attacks and other allergic responses.

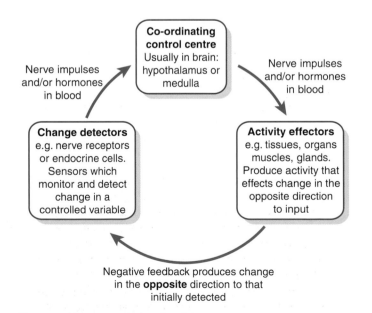

Fig. 3.1 Homeostatic feedback loop (from Montague et al 2005, with permission).

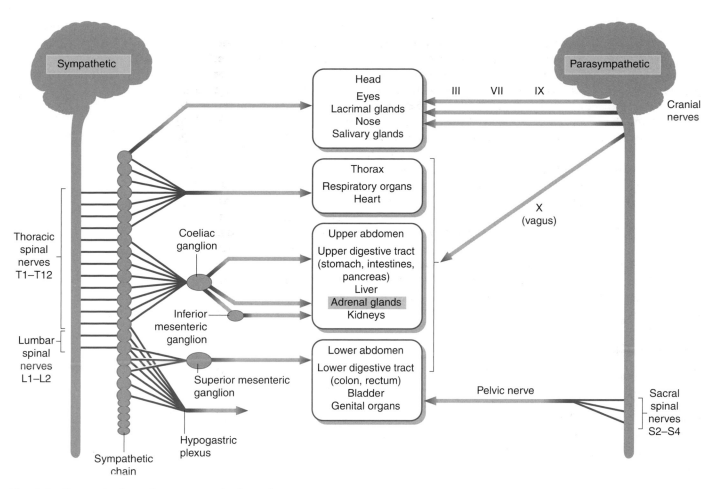

Fig. 3.2 Sympathetic and parasympathetic outflow (from Kindlen 2003, with permission).

Inflammatory process and tissue repair The inflammatory process is a locally initiated defence mechanism that responds immediately following damage to tissue caused by injury or infection. The process involves the production and release of a variety of chemicals that serve to defend the affected area, remove dead cells and promote the process of healing. The inflammatory process is essentially the first stage of the tissue repair process followed by a series of other stages. When damage is close to the surface of the skin the process can be directly observed as localised redness, swelling, reduced or loss of function, localised pain or irritation. Within a short space of time following the immediate inflammatory response the process of healing continues. The rate at which the process is completed depends upon the nature of the damage, which in some cases if chronic can take many years to be fully complete. The healing process is said to take place by primary and secondary intention (see Chapter 8).

Many factors play an important part in influencing the rate at which healing takes place, such as age, nutritional state, presence of infection and degree and location of the injury. For example, bones take considerably longer to heal and some tissue such as that found in the brain and spinal cord cannot repair itself, leading to permanent disabilities.

Exercise

Consider the physiological processes involved in the following scenarios and determine what factors will influence recovery and return to normal function:

1. A child with a scald to his left arm.
2. An elderly lady with a fractured neck of the femur.
3. A middle-aged gentleman who has suffered a severe subarachnoid haemorrhage.
4. A middle-aged woman with an abdominal incision from a hysterectomy.

Make notes on each one and use diagrams to explain what is happening to normal physiological function.

In each case the human body would have instigated a common series of steps that would be observable either directly or indirectly towards reacting to the injury or intervention. The rate at which the individuals will recover is less predictable due to age, fitness, speed and accuracy of medical intervention to reduce complications and degree of vital organ involvement and damage.

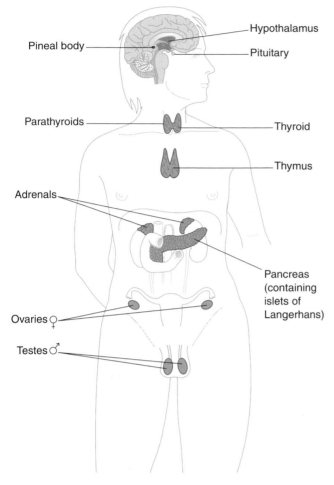

Pineal body

Hypothalamus

Pituitary

Parathyroids

Thyroid

Thymus

Adrenals

Pancreas (containing islets of Langerhans)

Ovaries ♀

Testes ♂

Fig. 3.3 Location of major endocrine structures (from Brooker & Nicol 2003, with permission).

External safe environment

The ability to interact with the external environment in order to avoid hazards and maintain safety is the concern of the somatic nervous system, which is made up of the following parts:

- central nervous system organisation and function
- skeletal muscle
- sensory organs.

Whilst each part has a distinctive role to play, together they provide a whole system that enables the body to be conscious of the surroundings and physiologically capable of responding to required changes. The system works by monitoring the external environment through sensory organs (eyes, ears, etc.). By making sense of the information received the body is then able to protect itself by initiating the appropriate response (see Fig. 3.9).

The complexity of the system explains how the body has the ability to respond simultaneously to both the external and internal environment in order to maintain

safety and also how appropriate responses can also be suppressed either by disease, impairment or choice (see Kindlen 2003, chs 20, 21, 25 and 29).

Understanding the systems in relation to the activity of maintaining a safe environment enables an appreciation of how important it is to preserve the ability to receive sensory information and how hazardous living can become when the ability to avoid danger is reduced either temporarily or permanently.

Exercise

Identify what hazards can be associated with a loss of sensation. What sort of hazards are the following people at risk from?

1. Through a works accident, Neil, aged 38 years, has lost all sensation in his right foot.
2. Jenny is totally blind and needs to come into hospital for minor surgery.
3. Beverly has had meningitis and lost her sense of smell and taste.
4. John is profoundly deaf and is embarking on a sailing holiday.

Make notes about each one and consider other similar situations you may have come across in your nursing practice.

This exercise demonstrates the extent to which disorders of the body's control and defence can impact upon daily lives, wellbeing and safety, causing patients to alter their lifestyles either temporarily or permanently.

Psychological factors

It is well recognised that psychological health and wellbeing is just as important as our physical health. Here the model acts as a guide to help consider what issues may be affecting the patient's ability to support or improve their quality of life.

Psychological factors are associated with the extent to which individuals are able to control and influence their own safety and circumstances and are central to the following:

- personality, mood and temperament
- knowledge, intelligence and competence
- attitude, motivation, confidence and personal experiences
- physical and mental impairment
- personal situations and stressors
- environment
- finances and resources.

This list demonstrates the complexity and the inter-relatedness between the ALs and the factors affecting

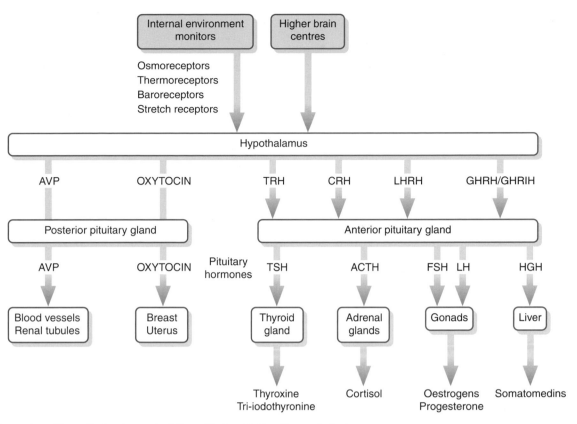

Fig. 3.4 Hierarchy of hypothalamic control (from Kindlen 2003, with permission).

health (FAH), highlighting the importance of ensuring that all components of the model are carefully considered in relation to addressing the individual needs of patients. The extent to which risks can be avoided depends upon many factors, some of which could on reflection have been avoided and others that simply cannot be imagined or foreseen until after the event. When applying the model into practice it is useful to identify the extent to which individuals are able to control and influence their own safety by determining their level of understanding and/or experience. The ability to avoid or minimise risk is primarily based upon personal understanding, experience and motivation, highlighting the importance that individual personality, intelligence, attitude and temperament play in the process. The ability to avoid danger starts with being able to recognise where risks may be present and then take appropriate action to prevent harm. In doing so the individual will be influenced by a whole variety of other factors in order to ensure safety as shown in Figure 3.10. Where there is an impairment in psychological wellbeing it is known that the risk of accidents are greater.

The following exercise helps to develop a greater understanding of the complexity of health and interrelatedness of the components of the model.

> **Exercise**
> The following scenarios are examples of individuals whose psychological safety is compromised. Using the diagram in Figure 3.10 consider the extent to which the other factors affecting health would influence their ability to improve their safety.
>
> 1. A person with a physical disability who accidentally sets the kitchen alight.
> 2. A woman who is suffering abuse.
> 3. An elderly person who is being intimidated by a group of children/youths.

In each case the degree of control is being influenced by a variety of factors such as physical ability, dependency and the environment. When caring for patients in clinical situations the nurse needs to consider the same factors.

Effects of stress
Stress is a term which everyone uses at some time in their lives to describe a state of disruption that is leaving them feeling threatened, uncomfortable or unwell, and this is known to contribute towards risks and accidents in all age

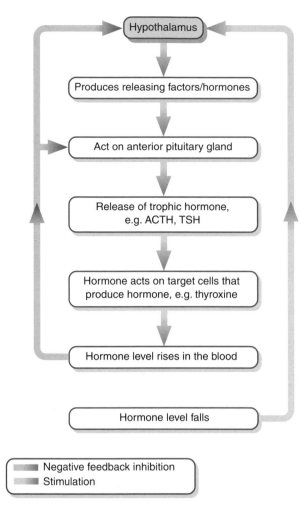

Fig. 3.5 Hormone negative feedback inhibition (from Brooker & Nicol 2003, with permission).

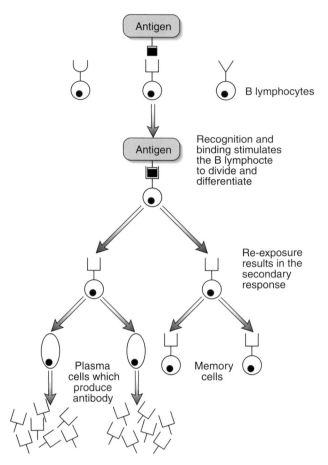

Fig. 3.7 The primary immune response (from Alexander et al 2006, with permission).

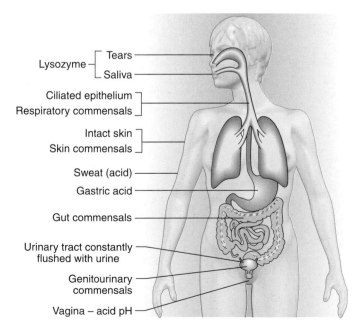

Fig. 3.6 Barriers to infection (from Alexander et al 2006, with permission).

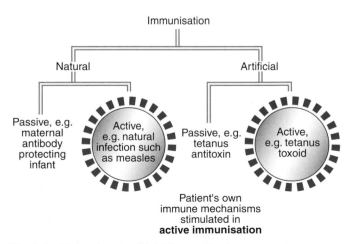

Fig. 3.8 Natural and artificial immunity (from Alexander et al 2006, with permission).

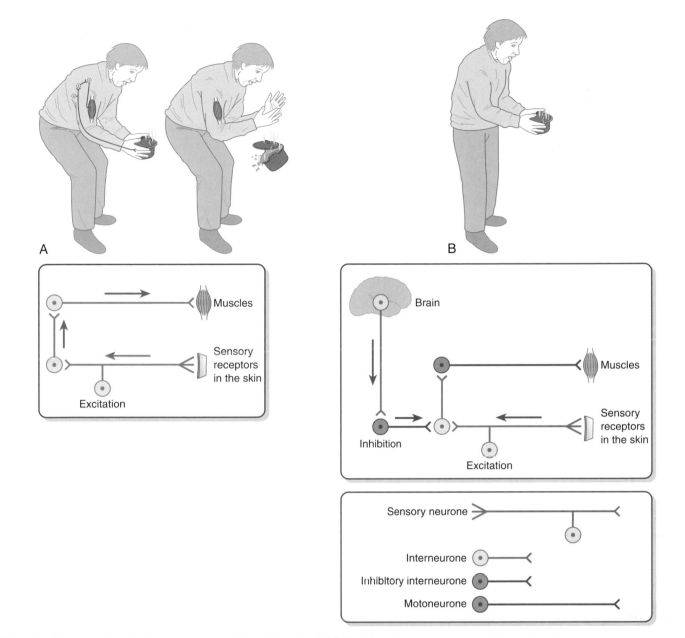

Fig. 3.9 An example of reflex response and how it can be inhibited (from Rutishauser 1994, with permission).

groups. The subject of stress is hugely complex and has been studied from many perspectives (biological/physiological, psychological, sociological and environmental) in an attempt to understand the causes and various effects. As such there are a variety of models available which describe these phenomena (see Brooker & Nichol 2003, ch. 6). Fundamentally the concept of stress is related to an excessive pressure or demand upon any of the body's systems, resulting in an effect upon emotional wellbeing, and thinking, reasoning and behaviour. A certain amount of stress is acknowledged as being a basic survival instinct that is followed by a process of recovery and adaptation. However, when stress becomes too great or prolonged then the symptoms become observable.

Exercise
1. Think about how you react and feel if any of the following happened to you:
   - you lose your purse or wallet
   - you are alone in your car at night and break down on the motorway
   - you have very noisy neighbours.
2. What happens to you physically?
3. What happens to your behaviour and your thinking and reasoning processes?

Through this exercise some of the effects of stress can be readily recognised. Feeling nauseous, agitated, terrified

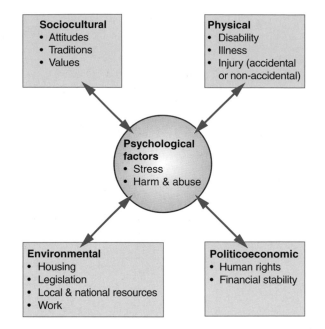

Sociocultural
- Attitudes
- Traditions
- Values

Physical
- Disability
- Illness
- Injury (accidental or non-accidental)

Psychological factors
- Stress
- Harm & abuse

Environmental
- Housing
- Legislation
- Local & national resources
- Work

Politicoeconomic
- Human rights
- Financial stability

Fig. 3.10 The interrelatedness of factors affecting health.

or angry, resulting in you crying, shouting and not being able to 'think straight' are some examples. Try to remember those reactions and relate them to how patients may feel or behave in any given circumstance.

Irrespective of the cause, whether real or imagined, the body's defence mechanisms become affected, leading to a range of physical illnesses and diseases, poor coping mechanisms, behavioural changes and disturbances. Individuality means that some people are more able to manage their stress than others and this is closely linked to personality, experiences and support mechanisms. From a nursing perspective it is important for the concept to be fully understood if it is to be managed effectively, not only in relation to patient care but also for oneself.

Exercise

In order to determine the range of reactions that other people have towards stressful situations consider the following scenario.

A patient on the ward where you are working develops severe pain during visiting time. The patient's relative is shouting and demanding that the consultant be called immediately. You are asked to stay with the patient, whilst your colleague who is in charge of the ward deals with the relative and tries to summon medical assistance.

1. Consider what physiological and psychological systems are reacting and describe how everyone might be feeling during this time:
   - the patient
   - the relative
   - your colleague
   - yourself
   - other patients.
2. Discuss your responses with colleagues.

Responses to this exercise will have illustrated that everyone would be acting differently to try and cope with the situation. In all of these situations good communication skills are essential (see Chapter 4).

Abuse and violence The problem of abuse and violence takes place throughout the world and is known to have devastating and lifelong effects on both physical and mental health. It is often brought to our attention through a combination of media coverage and action from pressure groups, which over time increase public and professional awareness about the scale of the problem. This has led to improvements in recognition and response mechanisms and support for victims through multi-agencies, legal frameworks, statutory and voluntary services. The problems are known to exist across the lifespan and in a variety of environments such as the home, the workplace and unfortunately even professional caregiving places such as residential care homes and hospitals (WHO 2002a). Research into the problem has demonstrated that there is a direct link between abuse and poor physical and psychiatric health (Arnow 2004). In an attempt to reduce the problem many national and international statutory and voluntary agencies exist to provide further research, awareness campaigns, literature, victim telephone helplines and support services. In Britain there is a national strategy that outlines the specific types of abuse and recommends how statutory and voluntary agencies can work together to help both victims and abusers (DoH 2006b).

Non-accidental injury (NAI) is a term that is used to describe a form of abuse that results from deliberate injury and harm caused by the self or another person. It is known to exist in varying degrees in all ages, in all societies and from all walks of life.

Children Sadly the abuse of children is an international problem. It is found in all societies and results in general neglect, physical injury, emotional and sexual abuse and even death. The problem has many related causes such as psychological predisposition, the surrounding environment, cultural and social conventions. Unfortunately the problem is also compounded by silence and secrecy. It is difficult to determine the cost of abuse, for beyond the cost of human pain and suffering, there are also the costs of related health and social care and law enforcement. For an abused child there is a high risk that their emotional development will be disturbed and an even greater chance that they themselves become abusers in later life (WHO 2002a, ch. 3). (Refer to Chapter 11 for information about bullying.) In the UK many statutory and voluntary agencies such as Social Services departments and the National Society for the Prevention of Cruelty to Children (NSPCC) work together to provide services, information, child protection training and research in an effort to reduce the problem. Following the tragic death of Victoria Climbie in 2000, national legislation and guidance was introduced to ensure that staff from all agencies work together to safeguard children and are capable of recognising abuse and responding appropriately (Children

Act 2004, Department for Education and Skills (DfES) 2003, 2005).

Women According to the WHO the abuse of women and girls is a major health and human rights concern. It occurs across the entire lifespan and can be physical and/or mental. Abuse can take place either privately or publicly, within the home, at work or in the wider community and can consist of direct violence, coercion or deprivation of liberty (WHO 2002a, ch. 6). The types of abuse women suffer encompass the following:

- battering
- sexual abuse
- dowry-related violence
- rape
- genital mutilation
- exploitation
- harassment and intimidation
- trafficking and prostitution
- punishments condoned by the state.

As a result women suffer a range of physical and mental health problems ranging from minor to severe injury, reproductive health problems, depression, anxiety and psychosomatic disorders. It is important to know that abuse is not only associated with physical violence but also takes place in the form of preventing access to legal/human rights, education, personal finance or even health care. Despite increased awareness of the problem some women will remain ignorant and powerless and unable to resolve or improve their situations. In many instances the women feel isolated and have a low self-esteem, living in fear of not only their own lives but also the safety of their children. As a result they are more likely to adopt unhealthy lifestyles or worse still become abusers themselves (Bornstein 2005).

Men It is generally acknowledged that men are more at risk of being assaulted by acquaintances or strangers and this risk is known to increase for gay men. However, the reality of domestic male abuse has been largely eclipsed by concern for the abuse of children and women, mainly due to social and cultural stereotypes that militate against acknowledgement, reporting and intervention. As a result there tends to be less agency support for victims who not unlike women suffer a range of physical, psychological, emotional and economic problems such as:

- stabbings, scalds and injuries to head, limbs and genitalia, and rape
- verbal and emotional abuse
- threat of attack during sleep
- threat of taking children away
- false allegations.

As a result men may experience loss of self-esteem and confidence, with social withdrawal, alcoholism, working long hours, separation or divorce as coping mechanisms. Although there is a lack of research and data about the experiences of domestic abuse experiences of gay men, it is known that they are at a greater risk of partner abuse than lesbian women and have to cope with some specific issues such as:

- the threat of 'outing' to family, friends and employers etc.
- expressing abuse as 'masculinity' in the relationship
- lack of services from which to seek help and support.

Increasingly there is recognition that action needs to be taken to acknowledge, accurately record and establish agencies to support male victims of abuse (DoH 2006b, Scottish Executive Central Research Unit 2002).

Elderly people Since the early 19th century, in the UK there has been a gradual increase in the number of older people and it is known that this trend will continue to rise due to improved health and lifestyles (DoH 2001a). Unfortunately in some societies this has led to the development of a prevailing image that older people have low social autonomy and are a burden to society. This dangerous stereotyping has perpetuated social and political discrimination and highlighted that older people have been subjected to the following types of abuse (WHO 2002a, ch. 5):

- financial exploitation (misappropriation of pensions and savings)
- physical abuse and neglect (withdrawal of food, fluids and overmedication)
- physical violence (by carers and intruders/thugs)
- psychological abuse (humiliation, ridicule and loss of dignity)
- sexual abuse.

It is important that the needs of a growing older population are recognised and that through good health and social policy, multi-agency professionals can work together with individuals and their families to maximise safe, independent living (Drennan et al 2005).

Exercise

1. Locate and browse the Age Concern website (www.ageconcern.org.uk) and consider how the information and links could help you support the needs of patients.

Disabled people It is estimated that nearly 650 million people throughout the world at all ages of the lifespan suffer from some form of disability and this figure is increasing due to the following (WHO 2005a):

- increasing populations, ageing societies and medical advances
- chronic diseases, genetic defects, injuries due to accidents, war and conflicts.

As a result a degree of dependency is created that leaves individuals vulnerable to abuse, and individuals with learning difficulties, severe or chronic mental illness and physical disability are thought to be more at risk (Evans 2004, Chaplin et al 2006). The abuse is known to take many forms ranging from withdrawal of care, neglect or injury. For example, Sullivan & Knutson (2000) identified that disabled school children were 3.4 times more likely to be abused than their non-disabled peers. The literature suggests that accident rates should be analysed more carefully in order to properly identify where non-accidental rates might be obscured in general accident reporting.

Self-harm Self-harm is a term that is used to refer to injury that is inflicted either by the individual themselves or through their consent/agreement, examples of which are self-poisoning, lacerations, gassing and hanging. However, in some cultures deliberate cutting, marking or piercing of the skin would signify a specific cultural/traditional rite or fashion trend. In England around 5000 people each year take their own lives. Although these rates have been falling they are known to be rising in young men aged between 19 and 34 years and there are also known links to certain socio-economic and occupational groups (DoH 2002a, National Institute for Mental Health in England 2005). The self-harm rates are measured by the attendance rates at accident and emergency departments and it is suggested that greater attention needs to be paid towards the assessment of the person's psychosocial needs in order to support the individual needs of patients (Barr et al 2005).

Sociocultural factors

Concern for safety differs throughout the world and the model urges us to acknowledge how social and cultural factors will influence the different behaviours that are found in societies. In the UK we take for granted the services that have been developed over many years to maximise personal and public safety. Indeed when those mechanisms fail to protect us we are at liberty to claim financial compensation for any inconvenience or injuries sustained. The degree to which individual safety can be influenced is dependent upon two main factors:

1. The extent to which the individual can take responsibility for their own safety be that within the home, public places or the workplace.
2. The amount of financial, political and legal support that is available within society.

Not all countries are able to fully support the safety of individuals as in the UK and even in societies where concern for safety is fairly comprehensive, cultural differences can influence the types of hazards that exist and present inequalities in the way in which health is promoted and risks prevented. For example, it is known that people of lower social economic groups and ethnic backgrounds are at greater risk of accidents (RoSPA 2004).

At a basic level, safety needs are met by the family, but in some instances cultural beliefs and values can be so strong

that they actually compromise safety. In many countries throughout the world there may be little education or political support for safety and people are forced to accept the degree of danger that they face, such as people living in poor or war-torn countries. Within all societies the daily lives of people are at some point influenced by religious and spiritual beliefs. The extent to which this occurs depends upon the degree of openness and freedom of choice that exists. Some societies have to abide by strict codes and traditions that to the onlooker may appear inappropriate, especially in relation to safety. In some instances people become willing to risk the safety of themselves and others and even die for their beliefs, e.g. suicide bombers. When the outside world attempts to influence change or intervene in the interests of safety this can create turmoil, acts of terrorism and even wars. Acts of terrorism and war have, sadly, become a common feature of our lives and have heightened concerns about our day-to-day safety.

The terrorist attack on America on 11th September 2001 was one of the most extensive acts of terrorism the world has ever seen. It caused the loss of thousands of lives and was a startling reminder of how vulnerable even the most developed countries in the world are to the beliefs held by others.

Internationally a growing number of people are prepared to place themselves in great danger in order to escape persecution or seek out a better life in another country. The risks that asylum seekers take are a reminder of the lengths that people will go to in order to protect themselves from danger. In some cases this has resulted in people tolerating terrible conditions or risking their lives to escape from the dangers they face in their home country. In relation to health it is important to recognise that many individuals will have been the victims of torture and organised violence and will have specific needs that will require expert attention (Burnett & Peel 2001, Carlsson et al 2005).

Exercise
1. Examine your own views about health and safety and social differences.
2. Consider the risks associated with the practice of female circumcision.
3. Consider the risks in countries which do not have seat belt laws.
4. Compare your views with other colleagues.

Knowledge of the risks will influence actions, highlighting the importance that education plays in maintaining safety. However, it is important to recognise how difficult it would be to change some of the practices that pose a risk to safety, because of tradition and strongly held beliefs.

As societies grow and develop it is inevitable that new hazards will emerge. Constant and rapid change, greater access to information and greater demand for services have seemingly speeded up the pace of life and work. As a result there appears to be a shortage of time and less tolerance, which is in turn creating new threats to our safety and well-being. In the UK alone, public service accidents and tragedies, racial tensions, riots, gun crime and antisocial behaviour are shaking public confidence in the ability of the state to maintain safety. Rising crime rates involving theft, assault and murder have caused people to take greater action to protect themselves and their property. In the UK, Victim Support is an independent national charity that offers free and confidential advice to over one million people per year who have been affected by crime. Even within schools and the workplace, bullying is known to cause health problems such as anxiety, depression and loss of self-esteem (Wolke et al 2001, Smith 2004). It is also acknowledged that people who are exposed to traumatic events either directly or indirectly can suffer from a range of physiological and psychological disturbances, known as post-traumatic stress disorder (PTSD). In recognition of the problem, it has become necessary to provide a range of services to support the immediate and long-term effects that individuals may suffer, such as mood swings, flashbacks and difficulty in sleeping or concentrating (Howard 2003). As a result the issue of who should accept responsibility and blame for accidents and other traumatic events has become exceedingly complex and has resulted in an increase in claims for compensation. Many legal firms now actively advertise their services widely to encourage individual claims.

Environmental factors

This aspect of the model is concerned with the surrounding (external) environment and the possible impact that certain conditions could have upon personal health and safety. The external environment can present many threats to public health at local, national and international levels and since the health of people is vital to the social economy, government initiatives are aimed at preventing and reducing risks wherever possible. Legislation outlines the responsibilities of governments, industries, groups and individuals in order to promote individual and public safety. In the UK, legislation and policies exist to ensure that improvements are made to the environment in order to ensure public safety and contribute towards reducing the environmental and health effects of global climate change. Through the United Nations many countries are working together to address the root causes and agree the measures necessary to reduce and cope with full effects of climate change. In the UK the Department of Health has already begun to develop strategies to cope with the effects that climate change may have upon changing health patterns and services (DoH 2001b). From an international health perspective the World Health Organization (WHO) is instrumental in working with other intergovernmental agencies to encourage the development of strategies related to improving the health of people by improving the environment. In 2002 a joint United Nations and WHO

report (WHO 2002b) published alarming facts that every day 5500 children the world over are dying from common preventable diseases such as diarrhoea (from polluted food and water) and acute respiratory infections. When issues are ignored, pressure groups, such as Greenpeace and Friends of the Earth, work to draw attention to the problems.

The Roper, Logan and Tierney model recognises that nurses are well placed in their daily work with patients to reinforce and incorporate health and safety information into their care, in order to promote health and safety. To be effective, however, nurses need to be able to present information in a creative and meaningful way and always ensure that the information is accurate, appropriate and up to date.

> **Exercise**
> 1. Access the World Health Organization website (www.who/int) and familiarise yourself with some of the current global environmental and health issues.

The subject of health and the environment is vast, but for the purposes of this chapter the following four areas will be used to explore the main health and safety issues:

- pollution (air, water and land)
- accidents
- infection
- fire.

Pollution

Pollution is considered to be a by-product of modern living, which at some point through a lack of understanding and/or provision of resources becomes a hazard for health. For example, in some countries where effective sewage systems are not available there is a huge risk to public health whilst in industrialised countries there are risks from emissions which may find their way into the air, land or rivers (WHO 2006a). The growing number of pollutants worldwide is a cause for concern, some of which will now be briefly discussed.

Water pollution Water is vital to human survival and has a range of functions within the body with an essential role in maintaining health, therefore the provision of clean water is recognised all over the world as being a basic health requirement. On a global scale the contamination of drinking water poses the most significant risk to humans, and throughout history there have been countless disease outbreaks resulting from untreated, poorly treated or polluted water. It is estimated that at least one-fifth of the Earth's population lacks access to safe drinking water and that the problem will worsen as the population grows. Water becomes polluted by microorganisms and chemicals, which when swallowed may result in a whole range of health problems, ranging from gastrointestinal diseases, infections and tumours to genetic disorders

(Eyles & Consitt 2004). Today even wealthy nations struggle to ensure that water sources are pollutant-free, but for poorer countries the inability to ensure the safety of drinking water or provide adequate health care when outbreaks occur means that death rates remain high.

Water contamination from industrial waste is a common factor of modern-day living and can occur accidentally or deliberately. When the risk of pollution is widespread it can affect the lives of not only humans but also marine life, wildlife and plant life. Ultimately there becomes a potential to disrupt the natural ecosystem, which in turn can interrupt the food chain. Humans who swim in polluted waters run the risk of contracting harmful infections (Nichols 2006). As well as chemical substances finding their way into waters, sewage and waste such as glass, plastic and metal objects can cause injury and even death for both humans and animals. Together voluntary, national and international agencies have raised awareness and introduced policies to reduce, prevent and reverse the damage caused by pollution.

Exercise

Using the World Health Organization and Department of Health website as a source of reference (www.who.int/ith and www.doh.gov.uk/traveladvice) consider what advice you would give to someone who is travelling abroad in relation to:

1. drinking water
2. swimming.

Air pollution   There are many pollutants that exist in the air and they have the potential to cause widespread damage. Many pollutants are invisible, which makes it difficult to deal with them, and often the first signs of air pollution will be changes in health patterns. The air naturally carries substances such as dust and pollen that are known to have an effect upon human health, such as asthma. Chemicals emitted into the air from cars, airplanes, factories, agricultural pesticides, insecticides and household aerosols are known to be responsible for damaging not only health, but also habitats, wildlife and even buildings. When such substances travel in cloud form they can cause damage many miles away from the point of origin, by polluting in the form of acid rain. On a global scale there has been growing concern regarding the role that pollutants play in changing conditions within the Earth's atmosphere, potentially threatening the very life of the planet itself. This is often referred to as global warming, evidence of which is believed to be in the form of increasing reports of floods, droughts, season changes and coastline alterations. It is believed that gases such as carbon dioxide, methane and chlorofluorocarbons (CFCs) are creating an imbalance in the Earth's natural ability to retain heat and protect itself via the ozone layer, by absorbing harmful rays from the sun. The predicted health risks are now beginning to be realised, some of which are described below (Brunkreef 2002, DoH 2006c):

- increasing number of deaths and injuries from 'natural' disasters
- changes in disease patterns
- increased mortality and morbidity caused by heatwaves
- increase in water and vector-borne diseases such as malaria
- increase in food contamination due to warmer climates
- increased dangers of exposure to ultra-violet (UV) radiation.

In the workplace a concentrated exposure to pollutants, such as in the mining, nuclear and chemical industries, is known to cause specific diseases and disorders, raising the importance of acknowledging the public health issues associated with the work environment (the effects of the work environment upon health are discussed in Chapter 11).

At a personal level, individuals take responsibility for being aware of the risks and are encouraged to take appropriate action to avoid hazards and maintain health. Health promotion and ill-health prevention information have been influential in raising awareness, particularly in relation to the increased risk of carcinoma through exposure to sunlight and cigarette smoking (smoking is discussed in Chapter 5). Health professionals can play an important role in influencing public and individual safety by not only ensuring that patients have access to appropriate information and care, but also through influencing changes in health policy through research and practice developments (Ewles & Simnett 2003).

Land pollution   Pollution of the land presents a number of immediate and long-term health and safety hazards to all living things. As a result many countries have introduced a number of initiatives to clean up the environment and recycle otherwise harmful waste. The soil can become contaminated through direct spillage of pollutants such as chemicals or from particles contained in the air (such as acid rain). When pollutants contaminate food or water supplies, the risk to the health of humans and wildlife is increased. Contamination can occur by accident or through the careless or illegal dumping of industrial or household waste which includes chemicals, discarded vehicles and appliances (such as refrigerators) and their associated by-products such as oil and petrol. As a result in the UK, the landfill regulations came into effect in 2002 in order to prevent and reduce the effects of landfill pollution (Landfill Regulations 2002).

Lead pollution   Lead is a natural substance found in the earth and was for many years used widely to make everyday products such as paint, plastics, petrol and water pipes. It is a serious pollutant (neurotoxin) which can be ingested, inhaled or absorbed and is capable of causing genetic disorders and widespread damage to the nervous, immune, reproductive, renal, cardiovascular, musculoskeletal and haematopoietic systems. Through increased awareness of the dangers many countries have considerably reduce the environmental and occupational exposure to lead, but even today throughout the world there are still national and international campaigns aimed at further reducing the harmful effects of lead, particularly in children (UNEP/UNICEF 1999, Health Protection Agency (HPA) 2006).

Noise pollution The subject of noise pollution is a difficult one to tackle because of individual levels of acceptance and tolerance. Noise is a product of modern living brought about by the need for transportation and communication for industrial, domestic and leisure requirements. However, the effects of noise are now known to cause a number of health problems and as a result the control of noise in the UK is governed by legislation and regulation (the Clean Neighbourhoods and Environment Act 2005 and the Control of Noise at Work Regulations 2005). In the workplace there are risks to hearing problems ranging from tinnitus to hearing loss. Around the home there are issues related to stress, anxiety, lack of sleep and concentration, causing accidents, violence and aggression caused by noisy vehicles, animals and general antisocial behaviour. It has also been recognised that young people are at risk from damaging their hearing through prolonged periods of listening to loud music at dance clubs. As a result music and entertainment industry regulations will come into force in April 2008 (HSE 2005).

The increased use of mobile phones has created both concern and controversy in terms of health risks. In the UK, the Department of Health in recognition that health risks are still not fully understood have issued further information and advice to enable individuals, parents and employers to make informed choices about safety (DoH 2000a). Because of the increased risk of road accidents resulting from the use of mobile phones whilst driving, in the UK a law prohibiting the use of hand-held mobile phones whilst driving was introduced in 2003 (RoSPA 2005b).

Preventing accidents

The potential for accidents to occur exists in all aspects of daily life, in the home, at work, during travel and at play. Many accidents are actually preventable and in recent years increasing attention has been given to accident prevention because of the personal and economic costs associated with them. It is estimated that in Britain 10 000 people die every year from accidental injury, caused by accidents in the home, at work, by falls, road accidents and fires. In 2000–01 it was estimated that the cost of accidents to the NHS was £2.2 billion, with the overall cost to society being a staggering £25 billion (DoH 2006d). However, the cost of pain, grief and suffering is incalculable. Research into accident patterns provides an understanding about the nature of accidents, which can inform prevention strategies. Surveys have also shown that the time of the day, days of the week and seasons also influence accident rates. Evenings, weekends and school holidays are known to record higher accident rates. Despite

this knowledge accidents continue to happen, resulting in death, physical and psychological injury on a global scale. In Britain the Government's strategy to reduce accidental injury and death was launched by the Department of Health in 1999 and as a result accident rates are falling (DoH 1999, 2002b). The strategy outlines how cross-government agencies, professionals, voluntary and community groups can work together to reduce accidents. Nurses play an important role in providing help and advice to patients and their families at all ages of the lifespan. It is also important for nurses to have an understanding of national strategy and work closely with other professionals and services such as schools and community groups in order to make an effective contribution to reducing injury and death. In addition it is important that manufacturers of household items and providers of facilities must also play a part towards ensuring safety.

Preventing accidents in the home It is known that people have more accidents in the home than any other environment; the kitchen, living/dining room, stairs, bedrooms and bathroom are extremely dangerous places. Accidents are related to everyday living activities such as playing, preparing food, carrying out household improvements or repairs or simply moving around the house. Different hazards can be linked to different family members, the most vulnerable groups being children, the elderly and those with learning disabilities and mental impairment (RoSPA 2004, 2005c).

Risks to children Accidents are known to be one of leading causes of death among children (DoH 2002b, CAPT 2006). Commonly children are known to suffer a range of accidents such as fractures, burns and scalds, drowning, choking and accidental poisonings, resulting from falls, road accidents, lack of appropriate supervision, secure storage of substances and equipment, particularly when in unfamiliar environments. The prevention of many accidents in essence relies upon adult supervision and intervention, particularly where very young children are concerned. It is, however, difficult for those caring for children to be vigilant at all times and the natural curiosity of children to explore their environment means that not all potential situations can be predicted.

Risks to the elderly At the opposite end of the lifespan, elderly people over the age of 75 years are known to be more susceptible to accidents in the home, due to falls caused by poor mobility, failing sensory ability and general health (Health Development Agency 2003, DoH 2001a). It is estimated that there are more people over the age of 65 years than under the age of 18 years with the population of people over the age of 85 set to double by 2020. Falls in older people are known to be the major cause of death and disability and also lead to the onset of many other physical, psychological, environmental, sociopolitical and socioeconomic problems (DoH 2006a). Many elderly people live alone and are further at risk from not being able to summon help, increasing the risk of complications such as dehydration and hypothermia in addition to their injury. Within the home, a range of health and social care professionals can help older people and their families assess the dangers that surround them and make the necessary changes to help them to live safely and independently. Simple measures such as removing obstacles, wearing sensible footwear, installation of alarm systems and ensuring regular communication with family, friends and neighbours are vital in preventing and responding early to accidents in the home. Even within professional care environments such as care homes, day centres and hospitals, the prevention of falls should be given the highest priority. In the UK the National Service Framework (NSF) for Older People specifically recognises the importance of reducing accidents as part of the overall strategy to improve the health and social care needs of older people and provide the most appropriate services that reflect the needs of an increasingly older population (DoH 2001a, 2006a).

Exercise
1. Identify how nongovernmental agencies contribute towards the health and safety of older people. Browse the Age Concern website (www.ageconcern.org.uk) for information regarding the safety of older people and current campaigns.

Risks to people with disabilities   In recent years more people with a range of disabilities have been encouraged to live independently within the community and gradual progress has been made to adapt living surroundings in order to maximise normality and safety. National statistics show, however, that accident rates amongst disabled people are increasing, particularly for people with learning disabilities and mental health problems (Office for National Statistics 2000).

People with a range of disabilities require resources and support appropriate to their needs in order to help them live independently and remain safe. With the introduction of the Disability Discrimination Act 2005, improvements have been made to enable greater access and inclusion in all aspects of society. At home and at work, people with disabilities will require adaptations to be made to the environment and appliances not only to enable access but also ensure safety. In the UK, house-building firms are encouraged to build homes that encourage independent living for disabled people, and government grants are available along with tax exemptions for building work that enables adaptations to be made (see Directgov/Disabled Living Centre Council websites for further information). A range of resources are also available for the home to aid communication such as hearing loop systems, personal emergency call systems and the use of flashing lights for telephones and door bells. The

Disability Alliance provides information, advice, training and research and heads up campaigns to ensure that improvements in the standard of living for disabled people can be made. Throughout the UK the Disabled Living Foundation has a network of centres that provide free and impartial information and advice about products, solutions and equipment to enable easier living.

Exercise
1. Browse the Disability Alliance and Disabled Living Foundation websites to increase your understanding of the resources that disabled people can access in order to maximise independent living and promote safety (www.disabilityalliance.org and www.dlcc.org.uk).

Preventing accidents at work   The importance of ensuring safety at work has two dimensions governed by the Health and Safety at Work Act 1974. One is the responsibility of the employer to protect employees and the other is the ability of the employee to act responsibly to ensure their own safety. In the UK the Health and Safety Executive (HSE) is a government agency that has statutory powers to monitor and investigate serious incidents. In 2005/6 the HSE estimated that a total of 30 million days of work were lost due to work-related injuries and illness, 2 million due to illness, 146 076 due to injury and 212 who were killed. It is worth noting that every job, regardless of physical effort involved, has some degree of health risk (HSE 2006a).

Through programmes of training for employers and employees and the provision of safety equipment and workplace standards and policies, many associated problems can be prevented. The HSE is just one organisation that collects information related to a number of occupations across a variety of industries such as agriculture, construction, leisure services, health services, manufacturing and retail services. The information enables trends to be identified and strategies to be developed to reduce health problems in the workplace.

Exercise
1. Locate and familiarise yourself with the Health and Safety Executive website (www.hse.gov.uk). You will find useful information regarding the work of the HSE and specific information for health-care-related topics.

In health care the risks associated with back injury, exposure to radiation and needle-stick injuries are just a few examples of accidents in the workplace, where both the employer and employee must take equal responsibility. In the UK there is a legal requirement for employers and self-employed people to report accidents and ill health at work under the Reporting of Injuries, Diseases and Dangerous Occurrences Regulations 1995 (HSE 2006b). Not all countries have legislation to protect the safety of workers and worse still, may risk the health and safety of whole communities or even neighbouring countries. As a result pressure is brought to bear upon countries and companies worldwide by action groups and international agencies such as the International Labour Organization (ILO) and the World Health Organization (WHO) who work to establish international standards of safe practice in the workplace.

Preventing accidents in play, sport and leisure   In the Western world, there has been a marked increase in the availability and pursuit of play, sport and leisure activities that, in turn, has brought about a variety of risks to health and safety. As a result it has become necessary to introduce new legislation in an attempt to prevent injury and death.

For children it is the responsibility of parents, schools and event organisers to assess the risks that may be present. To safeguard children the British Standards Institute has developed a number of quality standards to ensure the manufacture and of safe use of equipment (British Standards Institute 2003). During normal play, injuries associated with climbing, tripping, colliding, fighting and falling result in minor injuries such as skin cuts and grazes, sprains and more serious injuries such as fractures and head injuries. However, for children road accidents remain the greatest cause of accidental death (CAPT 2006, Department of Transport 2004).

More recently there has been growing concern for the safety of children at play, with an increasing number of reports related to street crime, drug taking, paedophile activity, abductions and even murders. Prevention of accidents related to sport essentially rests with the individual, although companies and organisers are be expected to take responsibility for ensuring the safety of buildings and equipment. Nevertheless sporting injuries are known to account for a number of emergency hospital admissions, days off work and even deaths (Department of Trade and Industry 2002, RoSPA 2005a).

Exercise
1. How many everyday sports can you identify and what types of injuries are associated with them?
2. What would be the impact upon other daily living activities?

The most popular sports such as football or racquet sports result in many musculoskeletal injuries, such as bruises and sprains (RoSPA 2005a). Fractured limbs can result in altered dependency in other ALs such as personal cleansing and dressing, eliminating and mobility. Some sports are even known to carry a high risk of injury or death and have been heavily criticised for the unnecessary cost of life and financial costs associated with ensuring safety or initiating rescue operations, for example outdoor pursuits such as mountain climbing, sailing, motor car and cycle racing and boxing. However, it is not only sport participants who are at risk, so too are spectators, particularly when the sport attracts large crowds. Over the years the importance of crowd safety has been heightened following a series of serious incidents related to stadium safety and violent behaviour, resulting in many regulations being put in place by event organisers to both prevent and respond to incidents.

This section has shown that whilst the importance of play and leisure is important, it is not without risk, whether it is a family outing or a high-profile sporting activity. Whatever the activity, individuals and organisers must take equal responsibility to ensure that safety regulations around supervision, food hygiene, buildings and equipment have been adhered to.

Accidents related to travel   The need to travel is an essential component of everyday living, and changes in lifestyles over time have witnessed an expansion of travel for both work and leisure purposes. As a result of a number of accidents and disasters related to air, coach, rail and sea travel, regulations have been enforced to establish standards of good practice in relation to safety checks and the provision of standard safety equipment. In Britain many manufacturers of products are expected to achieve a quality standard set by the British Standards Institute identified through a quality kitemark scheme. It is the responsibility of individual travellers, transport manufacturers and travel businesses to comply with safety standards arising from a number of laws and regulations such as the Railways Act 2005 and the Package Travel, Package Holidays and Package Tours Regulations 1992.

Although all types of travel carry an element of risk, road accidents in particular are commonplace in many countries. Over time a number of measures have been introduced in an attempt to reduce road accidents such as:

- improved street lighting
- traffic calming methods (e.g. speed bumps)
- speed restrictions in accident black spots
- breathalyser checks to reduce alcohol-related accidents
- compulsory wearing of seat belts for front and rear seat passengers and correct fitting of baby seats
- compulsory wearing of crash helmets for cyclists.

Despite these measures, with the number of vehicles on the roads ever increasing, the risk of road accidents and death remains high. In March 2000 the UK Government published an extensive Road Safety Strategy with the intention of dramatically reducing the number of deaths and serious injuries caused by all types of road accidents by the year 2010 (Department of Transport 2000, 2004). In addition there have been a number of national campaigns and the introduction of the Road Safety Act in 2006. To this extent

Roper et al (1996) point out the significance that changes in the law can have upon improving health and safety, highlighting the importance that pressure groups play in influencing government action. It becomes apparent that public safety is an extremely complex issue initially dependent upon the recognition and acceptance of personal responsibility. Nurses, however, have a variety of opportunities within their work at primary and acute care levels to support and influence individual behaviour in order to prevent accidents.

Preventing infection

Infection occurs when harmful pathogenic microorganisms invade the human body and cause disease and even death. Whilst not all microorganisms are harmful, under the right conditions infections can occur, highlighting the importance that preventing and controlling infection has in relation to the activity of maintaining a safe environment. To this extent advances in infection control need to be continually improving in order to address emerging challenges in infection control. Since the middle of the 20th century, advances in infection control have led to the introduction of many national and international guidelines in order to safeguard public health. The guidelines require health care organisations and individual professionals to take responsibility for adhering to agreed standard control of infection practices. In order to help maintain a safe environment against infection it is essential to have a basic understanding of how microorganisms behave, how infection is transmitted and how infection can be controlled. These can only be briefly described in this chapter and it is recommended that you refer to specialist texts to enhance your knowledge particularly when nursing patients with specific problems (see Ayliffe et al 2000, Horton & Parker 2002, Alexander et al 2006). It is essential that infection control care is always based upon an understanding of the patient's individual clinical and personal needs as well as informed infection control practice.

Microorganisms   Under normal circumstances the human body is host to many harmless microorganisms known as commensals, providing different parts of the body with protection against infection (see Table 3.1). Infection occurs when a disease-causing microorganism (pathogen) invades and damages body tissue. Microorganisms which cause infection do so by breaking through the body's defence mechanisms and affect specific body systems.

The chain of infection   The chain of infection illustrates the stages at which an infection develops and enters the body, outlining the sources of infection, sites of entry into and exit from the body, modes of transmission and host susceptibility (see Fig. 3.11). This simple cycle helps to identify the stages at which appropriate action and intervention contribute towards preventing and controlling infection.

Control of infection   Effective infection control consists of a variety of activities related to the infection chain.

Table 3.1 Normal commensal microorganisms

Site	Organism
Skin	Staphylococcus epidermidis Diphtheroids Corynebacterium sp.
Mouth and throat	Staphylococci Streptococci Anaerobes Neisseria sp.
Nose	Staphylococci Diphtheroids
Gut	Escherichia coli Klebsiella sp. Proteus sp. Streptococcus faecalis Clostridium perfringens Yeasts (Candida)
Kidneys and bladder	Normally sterile
Vagina	Lactobacilli Streptococci Staphylococci Anaerobes

From: Alexander et al (2006), p. 660.

Destruction of microorganisms   Preventing and destroying the cause of the infection is achieved with the use of antimicrobial agents which are used for sterilisation and disinfection processes. A range of techniques are utilised to minimise the spread of infection within the internal and external environment, through the use of chemicals such as liquids, gases and drugs and physical processes such as extreme heat and radiation. The use of antibiotics in modern medicine has revolutionised the control of infection, but misuse has encouraged the emergence of multiresistant strains of bacteria such as methicillin-resistant *Staphylococcus aureus* (MRSA). To this extent it is now recognised that prevention of infection cannot rely on antibiotics alone and that prevention and control of infection interventions are of equal and vital importance. Concern for increasing rates of infection has brought about the need for greater national surveillance and reporting of infection rates and trends, control of antibiotics and review of standard control of infection procedures, including the care environment (DoH 2005, 2006e).

Recognition of predisposing factors   It is known that there are several factors which influence an individual's susceptibility and resistance to infection. Very young people and older people have diminished immune systems, which reduces the ability to combat infection. Likewise drugs and other diseases which alter the body's immune response mechanisms are known to increase the risk of infection. Prolonged exposure to cold and damp environments and

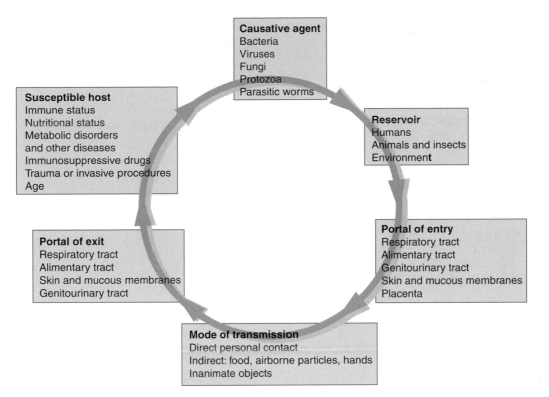

Fig. 3.11 The chain of infection (from Watson & Walsh 2002, with permission).

lack of adequate diet and exercise reduce the ability of the body to maintain natural body defences against infection and there is also a known link between psychological stress and infections. Where tissue damage occurs through trauma, disease or surgical intervention, the risk of infection is increased because skin defences are breached and tissue is exposed to microorganism invasion and multiplication.

Isolation Early isolation methods consisted purely of segregating and quarantining people in the belief that this would stop the spread of disease, as in the case of leprosy and bubonic plague sufferers. By the middle of the 20th century new understanding led to the development of more integrated approaches that concentrated upon prevention, treatment and cure and the provision of isolation hospitals was commonplace. As a result of new understanding and more integrated approaches many previously dangerous infective diseases such as smallpox have now been completely eradicated from the world and others have been dramatically reduced. Today it is well recognised that merely isolating the patient as a source of infection is insufficient, as it has implications for affecting individual mental wellbeing, confidentiality and human rights. The scope of informed control of infection is extensive. It begins with developing a greater understanding about the behaviour of specific diseases and includes surveillance of contacts and sources and monitoring the spread and containment of the infection. As a result many countries, although not all, are able to protect public health by implementing best practice guidelines for the notification and isolation techniques of certain

diseases. In England the control of health care associated infections (HCAI) is a national health care priority governed by the Health Act 2006 (DoH 2006e). The Department of Health issues policies and guidance and the Healthcare Commission inspects health care organisations to ensure that standards and national targets to reduce the number of infections are being achieved (DoH 2003, 2005, 2006e).

Immunisation Immunity to disease can be achieved either naturally or artificially. Natural immunity is achieved through exposure to disease microorganisms (toxins) that enable the body to develop internal recognition and resistance mechanisms (antibodies). Artificial immunity is achieved by the deliberate introduction (vaccination) of a safe amount of modified disease toxin into the body enabling an immune response to be created without suffering from the effects of the disease (see Fig. 3.8).

Over time immunisation programmes have played a key role in reducing the incidence and risks of some of the world's most common and dangerous infectious diseases such as diphtheria, tetanus, poliomyelitis, whooping cough, measles, mumps, rubella and more recently meningitis. The aim of an immunisation programme is to target the most susceptible groups of people who are likely to contract the disease, such as children, women of child-bearing age, pregnant mothers, health care workers and travellers to foreign countries. Immunisation programmes vary throughout the world, but unfortunately not every country is able to afford the resources to prevent or treat some of the most common diseases, which for a relatively small cost would save millions of lives. In 2006 it was reported that there has been a 60% reduction in global measles mortality as a result of a joint WHO and UNICEF campaign, far exceeding the campaign target (Wolfson et al 2007). In the UK a comprehensive vaccination programme is recommended by the Department of Health, referred to as the Green Book (DoH 2006f). The programme is generally available free of charge, but sometimes concerns arise about the safety of the vaccines, such as the scare that surrounded the measles, mumps and rubella (MMR) vaccine, which resulted in a reduction in the uptake of the vaccination. Any significant reduction in the uptake of vaccinations leaves individuals unprotected against the disease and a risk of an epidemic breaking out (Friederichs et al 2006). Without adequate protection, individuals increase the risk of contracting diseases, which may have serious consequences not only for themselves but also for whole communities. It is important to recognise, however, that whilst immunisation provides added protection for maintaining a safer internal environment, this needs to be complemented with improved social and economic conditions to minimise the prevention and spread of infectious diseases.

Control of epidemics   An epidemic occurs when there is a marked increase in the reported cases of a particular disease above the normal acceptable rate. Whilst each country must take responsibility for controlling its own epidemics, the WHO has a key role in monitoring infectious outbreaks, developing strategies and plans to deal with them as well as encouraging international collaboration to prevent worldwide spread. If an epidemic does extend across the world then it becomes known as a pandemic. The risk of epidemics is far greater in modern times due to the relative ease with which people and products can travel across land, sea and air, requiring the need for strict regulations to minimise the spread of infections. More alarmingly, following a number of incidences such as the anthrax attack in America in 2001 there are concerns that some countries have retained stocks of deadly diseases (such as smallpox), that could be used deliberately as part of a germ warfare strategy or bioterrorist attack.

Worldwide there are always new concerns about emerging diseases and the threats they bring to public health. Concerns linked to severe acute respiratory syndrome (SARS) and avian flu demonstrate how strategies and cooperation on an international scale will be required to cope with potential outbreaks on a pandemic scale. The WHO constantly surveys outbreaks and provides up-to-date information on the status of worldwide outbreaks.

Fire prevention

The devastating effects of fire are only too well known and increasingly it has become essential to understand the importance of safety not only in the home but also in public places. In 2002 the Fire Brigade attended 1 million fires and false alarms in the UK which resulted in 578 deaths and 16 400 non-fatal casualties (RoSPA 2005a). The importance of information being available in many forms enables individuals to not only gain knowledge and understanding but also practical skills in relation to raising the alarm, the use of extinguishers and the planning of escape routes.

Fire in the home   Despite major campaigns to increase public awareness house fires continue to cause many serious injuries and deaths caused mainly by kitchen fires (from chip pans), smoking, candles and faulty electrical appliances. In the UK individual householders are expected to take responsibility for the safety of their own homes and insure their homes in order to replace items destroyed by fire as the costs can run into thousands of pounds. In the home the correct fitting and regular checking of a smoke alarm is known to save many lives. In Britain as part of a national initiative to save more lives, in 2005 the Government launched a national fire safety campaign, publishing a free fire prevention handbook to increase public knowledge of how to improve prevention, detection and escape (Office of the Deputy Prime Minister 2005).

Fire in public places   In public places such as the workplace, shops, hotels, restaurants and entertainment centres, there are obligations to reach legal safety standards. Despite this every year there are reports of terrible tragedies, resulting in severe injury and loss of life due to the fact that escape routes were blocked, locked or inadequate. Throughout the NHS all health care premises are required to ensure fire safety by adhering to the *Firecode*. Health care organisations must provide an annual statement of safety to the Department of Health and severe legal penalties can be imposed where there is non-compliance (DoH 1994, Department for Communities and Local Government 2006).

Fire control   Having taken all necessary precautions to prevent a fire occurring, controlling a fire relies upon detection, raising the alarm, containing the fire and extinguishing it. Through community information programmes the Fire Brigade offers useful help and advice guiding people on how to prevent fires and ensure personal safety in the event of a fire both in the home and in public places.

Exercise

1. Find out how fire prevention is promoted within your community.
2. Locate the London Fire Brigade website and find out more about community fire safety programmes (www.london-fire.gov.uk).
3. Browse the Department of Health website to learn more about the *Firecode* (www.dh.gov.uk/PublicationsAndStatistics/LettersAndCirculars/Firecode/fs/en).

Individual effects of fire The effects of being injured in a fire can be long-lasting, resulting in both physical and psychological trauma including pain, stress, risk of infection and stigma from scarring. Loss of confidence may be encountered through a lack of desire to socialise or an inability to continue working during the healing process, which may cause additional anxiety not only for the individual but also for their family and social circle. Additional stress may be encountered where there has been a loss of property or an inability to make repairs either through physical disability or insufficient finances.

Politicoeconomic factors

Although the primary responsibility to maintain safety rests with the individual, it is evident that safety is enhanced with support from national and international policy, legislation and financial support.

Political responsibility

Actions taken by governments and international agencies are able to influence legislation and the provision of information and resources, but this does not happen throughout the world. In industrialised societies employers and service providers are expected to demonstrate regard for the safety of employees and customers. In developed countries public protection is supported through the provision of statutory and legal frameworks to such an extent that an official public enquiry would seek to identify the cause and make recommendations to prevent further incidents. In some cases persons found to be responsible for the death of an employee can expect to be found guilty of *corporate manslaughter* for failing to ensure that the health and safety prevention measures are in place. Every year throughout the world there are reports of tragic accidents that could have been prevented, enabling new lessons to be learned about health and safety. In health care it is estimated that 1 in 10 patients suffer adverse effects as a result of errors related to surgery, anaesthesia, medication, medical devices, investigations, diagnosis, complications and hospital acquired infections (Rohn et al 2000). Such is the magnitude of the problem worldwide, in 2004, the WHO launched the World Alliance for Patient Safety, urging countries to pay close attention to patient safety (WHO 2005b, 2006c). As part of the UK's 10-year programme of health reform the Department of Health introduced in 2001 the National Patient Safety Agency to help the NHS monitor and learn from actual and potential incidents (DoH 1998, 2000b, 2006g). As the health care reforms progress all health care organisations are required to have robust safety data collection and monitoring systems in place and all individual health care professionals must be able to demonstrate accountability for their actions. By way of monitoring the safety and effectiveness of health care organizations, periodic assessments are made against nationally agreed frameworks. In England, the Healthcare Commission monitors and rates the performance of health care organizations against a number of key indicators and publishes the *Annual Health Check Ratings* in October each year (see www.healthcarecommission.org.uk).

Individual responsibility

At every stage of the lifespan there is a need for individuals to take some form of action to maintain safety. To a certain extent this is politically supported through legislation and the provision of public services. At some point the responsibility to ensure safety rests purely at an individual level, but this may have cost implications that become unaffordable and consequently safety can become compromised. For example, individuals and families on low incomes may be forced to go without safety equipment or obtain it second-hand and run the risk of additional hazards because the equipment is not entirely safe. Often within society action or pressure groups have been successful in drawing attention to issues that are in the interests of the safety of the public at large, forcing politicians to introduce legislation and appropriate services.

Conflict and war

Unfortunately the threat of conflict and war for many people throughout the world has become an ever-present factor in their daily lives. Reports of new conflicts breaking out and slow progress toward peace have become regular news items, to the point that we are in danger of becoming immune to the actual misery, death and destruction that has taken place. Since the USA terrorist attacks on 11th September 2001 there have been a number of other events that have created an ongoing concern for individual safety in the midst of not knowing what future threats may be or when they may occur. It is the responsibility of all governments and individuals throughout the world to remain vigilant but more importantly to seek ways in which to promote tolerance and understanding, enabling people to live without fear and in safety.

CONCLUSION

The framework of the model of living has been used to demonstrate how the Roper et al (1996, 2000) model can be used to guide your understanding of the individual differences that exist when carrying out the AL of maintaining a safe environment. When planning and delivering care to individual patients it is vital that individual differences are taken into consideration and in doing so there is an acknowledgement that no one activity takes place without being interrelated with any of the other 11 ALs. Throughout the chapter exercises have been designed to show how important it is to:

- keep up to date with information
- base the assessment of your patient upon their individual habits and needs
- be mindful of how your own experiences and values might influence nursing care.

The last of the exercises in this section will now provide two brief scenarios to help begin the application of the model into practice. These exercises will help you gain an appreciation of how the AL of maintaining a safe environment can be influenced and how this can impact upon the other ALs.

FACTORS AFFECTING THE ACTIVITY OF MAINTAINING A SAFE ENVIRONMENT

> **Exercise**
> 1. Read through Case study 3.1 and consider how the activity of maintaining a safe environment is being influenced from a lifespan, dependency/independency and factors affecting health perspective.

> **Case study 3.1**
>
> **Scenario to identify MSE issues relating to the factors affecting health**
> A 24-year-old mother of two primary school age children has been discharged home from hospital following an assault by her husband, where she sustained facial and back injuries.

You may have considered the following points.

Lifespan
- expectation that she should be in good health and be able to care for and protect herself and her children.

Change in dependency
- dependency may increase upon family and close friends to support immediate physical, psychological, social, environmental and economic needs.

Factors affecting health
Biological
- injuries will need to heal
- risk of infection, concussion and pain
- difficulty eating, drinking, mobilising
- vision may be affected.

Psychological
- anxiety, fear, anger and distress
- low self-esteem and risk of depression.

Sociocultural
- concern for safety of self and children
- concern regarding reactions of others (friends, neighbours, school, work colleagues).

Environmental
- concern regarding safety in the home
- concern regarding leaving the home.

Politicoeconomic
- may have immediate and long-term financial concerns.

> **Exercise**
> 1. Read through Case study 3.2 and identify the impact that a change in health status would have upon the Activities of Living.

> **Case study 3.2**
>
> **Scenario to identify MSE issues relating to the Activities of Living (ALs)**
> A 76-year-old lady who lives alone has been discharged home following hip replacement surgery.

Impact upon Activities of Living
MSE
- home safety issues to be considered to prevent further accidents.

Communicating
- concern for ability to summon help if required
- need to ensure has access to information and support to meet physical and psychological needs.

Eating and drinking
- may be unable to fully meet needs due to reduced mobility
- at risk from malnutrition and dehydration
- poor diet may affect healing process.

Eliminating
- may require assistance and aids to carry out activity safely.

Mobilising
- at risk from slips, trips and falls
- reduced mobility in short and long term may impact on independency/dependency and other ALs.

Maintaining body temperature
- reduced activity may lower body temperature.

Sleep and rest
- loss of sleep may increase risk of accidents.

Dying
- at risk from accident or injury leading to death.

SUMMARY POINTS

The two exercises have helped to demonstrate the following:

1. MSE can be affected by all the factors affecting health.
2. MSE can be affected by all other ALs.
3. The lack of ability to engage fully in this activity can have detrimental affects upon health and the quality of life.

THE MODEL FOR NURSING

INDIVIDUALISING NURSING FOR THE ACTIVITY OF MAINTAINING A SAFE ENVIRONMENT

The application of the model for nursing is based upon integrating the components of the model of living (lifespan, dependence/independence and factors affecting health) with each of the four phases of the nursing process (assessing, planning, implementing and evaluating) as shown in Figure 3.12 (see also Chapter 1 for details of the model and the nursing process).

This part of the chapter will now concentrate on showing you how to link the framework of the model of living in relation to MSE, to nursing practice situations in order to determine individual patient needs. By using each of the components of the model of living as a main framework it becomes possible to appreciate how individuals normally carry out the activity of MSE. Whilst people are physiologically the same they may behave very differently depending upon individual circumstances. The model of living in health is briefly summarised in Box 3.1. When applying the

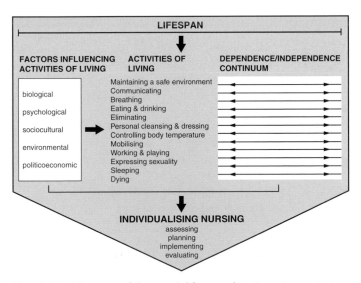

Fig. 3.12 Diagram of the model for nursing (from Roper et al 1996, with permission).

| Box 3.1 | Summary of the model of living in relation to MSE |

Lifespan
Acknowledge what is considered to be normal development, physiology and lifestyle activities in accordance with age.

Dependence/independence
Recognition of temporary or permanent issues related to age and states of ill health that create changes in independency.

Factors affecting MSE
Biological
- Internal – homeostatic systems are working correctly to ensure organ and system stability.
- External – there is ability to protect the body from external hazards.

Psychological
Emotional stability and intellectual capability affect the ability to cope with everyday life and identify dangers.

Sociocultural
Attitudes, beliefs and behaviour have a major influence upon maintaining safety.

Environmental
Dangers exist in the environment and measures can be taken to avoid them.

Politicoeconomic
Legislation, national and local resources and financial support is required to maximise safety.

model for nursing it is necessary to transfer this knowledge and understanding to each individual patient in order to determine the extent to which the activity has altered as a result of injury or ill health. Only then can individualised care using the model be achieved.

This information will now form the basis upon which patients' needs can be assessed. By comprehensively and systematically integrating the MSE information within each stage of the nursing process, the individual needs of the patient can be identified in order to maximise the individuality of the care plan. Whilst using the book and when encountering individual patients in practice, you may find it useful to refer back to the information contained within the MSE model of living, recognising the importance of keeping up to date with related information in order to ensure that patients always receive the highest standard of care. By using the model a broad range of nursing interventions will be identified that are appropriate to the AL such as:

- teaching patients about health and safety
- preventing accidents and ill health

- supporting patients to cope with altered health states
- providing care to support individual needs
- helping patients to adopt healthier lifestyles.

In order to help develop skills this section of the chapter will continue to provide a series of case scenarios and reflective exercises.

ASSESSMENT

Assessing the individual using the model for nursing

The aim of the assessment phase in relation to MSE is to utilise the components of the model of living to carry out the following:

- collect specific information related to the AL of MSE
- interpret information to determine the degree to which the AL is altered
- identify actual and potential problems related to the AL.

It is important to recognise that whilst the process of nursing begins with an initial assessment, it is a continuous activity, which supports the changing needs of patients through their entire period of care. This section of the chapter will now begin by describing how the model can be integrated to support the full range of patient assessment activities.

Collection of specific information related to the AL of MSE

Prior to the assessment

The assessment begins with using the components of the model of living to assess the patient's normal habits and routines in order to identify the extent to which ill health is influencing the ability to carry out the activity of MSE. When undertaking the assessment, it is important to remember the interrelatedness of the AL of MSE in order to identify:

1. whether actual or potential problems identified may be more readily aligned to another AL
2. the extent to which other professional groups or agencies may be required to help solve or alleviate the problems.

What matters most is that through the assessment process, problems are firstly identified and that a realistic plan of nursing care is designed to meet the individual needs of the patient (see Chapter 1). It is important to remember that the accuracy of the assessment is based upon having a sound understanding of related normal health needs, particularly those related to vital body functions such as homeostasis and you are advised to make reference to other chapters and the recommended reading listed at the end of this chapter.

Identification of health problems associated with MSE

Before undertaking an actual patient assessment, it is important to have a good understanding of the range of health problems that are associated with MSE. The components of the model of living enable the identification of common illnesses that are associated with the activity of MSE and are shown in Box 3.2. When assessing patients this will enable a judgement to be made about the extent to which the activity of MSE can be altered in different states of ill health and how this may manifest in individual patients.

Exercise

1. You may wish to check your knowledge and experience against the issues listed in Box 3.2 and consider them against your clinical experience to date. Consider what your learning needs might be, discuss these with your mentor and develop a learning plan.

The patient assessment

The ability to provide individualised nursing care is based upon the knowledge gained about a person's individuality in living. As demonstrated in the model of living, individuals carry out numerous activities to maintain a safe environment, some of which are similar and some of which are different. The purpose of undertaking an assessment of MSE is to determine what a particular patient's normal habits and routines are and identify where they may be vulnerable within the AL, given their current health state. Hence a thorough assessment is vital in order to ensure that the subsequent care plan is relevant to what the patient can realistically achieve and should reflect the following:

- how actual problems may be solved
- how to prevent potential problems becoming actual ones
- how to prevent solved problems from recurring
- how to alleviate problems which cannot be solved
- how to help the person cope with temporary or permanently altered states.

Data collection

In relation to MSE the assessment should be based on the following:

- What are the individual's attitudes to maintaining health and safety of self and others?
- What activities does the person engage in to maintain health and safety of self and others?
- What factors are influencing the individual's approach to maintaining a safe environment (ability, knowledge, experience, resources)?
- How does the individual normally cope with the ability to maintain a safe environment?
- What identifiable problems or difficulties is the individual currently experiencing?

When undertaking an assessment ensure that the following skills are utilised:

- interviewing skills
- observation skills
- listening skills.

| Box 3.2 | To show identification of common health problems within the framework of the model |

Lifespan

Consider health problems commonly associated with the stages of the lifespan, i.e. childhood illnesses and accidents, illness associated with lifestyle, disability and the ageing process.

Dependency/independency

Consider how dependency is altered in the presence of disease, trauma, medical intervention (i.e. anaesthesia or chemotherapy), trauma, disability and ageing.

Factors affecting health

Begin by identifying if the problem is being caused by an internal or external factor and consider the effect this may be having on other ALs. This demonstrates the interrelatedness and complexity of the AL.

Biological
- abnormality or damage to internal organs and systems that can lead to minor instability or life-threatening situations such as shock or haemorrhage
- problems associated with all known diseases affecting body organs and systems that are disrupted or failing
- infection

- trauma (haemorrhage, fractures)
- medical intervention (anaesthesia, surgery, reactions to investigations and treatments, i.e. pharmacological).

Psychological
- anxiety and stress
- disability
- abuse by self or others
- inability to recognise and avoid hazards.

Sociocultural
- trauma and injury associated with taking risks
- diseases associated with beliefs, behaviours or lack of understanding (infectious diseases).

Environmental
- trauma causing minor or major disabilities
- diseases associated with exposure to hazards, such as lung diseases, widespread tumours.

Politicoeconomic
- injuries and diseases associated with lack of ability to protect oneself in the home, in the workplace and in public places.

In addition there will also be a need to determine the extent to which the assessment is affected by physiological changes that are associated with MSE. For example, patients who are severely ill/injured, semiconscious or in a state of shock may be unable to provide information accurately, but this may also indicate that certain body systems are failing.

Using the components of the model of living in a systematic way will help structure the assessment. Regular use

of the components will help to develop an effective assessment style and ensure that patients receive a thorough and professional assessment. The components of the model in relation to conducting an assessment of MSE will now be considered as shown in Box 3.3.

Patient assessment exercise

Using the assessment guide outlined in Box 3.3 consider the information that might be gathered from Case study 3.3. Record the information on the Patient Assessment Sheets provided in Appendix 3. This case scenario will be used as

---

Exercise

Consider what assessment skills you have and the ones you need to develop when undertaking an assessment of MSE in the following areas:

1. Interviewing:
   - asking open and closed questions appropriate to the health status of the patient
   - determining the priority of questions to be asked
   - giving information and checking understanding
   - involving relatives.
2. Observation:
   - verbal and nonverbal responses
   - body language
   - neurological and vital signs
   - stress, pain and anxiety.
3. Listening:
   - acting on verbal and nonverbal cues
   - use of own body language to reassure and encourage the patient.

| Case study 3.3 |

Maintaining a safe environment

Frank is a 47-year-old man who has been admitted to the surgical ward following a diagnosis of a perforated gastric ulcer and is scheduled for emergency surgery. Frank has had a history of epigastric discomfort for some time and has been under the care of his GP, who has prescribed medication to relieve his symptoms. Frank has a hectic lifestyle and is under considerable stress at work. His eating habits are erratic, he smokes about 15 cigarettes a day and he admits to drinking heavily at times. Frank is married with two daughters who are both at university. On admission Frank is quite shocked, in pain and extremely agitated. His wife is upset as she has been trying to encourage Frank to slow down and change his lifestyle.

Box 3.3	MSE assessment guide

Lifespan
- At what stage of the lifespan is the patient?
- Does the patient have an understanding of risks/hazards associated with age and current situation?
- How vulnerable is the patient?
- By comparison with the expected normal lifespan how healthy/unhealthy is the patient?

Dependency/independency
- What constraints are influencing dependency (age, ill health)?
- Is the level of dependency high, average or low (upon other people or aids)?

Factors affecting health
Biological
- Is the patient in good physical health?
- Is there presence of a disability?
- Is there a risk of infection, shock, altered consciousness or haemorrhage?
- Are all senses responding appropriately?

Psychological
- Is the patient stressed or anxious?
- What is the patient's mood or temperament?

- Is the patient confident/motivated?
- Does the patient lack knowledge or understanding?
- What is the patient's experience or attitude to personal safety?

Socioeconomic
- What are the patient's personal beliefs/values regarding health and safety?
- Are there any social difficulties affecting health and safety?
- Is the patient at risk from exposure to any social hazards which may affect safety, health or recovery?

Environmental
- Is the patient able to recognise hazards within their environment (home, work and hospital)?
- Is the patient able to take appropriate action to maintain safety?

Politicoeconomic
- Are there any economic circumstances inhibiting the patient's health/lifestyle?
- Is a lack of resources/facilities compromising health, recovery and safety?
- Is the patient aware of support services that are available?

---

the main study for the chapter. Other short scenarios will be used to help transfer understanding of MSE to other individual patients.

Using the knowledge and experience along with the assessment guide in Box 3.3 identify what Frank's individual MSE needs are as follows.

1. Identify the normal lifespan stage/lifestyle expectations, level of dependency and the factors which have led to the health breakdown.
2. Identify the actual and potential needs/problems associated with the AL of MSE.
3. Identify which other ALs are affected.

Assessment of lifespan, dependency and factors contributing to health breakdown

By using these three components of the model it is possible to determine the individual's normal habits and routines and identify where the patient is vulnerable within the AL. This aspect of assessing MSE focuses upon the following:

- health expectation against stage in the lifespan
- usual routines and habits
- normal dependency capability
- previous coping mechanisms.

Box 3.4 outlines the kind of assessment information you might identify in relation to Case study 3.3.

From this exercise it is possible to determine that as an individual Frank has the following problems that have resulted in him becoming a surgical emergency:

- an acute shock and haemorrhage problem
- a longstanding peptic ulcer problem
- a health education need in relation to his diet, alcohol and smoking
- a health promotion need to adopt a healthier lifestyle.

Identification of actual and potential problems associated with MSE

Having identified the number of problems that are individual to Frank, the next stage is to determine which of the problems are actual and require solving and those which are potential and require prevention. By continuing to use the factors affecting health as a framework it becomes possible to apply knowledge of health to the patient's individual situation and determine the extent to which safety is threatened. Each of the factors will now be explored and Box 3.5 will illustrate how this can be applied to Case study 3.3.

Physical problems

As outlined in the model of living, many activities associated with the AL of MSE are associated with mobility and sensory responses. When problems occur they can result in temporary or permanent changes. The degree to which the activity is altered ultimately has an effect upon complete

Box 3.4	Assessment of lifespan, dependency and factors contributing to health breakdown

Lifespan
- common problem in adult life – exacerbated by adopted lifestyle
- under pressure at work and at home to provide for family needs
- need to identify why Frank has been unable to alter his lifestyle to prevent/reduce health breakdown.

Dependency
- currently in a high-dependency state – dependent upon surgical intervention to prevent life-threatening situation
- normally very independent with responsibilities for work and family.

Factors leading to health breakdown
Physical
- damage to digestive anatomy and function through poor eating habits, alcohol intake and smoking – has been

taking antacid medication to relieve symptoms and visiting GP as required.

Psychological
- stress and anxiety affecting ability to adopt a healthier lifestyle
- has not been able to adjust lifestyle to cope with symptoms.

Sociocultural
- has strong values of being the family provider and need to achieve at work.

Environmental
- nature of work routine has not helped to improve eating and drinking habits – has support from wife to eat sensibly.

Politicoeconomic
- pressure to remain in employment and to fund mortgage and university fees.

Box 3.5	Actual and potential problems identified for Case study 3.3	
Maintaining a safe environment	**Actual problems**	**Potential problems**
Physical	The patient is shocked due to haemorrhage and peritoneal contamination from a perforation of the gastric wall caused by a peptic ulcer	The patient is at risk of loss of consciousness/cardiac arrest due to shock and haemorrhage The patient is at risk from injury due to bed rest, weakness and being in a strange environment
Psychological	The patient is agitated, anxious and in severe pain around the epigastric region	
Sociocultural		The patient may be concerned about his family and work
Environmental	The patient is at risk from accidents, being in an unfamiliar environment	The patient may be concerned about his ability to change his lifestyle
Politicoeconomic		The patient may have concerns about employment and financial commitments

independency and the ability to fully ensure safety. By considering the internal and external environments separately the nurse is able to plan in detail the care that is required to:

- detect and ensure early intervention for life- and safety-threatening situations
- prevent risks and accidents from occurring.

Prevention of life-threatening situations – shock Shock is one of the main causes of death in seriously ill patients and it is important that nurses have both the knowledge and the skills to ensure that appropriate and early intervention takes place. Caring for the patient with symptoms of shock requires an understanding of the pathophysiological processes that are taking place within the body and also the psychosocial effects that this may have upon the patient.

Shock occurs when the body's ability to distribute oxygen and nutrients to body tissues becomes diminished due to the following:

- a reduction of blood volume (hypovolaemic)
- damage to the heart (cardiogenic)
- altered vascular resistance (distributive); this includes septic shock, neurogenic shock, spinal shock and anaphylactic shock.

Clinical signs and symptoms of shock The clinical signs of shock vary depending upon the underlying cause and are generally divided into four stages. Essentially the stages are indicators of the internal physiological mechanisms that are taking place in an attempt to restore homeostasis as described earlier in the model of living. All types of shock are characterised by the following:

- fall in blood pressure
- initial increase in the pulse rate
- pale, cool and clammy skin
- reduction in urinary output
- confusion
- mottling of the skin (particularly the lower extremities).

This is brought about by an early response by the sympathetic nervous system, triggered by a fall in blood pressure. Tissue hypoxia causes the heart rate to increase and a generalised vasoconstriction in an attempt to direct blood from less vital organs to the heart and the brain.

Stages of shock

1. *Initial stage:* Initially there are no visible changes, but internally the cellular environment is responding and producing a metabolic acidosis.
2. *Compensatory stage:* At this stage the body is trying to correct the physiological disturbance.
3. *Progressive stage:* The body enters this stage when the compensatory mechanisms begin to fail and start to produce adverse effects.
4. *Refractory (irreversible) stage:* Damage to body tissues and organs cannot be stopped or reversed and death is imminent.

It is important to understand that the stages of shock are complex and it is not always possible to detect transition from one stage to another. It is recommended that you read further to increase your understanding around the distinguishing features of the different types of shock (see Alexander et al 2006, ch. 18).

Haemorrhage A haemorrhage may be external and observable or internal and hidden. Where bleeding is external it may be arterial, venous or capillary. Arterial blood will be oxygenated and bright red, spurting rhythmically and blood loss can be considerable. Venous blood is bluish in colour and flows more evenly from the injured vessel, whilst capillary blood is reddish and tends to ooze from the area. When a vessel is injured the body initiates a response to reduce the bleeding (see Kindlen 2003, ch. 3). When bleeding is external, first-aid treatment will be to apply pressure directly over the injured site. Where major vessels are involved surgical intervention will ultimately be required to repair the vessel. Where considerable blood loss takes place the patient will display signs of hypovolaemic shock.

Altered consciousness and mobility Through the onset of illness, injury or medical/surgical/pharmacological intervention, consciousness and mobility can become altered. Even minor problems can create an increased level of individual dependency, which can result in an inability to maintain a safe environment either temporarily or permanently. These will be further discussed in Chapters 10 and 13, but because of the interrelatedness of the issues with MSE they are briefly outlined in this chapter. Unconsciousness presents a major threat to the patient's ability to maintain a safe environment. It is essential that the nurse is able to distinguish the difference between sleep and unconscious states which are indicative of altered physiology that can be potentially life-threatening.

Sensory impairment The model of living highlighted the importance that the five senses play in maintaining safety within the body's internal and external environment. Loss or impairment can be either temporary or permanent and will create a degree of dependency that requires adjustment. Loss of vision and hearing can be caused by ageing, disease or injury, which may not only affect the ability to communicate effectively but also increase the risk of accidents occurring. Loss of sensation means that individuals cannot feel pain, heat, cold or pressure. Paralysis is a term which describes a loss of sensation that is accompanied with a loss of movement and can cover large areas of the body as shown in Figure 3.13.

Different types of paralysis can make it difficult for patients to avoid hazards and ensure their own safety without the use of a range of living aids and resources to support normal activity. Loss of smell and taste can be commonly experienced by individuals of all ages, caused by temporary minor ailments such as upper respiratory tract infections or through disease or ageing processes. Localised injury, medical treatment, medication and generalised disorders can also affect normal sensory function, putting patients at risk from a range of accidents such as burns and scalds, ingestion of poisons or an inability to smell fire or other noxious substances.

Risk of infection The risk of infection during illness is potentially greater due to a lowered resistance to infection and an increased exposure to a large number of microorganisms. When patients are admitted to hospital the risk of exposure to an even greater number of microorganisms is further increased. It is vital that the spread of infection is rigorously controlled in order to prevent the patient from developing a health-care-associated infection (HCAI) An HACI is defined as an infection that has been acquired whilst receiving hospital care and results in considerable costs for both patients and health care providers. For patients an infection becomes an added complication resulting in anxiety, discomfort, disability, delayed recovery and personal economic costs. Even worse, it is reported that at least 5000 patients die every year. It has been estimated that the national costs of infection rates are £1 billion resulting from increased length of stay in hospital and additional investigations, medications and provision of continuing care services (National Audit Office 2004).

Psychological problems

When patients become unwell their mental health and intellect may become impaired due to infection, disease, injury or stress and anxiety. The effects of ill health may prevent

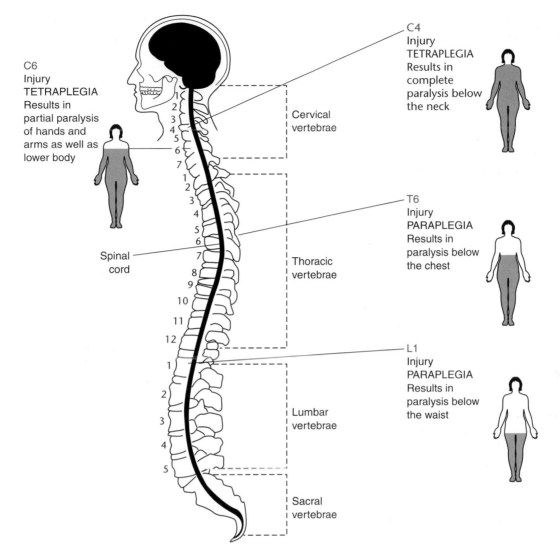

Fig. 3.13 Motor and sensory loss in paralysis (from Walsh 2002, with permission).

the individual from being able to reason or make appropriate decisions regarding personal safety and it may be difficult to identify their normal individual state of dependency. It is important to recognise that patients who already have limitations, which are a part of their individuality, such as patients with learning difficulties or mental health illness, have these taken into consideration in order to ensure that their safety is maximised (Thompson 2001, Norman & Ryrie 2004).

Sociocultural problems

Safety issues related to sociocultural needs are generally central to three areas of concern:

- the degree to which sociocultural issues may have contributed towards ill health
- the degree to which normal habits and routines may be disturbed by illness or injury
- the degree to which safety can be influenced due to individual beliefs and values.

Having established the issues that may have contributed to the health breakdown, it is also important to determine how the patient might be supported in the recovery phase. Assessment in this area may also give an indication of how the patient might manage their own personal safety during their stay in hospital and identify any specific individual needs that they may have in relation to personal beliefs and values. For example, it may be important for the patient to carry out specific religious practices which if restricted may cause them anxiety (Holland & Hogg 2001, Henley & Schott 1999).

Environmental problems

It is important that all health care professionals recognise the hazards that exist in the health care environment. It is known that throughout the world, even in developed countries, patients are dying needlessly or suffering from avoidable exposure to infections, accidents and medical errors. As such there is worldwide attention to improve the quality and the safety of health care in order to ensure that patients have confidence in health care services (Institute of Medicine 1999, Rohn et al 2000, WHO 2006b). It is the responsibility of all health care professionals to recognise and respond appropriately to hazards, and continuously seek to improve the quality and safety of care by keeping up to date and sharing best practice.

> **Exercise**
> 1. Browse the Institute of Healthcare Improvement (IHI) website (www.IHI.org) and find out about the Saving Lives campaigns. This site also contains several white paper publications to help nurses understand how they can contribute towards saving lives by transforming care at the bedside.

Unfamiliar environment When patients are admitted to hospital they are often anxious and frightened, indeed it may be the first time they have been an inpatient. They may not be familiar with the routine, equipment or the environment and this has the potential to lead to accidents. The age and dependency of the patient must be taken into consideration in order to provide the patient with the correct information, orientation, equipment, support or supervision.

Risk of accidents in hospital For the patient the care environment is unfamiliar and there are many potential hazards associated with the following:

- reduced mobility through age, illness, medication or medical intervention
- altered mental/conscious state
- impaired vision, hearing and speech
- lack of awareness or understanding of the need for safety precautions.

The hazards within the care environment can result in a number of accidents, most commonly:

- slips, trips and falls
- drug administration errors
- medical negligence.

In the UK, NHS organisations are required to have risk management policies and procedures in place to assess, prevent and manage risks on behalf of patients, visitors and staff within the scope of legal requirements and best clinical practice. Because of the rising costs of clinical claims the NHS established the NHS Litigation Authority (NHSLA). The authority governs a series of clinical and non-clinical risk management standards, against which NHS organisations are regularly assessed, measuring how well an organisation prevents, monitors and reports actual and potential (near miss) incidents.

Noisy environment Hospitals are known to be busy and noisy environments. Noises originate from people within the environment such as staff, other patients and visitors talking, shouting out and moving around. Equipment such as telephones, trolleys, sinks, toilets, oxygen administration, ventilators, alarms and monitors create additional noises. Noise not only inhibits the patient's ability to rest and sleep, but may also increase the risk of accidents occurring due to tiredness, distraction or an inability to hear surrounding dangers. Particular attention should be paid to patients who have reduced sensory function or who are sedated, in pain, anxious or depressed. It is important that nurses recognise the impact that a noisy and unfamiliar environment may have upon patients both during the day and at night and seek to minimise this where possible (Topf 2000) (see also Chapter 13).

Medication risks Under normal circumstances individuals and their families take personal responsibility for correctly administering their own medication. Upon admission to hospital, patients become dependent upon medical, nursing and pharmacy staff to prescribe and administer medication, except in places where self-medication schemes are in operation. Because of the potential dangers associated with medication, administration is strictly governed by legislation and nurses are required to adhere to a number of laws, guidelines and policies such as (NMC 2002):

- The Medicines Act 1968 and Misuse of Drugs Act 1971
- Medicinal Products Prescription by Nurses, Midwives and Health Visitors Act 1992
- professional standards
- local organisational policies.

Risk of fire Hospitals are large buildings that have the potential for fire to break out. This is a serious matter since many patients may not be able to escape without help and some would also require continuing medical attention during the process. Some patients may express concern about their safety during their stay in hospital and will require reassurance in the form of being shown what to do in case of a fire. The Health and Safety at Work Act 1974 places the responsibility for organisations and their staff to take personal responsibility for observing and adhering to safety policy and keep continually up to date on how to raise the alarm and begin evacuation procedure. In the NHS the Department of Health issues additional fire safety guidelines known as the *Firecode* (Department for Communities and Local Government 2006).

Anaesthesia An anaesthetic is used to block any sensations of pain caused by a medical or surgical intervention. It can be applied locally or regionally to a specific area of the body or generally. A general anaesthetic not only reduces pain but also induces unconsciousness as muscles become relaxed and normal reflexes are lost. During this time the patient will be unable to maintain an airway and is dependent upon medical intervention to prevent risks occurring. Patient safety in the operating theatre is aimed at minimising the risks of infection, haemorrhage, allergic reactions, limb and posture damage, burns and retention of foreign bodies from the surgical procedure. It is vitally important to ensure that patients are correctly prepared for surgical procedures in order to minimise the risks from anaesthesia.

Politicoeconomic problems

Potential and actual problems related to MSE are often associated with the ability to afford the necessary resources to maintain health and prevent accidents, whether this is at a personal, local community or national level. Without support, a lack of personal finance may reduce a person's ability to maintain health, or protect themselves from injury, for example the need to purchase medicines, special diets or home safety equipment. When advising patients about safety it is important to sensitively determine whether the advice is realistically affordable, and where necessary support the patient's needs by making appropriate referrals to other agencies who may be able to arrange access to benefits and resources.

By using the factors affecting health as a framework, it has been possible to identify a range of actual and potential problems associated with MSE. Box 3.5 describes how the framework can help identify the problems related to Case study 3.3.

Identification of the impact on other ALs

In reality rarely would one AL be affected in isolation. Whilst this chapter concentrates upon MSE it is important to consider the impact that an altered dependency in MSE might have upon the other ALs, particularly in relation to the internal environment. Box 3.6 demonstrates how the problems identified from Case study 3.3 may impact upon the remaining ALs.

Box 3.6	Impact of the MSE problem on other ALs	
Activity of living	**Actual problems**	**Potential problems**
Communicating	• Has epigastric pain and is restless and anxious due to perforation • Has difficulty communicating due to oxygen therapy, nasogastric tube • Will be anxious about current health state and require information and reassurance	• May develop dry mouth and lips which may affect ability to communicate
Breathing	• Has difficulty breathing due to pain	• Respirations may deteriorate due to increased level of shock
Eating and drinking	Unable to eat or drink due to: • Nil-by-mouth requirement in preparation for surgery • Is nauseous and is vomiting • Has unpleasant taste in the mouth	• At risk of haemorrhage and haematemesis
Eliminating	• Unable to pass urine normally due to bed rest and urinary catheter	• At risk of diminished urinary output due to shock • May develop malaena due to gastrointestinal bleeding
Personal cleansing and dressing	• Has difficulty maintaining own hygiene needs due to current physical state	• At risk from developing pressure sores
Mobilising	• Unable to mobilise normally due to current physical state, pain, weakness and medical intervention	
Sleep and rest	• Experiencing difficulty due to pain and anxiety	
Work and play	• Unable to engage in normal activities due to current health state	
Expressing sexuality		• May be anxious about body image and self-esteem
Maintaining body temperature		• May develop an infection
Dying		• At risk of collapse due to shock and haemorrhage

Exercise

Using the information presented so far in this chapter consider how different your assessment and identification of MSE might be in relation to the following scenarios.

1. A 72-year-old lady with diabetes and failing eyesight who lives alone has fallen at home and sustained a severe pretibial tear.
2. A 20-year-old man who has epilepsy has not been taking his medication regularly; he is admitted in a semiconscious state following a series of grand mal seizures over the last 3 hours.
3. A 36-year-old lady has developed MRSA following a routine surgical operation.

Check your answers with the information in Boxes 3.7, 3.8 and 3.9.

PLANNING NURSING ACTIVITIES

Planning nursing activities involves the following:

- identifying the priorities
- establishing short- and/or long-term goals
- determining the nursing actions/interventions required
- documenting the nursing care plan.

Planning nursing care accurately and effectively begins with exploring the actual and potential problems that have been identified and determining the nursing interventions that are required to achieve the following:

Box 3.7	72-year-old lady with diabetes

Physical
- How long has she suffered from diabetes?
- How is the diabetes managed?
- When did the fall occur?
- How long has eyesight been poor?

Psychological
- What is the patient's mood?
- Does the patient seem alert?
- What are the patient's concerns regarding the injury?

Sociological
- What personal support is available?

Environmental
- Awareness of safety in the home?
- Availability of support/resources to promote safety?

Politicoeconomic
- Is there a lack of resources which have contributed to the problem?
- What might be preventing the patient from taking care of herself?

Box 3.8	20-year-old man with epilepsy

Additional information may need to be obtained from whoever is in attendance with the patient, for example: family, friends, neighbour, work colleague or passerby.

Physical
- How long has he suffered from epilepsy?
- When did the seizures start?
- Has the patient experienced grand mal seizures before?
- Has the patient sustained any other injuries?
- What are the patient's neurological observations indicating?

Psychological
- How has the patient been behaving?
- What has the patient's mood been like?
- Has the patient been suffering from stress or anxiety?
- How compliant normally is the patient in taking his medication?

Sociological
- What support does the patient have at home?
- How does the patient normally cope with having epilepsy in everyday living (at home or at work)?
- Does having epilepsy restrict life and normal activities?

Environmental
- What are the risks for the patient at work?
- What are the risks of further injury by admission to hospital?

Politicoeconomic
- Does the patient require any resources to carry out normal living activities?
- Does the patient's health problem affect economic independency?

Box 3.9	36-year-old lady with MRSA

Physical
- What observable symptoms are to be recorded?
- What potential problems is the patient at risk from?

Psychological
- How is the problem affecting mood and personality?
- How is the patient coping with the situation?
- Is the patient irritable or anxious?

Sociological
- What restrictions/effects will isolation have upon lifestyle, individuality and independency?

Environmental
- Is the patient aware of the safety precautions required?
- Does the patient understand the reason for isolation?

Politicoeconomic
- What economic difficulties might arise from prolonged hospitalisation?

- to solve actual problems
- to prevent potential problems occurring
- to prevent solved problems from re-occurring
- to develop positive coping strategies for any problem which cannot be solved.

Throughout the planning phase it is important that the nurse remains focused upon the patient's problems and what is appropriate to the patient's recovery in the immediate, short and long term.

Factors influencing the planning stage

It is important to recognise that certain factors may exist to influence the planning stage. In relation to MSE these may be as shown in Box 3.10. Check the information contained within Box 3.10 to determine what your own personal development needs might be.

Identification of priorities

Having undertaken a comprehensive individualised assessment the next stage is to plan the nursing care. This begins with the following:

- making a judgement about the priority order of the actual and potential problems.
- identifying the impact that the health problem is having on all of the ALs.

By using the dependency/independency component of the model it is possible to develop criteria which describe the degree of altered dependency that the patient is experiencing, particularly where this is causing a life-threatening

Box 3.10	Factors influencing planning nursing care for the AL of MSE
Nurses	**Patients/clients**
• Knowledge of normal physiology and specific pathophysiological processes • Knowledge of normal living and dependency across the lifespan in various cultures • Knowledge and skill in required evidence base for nursing interventions • Skill in observation and assessment • Skill in determining priorities • Staffing levels, skill mix, supervision and ongoing professional development	• Understanding of the need for safety • Personal beliefs, values and experiences • Ability to communicate needs and describe symptoms and feelings • Anxiety, pain and concern about coping mechanisms

situation. In clinical practice it is possible to use the criteria to score or measure individual patient or ward levels of dependency (see Box 3.11).

It is important to recognise that dependency/independency can change very rapidly and this requires continuous assessment.

The priorities identified amongst the other ALs are described in Table 3.3.

Exercise

1. In relation to Case study 3.3 review the actual and potential problems identified and determine the priority against them (see Table 3.2).

From this exercise it can be identified that Frank's problems are not only serious, but are complex and initially much of the care he will require is central to the following:

- continuous observation of actual problems to detect for signs of his condition worsening prior to surgery
- supporting medical intervention to stabilise and improve his condition in preparation for surgery
- preventing potential problems from occurring.

This exercise demonstrates that by using the model it is possible to identify a number of problems and the effect these are having upon Frank as an individual. Planning care in this way also highlights that, in some instances, preventing potential problems from occurring may take priority over actual problems, depending upon the threat that is posed to life. Tables 3.2 and 3.3 demonstrate how the main problem of shock is actually presenting, not only in relation to MSE but also by the impact this is having on all other ALs. The rationale for identifying problems using the model is to increase the understanding of the individuality in

Box 3.11	Dependency/independency priority criteria
Priority 1	Completely independent in the AL/independence maintained
Priority 2	Potential problem in the AL/remains mostly independent
Priority 3	Actual problems identified within more than one AL/some independency noted but remains mostly independent
Priority 4	Existence of actual and potential problems/ a number of other ALs with associated increasing dependence
Priority 5	Life-threatening actual and potential problems/ total dependence

Table 3.2 Prioritising MSE actual and potential problems related to Case study 3.3

Maintaining a safe environment	Actual problems	Priority	Potential problems	Priority
Physical	The patient is shocked due to haemorrhage and peritoneal contamination from a perforation of the gastric wall caused by a peptic ulcer	5	The patient is at risk of loss of consciousness/cardiac arrest due to shock and haemorrhage	5
			The patient is at risk from injury due to bed rest, weakness and being in a strange environment	4
Psychological	The patient is agitated, anxious and in severe pain around the epigastric region	4		
Sociocultural			The patient may be concerned about his family and work	3
Environmental			The patient may be concerned about his ability to change his lifestyle	2
Politicoeconomic			The patient may have concerns about employment and financial commitments	2

illness. By alleviating and supporting the main problem(s) it is also possible to observe the effect this has on other ALs. Coupled with a comprehensive assessment, focused upon the individual lifestyle, normal habits and routines of the patient, the setting of realistic short- and long-term goals becomes enhanced.

Goal setting

Goal setting in relation to MSE can be immediate term (hourly), short term (less than 1 week) or long term (for a longer period). When setting goals, the seriousness of the problem and its identified priority must be taken into consideration. The goal statement is important, as it describes what the patient is expected to, or has agreed to, achieve (see Chapter 1). The more realistic, measurable and observable the goal the easier it becomes to monitor and evaluate the progress the patient is making. Table 3.4 gives an example of the short- and long-term goals that might be set for Frank. It is important to recognise that whenever possible, patients should be involved in the goal-setting process, as it provides an opportunity to promote independence, motivation and a greater understanding of personal health, safety and recovery (refer to Chapter 1 for further details on goal setting). Essentially the short- and long-term goals for Frank will be central to the following:

1. alleviate his immediate life-threatening problems
2. support his recovery from surgery
3. help him to adopt an altered lifestyle.

Table 3.4 shows the short- and long-term goals that could be set for Frank during his hospital stay in relation to MSE.

Once the short- and long-term goals have been set the appropriate nursing actions can be planned to enable the goals to be achieved.

IMPLEMENTING CARE TO MEET MAINTAINING A SAFE ENVIRONMENT NEEDS AND PROBLEMS

This section of the chapter will show how, by using the factors affecting health components of the model, nursing actions associated with MSE can be broadly outlined in order to guide professional nursing practice. It is essential that the nurse constantly updates knowledge and skills in the areas outlined in order to ensure that patients receive quality care.

Nursing interventions related to physical factors affecting ill health

The object of nursing actions related to physical factors affecting health are in relation to promoting and maintaining health and preventing disease irrespective of the health care setting. Nursing actions must be based upon full understanding of biological systems across the lifespan as described in the model of living and linked closely to sound knowledge and understanding of anatomical and physiological systems. It is also increasingly essential for nurses to communicate and work closely with fellow medical and non-medical health care professionals who make up the multidisciplinary team, such as therapists, scientists, technicians and specialists who work in acute and primary health and social care settings.

Health education

Health education plays an important role in maintaining health and preventing disease (Ewles & Simnett 2003). In order to ensure social and economic wellbeing, nurses should seize every opportunity to promote health where it is deemed appropriate to the individual needs of the patient. Health promotion should be aimed at:

- preventing diseases and reducing mortality rates
- reducing the risks associated with disease (i.e. diet, smoking and exercise)
- improving healthy lifestyles.

Table 3.3 To show identification of priorities in all other ALs

Activity of living	Actual problem	Priority	Potential problems	Priority
Communicating	Has epigastric pain and is restless and anxious due to perforation	4	May develop dry mouth and lips which may affect ability to communicate	3
	Has difficulty communicating due to oxygen therapy, nasogastric tube	4		
	Will be anxious about current health state and require information and reassurance	3		
Breathing	Has difficulty breathing due to pain	3	Respirations may deteriorate due to increased level of shock	3
Eating and drinking	Unable to eat or drink due to: • Nil-by-mouth requirement in preparation for surgery • Is nauseous and is vomiting Experiencing: • Has unpleasant taste in the mouth	4	At risk of haemorrhage and haematemesis	3
Eliminating	Unable to pass urine normally due to bed rest and urinary catheter	4	At risk of diminished urinary output due to shock	3
			May develop malaena due to gastrointestinal bleeding	3
Personal cleansing and dressing	Has difficulty maintaining own hygiene needs due to current physical state	3	At risk from developing pressure sores	2
Mobilising	Unable to mobilise normally due to current physical state, pain weakness and medical intervention	3	At risk from developing pressure sores, deep vein thrombosis	3
Sleep and rest	Experiencing difficulty due to pain and anxiety	3		
Work and play	Unable to engage in normal activities due to current health state	3		
Expressing sexuality			May be anxious about body image and self-esteem	3
Maintaining body temperature	Has difficulty in maintaining body temperature due to shock and haemorrhage	3	May develop an infection	3
Dying			At risk of collapse due to shock and haemorrhage	4

Table 3.4 Short- and long-term MSE goals set for Frank

Problem	Short-term	Long-term
The patient is shocked due to haemorrhage and peritoneal contamination from a perforated gastric ulcer	The patient's physical condition will be stabilised prior to surgery	The patient will recover from surgery without complications

Observation of vital signs

As outlined in the model of living the human body is highly complex. For the purpose of understanding how the body functions, body systems are studied separately, and in the model the systems are aligned to specific ALs. In reality, however, body systems are very closely interrelated, hence the appreciation of why, during ill health, rarely is an AL altered on its own. The object of enabling the patient to maintain a safe internal environment depends upon being able to make accurate essential observations of the cardiovascular and neurological systems, as described within the model of living. In the model described by Roper et al (1996), vital signs are discussed under the AL of breathing (see Chapter 5); however, it is important to acknowledge the importance of observation of vital signs as related to the AL of MSE. These include the measurement of vital signs that are related to the cardiovascular and central nervous systems as follows:

- blood pressure
- pulse rate
- circulation
- sensory and motor responses (neurological observations).

Vital signs also include observation of respirations and body temperature and these will be discussed in Chapters 5 and 9. The process of diagnosing pathophysiological disorders will also involve many other specialised observations/investigations that will be specific to the preliminary diagnosis (e.g. blood tests, electronic and radiological investigations). When working in clinical practice it is important that nurses develop their understanding of specialised investigations and ensure patients' needs are fully supported and that practice is safe. When carrying out observations of vital signs, it is important that measurement is both consistent and accurate (Wheatley 2006). Since the patient's medical treatment and ultimate safety often relies upon vital-sign information, the competency and accuracy of observation, recording and reporting cannot be stressed enough. In the UK, a method of detecting early changes in a patient's vital signs is known as the Early Warning Score (EWS), which has been widely implemented in order to ensure that patients do not unnecessarily deteriorate, especially when being nursed in general medical and surgical wards (Goldhill et al 1999). The scoring system includes the continuous assessment, scoring and reporting of a collection of baseline physiological measurements that deviate from normal values such as:

- respiratory rate
- systolic blood pressure
- heart rate
- temperature
- conscious level
- oxygen saturation
- urine output.

In clinical practice it is important you are competent in the use of a variety of devices and ensure that observations are *always* accurately made and promptly recorded and reported.

Blood pressure

Accurate recordings of the blood pressure and pulse provide information about changes in the patient's physiological state in relation to:

- diagnosis of the disease
- assessment of normal cardiovascular function
- assessment of cardiovascular recovery following disease, surgery or trauma.

The importance of making an accurate recording is essential in order to determine if homeostasis is being restored. Generally, alterations in systolic blood pressure indicate problems with cardiac output, whilst diastolic recordings enable venous return and cardiac inflow to be assessed. Individual patients can have very different blood pressure readings, therefore it is important to establish as early as possible each patient's normal reading. To ensure patient safety all staff should adhere to local policies and guidelines, which govern accurate recording (see Dougherty & Lister 2004 for practice guidelines).

Pulse rate

The purpose of assessing the pulse rate is to determine heart rate, rhythm and strength. The pulse rate is most commonly assessed at the radial site but there are many other sites as shown in Figure 3.14.

The pulse can be measured either by palpation or by simultaneous sound and palpation, as used when measuring

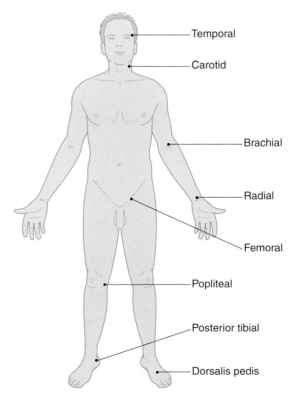

Fig. 3.14 Major pulse points (from Jamieson et al 2002, with permission).

Labels: Temporal, Carotid, Brachial, Radial, Femoral, Popliteal, Posterior tibial, Dorsalis pedis

the apical–radial pulse. This requires two nurses to observe for deficits in the heart rate. It is important that the rate is measured for a full 60 seconds in order to:

- determine normal baseline range for lifespan
- estimate altered range caused by disease, medication, medical intervention
- correlate information with other observations, i.e. pulse and temperature.

Circulation Circulation can be observed visually or through palpation in several ways:

- *Capillary refill:* By applying pressure to the nail bed the skin becomes white (blanched). When the pressure is released quickly the skin should return to being pink within 3 seconds.
- *Temperature:* By touching the skin it is possible to detect areas of warmth and coolness.
- *Colour:* General observation of the patient's skin can indicate cyanosis, pigmentation, redness, pallor, jaundice or signs of bleeding such as bruising, petechiae or haematoma.
- *Moisture:* The skin can display signs of dryness and turgor caused by dehydration or sweating due to shock and anxiety.
- *Oedema:* Assessment of swollen areas around the feet, ankles, lower arms and sacrum can indicate circulatory dysfunction.

Neurological observations Assessment of the patient's conscious level is necessary in order to support the maintenance of a safe environment, particularly where there is increasing dependency caused by various states of ill health. Neurological observations are carried out in conjunction with blood pressure, pulse and respiratory rate measurement, enabling changes in the patient's condition to be detected and acted upon. In the UK the Glasgow Coma Scale observation chart (Fig. 3.15) is used to record the full range of vital and neurological signs, incorporating three aspects of consciousness:

- visual responses
- verbal responses
- motor/sensory responses.

Preoperative nursing care

The aim of preoperative nursing care is to maximise the safety of the patient's internal and external environment in the days or hours prior to surgery. Surgical operations are classified as being either elective (planned) or emergency. An emergency operation is carried out without delay in the interest of the patient's immediate survival. In either case, the aim is to ensure that the patient is as physically fit as possible, by conducting a thorough assessment of the patient through a range of medical and nursing observations and laboratory tests and investigations.

In preparing patients for surgery irrespective of the complexity of the surgery, a number of core procedures must be carried out in order to prevent potential risks/complications from occurring. The preoperative phase begins as soon as the decision for surgery has been identified and care is central to the patient being in the best possible health from a holistic perspective. The nurse must be constantly alert to any physiological changes that might occur in the preoperative phase for both emergency and elective patients, and report them promptly. Boxes 3.12 and 3.13 provide an overview of preoperative preparation, which whilst being essentially related to the AL of MSE, highlights once again the interrelatedness to other ALs. Table 3.5 shows how this would relate to the care of Frank (Case study 3.3).

In order to ensure the safety of the patient immediately prior to going to theatre the checks listed in Box 3.13 would need to be undertaken.

Intraoperative care

Operating theatres are specifically constructed and operated to maximise patient safety at every stage of the patient's journey from reception through to the recovery room. Every aspect of care in the intraoperative phase is focused upon maintaining the safety of the patient from collapse, infection, complications and injury. Strict asepsis is maintained and precautions are taken to minimise the transmission of microorganisms from the air, equipment and personnel. Upon arrival at the operating theatre the following details are double-checked by the ward and theatre nurse in order to ensure safety:

- conscious level
- identification band, patient's notes and theatre list details
- operation consent form
- paired limb or organ site clearly marked and identified
- special problems highlighted, e.g. allergic reactions
- laboratory/investigation reports handed over
- preoperative medication amounts and effects
- vital sign status.

Throughout the time spent by the patient within the operating theatre from the induction of anaesthesia to recovery, the focus of nursing care is to maintain the patient's vital functions. The patient will only return to the ward when the vital functions are sufficiently recovered and the patient is no longer dependent upon life-supporting machinery (Iggulden 2006).

Postoperative nursing care

All surgical interventions have a common series of problems that the patient may experience such as pain, tissue trauma, infection, shock and haemorrhage. As in the preoperative phase, MSE nursing actions focus upon supporting the vital body functions and minimising risks, to ensure that the patient makes a timely and uneventful recovery. Dependent upon the type and nature of the surgery there will be some general and specific physiological disturbances. Care of the patient must be central to the particular type of surgery and the ongoing individual needs of the patient.

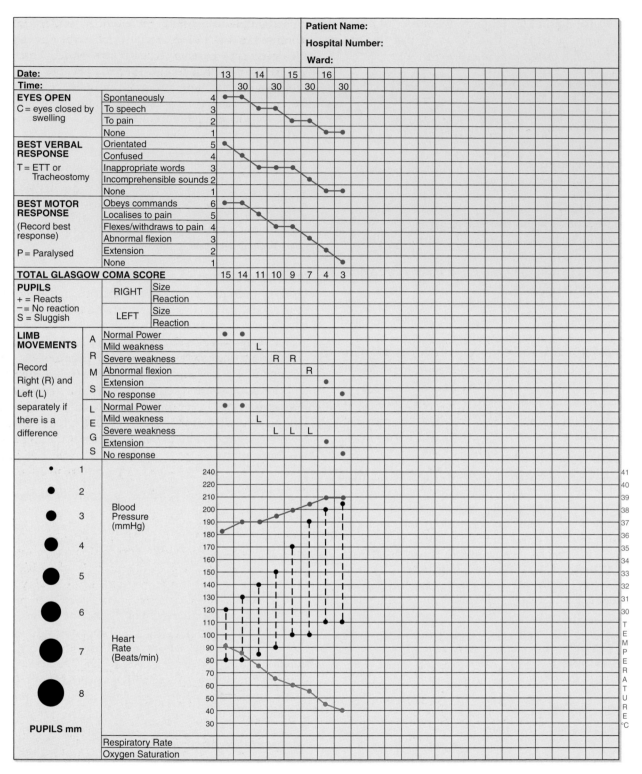

Fig. 3.15 Glasgow Coma Scale chart (from Alexander et al 2006, with permission).

From the moment that the patient returns from the operating theatre nursing actions are central to constantly monitoring the patient's recovery in terms of:

- monitoring vital physiological signs
- recording, interpreting and reporting any significant changes

- supporting patient comfort and pain
- providing information and encouragement to support recovery.

Table 3.6 illustrates the nursing interventions associated with the physical aspects of MSE care for Frank (Case study 3.3).

Box 3.12	Overview of physical preoperative patient preparation

1. Patient history
- Information regarding lifestyle, normal health state and normal habits and routines specific to the individual that may be significant to surgery or recovery (i.e. history of previous illness and surgery)
- Drug history (prescribed and nonprescribed)
- Allergic reactions.

2. Physical assessment
- Cardiac, respiratory and renal functions
- Blood volume and composition
- Nutritional, fluid and electrolyte status
- Electrocardiogram, X-rays and laboratory tests
- Routine observations of temperature, blood pressure, pulse, respirations, conscious levels and circulation
- Urinalysis
- Other observations such as menstruation, diarrhoea, nausea, vomiting, dehydration, sore throat, bleeding gums or dental caries, discharges and wounds.

3. Health promotion
- Encourage patients who smoke to stop or reduce smoking to prevent complications
- Discuss pre- and postoperative safety requirements and rationale in relation to other ALs such as skin preparation, leg and chest, exercises, fasting, bowel and bladder preparation, premedication, bed rest, sleep, pain and identification checks.

For example, pain may be described under the AL of communicating and wound care under the AL of personal cleansing and dressing. It is not the model's intention to be prescriptive, but to ensure that aspects of care are not overlooked. Through good clinical leadership, teams can agree how best to standardise key aspects of care to the most appropriate AL.

> **Exercise**
> 1. In relation to Case study 3.3 consider what the postoperative care would be required in all other ALs.

Day surgery

Day surgery involves admission, pre- and postoperative surgery and discharge in the same day and is being increasingly used for a variety of general and specialist surgical interventions, mainly due to advances in techniques and technology. As such, day surgery is now regarded as a specialism and hospitals have targets to increase day surgery access (Morris & Ward 2006). Success lies in transferring good practice from traditional pre- and postoperative care with a range of specific knowledge and skills in order to ensure the safety of the patient. Whilst not all patients will be suitable for day surgery, there are many benefits for both patients and health care providers in terms of reducing waiting times, length of hospital stay, exposure to infection and of course health care costs.

Impact of surgery on other ALs

All of the operative phases identified will have some kind of impact upon other ALs, depending upon the age, general fitness of the patient and type of surgery that is performed. This may lead to the identification of 'problems' that may be more suitably aligned to another AL.

Administration of medicines

Administering medicines is an important role of the nurse and the practice is strictly governed by legislation, professional guidelines and local policy. In the UK, nursing practice is guided by the Nursing and Midwifery Council (NMC 2007), whereupon individual nurses are personally

Box 3.13	Example of preoperative checklist

- Pre- and postoperative procedures explained
- Check consent form has been signed
- Check preanaesthetic assessment has been undertaken
- Check operation site is correctly marked
- Record temperature, pulse, respirations and blood pressure (T, P, R & BP)
- Record urinalysis
- Administer bowel preparation
- Check if patient needs to micturate prior to premedication
- Administer preoperative medication
- Skin preparation
- Remove make-up and restrictive clothing
- Note dentures/crowns, etc
- Note prosthesis, i.e. contact lenses, hearing aids, false limbs

- Ensure dentures and prosthesis are removed
- Tape/remove jewellery
- Ensure valuables are securely stored
- Check identification band
- Check when patient last had food or drink
- Ensure all investigation reports are present (i.e. blood and X-ray reports)
- Promote rest.

Immediately prior to theatre
- Continue to reassure and support the patient
- Empty bladder prior to theatre
- Check identification band and case notes
- Escort patient to theatre
- Hand over patient correctly to theatre staff.

Table 3.5 Preoperative nursing interventions for Frank (Case study 3.3)

Problem	Goal	Nursing intervention
Frank is to undergo abdominal surgery to repair a perforated gastric ulcer	Ensure Frank is physically fit for surgery to minimise the risk of complications	• Record baseline observation of vital signs (T, P, R & BP and conscious level) • Record urinalysis • Record results of blood tests, crossmatching • Record results of cardiovascular investigations • Record results of radiological investigations • Ensure Frank is fasted • Assess patient's allergic responses • Complete preoperative checklist
Frank is at risk from developing pre- and postoperative complications such as: • Shock • Haemorrhage • Chest infection • Thrombosis • Dehydration		

Table 3.6 Postoperative nursing interventions associated with the physical aspects of MSE

Problem	Goal	Nursing intervention
Frank has undergone surgery for the repair of a perforated gastric ulcer and is at risk from: • Shock • Primary haemorrhage • Blood loss from the wound • Respiratory problems • Wound infection • Postoperative complications (chest infection, thrombosis, renal failure)	To return Frank to a normal conscious and physiological state and prevent the onset of postoperative complications	Monitor vital signs ½ hourly until stable Monitor vital signs 2–4 hourly for 12–14 hours when stable Monitor conscious level Observe skin for signs of shock and circulatory problems Observe fluid intake and output for reduced output until normal intake resumes Provide oxygen as prescribed Position patient carefully to promote recovery to prevent injury and complications Record and report any significant changes Observe wound site for bleeding, drainage or swelling Maintain strict asepsis to prevent wound infection Encourage deep breathing and leg exercises to prevent postoperative complications

accountable for their practice and responsible for keeping themselves up to date. Where mistakes are made there is a requirement for the employing organisation to investigate the incident and determine the cause of the error and if necessary refer the person to the NMC for professional disciplinary action. It is imperative that nursing care is focused upon the following:

• knowledge of the patient's condition and treatment regime
• knowledge of the patient's compliance and understanding
• knowledge of the medication action and potential side-effects
• knowledge of legal, professional and local policy for checking and administration
• knowledge and skill in correct storage and preparation
• knowledge and skill in using the correct route of administration
• knowledge of correct procedure for recording administration

• knowledge of prescribing principles
• knowledge of the management and reporting of errors and incidents.

In the UK through the introduction of The Medicinal Products Prescription by Nurses, Midwives and Health Visitors Act 1992 it is possible for some nurses to prescribe a limited number of drugs. The practice is strictly underpinned by an educational programme and employer approval (DoH 2006h). Despite rigorous training, unfortunately mistakes are made which cause serious side-effects and even death, therefore it is imperative that correct dosages are given, by the correct route and regular observations are made to detect side-effects.

Nursing interventions related to psychological factors affecting ill health

The model of living highlighted the importance of nursing care being available to support the intellectual and emotional needs of the patients in relation to their individual needs. Very often this requires additional specialist health care professionals to be involved, for example specialist nurses, doctors, mental health professionals, therapists and social workers. As a basic survival instinct the human body is naturally equipped to cope with a certain degree of stress, but the extent to which individuals are able to cope varies immensely.

In relation to surgery, it is important to be able to determine the patient's level of understanding of pre- and postoperative procedures and identify any anxieties that are present. This helps the nurse to support the individual needs of the patient, to provide accurate information, relieve anxiety and ensure sufficient rest before surgery. Table 3.7 illustrates the nursing care that Frank would require to meet his psychological needs.

Nursing interventions related to sociocultural factors affecting ill health

Nursing actions in relation to sociocultural factors are central to integrating the patient's individual beliefs and values into the planned nursing care and providing support for any health inequalities that may have been identified. There is, however, a degree of complexity involved because of the vast differences that can exist between individuals. It is important that this is not overlooked at the expense of more medically orientated issues, as failure to do so can result in the following:

- unpleasant/uncomfortable care experience (leading to complaints)
- delayed recovery
- preventable risks/hazards not being identified.

In a multicultural society it is increasingly important for nurses to consider how to preserve the individual patient's social, cultural, spiritual, religious and ethical needs in order to help the patient understand, agree and cooperate with any planned care. There are many traditions and beliefs associated with health and illness that can alter a person's behaviour when they become ill and the nurse must seek to understand how this may be observed in their patients (Holland & Hogg 2001, Henley & Schott 1999). Every patient will have a different level of knowledge and understanding of their problems and different expectations regarding their treatment and involvement. For example, through the internet a growing number of people have greater access to information regarding ill health and treatments and need to be informed and involved in their care. However, other patients may have little understanding or no information. In relation to MSE it is important that the safety of the patient is ensured without infringing upon their personal beliefs, therefore nursing actions will be central to the following:

- determine the patient's level of understanding
- explain the rationale for procedures
- identify the difficulties this may pose for the patient/family
- report concern immediately
- negotiate and seek to provide an agreed safe level of care.

Informed consent

Prior to treatment, patients (or in the case of children, parents and guardians) are required to give their consent. In the UK any person over the age of 16 years can legally give consent. In emergency situations such as unconsciousness the law allows medical intervention without the patient's consent in order to preserve life. Exceptions to this would be when the patient has given advanced refusal of treatment (NMC 2006a). Consent must only be given on the understanding that sufficient detail and information regarding the procedure has been received from the doctor. It is important that the details given enable the patient or guardian to understand the procedure and make an informed decision to proceed, having had the potential risks and complications pointed out. The purpose of gaining consent is to protect the patient from undergoing any unauthorised procedures and also to safeguard the medical practitioner and the health care organisation. The consent form is validated by the presence of signatures from the patient or guardian and the doctor.

There is a professional and legal requirement to ensure that consent is properly obtained in recognition of the individual needs of patients. Nurses must always act in the best interests of the patient and take professional responsibility

Table 3.7 Illustration of psychological needs for Case study 3.3		
Problem	**Goal**	**Nursing intervention**
Frank may be anxious about his ability to cope with: • Surgery and/or anaesthesia • Pain	Ensure Frank is psychologically fit for surgery	• Ensure Frank has sufficient information according to individual needs • Continuously assess the patient and family anxiety and provide information and support as required • Support patient rest and relaxation and report any difficulties/concerns • Administer sedatives as prescribed and monitor effectiveness

for ensuring that the consent process is rigorous, transparent and accurately recorded (Steevenson 2006). With the introduction of the Mental Capacity Act 2005, nurses must also take into consideration the needs of vulnerable patients who are unable to make their own decisions.

Nursing interventions related to environmental factors affecting ill health

Safe practices in infection control

Although infections in health care settings are a common world-wide problem, they are largely preventable (WHO 2005b). In the UK, infection rates in the NHS are known to be higher than in some other countries and in order to reduce current unacceptable rates a national strategy was introduced by the Department of Health (DoH 2003, 2005, 2006e). The strategy is based upon the adoption of best evidence-based measures such as:

- the development of high-quality surveillance systems
- setting clear standards for infection control
- concentration on clean hospital environments and hygiene practice
- strict antibiotic prescribing policies
- isolation procedures for infected patients
- raising the profile of health-care-associated infections as a key feature of patient quality and safety.

All nurses have a professional responsibility to keep up to date with the most effective practices and promote the control of infection at both a personal and patient level (DoH 2003, NMC 2006b). As part of a national development programme the Department of Health and the National Patient Safety Agency (NPSA) have launched a series of campaigns and training programmes, including an on-line training programme (DoH 2005, NPSA 2005), covering the range of safe practice in the control of infection such as:

- knowledge of microorganisms and the spread of infection
- maintaining cleanliness of the hospital environment
- good hand hygiene technique
- cleaning and disinfecting procedures for *all* patient, nursing and medical equipment (for example meal time utensils, toileting equipment, medicine pots, mattresses, bed linen and trolleys)
- use of personal protective equipment
- correct use and disposal of sharps
- safe handling and disposal of clinical waste and spillages
- safe management of blood and body fluids
- correct handling of specimens.

Health-care-associated infections (HCAIs) commonly occur in surgical wounds and urinary and lower respiratory tracts, and are caused by *Staphylococcus aureus* and Gram-negative bacilli that are normally present in the nose and on the skin. To this extent it is imperative that all members of the medical and non-medical multidisciplinary team are aware of their individual responsibilities and are encouraged to utilise safe control of infection practices.

Failure to control infection effectively increases the opportunity for contamination either by direct contact, droplet or airborne routes, the most common being *Staphylococcus aureus*. There are a variety of *S. aureus* strains, some of which are highly resistant to antibiotics; these are referred to as 'superbugs', and are associated with HCAIs.

Antibiotic-resistant organisms commonly seen in the UK are methicillin-resistant *Staphylococcus aureus* (MRSA), vancomycin-resistant *Enterococcus* (VRE), *Clostridium difficile*, multidrug-resistant tuberculosis (MDRTB) and more recently an increase in the very resistant *Escherichia coli* known as extended-spectrum beta-lactamase (ESBL). Table 3.8 provides an overview of sources of the commonest bacteria and their effects upon health.

Isolation management

There are two types of isolation management. *Source isolation* (previously known as barrier nursing) involves putting the patient who is the source of the infection into a single room or isolation area in order to prevent the spread of the infection to other patients. Alternatively *protective isolation* is used to protect patients who have a greater susceptibility to infection because of their current health condition, such as patients who are immunosuppressed. Care of the patient is central to the following:

- determine the infective source
- determine the transmission modes
- determine the communicability risks of the infection
- determine the psychological support the patient may require
- ensure strict adherence to standard infection control precautions.

In the UK as a minimum, standard infection control precautions (SICPs) must be followed as recommended by the Hospital Infection Control Practices Advisory Committee (HICPAC) (see Table 3.9). In relation to individualising the care of the patient, isolation can be a very stressful experience requiring sensitive understanding. The nurse will need to address all the related factors affecting the care of the patient, providing information to the patient and family and support to meet physical, psychological and sociocultural needs.

Hand hygiene

Hands are known to be the main vehicle for the transmission of microorganisms between people and equipment and therefore good handwashing techniques are vital in controlling the spread of infection. Handwashing techniques have been the subject of many studies over time that have led to the development of guidelines for good practice (Ayliffe et al 2000, DoH 2003, 2005). Handwashing guidelines are based upon the principle of seeking to reduce, remove or destroy potentially harmful microorganisms that may be present on the hands and are at risk of being transmitted to the patient (see Table 3.10). In the UK there are national guidelines which govern handwashing techniques

Table 3.8 Examples of common bacteria encountered while providing health care

Organism	Main sources	Main mode of spread and means of entry	Examples of resulting disease/conditions
Staphylococcus aureus including MRSA	People, skin, wounds, and at times in sputum Environmental dust	Direct and indirect contact with persons carrying the organism or from the environment. Entry through e.g. open wounds	Wound and skin infection Bacteraemia, endocarditis Osteomyelitis and septic arthritis
Clostridium difficile	In the animal and human lower bowel, therefore faeces and any faecally contaminated areas. Especially found in hospitalised patients who have received antibiotic therapy that has disturbed their normal bowel flora Also soil	Direct and indirect contact with persons carrying the organism or from the environment, especially as it can form spores that survive for long periods in the environment. Often also called faecal–oral spread if ingestion occurs resulting in further GI upset/infection	GI infection, characterised by loose, foul-smelling green stools and abdominal pain The most common cause of HCAI diarrhoea Can lead to pseudomembranous colitis
Streptococcal infections	Found in humans, at various sites, and in the environment	Direct and indirect contact with persons carrying the organism or from the environment Through droplets from infected respiratory tracts	Pharyngitis Wound infection, rarely necrotising fasciitis Septicaemia Toxin-mediated disease, e.g. scarlet fever, toxic shock syndrome Pneumonia and associated bacteraemia
Enterococci, including vancomycin-resistant enterococci (VRE) *Pseudomonas aeruginosa*	Mainly environmental sources but also in the human GI tract. In the lower bowel of animals and humans, most commonly in hospitalised patients who have received antibiotic therapy Moist sites in the environment, but especially poorly draining shower areas and open fluid containers Also soil	Direct and indirect contact with persons carrying the organism or from the environment	Urinary tract infection Wound infection Endocarditis Eye and ear infections Wound infections, e.g. in burns Septicaemia Respiratory infections, especially in the immunocompromised, e.g. cystic fibrosis patients
Mycobacterium tuberculosis (TB)	Found in humans, animals and in the environment	Through the airborne route when respiratory infection is present Through direct contact when other systems are infected	Respiratory or pulmonary TB; can be termed as open TB or closed TB, where another system or site of the body is infected. It can infect any organ in the body
Escherichia coli	Found in humans, particularly the GI tract, and in the environment	Direct and indirect contact with persons carrying the organism From the environment or from food From poor hand hygiene	GI infection Urinary tract infection

From Alexander et al (2006), p. 662, Table 16.2.

and recommended cleansing agents. Box 3.14 provides an overview of best practice in hand hygiene and Figure 3.16 shows the recommended standard technique that should be used (Horton & Parker 2002).

Use of gloves Gloves are used to protect both patients and staff in order to reduce the risk of cross-infection when carrying out a variety of procedures. They are made from a variety of different materials such as latex, vinyl and plastic, for specific purposes and can be coated inside with a powder to make application and removal easier. The wearing of gloves is known to cause problems for some staff who may be allergic to either the material (such as latex), or the powder coating. Patients too are at risk from allergic reactions

Table 3.9 Standard infection control precautions

Element	Action/timing	Rationale
1. Hand hygiene	At the right times In the most appropriate way for the situation (see Table 3.10)	Frequently called the single most important action to prevent, control and manage infection
2. Personal protective equipment (PPE)*	Gloves (powder-free): • non-latex alternatives should be available and their use is being increasingly encouraged due to the adverse affects of latex Aprons, gowns, footwear Eye and mouth protection	To protect mouth and eyes in particular, and the skin of the face, hands and the rest of the body with the use of clothing and equipment in order to avoid contamination/soiling/splashing and potential exposure to harmful microorganisms, originating from patients, the environment or even live vaccinations The use of gloves does not negate the need for hand decontamination and all PPE must be disposed of safely and properly immediately after being removed Often this is into clinical waste
3. Prevention of occupational exposure to infection	Cover all breaks in skin Avoid sharps injuries: • never resheath sharps such as needles • utilise sharps receptacles close to the point of use • never try to retrieve any items from sharps receptacles Avoid splashes with blood or body fluids by using PPE when exposure is anticipated Report any exposure incidents following local policies (see www.riddor.gov.uk/info.html)	To additionally protect health care workers, carers and others from exposure to microorganisms that cause infection, e.g. hepatitis B, C, HIV, MRSA
4. Management of blood and body fluid spillages	Utilise cleaning products and disinfectants (often found in 'spillage kits') immediately spillages occur, following local policies	To protect all of those in the surrounding area from exposure to microorganisms found within spillages that could cause harm and to protect the environment from contamination
5. Management of equipment utilised during care	Prevent reuse of single-use devices Prevent single-patient use devices being used on other patients Ensure reusable devices are handled safely and decontaminated between use on the same patient and before use on others, following local policies: • basic cleaning measures are a vital part of health care and should also be performed before any required disinfection processes	To ensure that items used during care are not a factor in the spread of potentially infectious microorganisms directly to patients or a factor in the contamination of patients' environment leading to indirect spread of infection
6. Environment control	At the right times and in the most appropriate way for the situation Cleanliness and maintenance must be kept at the optimum level	To ensure that the care setting, its fixtures and fittings and other items within it are adequately decontaminated and maintained to prevent cross-infection occurring through this route
7. Safe disposal of waste, including sharps	Waste is categorised by regulations so that it will be segregated and subsequently destroyed safely and effectively: • clinical waste generated in the home and community is often dealt with differently from that generated in hospital settings; local policies reflecting current regulations must be followed • the area around the opening of clinical waste bags and sharps containers is often the most contaminated in health care settings and should never be touched. 'Hands-free' waste sack holders, e.g. foot-operated, must always be in place Attaching waste bags to other pieces of furniture, e.g. trolleys, is not generally acceptable, nor is overfilling of bags	To prevent the risk of inappropriate, avoidable exposure to the microorganisms found contaminating clinical waste in particular, thus protecting all health care workers and others The use of PPE when handling waste is essential

Table 3.9 *(continued)*

Element	Action/timing	Rationale
8. Linen	Safe handling, transport and processing of bags: • linen should never be held against the body or shaken, even if protective clothing is worn • linen should always be disposed of into appropriate receptacles immediately after being removed and never placed on the floor	To prevent the risk of inappropriate, avoidable exposure to microorganisms when linen is being handled or reused, thus protecting health care workers and others and preventing contamination of the environment Linen can be heavily contaminated with potentially pathogenic microorganisms; items such as urinary catheters, needles, etc. are often found in linen by laundry staff, putting them at unnecessary risk Use of PPE when handling used linen is essential
9. Appropriate patient placement	Choosing the most appropriate site/area to care for a patient must be considered using a risk management approach at all times, e.g. consider the route of transmission of any known or suspected infections/colonisation, how these might then spread to others, the potential outcomes of this spread, the availability of resources to site patients in the best place	To prevent exposure of others and the environment to potentially infectious microorganisms and to protect the patient as far as possible

* Also known as protective clothing.
From Alexander et al (2006), pp. 665–666.

Table 3.10 Hand hygiene

	Action	Rationale
Provision of hand decontamination facilities	Access to adequate hand hygiene facilities and supplies is an essential element of SICPs in all settings where exposure to microorganisms might occur The use of 'hands-free' tap systems, e.g. elbow taps, is recommended wherever possible in health care as this ensures that hands are not contaminated during the process of turning taps on or off and potentially becoming a source for further contamination of patients or the environment Also important is the use of mixer taps to ensure water of the right temperature can be provided as well as the absence of plugs to discourage washing in filled sinks where microorganisms can harbour Where running water cannot be accessed, the use of alcohol hand decontamination products, e.g. gels, is a useful alternative	By providing adequate facilities, hand decontamination should be carried out in the correct manner at the correct times to prevent cross-infection from occurring Alcohol gel is appropriate if hands are not soiled; it is inactivated by organic matter

	Level 1 Social handwash	Level 2 Hygienic handwash	Level 3 Surgical scrub
***When* to wash or decontaminate**	**Before** commencing/leaving work, eating/handling of food/drinks, preparing/giving medications, general patient/client contact **After** visiting the toilet; patient/client contact, handling laundry/equipment/waste, blowing/wiping/touching nose *NB* even if gloves have been worn	**Before** aseptic procedures, contact during all patient/client care procedures, leaving isolation rooms (all levels of transmission-based precautions) **After** contact with isolated patients/clients, any potential contact with body fluids/excretions/secretions, etc. *NB* even if gloves have been worn **Between/within** the above described procedures if any contamination occurs **In high-risk areas at all times:** infant nurseries/special care baby units, infectious disease units/intensive care/therapy units, wards/ departments during outbreaks of infection	**Before** surgical/other invasive procedures **Between/within** the above described procedures if any contamination occurs

(continued)

Table 3.10 *(continued)*

	Level 1 Social handwash	Level 2 Hygienic handwash	Level 3 Surgical scrub
Why decontaminate	To render the hands physically clean and to remove microorganisms picked up during activities (transient microorganisms)	To remove or destroy transient microorganisms and to provide residual effect	To remove or destroy transient microorganisms and also to substantially reduce those which normally live on the skin (resident microorganisms)
How to decontaminate When washing hands for whatever purpose, the tap should first be turned on and the hands wet before applying the soap. A good lather should be evident for undertaking the steps, with all areas of the hands being covered (and forearms when surgical scrub is being undertaken). Following this, hands should be rinsed well Cleansing solutions' instructions should give guidance as to the volume of solution to be used; this also applies to alcohol hand products	Using soap, preferably liquid, wash hands Alternatively, where hands are not soiled, utilise alcohol hand products using the same steps	Using an approved antiseptic hand cleanser or soap, wash hands If hands have any contact before or during a procedure, but are not soiled with any body fluids and, therefore, do not require hand washing with soap or an antiseptic hand cleanser, alcohol hand-rub can be used, using the same technique Any soilage can inactivate the activity of alcohol and therefore hand washing in these circumstances is essential *NB* Alcohol hand-rubs/gels can also be used following hand washing, e.g. when performing aseptic techniques	Using an antiseptic hand cleanser carry out Level 2 hygienic hand wash for 2 to 3 min, ensuring all areas of hands and arms are covered (The time used for surgical scrub is often debated and local policies must be followed)

	Action	Rationale
How to dry	Using clean disposable towels, dry each area of the hand thoroughly each time after washing. This should be done by drying each part of the hand, remembering all of the steps included in the hand washing process If 'hands-free' taps are not available, the disposable towels should then be used to turn off the tap	Hand drying is an important process in removing any remaining transient microorganisms on the hands and hands that are not dried properly can become dry and cracked, leading to problems Recontamination of the hands following drying should be avoided as far as possible Other forms of hand drying, e.g. hot air driers or reusable towels, are available but are not considered acceptable in ensuring that the whole hand decontamination process is effective Reusable towels that are freshly laundered are sometimes acceptable in the home
Additional points Gloves	It may be necessary to change gloves and decontaminate hands between tasks on the same patient	To ensure that contamination of gloves/hands does not lead to microorganisms coming into contact with an area/site of the body where they would not normally be present and might cause infection
Cuts and abrasions	Cover all cuts and abrasions with a waterproof dressing, even when gloves are being worn	To prevent inadvertent exposure to blood or body fluids and to protect the patient from exposure to the blood or body fluids of the health care worker

Table 3.10 *(continued)*

	Action	Rationale
Soap	Liquid soap dispensers should be kept clean and the 'topping up' of solutions into bottles should not take place If bar soap must be used in home care settings, it should be kept on a rack that facilitates drainage	To prevent microorganisms from harbouring in dispensers and spreading to those using them and subsequently to patients Liquid soap solutions can become contaminated when a 'topping up' system is used
Nail brushes	Do not use nail brushes to scrub nails or any part of the hands during social or hygienic hand washing	Most microorganisms can be easily removed by hand washing and scrubbing can break the skin, leading to increased risk of picking up microorganisms or dispersing skin scales that may cause harm to others
Nails	Nails must be kept short and clean Nail polish or artificial nails should not be worn	To prevent the harbouring of microorganisms which may then be spread It has been shown that nails and chipped nail polish can harbour potentially harmful bacteria
Hand creams	Communal hand creams should not be used unless in a wall-mounted pump dispenser that undergoes a maintenance and cleaning regimen If a particular skin problem is experienced, advice should be sought from your GP or Occupational Health Department	To protect skin from drying and cracking, where bacteria can harbour Communal tubes or tubs of hand cream can become contaminated with microorganisms from the hands of those using them, therefore only individual tubes of hand cream should be used or those that are in contained dispensers Hand skin problems should be appropriately treated to try to ensure broken skin is not a problem when being potentially exposed to microorganisms in the workplace
Jewellery	Wrist and hand jewellery should be removed at the start of each shift if there will be close personal contact with patients during this time	To prevent contamination of jewellery, particularly those with intricate parts such as stones, with microorganisms and subsequent spread to health care workers or patients

SICPs, standard infection control precautions.
From Alexander (2006), pp. 666–668.

Box 3.14 Handwashing guidelines

Handwashing should be carried out
- on arrival and on completion of duty
- after using the toilet (self or assisting patients)
- before and after preparing, serving or eating food or medicines
- before and after attending each individual patient
- before and after aseptic procedures
- before and after removing protective clothing (masks, gloves or aprons)
- after handling contaminated laundry/equipment
- when hands are visibly soiled
- after contact with body secretions/excretions.

Procedure
- remove jewellery, wristwatches, bracelets and rings (except wedding rings)
- all surfaces of the hands must be washed
- pay particular attention to thumbs, fingertips and finger webs
- begin by wetting the hands with warm running water
- apply recommended soap/antiseptic cleansing agents
- use alcohol gel in situations where time or facilities inhibit handwashing
- use the technique outlined in Fig. 3.16 to rub agent into all areas
- rinse thoroughly under running water
- turn off taps with elbows or wrist or clean paper towel
- dry hands thoroughly using two clean paper towels
- take care not to recontaminate hands when throwing paper towel away
- use hand creams provided to prevent skin irritation.

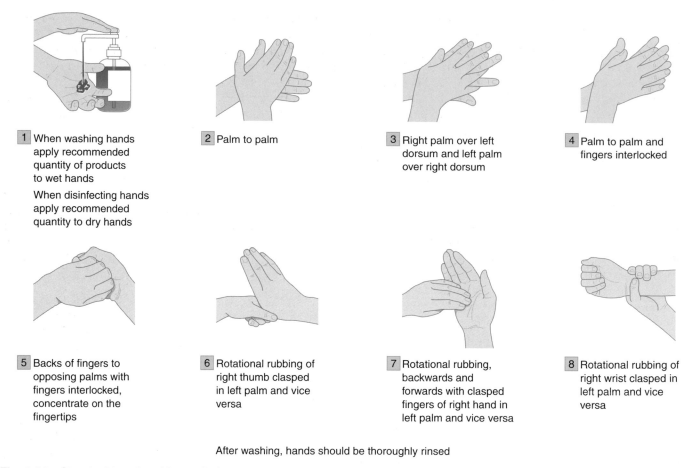

1. When washing hands apply recommended quantity of products to wet hands

   When disinfecting hands apply recommended quantity to dry hands

2. Palm to palm

3. Right palm over left dorsum and left palm over right dorsum

4. Palm to palm and fingers interlocked

5. Backs of fingers to opposing palms with fingers interlocked, concentrate on the fingertips

6. Rotational rubbing of right thumb clasped in left palm and vice versa

7. Rotational rubbing, backwards and forwards with clasped fingers of right hand in left palm and vice versa

8. Rotational rubbing of right wrist clasped in left palm and vice versa

After washing, hands should be thoroughly rinsed

Fig. 3.16 Standard handwashing technique (from Brooker & Nicol 2003, with permission).

and there is some concern that the powder may increase the risk of wound infections. In order to prevent risks occurring it is important that patients are accurately assessed and that gloves are appropriately selected for the task (Beckford-Ball 2005). It is recommended that gloves are always used when handling blood and body fluids. Sterile gloves should be worn to protect the patient from infection and non-sterile gloves should be worn to protect practitioners when conducting non-sterile procedures. It is also recommended that hands should still be washed after gloves have been removed (Hunte 2004).

Needle-stick and risk from other injuries Essentially, all patients are a source of infection and the nurse must carefully balance the quality of individual care against the need to reduce the risks associated with the occupational transmission of infection. It is not always possible to know what the infection status of a patient is and all health care workers are advised to take universal precautions to minimise the risk of infection caused by either certain procedures or by patients themselves. These are categorised as being needle-stick or sharp injuries or patient-related injuries, e.g. being bitten by a patient, which may result in contamination of the health care worker from bloodborne infections.

To protect staff all care organisations should have a policy and clear guidelines that must be followed governing the process for reporting and recording any incident irrespective of the patient's infection status. Policies will outline the action to be taken to ensure that appropriate attention is given to the injury site, blood investigations, prophylactic treatment, counselling and follow-up care. Through the occupational health department, staff should also have access to an immunisation programme in order to reduce infection amongst staff.

Aseptic technique This is a technique which is used to reduce the risk of introducing pathogens into the body, based upon the principle that only uncontaminated objects or solutions make contact with the area and that the risk of airborne invasion is kept to a minimum. The technique should be carried out in a clean environment, using only sterile equipment and is used for dressing wounds, removing sutures, drains, etc., or carrying out other invasive procedures such as urinary catheterisation. It is important that hands are thoroughly washed, trolleys and surfaces correctly prepared and only sterile cleansing and dressing materials used (see Doherty & Lister 2004 for practice guidelines).

Control of the external environment Nursing actions central to controlling the care environment in relation to MSE focus upon taking a risk management approach to preventing accidents, reducing infection and ensuring that patients receive sufficient rest and sleep. If it has been identified that a patient is at risk from falling or sustaining any other injuries because of their age or health state, then appropriate action should be taken. It is important to recognise that equipment used within the health care setting may have hidden dangers for patients such as trolleys and tubing. In addition unfamiliar environments and limited or shared facilities may cause the patient some anxiety and result in accidents. If the patient is receiving care as a result of a fall at home then the focus of care would be to discuss safety measures to be taken upon returning home, with a possible referral to another health or social care professional for further assessment. Controlling noise within the care environment can be difficult to achieve, particularly when noises are coming from other patients. Increasing use of technology has resulted in a greater use of electronic equipment, which adds to the total volume of noise in any given environment. To this extent the nurse should consider regularly the effects this may have on individual patients and take appropriate individual or team action to minimise noises, particularly at night.

Control of infection environment Infection is known to spread more quickly in large open spaces and this understanding has influenced the way in which care facilities are being designed and provided. To reduce infection rates, greater consideration is now given to installing more single rooms with en-suite facilities, subdivided wards, more toilets and showers, and dedicated rooms for wound dressing and invasive procedures and spaces for correct storage of equipment and substances.

Medical devices and products
In all health care settings practitioners use a wide range of medical devices for diagnosis, prevention, monitoring or treatment for which they must take responsibility for ensuring safe use. In England, the use of medical devices is regulated by the Medicines and Healthcare products Regulations Agency (MHRA), which provides guidance for health care organisations, professionals and manufacturers in line with legal requirements issued under European directives (MHRA 2006).

Nursing interventions related to politicoeconomic factors affecting ill health
It is important to recognise that for some patients an episode of illness or injury can create financial hardship. Not all patients enjoy the protection of employer sickness schemes. The nurse must be sensitive to the issue and consider that from the patient's perspective a financial anxiety may be greater than that of concern for physical wellbeing. In Britain, the Department of Health publishes an information booklet that explains how patients can get help with NHS

costs (DoH 2006i) (see also Chapter 11). To support patient care responsibly, it is important that nurses have a good understanding of how political and economic factors influence individual and community health. In doing so it is essential that nursing actions are central to the patient's individual circumstances and that the support of other health and social care professionals and agencies is sought in the most appropriate way.

Delivery of MSE nursing interventions
The delivery of quality care is dependent upon the quality of the information detailed within the care plan. In the care setting a variety of health professionals will need to refer to the care plan and it is essential that the plan is conducive to the delivery of consistency in care standards. Prior to the implementation of nursing activities the following must be in place:

1. A detailed written care plan and verbal handover to ensure that all staff are aware of patient progress, goals to be achieved and skills required to deliver the care.
2. Competent practitioners are identified to safely deliver the planned care.
3. Nursing actions and patient progress are recorded and goals are evaluated.

The nursing plan is a document that guides the required nursing activities to help the patient achieve the identified goals (see Chapter 1). The plan should be constantly reviewed and updated to record the following:

- when a goal/desired outcome has been achieved
- when nursing intervention has been changed to support goal achievement
- when the goal needs to be modified
- when the evaluation date needs to be changed
- when problems change or develop.

Factors influencing implementation of MSE nursing interventions
To ensure the effectiveness of implementing the MSE plan it is important to identify the factors which can influence this.

Knowledge
- normal anatomy and physiology and pathophysiological states and processes
- related psychological effects associated with ill health
- social and cultural implications for poor health or recovery
- environmental influences and concerns
- political and economic influences and concerns.

Skill and competency
- philosophy of care and attitudes to patient care
- communication/interpersonal skills
- observation skills
- problem-solving skills
- technical/caring skills

- management/leadership skills (directing, coaching, delegating, supervising skills)
- teaching skills
- research skills.

Resources
- appropriate skill mix
- sufficient equipment
- sufficient support services.

MSE and medically derived care

In addition to the identified nursing care plan, it is also important to consider the impact that medical or other health care intervention can have and should where possible be integrated into the plan as shown in Table 3.11.

EVALUATING CARE

The evaluation stage provides the basis by which to determine if the patient is making the desired progress and the mechanism to judge the effectiveness of the nursing actions. Evaluation of the patient's progress should be ongoing and undertaken on a continuous, hourly, per shift, daily or weekly basis, depending upon the patient's problem and timescale for achieving the goals. To evaluate effectively the following skills are required:

- observing
- interviewing
- listening
- analysing
- measuring.

The steps in evaluating are detailed as follows. It is recommended that where possible the patient is involved in describing the progress/achievement made.

1. Check the identified goals against patient progress:
   - Have the goals been partially or completely met?
   - Have the goals been unmet?
2. Is the timescale realistic?
3. Record the progress as follows:
   - Goal completely met – state the evidence to support this and discontinue the problem.

Box 3.15	Factors influencing the evaluation of care

- Quality of the assessment and planning stages
- Accuracy of the goals set
- Standard and quality of the care delivered
- Timing of the evaluation(s)
- Knowledge and skills of the nurse
- Abilities of the patient.

- Goal partially met – decide if there is a need to extend the timescale or modify the plan.
- Goal not met at all – decide if there is a need to extend the timescale, change the plan or reassess the whole problem.

It is important to recognise that the evaluation stage can be influenced by a number of factors, which must be taken into consideration (see Box 3.15). Consider the skills that underpin these factors in relation to personal development needs.

Plan review

If the goals are achieved, nursing actions effectively become redundant. Where goals are not achieved the following questions need to be asked:

1. Is more information required to determine goal achievement?
2. Should the nursing plan be adapted to enable the goal to be achieved?
3. Has the problem changed?
4. Can the nursing care planned be stopped?
5. Has the problem worsened?
6. Should the goal and intervention be reviewed?
7. Was the goal inappropriate?
8. Does the plan require intervention from other health care professionals?

Upon discharge, there will usually be some continuing care needs that the patient requires. Often the patients themselves can meet the identified needs, providing that sufficient information is given. Planning an effective discharge should begin at the point of admission as increasingly it involves working collaboratively with a range of other health and/or social care professionals. Failure to collaborate and

Table 3.11 Identification of medically derived care and its impact upon nursing care

Medically derived care	Nursing intervention/support
Specific medicotechnical intervention	Knowledge, skill and competency to manage equipment, observe results and report changes
Specific pharmacological intervention	Knowledge and skill regarding action and side-effects
Specific nutritional intervention	Knowledge and skill to support patient information
Specific physiotherapy intervention	Knowledge and skill to provide 24-hour continuing care

Table 3.12 Evaluation and plan review

Goal	Evaluation	Plan review
Frank's physical condition will be stabilised prior to surgery	Frank's physical condition was satisfactorily stabilised prior to surgery	No further preoperative intervention required
Frank will recover from surgery without complications	Frank made a successful recovery with no immediate complications noted	Continue to observe vital signs twice daily until discharge from hospital
Ensure Frank is psychologically fit for surgery	Frank is fully aware of the need for surgery and received information and support to reduce anxiety	Frank has some concerns regarding his recovery
Frank will need to adapt lifestyle to promote full recovery and prevent further problems following discharge	Frank will need further advice and support prior to discharge to help adjust lifestyle	Refer to appropriate health professionals • Dietitian • Counselling services • Medical team and GP

communicate with other services and professionals can lead to delays in discharge, recovery and unnecessary exposure to risks as outlined in this chapter. Such is the importance of a well-planned discharge the Department of Health has issued multidisciplinary guidance (DoH 2004b). Table 3.12 illustrates the extent to which Frank (Case study 3.3) has achieved the goals set prior to discharge and indicates his continuing care needs.

SUMMARY POINTS

1. Maintaining a safe environment is essential for an individual's health and wellbeing.
2. Using a model framework together with the nursing process, the nurse can identify the way in which the AL is interdependent with all the other ALs.
3. Assessment of patient needs associated with the AL of maintaining a safe environment involves taking account of both internal (within the body) and external (outside the body) environments.

References

Alexander M, Fawcett JN, Runciman PJ 2006 Nursing practice hospital and home, the adult, 3rd edn. Churchill Livingstone (Elsevier), Edinburgh

Arnow BA 2004 Relationships between childhood maltreatment, adult health and psychiatric outcomes and medical utilization, Journal of Clinical Psychiatry 65(suppl 12):10–15

Ayliffe GAJ, Fraise AP, Geddes AM et al 2000 Control of hospital infection – A practical handbook, 4th edn. Arnold, London

Barr W, Leitner M, Thomas J 2005 Psychosocial assessment of patients who attend an accident and emergency department with self harm. Journal of Psychiatric and Mental Health Nursing 12(2):130

Beckford-Ball J 2005 Tackling latex allergies in patients and nursing staff. Nursing Times 101(24):24–27

Bornstein RF 2005 Interpersonal dependency in child abuse perpetrators and victims: a meta-analytical review. Journal of Psychopathology and Behavioural Assessment 27(2):67–76

British Standards Institute 2003 British Standards related to childcare provision information sheet. BSI, London (www.bsieducation.org/Education/downloads/publications/ChildcareleafletIssue3.pdf)

Brooker C, Nicol M 2003 Nursing adults: the practice of caring. Mosby, Edinburgh

Brunkreef B 2002 Air pollution and health. Lancet 360(9341):1233–1242

Burnett A, Peel M 2001 Asylum seekers and refugees in Britain. The health of survivors of torture and organised violence. British Medical Journal 10(322)/(97286):606–609

Campbell O, Graham W 2006 Strategies for reducing maternal mortality: getting on with what works. Lancet 368(9543):1284–1299

Carlsson JM, Mortensen EL, Kastrup M 2005 A follow-up study of mental health and health-related quality of life in tortured refugees in multidisciplinary treatment. Journal of Nervous and Mental Disease 193(10):651–657

Chaplin R, McGeorge M, Lelliott P 2006 Violence on inpatient units for people with learning disability and mental illness: the experience of service users and staff. British Journal of Developmental Disabilities 52(2):105–115

Child Accident Prevention Trust 2006 Child accident facts. (www.capt.org.uk/FAQ/default.htm)

Children Act 2004. HMSO, London (www.opsi.gov.uk/acts/acts2004/20040031.htm)

Clean Neighbourhoods and Environment Act 2005. HMSO, London (www.opsi.gov.uk/acts/acts2005/20050016.htm)

Control of Noise at Work Regulations 2005. HMSO, London (www.opsi.gov.uk/si/si2005/20051643.htm)

Department for Communities and Local Government 2006 Fire Safety risk assessment – healthcare premises. Department for Communities and Local Government publications, London (www.communities.gov.uk/pub/258/Healthcarepremisesfullguide_id1503258.pdf)

Department for Education and Skills, Department of Health, Home Office 2003 Keeping children safe: the Government's response to the Victoria Climbié inquiry report and the Joint Chief Inspectors' report safeguarding children. HMSO, London

Department for Education and Skills 2005 Every child matters. Change for Children Statutory Guidance on making arrangements to safeguard and promote the welfare of children under section 11 of the Children Act 2004. DfES, London (www.everychildmatters.gov.uk/_files/FF30C3EA825087134 5738CFA44EA3197.pdf)

Department of Health 1994 Firecode, Health Technical Memorandum 83, Fire safety in healthcare premises – General fire precautions. DoH publications, London (www.dh.gov.uk/assetRoot/04/11/92/72/04119272.pdf)

Department of Health 1998 A first class service: quality in the new NHS. HMSO, London

Department of Health 1999 Saving lives: our healthier nation. DoH publications, London (www.dh.gov.uk/assetRoot/04/04/93/29/04049329.pdf)

Department of Health 2000a Mobile phones and health, 2000 edition, DoH Leaflet, London (www.dh.gov.uk/assetRoot/04/12/39/81/04123981.pdf)

Department of Health 2000b The NHS plan: a plan for investment – a plan for reform. DoH Publications, London

Department of Health 2001a National service framework for older people. DoH Publications, London (www.dh.gov.uk/assetRoot/04/07/12/83/04071283.pdf)

Department of Health 2001b Health effects of climate change in the UK. DoH Publications, London (www.dh.gov.uk/assetRoot/04/10/80/61/04108061.pdf)

Department of Health 2002a National suicide prevention strategy. DoH Publications, London (www.dh.gov.uk/assetRoot/04/01/95/48/04019548.pdf)

Department of Health 2002b Preventing accidental injury: priorities for action, report to the Chief Medical Officer. DoH publications, London (www.dh.gov.uk/assetRoot/04/06/49/50/04064950.pdf)

Department of Health 2003 Winning ways – working together to reduce healthcare associated infections in England. DoH Publications, London (www.dh.gov.uk/assetRoot/04/06/46/89/04064689.pdf)

Department of Health 2004a The national service framework for children, young people and maternity services. Change for Children – Every Child Matters. DoH Publications, London (www.dh.gov.uk/assetRoot/04/09/05/52/04090552.pdf)

Department of Health 2004b Achieving timely 'simple' discharge from hospital: A toolkit for the multi-disciplinary team. DoH Publications, London (www.dh.gov.uk/assetRoot/04/08/83/67/04088367.pdf)

Department of Health 2005 Saving lives: a delivery programme to reduce healthcare associated infection including MRSA. DoH publications, London (www.dh.gov.uk/Publications AndStatistics/Publications/PublicationsPolicyAndGuidance/PublicationsPolicyAndGuidanceArticle/fs/en?CONTENT_ID=4113889&chk=Uz2v2Q)

Department of Health 2006a A new ambition for old age: next steps in implementing the national service framework for older people, DoH Publications, London (www.dh.gov.uk/assetRoot/04/13/39/91/04133991.pdf)

Department of Health 2006b Tackling the health and mental health effects of domestic and sexual violence and abuse. DoH Publications, London (www.dh.gov.uk/assetRoot/04/13/66/11/04136611.pdf)

Department of Health 2006c Cardiovascular disease and air pollution – A report by the Committee on Medical Effects of Air Pollution, DoH Publications. London (www.advisorybodies.doh.gov.uk/comeap/statementsreports/CardioDisease.pdf)

Department of Health 2006d Accidents. DoH Publications, London (www.dh.gov.uk/PolicyAndGuidance/HealthAnd SocialCareTopics/Accidents/fs/en)

Department of Health 2006e The Health Act 2006 Code of Practice for the prevention and control of healthcare associated infections. DoH Publications, London (www.dh.gov.uk/assetRoot/04/13/93/37/04139337.pdf)

Department of Health 2006f Immunisation against infectious disease. The Stationery Office, London (www.dh.gov.uk/assetRoot/04/14/17/61/04141761.pdf)

Department of Health 2006g Our health, our say: making it happen. DoH Publications, London (www.dh.gov.uk/assetRoot/04/14/00/65/04140065.pdf)

Department of Health 2006h Improving patient's access to medicines: a guide to implementing nurse and pharmacist independent prescribing within the NHS in England. DoH publications, London (www.dh.gov.uk/assetRoot/04/13/37/47/04133747.pdf)

Department of Health 2006i HC11 Help with health costs. DoH publications, London (www.ppa.org.uk//pdfs/ppc/HC11_Sep_06.pdf)

Department of Trade and Industry 2002 24th (Final) Report of the Home and Leisure Accident Surveillance System (2000, 2001 & 2002 data). HMSO, London (www.hassandlass.org.uk/query/reports/2000_2002.pdf)

Department of Transport 2000 Tommorrow's roads: safer for everyone. The Government's road safety strategy and casualty reduction targets for 2010. HMSO, London (www.dft.gov.uk/stellent/groups/dft_rdsafety/documents/page/dft_rdsafety_504644.hcsp)

Department of Transport 2004 Tommorrow's roads: safer for everyone. The Government's road safety strategy and casualty reduction targets for 2010. The first three year review. HMSO, London. (www.dft.gov.uk/stellent/groups/dft_rdsafety/documents/downloadable/dft_rdsafety_028169.pdf)

Disability Discrimination Act 2005. HMSO. London (www.opsi.gov.uk/acts/acts2005/20050013.htm)

Dougherty L, Lister S 2004 The Royal Marsden manual of clinical nursing procedures, 6th edn. Baillière Tindall, London

Drennan V, Iliffe S, Haworth D 2005 The feasibility and acceptability of a specialist health and social care team for the promotion of health and independence in 'at risk' older adults. Health & Social Care in the Community 13(2):136–144

Evans G 2004 Vulnerable adults: the challenge for health and social care practitioners. Nurse 2 Nurse 4(4):49–50

Ewles L, Simnett I 2003 Promoting health: a practical guide. Baillière Tindall, Edinburgh

Eyles J, Consitt N 2004 What's at risk? Environmental influences on human health. Environment 46(8):24–39

Frederick K, Barlow J 2006 The Citizenship Safety Project: a pilot study. Health Education Research 21(1):87–96

Friederichs V, Cameron JC, Robertson C 2006 Impact of adverse publicity on MMR vaccine uptake: a population based analysis of vaccine uptake records for one million children, born 1987–2004. Archive of Diseases in Childhood 91(6):465–468

Goldhill D, White S, Sumner A 1999 Physiological values and procedures in the 24 hours before ICU admission from the ward, Anaesthesia 54:853–860

Health Development Agency 2003 Prevention and reduction of accidental injury in children and older people, evidence briefing. NICE, London (www.nice.org.uk/page.aspx?o=502597)

Health Protection Agency 2006 HPA Compendium of chemical hazards. HPA, London (www.hpa.org.uk/chemicals/compendium/lead/PDF/LEAD_full_version.pdf)

Health and Safety at Work Act 1974. HMSO, London

Health and Safety Executive 2005 Noise at work: Guidance on the Control of Noise at Work Regulations 2005, HSE Publications, Suffolk (www.hse.gov.uk/pubns/indg362.pdf)

Health and Safety Executive 2006a HSE statistics. HSE Publications, Suffolk (www.hse.gov.uk/statistics/index.htm)

Health and Safety Executive 2006b RIDDOR explained. HSE Publications, Suffolk (www.hse.gov.uk/pubns/hse31.pdf)

Henley A, Schott J 1999 Culture, religion and patient care in a multi-ethnic society: a handbook for professionals. Age Concern, London

Holland K, Hogg C 2001 Cultural awareness in nursing practice: an introductory text. Arnold, London

Horton R, Parker L 2002 Informed infection control practice. Churchill Livingstone, London

Howard D 2003 Stress. In: Brooker C, Nichol M (eds) Adult nursing: the practice of caring, p. 102. Mosby, London

Hunte SC 2004 Choosing the right glove for the right purpose. Professional Nurse 20(3):43–47

Iggulden H 2006 Care of the neurological patient. Essential Clinical Skills for Nurses Series. Blackwell, Oxford

Institute of Medicine 1999 Crossing the quality chasm: a new health system for the 21st century. National Academy Press, Washington DC

Jamieson EM, McCall JM, Whyte LA 2002 Guidelines for clinical nursing practices, 4th edn. Churchill Livingstone, Edinburgh

Kindlen S 2003 Physiology for health care and nursing, 2nd edn. Churchill Livingstone, Edinburgh

Kumar S, O'Brien A 2004 Recent developments in fetal medicine. BMJ(Clinical research ed) 328(7446):1002–1006

Landfill Regulations 2002 HMSO, London (www.opsi.gov.uk/SI/si2002/20021559.htm)

Medicinal Products Prescription by Nurses, Midwives and Health Visitors Act 1992. HMSO, London (www.opsi.gov.uk/ACTS/acts1992/Ukpga_19920028_en_1.htm)

Medicines Act 1968 Amendment Regulations 1992. HMSO, London (www.opsi.gov.uk/si/si1992/Uksi_19920604_en_1.htm)

Medical and Healthcare Regulations Agency 2006 Device Bulletin. Managing medical devices, guidance for healthcare and social services organisations, DB2006(05). DoH Publications, London (www.mhra.gov.uk/home/idcplg?IdcService=SS_GET_PAGE&useSecondary=true&ssDocName=CON2025142&ssTargetNodeId=572)

Mental Capacity Act 2006. HMSO, London (www.opsi.gov.uk/acts/acts2005/20050009.htm)

Misuse of Drugs Act 1971 (modification order) 2001. HMSO, London (www.opsi.gov.uk/si/si2001/20013932.htm)

Montague SE, Watson R, Herbert RA 2005 Physiology for nursing practice, 3rd edn. Elsevier, Edinburgh

Morris D, Ward K 2006 Perioperative nursing. In: Alexander M, Fawcett JN, Runciman PJ (eds) Nursing practice hospital and home. The adult, 3rd edn. Churchill Livingstone (Elsevier), Edinburgh

National Audit Office 2004 Improving patient care by reducing the risk of hospital acquired infection: a progress report by thee controller and auditor general HC 876 session 2003–2004. The Stationery Office, London (www.nao.org.uk/publications/nao_reports/03-04/0304876.pdf)

National Institute for Mental Health in England 2005 National suicide prevention strategy for England: Annual report on progress 2004. Department of Health, London (www.dh.gov.uk/assetRoot/04/10/16/69/04101669.pdf)

National Patient Safety Agency 2005 Clean your hands campaign (www.npsa.nhs.uk/cleanyourhands/campaign/background)

NICE 2006 Interventions to prevent accidental injury to young people aged 15–24, Evidence briefing summary. NICE, London (www.nice.org.uk/page.aspx?o=346187)

Nichols G 2006 Infection risks from water in natural and man-made environments. Euro Surveillance 11(4):76–78 (www.eurosurveillance.org/em/v11n04/1104–221.asp?=&langue=02)

Norman I, Ryrie I 2004 Art and science of mental health nursing: a textbook of principles. Open University Press, McGraw-Hill Education, Berkshire

Nursing and Midwifery Council 2007 Standards for medicine management. NMC Publications, London (www.nmc-uk.org)

Nursing and Midwifery Council 2006a Consent advice sheet. NMC Publications, London (www.nmc-uk.org/aFrameDisplay.aspx?DocumentID=1563)

Nursing and Midwifery Council 2006b Infection control advice sheet. NMC Publications, London (www.nmc-uk.org/aFrameDisplay.aspx?DocumentID=1577)

Office for National Statistics 2000 National health activity for sick and disabled people: accident and emergency and acute outpatient and day cases 1981–98: social trends 30. The Stationery Office, London

Office of the Deputy Prime Minister 2005 The fire prevention handbook: Essential fire safety information for your home (www.firekills.gov.uk/handbook/pdf/handbook-english.pdf)

Package Travel, Package Holiday and Package Tours Regulations. 1992 HMSO, London (www.opsi.gov.uk/si/si1992/Uksi_19923288_en_1.htm#end)

Railways Act 2005. HMSO, London (www.opsi.gov.uk/acts/acts2005/20050014.htm)

Road Safety Act 2006. HMSO, London (www.opsi.gov.uk/acts/acts2006/20060049.htm)

Rohn LT, Corrigan JM, Donaldson MS 2000 To err is human: building a safer health system. National Academy Press, Washington DC

Roper N, Logan W, Tierney AJ 1996 The elements of nursing: a model for nursing based on a model of living. 4th edn. Churchill Livingstone, Edinburgh

Roper N, Logan W, Tierney AJ 2000 The Roper–Logan–Tierney model of nursing based on activities of living. Churchill Livingstone, Edinburgh

Royal Society for the Prevention of Accidents 2002 Home and leisure accident surveillance system – annual report. RoSPA, Birmingham (www.hassandlass.org.uk/query/reports/2002data.pdf)

Royal Society for the Prevention of Accidents 2004 Home accident prevention strategy and action plan 2004–2009, England (www.rospa.com/ni/info/hap_strat_04.pdf)

Royal Society for the Prevention of Accidents 2005a Home and leisure statistics, RoSPA home and leisure accident web page. RoSPA, Birmingham (www.hassandlass.org.uk/query/index.htm)

Royal Society for the Prevention of Accidents 2005b Mobile phones and driving: road safety information leaflet. RoSPA, Birmingham (www.rospa.com/roadsafety/info/mobile_phones.pdf)

Rutishauser S 1994 Physiology and anatomy: A basis for nursing and health care. Churchill Livingstone, Edinburgh

Royal Society for the Prevention of Accidents 2005c Accident statistics – brief overview. RoSPA, Birmingham (www.rospa.co.uk/factsheets/accidents_overview.pdf)

Scottish Executive Central Research Unit 2002 Domestic abuse against men in Scotland. The Stationery Office, Edinburgh (www.scotland.gov.uk/cru/kd01/green/dvam.pdf)

Smith PK 2004 Bullying: recent developments. Child and Adolescent Mental Health 9(3):98–103

Sullivan PM, Knutson JF 2000 Maltreatment and disabilities: a population-based epidemiological study. Child Abuse and Neglect 24(10):1257–1273

Steevenson G 2006 Informed consent. Journal of Perioperative Practice 16(8):384–388

Thompson J 2001 Health needs of people with learning disabilities. Baillière Tindall, London

Topf M 2000 Hospital noise pollution: an environmental stress model to guide research and clinical interventions. Journal of Advanced Nursing 2000, 31(3):520–528

UNEP/UNICEF 1999 Childhood lead poisioning information for advocacy and action (www.chem.unep.ch/irptc/Publications/leadpoison/lead_eng.pdf)

Walsh D 2006 The challenge of interdisciplinary collaboration: midwifery needs a model. British Journal of Midwifery 14(9):549

Watson JE, Walsh M 2002 Watson's clinical nursing and related sciences. Baillière Tindall, London

Weinert BT, Timiras PS 2003 Invited review: theories of aging. Journal of Applied Physiology 95:1706–1716

Wheatley I 2006 The nursing practice of taking level 1 patient observations. Intensive Critical Care Nursing 22(2):115–121

Williams C 2006 Dilemmas in fetal medicine: premature application of technology or responding to women's choice. Sociology in Health & Illness 28(1):1–20

Wolfson LJ, Strebel PM, Gacic-Dobo M et al 2007 Has the 2005 measles mortality reduction goal been achieved? A natural history modeling study. The Lancet 369:191–200

Wolke D, Woods S, Bloomfield 2001 Bullying involvement in primary school and common health problems. Archives of Disease in Childhood 85(3):197–201

World Health Organization 1999 Integrated management of childhood illness – a joint WHO/UNICEF initiative (www.who.int/child-adolescent-health/New_Publications/IMCI/imci.htm)

World Health Organization 2002a World report on violence and health. WHO, Geneva (www.who.int/violence_injury_prevention/violence/world_report/en/full_en.pdf)

World Health Organization 2002b Children in the new millennium: environmental impact on health. WHO, Geneva (www.who.int/water_sanitation_health/hygiene/settings/ChildrenNM1.pdf)

World Health Organization 2005a Disability and rehabilitation. WHO, Geneva (www.who.int/nmh/donorinfo/vip_promoting_access_healthcare_rehabilitation_v2.pdf)

World Health Organization 2005b Global patient safety challenge 2005–2006, cleaner care is safer care. World Alliance for Patient Safety. WHO, Geneva (www.whqlibdoc.who.int/publications/2005/9241593733_eng.pdf)

World Health Organization 2006a Goal 5: Improve maternal health. WHO, Geneva (www.who.int/mdg/goals/goal5/en/index.html)

World Health Organization 2006b Preventing disease through healthy envrionments: towards an estimate of the environmental burden of disease. WHO, Geneva (www.who.int/quantifying_ehimpacts/publications/preventingdisease.pdf)

World Health Organization 2006c Promoting patient safety at health care institutions (working paper for the technical discussion). WHO, Geneva (www.who.int/patientsafety/events/06/Searo_PS_workingpapers.pdf)

Further reading

Alexander M, Fawcett JN, Runciman PJ 2006 Nursing practice hospital and home. The adult, 3rd edn. Churchill Livingstone (Elsevier), Edinburgh

Brooker C, Nicol M 2003 Nursing adults: the practice of caring. Mosby, Edinburgh

NHS Infection Control Learning Programme (www.infectioncontrol.nhs.uk/lms/nhs_splash/nhs_splash.asp)

Watson JE, Walsh M 2002 Watson's clinical nursing and related sciences, 5th edn. Baillière Tindall, London

Useful websites

www.ageconcern.org.uk (Age Concern)
www.bsi-glogal.com (British Standards Institute)
www.capt.org.uk (Child Accident Prevention Trust)
www.childline.org (Childline)
www.doh.gov.uk (Department of Health)
www.dti.gov.uk (Department for Trade and Industry)
www.directgov.uk (Directgov)
www.disabilityalliance.org (Disability Alliance)
www.dlcc.org.uk (Disabled Living Centre Council)
www.environmentagency.gov.uk (Environment Agency)
www.hse.gov.uk (Health and Safety Executive)
www.healthcarecommission.org.uk (Healthcare Commission)
www.icna.co.uk (Infection Control Nurses Association)
www.IHI.org (Institute of Healthcare Improvement)
www.ilo.org (International Labour Organisation)
www.nspcc.org.uk (National Society for the Prevention of Cruelty to Children)
www.nhsla (NHS Litigation Authority)
www.thinkroadsafety.gov.uk (Road Safety)
www.rospa.co.uk (Royal Society for the Prevention of Accidents)
www.unicef.org (UNICEF)
www.who.int/peh (World Health Organization)

Communicating

Helen Iggulden

INTRODUCTION

Human communication evolved over thousands of years, influenced and motivated by survival and safety needs, bonding needs, social and cultural factors and technological changes. We communicate thoughts and feelings by the activity of nerves and muscles that enable us to speak, write, hear, see, touch and gesture in a range of different personal, social and formal situations.

The first part of this chapter (the model of living) will explore:

- the process of communication
- communication across the lifespan
- biological features of communication rooted in the nervous system
- the role of emotion and other psychological factors involved in the act of communicating
- the influence of social, cultural and educational factors in communicating in different situations
- how the environment influences our communication abilities and patterns
- how legislation and economic factors have influenced the development of human communication.

Each of these sections has exercises, activities and reflective triggers to help you to relate these general aspects to clinical situations.

The second part of this chapter (the model for nursing) then focuses on some case studies, highlighting how communication is affected when people become ill. The discussion uses the nursing process and the application of biological, psychological, social, cultural, environmental and economic aspects.

THE MODEL OF LIVING

The following exercise draws attention to aspects of personal life and professional role. In all aspects three modes contribute to the communication that takes place:

Exercise

1. Think of a practice situation when you needed to communicate with some or all of the following: a patient, nursing colleagues, medical staff, a physiotherapist, an occupational therapist, a pharmacist, a relative, a social workers, a porter and a cleaner.
2. Does your style of communication alter when interacting with others in your professional role?
3. How do your communication styles differ when you are interacting with family, friends and loved ones and when you are interacting professionally?

1. what you say, the words you choose and the tone of your voice
2. the facial expressions and the body language that accompany the words, or the body language used instead of words
3. What you write, the vocabulary you use and its level of formality.

In developing communication patterns as a student nurse, some of the patterns you use will be ones you use already, some will be new to help you in new situations and some will be learned from role models you come across in practice. Students learn this by observing how nurses respond to patients' needs in their interactions with them and facilitate care through interactions with colleagues. The complexities and subtleties of this skilled communication can be made more explicit through models of communication.

MODELS OF THE PROCESS OF COMMUNICATION

Models of communication graphically illustrate both simple and complex communication activity. Consider the following.

Example

Laura is a staff nurse with an 8-month-old baby and she is keen to spend Christmas at home with her. Gina, the ward manager is finding it very difficult to cover the ward over Christmas.

Face-to-face communication

Laura: Hi Gina [*smiles*]. Could we meet up sometime today to sort out the Christmas off-duty [*pulls a face and laughs*].

Gina: [*Lips tighten, eyebrows lower, no eye contact with Laura, stares at the desk*] Yes of course although I do not know what everyone wants [*with sarcastic emphasis*] yet.

In this situation Laura is getting nonverbal responses from Gina as she speaks and she will probably (assuming she has commonsense and empathy) modify her response when she realises that Gina is feeling quite stressed and anxious about the issue of the Christmas off-duty.

Email from Laura to Gina

Hi Gina, I would be grateful for an early Christmas Eve, day off Christmas and any shift you like on Boxing Day. Please could you let me know ASAP so I can make my arrangements?
See you, Laura

In this situation the email is delivered instantaneously, but Gina cannot give Laura the simultaneous responses. Thus, while a simple communication model will serve for the email communication, a transactional model is more suitable for face-to-face contact and more situations where the subtleties of communication become apparent. A transactional model of communication shows how we make ongoing adjustments to the content, style and manner of our communication. Laura's face-to-face communication with Gina enables her to receive, decode and respond to Gina's verbal and nonverbal behaviour, while at the same time Gina is responding to the fact that Laura has registered

that she (Gina) is feeling bad tempered about the off-duty. Laura is modifying her tone and facial expression as a result (see Fig. 4.1).

Written communication

Written communications can compensate for the absence of nonverbal indicators by using levels of formality, layout, vocabulary, certain conventions of greeting and leave-taking and punctuation. Both formal and informal writing also make use of features such as emboldening, underlining, and italicising to add emphasis. Consider how the meaning is made clear by the use of these conventions in the second of these sentences.

1. pleasedonothaveanythingtoeatordrinkaftermidnightthe nightbeforetheinvestigationbringaurinesamplewith youandbeawarethatyoumayfeeldrowsyaftertheinvestiga- tionandmaynotbeabletodriveacarimmediatelyafterwards.

2. Please do **not** have anything to eat or drink after **midnight** the night before the investigation. Please bring with you a sample of urine.

   BE AWARE that you may feel drowsy after the investigation and may not be able to drive a car immediately afterwards.

> ### Exercise
> 1. What do you think of the overall tone of these instructions?
> 2. Are they clear and unambiguous?
> 3. What questions might still be in the patient's mind?

Although these instructions are perfectly clear when the word spaces, full stops, capital letters and emboldening have been added, they lack a human factor. It would help to have a contact name and details of someone who can answer

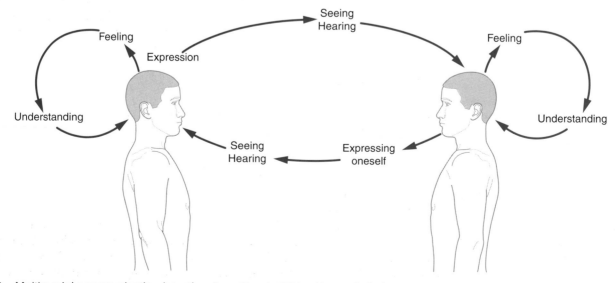

Fig. 4.1 Multimodal communication in action (from Moonie 2000, with permission).

any queries, and it may also help to give some idea of how long the person is likely to be having the investigation so that they can make arrangements to picked up. The instructions, although clear, are written from the perspective of the needs of the investigator rather than the patient.

Electronic communication

The more modern forms of written communication such as emailing and text messaging are already influencing and changing the formality and conventions of paper-written communication. However, the rules governing this form of communication are still in the making, although email packages will often give an e-etiquette guide in the Help menu, and there are 'emoticons' on many packages that show stylised happy, sad or puzzled faces.

Oral communication

The invention of the telephone created a new medium of communication that has developed a technique and style of its own to compensate for the lack of visual nonverbal information. On the telephone, we pay extra attention to the manner of speaking, the tone of voice, the pitch, and the breathing patterns to gain information about the person to whom we are speaking. Telephone contact with patients and their relatives is a daily part of most nurses' lives, and experienced nurses will often perceive and respond to these nonverbal indicators. Blind people also become highly skilled in interpreting the more subtle qualities of voice, whilst someone who is deaf develops a keen eye for facial expression, gesture and lip movements.

Face-to-face communication

Face-to-face communication offers the richest scope for multimodal communication. However, the formal conventions governing board meetings or meetings between heads of state differ very much from those operating in the relationship that develops between nurses and patients. At its best this relationship balances human closeness and professional integrity and is the subject of many nursing theorists such as Hildegard Peplau, Patricia Benner and Pam Smith. Government legislation and regulation by the Nursing and Midwifery Council (NMC 2004) ensure a level of formality and code of professional conduct that clearly indicate the professional role responsibilities (see Chapter 2). Thus, a professional relationship with a patient may be a close one, but clearly differs from the informal relationships with friends and family.

Universal and culture-specific communication

Verbal and nonverbal communication, oral and written communication involve several different parts of our nervous system that help us assimilate overall meaning. There are primitive, instinctive nonverbal behaviours such as crying, frowning, laughing or smiling in all human societies. In fact, some of these may also be seen in creatures fairly close to us in the evolutionary chain such as apes and chimpanzees.

Nonverbal communication can also develop as an integral part of a specific culture within a social group. Some societies (e.g. Italians) use many gestures and facial expressions, while others (e.g. Japanese) use very few. Also and unfortunately, a nonverbal gesture may mean one thing in one society and something very different in another. For example, in France using a finger to pull down the eyelid means that the speaker is aware of something going on, whilst in Italy the same sign means that the listener must become aware. Cultural variations in facial expression, eye contact, gesture and body posture are among the first things a 'foreigner' notices, and it can be very difficult working out what they mean and even more difficult deciding whether one is permitted to use them.

Exercise

Consider the ways in which people communicate when they are angry, sad, confused or excited.

1. What kind of facial and body movements do they make in each situation?
2. Draw figures of facial expressions and body movements to represent these. Compare yours with fellow students/colleagues.

Drawing talent aside, most people will be able to draw a circle with an upturned mouth for a smile and a downturned mouth for sadness. The angry face might have had a few squiggles for frowns and the eybrows flattened or slanted towards the nose and downwards. The confused face might have had a lop-sided or squiggly mouth and a furrowed brow with eyebrows drawn together. While these line drawings are clearly exaggerated, like all cartoons they make a serious point. Nonverbal communication cannot really be taught as a language can – it is more caught than taught and we have all probably developed our unique blend of expressions and mannerisms from childhood, although nevertheless retaining a universally recognisable human component.

Exercise

Now consider the crying of babies.

1. Are there different kinds of crying?
2. How do mothers and others learn to interpret a baby's cry?

A healthy baby may cry between 1 and 3 hours a day, and it takes a new mother about a fortnight to begin to pick out different types of crying in the new baby. At first the cries will usually indicate hunger, boredom or pain. Young babies may also cry when feeling too hot or too cold, they have colic or wind, need a nappy change, are feeling bored and want company, are upset and want a cuddle, or have got overstimulated. Mothers will often explain the timing and the sound of different types of crying, a grizzling sort of cry indicates tiredness and crossness, whereas a higher-pitched screaming type of cry may indicate colic. In fact there is, on the market, a cry analyser. This sound-sensitive device is programmed to recognise different pitches and then digitally analyse and transmit the baby's cry into one of five simple expressions – hungry, bored, annoyed, sleepy or stressed.

Transition from verbal to nonverbal communication

Although primitive man made simple sounds to convey simple messages, as human life became more complex it outstripped the capabilities of this simple system and a pictorial writing developed. Later, alphabetic systems developed which made economic use of symbols. Today there are over 100 major languages (each spoken by at least one million people), and thousands of other languages and dialects. Yet for political and economic reasons English has become the major world language. This is because of its dominance in its former empire outside England, in India, Africa and particularly because of the economic dominance of the English-speaking United States of America. However, in today's multicultural society there are significant trends towards meeting people's language needs in the community, and interpreters are used in health care whenever possible, and signs and notices in hospitals and health centres are presented in the languages spoken in the local community.

The importance of communication between patients, carers and health care personnel has been benchmarked to a standard in the UK and is included in *Essence of Care* (Department of Health (DoH) 2003b). In addition, the UK policies that advocate interprofessional working to achieve good communication are outlined in *The New NHS* (DoH 1997), *A First Class Service* (DoH 1998c) and *Clinical Governance* (NHS Executive 1999). The underlying assumption is that a greater degree of structural integration benefits service users, cuts down on duplication and overlap, prevents gaps in the service delivery, and helps to clarify roles and responsibilities (Kenny 2002, Masterson 2002, Leathard 1994, Ovreteit et al 1997).

Communication, joint working and community care

The increased emphasis on interprofessional working extends to joint working between social services and primary health care, with financial incentives to local councils and health authorities to encourage joint working and help break down barriers between health and social services that can be seen as preventing service users getting the care they need. Joint working has also been encouraged by the development of National Service Frameworks (DoH 1999, 2000a, 2001, 2003a, 2004a, 2004b, 2005a) and integrated care pathways, also known as collaborative care plans. Care pathways began in the USA in the early 1980s, and are used in the UK to facilitate the development and implementation of multidisciplinary guidelines, minimise delays, make the best use of resources and enhance patient care. Through collaborative care the hoped-for benefits include increased collaboration, increased professionalism, more effective clinical care, and improved patient–clinician communication and patient satisfaction.

The skills nurses need to be effective in communicating with patients, relatives and colleagues include the ability to reflect on experiences, develop new perspectives as a result of that reflection and identify what actions to take to develop communication skills further. For many students this activity will be part of portfolio development, or personal development planning, and will help in developing a repertoire of communication styles for different situations. For example, as exposure to other branches it would include using age-appropriate language and nonverbal communication with young children. A further example would be using appropriate pace, tone and verbal style, together with appropriate nonverbal written and graphical supplements with patients whose first language is not English. Good communication skills also involve common courtesy, empathy and comforting skills. This in turn presupposes high levels of self-awareness, listening skills, sensitive and appropriate use of touch and gesture, the ability to summarise and paraphrase information in an appropriate style, and skill in negotiating personal space and proximity.

Such skills are just as important when working as a team member and communicating with colleagues in nursing and other health care disciplines. The strength of true collaboration lies in its ability to overcome traditional barriers such as hierarchies, power bases, professional boundaries, jealousies and insecurities. For nurses to participate effectively in the successful implementation of collaborative care and its associated documentation, benchmarks and audit criteria, interpersonal skills are needed in developing rapport, recognising and addressing conflict, giving and receiving feedback, assertiveness, advocacy and negotiation skills and boundary making skills. The work of Sully & Dallas (2005) is an excellent communication resource.

THE ACTIVITY OF COMMUNICATING ACROSS THE LIFESPAN

Childhood

Theoretical explanations of how babies learn to speak and communicate are mainly the province of psychology and linguistics, but the biological substrate is crucial. Before birth virtually all the neurones and some synapses are formed, and in the first weeks of life babies use them to announce hunger or discomfort and to explore their own bodies. A little later, babies explore two-way linguistic communication. This two-way language is acquired in stages.

The babbling stage occurs spontaneously and babies try out a variety of sounds, some of which are the sounds of human language. In the second stage single words appear, followed by a two-word communication, which can usually be understood by an adult. Longer 'telegraphic' sentences then emerge, which are refined in childhood, and depend on innate language ability and the richness of the child's communicative environment. Deaf children exposed to sign language show the same stages of language acquisition as do hearing children exposed to spoken language (Fromkin & Rodman 1983). Imitation theory argues that children learn their language by imitating an adult. Speech and reinforcement theory suggests that children are conditioned by positive, negative or corrective reactions to their attempts at speech. Neither on its own can fully explain this complex process.

> **Exercise**
>
> In the 13th century the German Emperor Frederick II, curious to know what language children would speak if they were raised without hearing any words at all, decided to conduct some empirical research. Seizing a number of newborn children from their parents, he handed them to nurses with strict instruction to feed them, but not to talk to them or to hold them. The babies never learnt a language. They all died before they could talk. Frederick's experiment whilst failing to find the answer to his desired question had nevertheless made an important discovery.
>
> 1. What do you think that important discovery was? Discuss with colleagues.

You probably guessed right – communication is much more than talking – if true this horrible story illustrates how important the other elements of human communication are – and modern paediatric wards, outpatient centres, clinics and day units all now take into account the child's need for loving, protective human companionships and a rich environment.

Adolescence

One of the marked features of many adolescents is a great need to communicate with their peers, and an increasing withdrawal from communicating with adults. During this phase of development, adults may see adolescents as increasingly 'uncommunicative', or sullen. Adolescents often need more privacy, yet need more social contact with their peers. They develop peer-bonding behaviour such as using their own 'crowd's' jargon, dress code and values. The use of slang, taboo words and cursing reaches a peak in this period of development. Adolescents may take up extreme positions on certain issues and defend those positions with strong emotions, a combination with which it is difficult to reason. Adolescents also begin to learn decision-making through experience rather than someone telling them which way to do things to achieve the best outcome, their attention span grows and their intellectual curiosity strengthens.

> **Exercise**
>
> Greg is 17 and very bright in English, History and German, and he is expected to do well in his A levels. However, at the dermatology clinic, which he attends for treatment of his severe acne, he uses vague words, 'I've done what you said and stuff' and instead of answering the nurse's questions directly, he says 'Well you know what I mean like'.
>
> 1. What skills and techniques might elicit a more specific response? Discuss with colleagues.

It is not always easy to establish rapport with an adolescent during the first visit or several visits. Greg may have a lot of embarrassment about the spots on his face; there may be a number of physiological and psychological factors that contribute to his acne, which may be affecting his social life and his self-concept. Skilful techniques to help establish rapport with him will help him overcome some of his negative feelings. Rapport can be fostered by a range of fairly simple communication techniques. These include introducing yourself, offering to shake his hand, whilst asking a couple of 'small-talk' introductory questions that you know will elicit the answer 'yes', such as ' So you found your way here OK then?' Also a general chat about other topics such as school work, hobbies, interests, etc. will give Greg the chance to talk for a while on topics where he feels more confidence. Listening closely to Greg can be a key to developing rapport, responding to show that his comments and perspective are be taken seriously, and taking opportunities to explore the issues that concern him without lecturing and admonishing him.

Adulthood

In early adulthood people are more likely to interact with people of all different ages through their work, leisure and family activities. Communication skills develop from this as well as from formal training and from experience in applying for jobs and attending interviews. In addition, young adults meet for the first time the intricacies of completing commercial, social, governmental and legal documentation in relation to making claims, purchasing goods, taking out a mortgage and deciding on a pension scheme. It is estimated that 7 million adults who are native speakers have literacy problems, whilst another half a million adults need help with speaking and writing English as a second language (Department for Education and Skills (DfES) 2001).

In early adulthood, the loss of the tremendous physical growth spurt is counterbalanced by the increased strength of maturity and experience and in many cases a liberating financial independence. Early adulthood is often a time when people will travel widely, which may bring them into contact with a range of different cultures and values. In addition, being able to use computers has become a basic requirement for employment in many jobs, and middle adulthood may be a time of mastering new skills. It is also in this period that pressures of caring for elderly relatives, supporting adolescents or child-minding grandchildren can reduce the time and opportunity to go to an evening class to learn a language or pursue hobbies that bring in social contact and interpersonal communication. Nevertheless, the communicative range of people in middle adulthood is probably at its peak, blending all the advantages of experience, education and work.

Later life

Growth and decline are such individual variables that it is unwise to make generalised or sweeping statements of the effects of ageing on communication ability. As a group, however, elderly people are more vulnerable to stereotyping by others than any other age group. Carers may assume that older people have a far greater degree of hearing and comprehension impairment than they actually have. This can lead to inappropriate and mismanaged communication, with a corresponding decline in their psychological and physical wellbeing.

Social contacts often diminish as people get older, as relatives and friends become ill or die, or as other problems such as mobility limit an active social life. Even in residential care it can be difficult to form new relationships, although the social climate and the regular company of nurses and carers can considerably benefit an elderly person's quality of life.

> **Exercise**
>
> Margaret is 88 years old, lives alone and manages to get from the kitchen to the living room using two sticks. She has had a leg ulcer, which has now healed, and you are about to discharge her from community nurse visits. You feel that she might deteriorate emotionally and psychologically once the visits stop.
>
> 1. What kind of questions could you ask to help make a nursing assessment of her communication needs and abilities?
> 2. Consider how you would ensure that her communication needs are met following discharge from community nursing care services.

It may be helpful here to refer to the *Essence of Care* (DoH 2003b) benchmarks on communicating, to the *National Service Framework for Older People* (DoH 2001), and the role of the Primary Care Group or Trust in facilitating seamless care between health and social services.

FACTORS INFLUENCING THE AL OF COMMUNICATING

Biological factors

Despite differentiating cultural, psychological, social and political features, the basic biological equipment is similar in all humans. The nervous system provides the human organism with the ability to:

- survive
- express emotions
- exchange information
- develop and maintain interpersonal and social relationships
- enjoy and share creative and recreational activities.

Neurones

Along with all but the most primitive organisms, the basic communicative unit of the human nervous system is a nerve cell, or neurone (see Fig. 4.2).

Some neurones are sensory (afferent) which transmit sensations such as heat, pain, pleasure, danger or discomfort. Other neurones are motor (efferent), which enable us to act, either consciously or unconsciously, in response to different sensations (see Fig. 4.3).

The millions of neurones in the nervous system are organised into 'neuronal pools' and pathways and are connected by association or interneurones that help process information. These pools and pathways process and integrate incoming information from other pools or from simple sensory receptors in the skin, the eyes, the ears or the mouth (see Fig. 4.4).

Central nervous system

The central nervous system develops from the neural tube. It grows to form the spinal cord, lower brain, mid brain and higher brain. The most primitive reflexes emerge from the spinal cord and lower brain. The mid brain acts as a kind of relay station between the lower brain and the higher brain, and gives rise to emotions. The higher brain analyses symbolic information and gives rise to cognitive and intellectual abilities (see Figs 4.5, 4.6 and 4.7).

The peripheral nervous system

Communication between the brain, spinal cord, trunk and limbs of the body is achieved through the peripheral nervous system. It is made up of 12 pairs of cranial nerves and 32 pairs of spinal nerves (see Fig. 4.8). These nerves are sensory and motor and connect the limbs, trunk, head and neck with the central nervous system. They may operate as a reflex, such as the knee jerk elicited by a tendon hammer, or voluntarily, for example when kicking a ball.

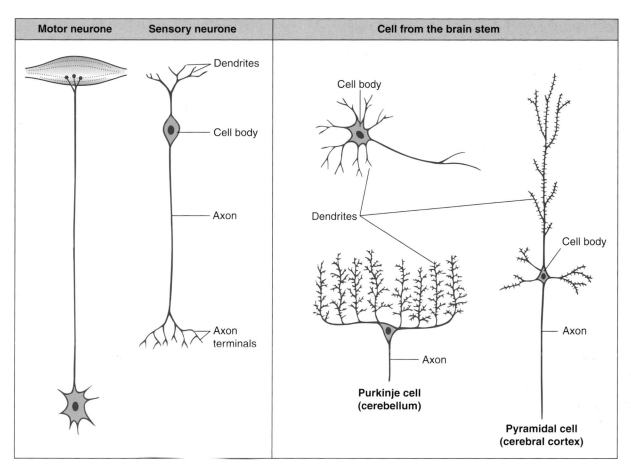

Fig. 4.2 Sensory and motor neurones – the basic unit of communication (from Kindlen 2003, with permission).

Thus the links may be very primitive at the level of reflex action (see Fig. 4.9) or may be part of a chain of complex responses that involve a whole range of neuronal pools and pathways as part of the 'decision tree'. This is best illustrated in Fig. 4.10.

The autonomic nervous system

The autonomic nervous system is part of the central nervous system and the peripheral nervous system, although it is often described separately. It regulates unconscious processes such as heart rate, smooth muscle contraction, blood pressure, respiration rate and glandular secretion, keeping these processes balanced. It does this by either increasing activity through stimulation of the structures by the sympathetic branch or by decreasing activity in the structures through inhibition by the parasympathetic branch. The main exception is that the parasympathetic branch actually stimulates digestive processes (see Fig. 4.11).

Blushing is a good example of the autonomic system in action. When people are embarrassed they may find verbal ways of trying to alleviate the uncomfortable situation, but nothing can stop the sympathetic system from dilating the blood vessels in the face and neck, giving the tell-tale red hue.

Exercise

Pain is the result of damage to or pressure on a part of the body and can be managed very effectively if the care team have a good understanding and a range of potential interventions to choose from.

1. On a scale of 1–10, with 10 being excellent, how good is your current understanding of pain theory, assessment and management?
2. If you do not score yourself well, refer to the Further Reading list at the end of this chapter and compile an action plan to read and apply the principles and practices of pain management.
3. Undertake a literature search and review of the literature on pain assessment and management.

Vision and the eye

The eyes allow us to learn more about the surrounding world than any of the other four senses and much of the brain is designed to interpret visual information. We see by processing the light that colours, shapes and objects give off, even in dim light (see Figs 4.12 and 4.13).

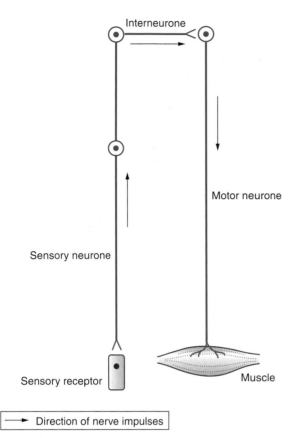

Fig. 4.3 Sensory neurones transmit information to motor neurones, which can then activate muscles (from Kindlen 2003, with permission).

Exercise

Bill has suffered from blurred and dim vision in his left eye. He complains of feeling as if a shadow is passing across this eye, and sometimes experience flashes of light or showers of dark spots.

1. Look up the structure and function of the eye and then explain briefly what a 'detached retina' is and how it might affect someone in the Activities of Living.
2. Write down ways in which nurses can help in communicating with him in view of his sudden loss of vision.

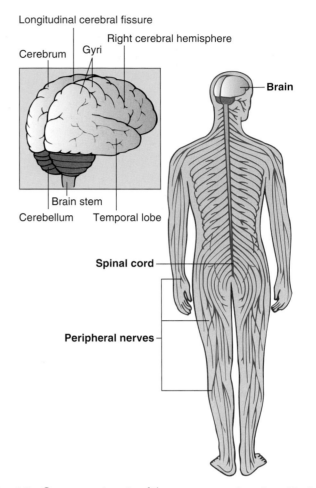

Fig. 4.5 Component parts of the nervous system (from Kindlen 2003, with permission).

A retinal detachment occurs when the retina is pulled away from its normal position in the back of the eye. The retina sends visual images to the brain through the optic nerve. When detachment occurs, vision is blurred. A detached retina is a very serious problem that almost always causes blindness unless it is treated.

When nurses attend to people with an eye injury or problem they may need to overcome the fear many people have of having their eyes touched. Sudden loss of vision can make

---

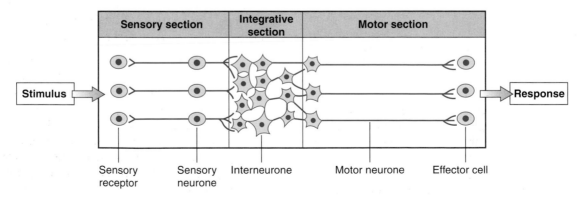

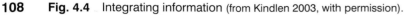

Fig. 4.4 Integrating information (from Kindlen 2003, with permission).

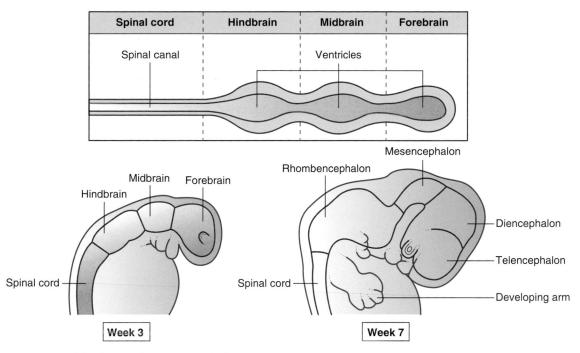

Fig. 4.6 Development of the human brain and spinal cord (from Kindlen 2003, with permission).

people lose confidence and feel vulnerable. They will also have lost visual aspects of nonverbal communication and need thoughtful and considerate help to compensate for this sensory loss. This can be done in simple ways:

- tell the person when you have entered the room or are about to leave
- say who you are
- don't raise your voice, but speak clearly
- approach and leave the patient from the side where vision is best
- put things at the side where the vision is best and in the same place each time
- at mealtimes use a clock face metaphor to describe where food is on the plate
- ask whether they would prefer to eat alone or with assistance.

Hearing and the ear

Although a huge part of the human brain is given over to analysing visual information, auditory information contributes to that analysis. Hearing is the sense used in decoding emotional messages conveyed through voice tone, modulation, pitch and rhythm, which the brain then matches against visual information. Sound enters the system through the external ear (see Fig. 4.14) through to the brain where the sound is perceived, and either understood or not as the case may be. This whole process takes less than half a second. Consider the following case study.

In this scenario the nurse has a responsibility to ensure that the communication environment takes into account Hannah's needs. Her first task would be to find a British

---

Case study 4.1

Communicating with someone who uses British Sign Language

Hannah Jones is 16 years old and is considering embarking on her first sexual relationship with her boyfriend, Phillip. They have known each other for 2 years, are happy together, and are aiming to attend the same college after the summer break. Hannah, who is prelingually profoundly deaf, uses British Sign Language as her first and preferred language.

Hannah has been a patient at the same GP Practice since she was a child. Hannah has rarely needed to visit her GP, and her mother was always on hand to interpret for the GP and Hannah. Hannah now wants to discuss contraception with the Practice Nurse. Hannah has asked her mother not to be informed of the appointment and therefore mum is not available to assist in interpreting at the appointment. The Practice Nurse recognises there is a lot of information to convey to Hannah, and it is imperative that Hannah understands this information.

1. What rights does Hannah have in the situation that could assist her?
2. What ethical issues might arise when a mother interprets for her daughter in a situation like this?
3. What should the Practice Nurse do first?
4. Consider the barriers to effective communication in this case study. Discuss with colleagues and identify your learning needs in communicating with people who have hearing difficulties.

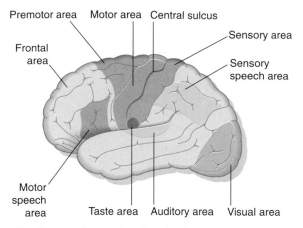

Fig. 4.7 The cerebrum showing the functional areas (from Waugh & Grant 2006, with permission).

Sign Language interpreter for the appointment. The interpreter's role is to enable the nurse and Hannah to converse. The interpreter has a responsibility to ensure that the communication meets the needs of everyone present. They also facilitate understanding across English-speaking and -signing cultures's

Using an interpreter is a process that some nurses find initially difficult because of the third-party involvement. However, some fundamental guidelines can quickly assist the situation.

1. Make sure you can see everyone involved in the discussion.
2. Speak directly to the deaf person not to the interpreter.
3. Speak at your normal speed and in full sentences, do not raise your voice.
4. The interpreter will be signing what you are saying, just after you have said it, so there will be a time delay in the responses from the deaf person.
5. It is good practice to prepare the interpreter in advance of the session, inform them of what they will be interpreting, where it will be, and start and finish times.
6. Be gender aware. In health situations it is good practice to ensure gender-appropriate interpreters are used though the deaf person may have their own preference.

Using a family member for interpreting may place too much responsibility on the relative and may affect the quality of care given to the patient. In addition, the family member filtering the information or not having the requisite signing skills to provide sufficient information to the nurse, doctor or patient could seriously undermine the deaf person's

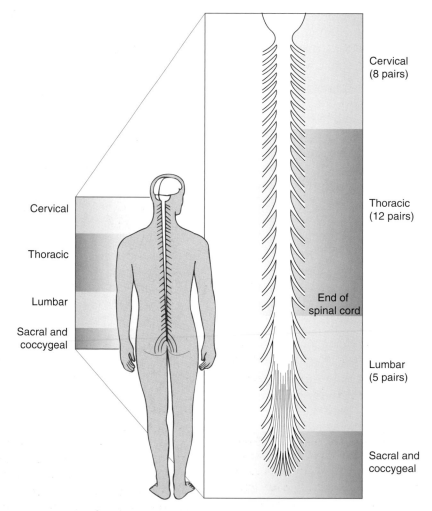

Fig. 4.8 The spinal nerves (from Kindlen 2003, with permission).

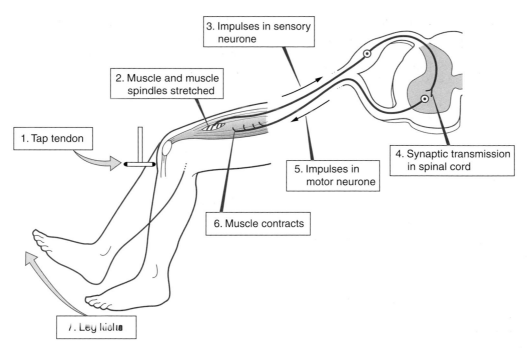

Fig. 4.9 The knee jerk (from Kindlen 2003, with permission).

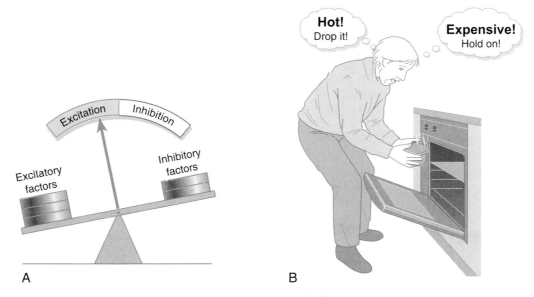

Fig. 4.10 How we respond to a stimulus depends on the balance between excitatory and inhibitory factors (from Rutishauser 1994, with permission).

access to their health information. Refer to the Further Reading for more sources on understanding the rights of deaf people, British Sign Language, the role of interpreters and the British deaf community (Sharples 2002).

Smelling and the nose

Whilst seeing and hearing are highly prized sensory experiences, olfaction (smelling) also exerts a very powerful influence on communication activities at a very fundamental and primitive level (see Fig. 4.15). The sense of smell adds a richness to life that we aren't always conscious of, and as well as giving great pleasure, it can warn of danger,

such as burning or leaking gas, or in food stuffs. Smells are processed very close to the 'emotional brain' (the limbic system) and can have strong emotional associations.

Exercise

1. Think back over your life and jot down any smells that you can remember from your past.
2. With what do you associate these smells?
3. Are the smells pleasant or unpleasant?
4. Do you have a favourite perfume/aftershave?
5. Why is it a favourite and how does it make you feel?

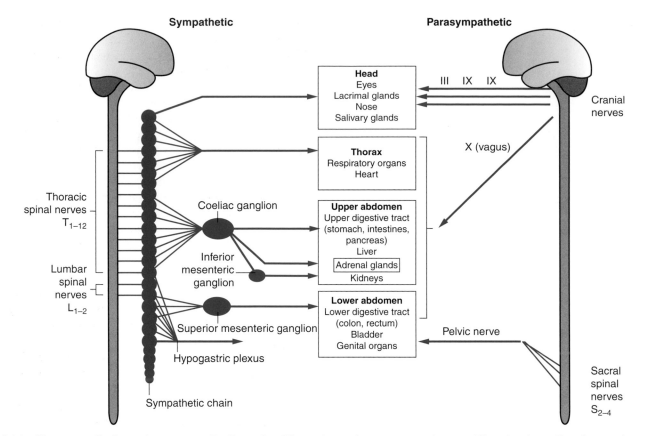

Fig. 4.11 The sympathetic and parasympathetic parts of the autonomic nervous system and the structures they innervate (from Kindlen 2003, with permission).

Perception of smell is of the smells themselves, the experiences and the emotions associated with the smell. In surveys on reactions to odours, responses show that many of our olfactory likes and dislikes are based purely on emotional associations (Millot & Brand 2001). You must have heard people say 'I don't like the smell of hospitals'. Many of us still experience feelings of anxiety at the smell of the spirit that used to be used in spirit duplicators to produce school exam papers (Herz 1997). Pleasant fragrances, however, have been found to have positive effects on mood in all age groups. The thought of pleasant fragrances may be enough to make us a bit more cheerful, but the actual smell can have dramatic effects in improving our mood and sense of wellbeing (Millot & Brand 2001).

In addition to this personal role that smell plays in people's lives, nurses also need to develop a professional 'nose' to help them develop clinical data collection methods. Waste body products of a gaseous, fluid or solid nature have their own normal odour that can change when abnormal. Bad breath, for example, can be indicative of dental caries or gastrointestinal problems, and smell of many toxins and metabolites, such as ethanol and ketones, can be detected on exhalation as the body tries to rid itself of the unwelcome substance. Wounds that are described as 'malodorous' may be infected, ischaemic or sloughing, and should prompt a nurse to establish the cause and

select an appropriate intervention. Faecal matter becomes particularly offensive when there are abnormal constituents or infection. Bad smells are indeed a daily part of most nurses' lives, and in addition to providing valuable clinical data, nurses need to assess how far this impacts on the general environment and whether odour neutralising measures need to be taken.

The sense of touch

When changes occur in the external and internal environments sensory receptors are stimulated. These enable the experience of touch, temperature, pain and pressure from receptors in the skin (see Fig. 4.16).

All these sensations are processed by the brain through the limbic structures, which label them as pleasant, unpleasant, soothing or arousing. The sensation experienced then activates the sympathetic system if the experience is arousing or the parasympathetic system if the experience is calming. General senses are distributed throughout the body and include tactile ones of touch, pressure, vibration, tickle, itch, and thermal ones of hot and cold, and acute and chronic pain receptors. Deeper sensory receptors enable the monitoring of the position of muscles, bones and joints (the sense of proprioception) (see Fig. 4.17). The other senses, sight, hearing, smell and taste, have specialised receptors unique to that organ. Nursing involves

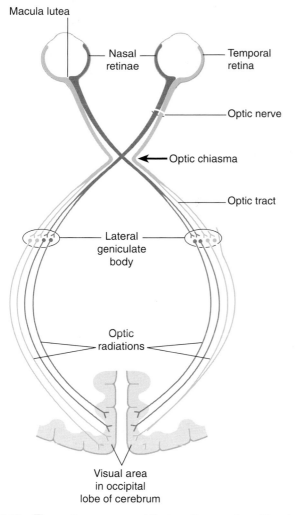

Fig. 4.12 The optic nerves and their pathways (from Waugh & Grant 2006, with permission).

both instrumental touch and non-instrumental touch. For example, palpation of the abdomen may indicate a full bladder or detect a swelling and touch can also establish whether a reddened area is also hot, or to help locate the site of pain. In clinical care it is the sense of touch that over time leads experienced nurses to apply bandages to the correct tension, apply a sphygmomanometer cuff efficiently, pass a nasogastic tube with ease and know how to use touch therapeutically and appropriately.

Speaking and the larynx

The quality of a person's voice communicates a great deal to listeners. A voice is often as unmistakable a signature as a face or laughter. Whether we intend to let people know what we are feeling or not, our voices often give us away. The larynx, or voice box, is an organ in the neck that plays a crucial role in speech and breathing (see Figs 4.18 and 4.19) and is the point at which the respiratory and digestive tract splits into two separate pathways. It is very sensitive to touch, and foreign bodies such as crumbs, produce a protective cough, a response which can be damaged by brain injury or stroke. Nurses will often use clues in a person's voice to infer what kind of emotional state the person is in, and again also to collect clinical data and give clinical care. For example, a wet or gurgling sounding voice may indicate a swallowing problem, which if not detected quickly could lead to a chest infection through aspiration pneumonia, and a very weak voice may indicate respiratory problems or neurological problems as well as an emotional state. In either case, good interdisciplinary care would indicate that these nursing observations be referred on to the speech and language therapist and the physiotherapist for assessment and hopefully thereby avert a worsening of the symptoms. In interacting with patients

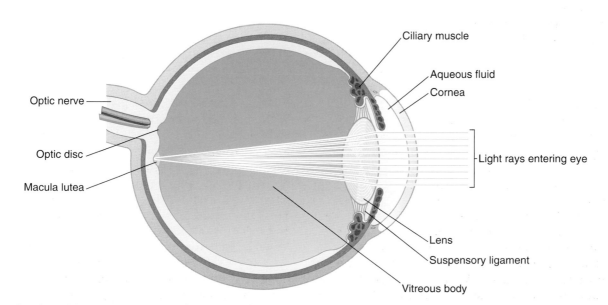

Fig. 4.13 Section of the eye showing the focusing of light rays on the retina (from Waugh & Grant 2006, with permission).

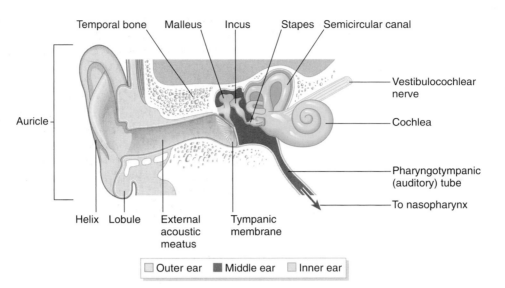

Fig. 4.14 Structures through which sound passes before entering the brain (from Waugh & Grant 2006, with permission).

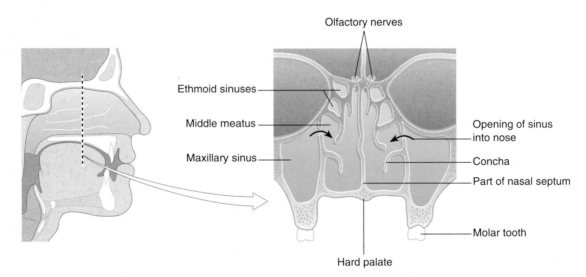

Fig. 4.15 Structures involved with sense of smell (olfactory receptors) (from Kindlen 2003, with permission).

and relatives, nurses can also use their voice quality to communicate care and empathy, and invite discussion and negotiation on care.

Exercise

Consider the structure and function of the larynx.

1. In what ways do you think communication might be affected in a person with a tracheostomy?

A tracheostomy is a surgical opening in the trachea by cutting the neck below the Adam's apple, below the vocal cords. A tube is placed in the opening, and air is inhaled and exhaled through the tube rather than through the mouth and nose. If the tube allows some air to escape and pass over the vocal cords, the patient may be able to speak by holding a finger over the tube or a specially designed speaking tube may be inserted.

Carers and family members may become frustrated because they do not know the needs and wants of the patient. The patient can feel isolated and alone at a time when his or her life is undergoing dramatic change. Choosing the options that best meet the whole needs of the patient is an interdisciplinary matter. Physicians, nurses, respiratory therapists, dietitians, speech and language therapists and others work together to choose the options that best meet the patient's total health needs. The speech and language pathologist can assess the patient's cognitive and language abilities to determine communication potential, evaluate swallowing functions, and assess the patient's ability to produce voice in different situations that may include using a speaking valve. Many health care trusts already have

inefficient. This happens because high arousal interferes with communication between the analytical and emotional parts of the brain. People in these situations may appear 'stupid' or irrational.

Most people have experienced this phenomenon when, for example, sitting an exam, going for a job interview or taking a driving test. Until the 1990s, intelligence was measured solely by cognitive outputs. Emotional intelligence as defined by Goleman (1996, p. 317) refers to 'the capacity for recognising our own feelings and those of others, for motivating ourselves and for managing emotions well in us and in our relationships'. He identifies five basic emotional and social competencies and argues that people with emotional intelligence demonstrate particular qualities to a high degree (see Box 4.1).

The more traditional meaning of intelligence, which used to be measured by IQ tests, is closely related to deductive reasoning based on symbolic knowledge such as numbers for numerical reasoning, words for verbal reasoning, and formal shapes and representational pictures for perceptual reasoning. These tests are also used to assess cognitive and perceptual states following a brain injury of some kind. There are dangers in relying solely on test batteries as indicators of cognitive intelligence. It is more common now to appraise how a person's mind processes information

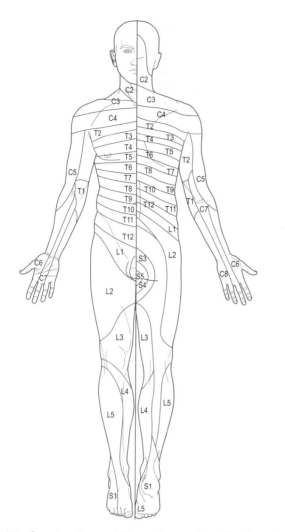

Fig. 4.16 Sensing the world through our skin – the dermatome area (from Kindlen 2003, with permission).

an integrated pathway or a collaborative care plan for all patients with a tracheostomy, regardless of the cause for which it has been performed to ensure this interdisciplinary approach.

Psychological factors

Psychological factors in communication include both cognitive and emotional components. The cognitive rational mind works through words and the emotional mind generally works nonverbally. One rule of thumb used in communications is that probably as much as 90% of an emotional message is communicated through tone of voice, facial expression, gestures and subtle differences in body posture and movement. People receive and respond to these messages almost unconsciously. Good nurses are particularly skilled in noticing nonverbal signs of anxiety for example, and may give more weight to these if a person denies feeling anxious. Even if a patient's first language is English, the high level of emotional arousal can render processing information at a cognitive level

---

Box 4.1	Five basic emotional and social competencies

Self-awareness
Knowing what we are feeling in the moment, and using those preferences to guide our decision making having a realistic assessment of our own abilities and a well-grounded sense of self-confidence.

Self-regulation
Handling our emotions so that they facilitate rather than interfere with the task at hand; being conscientious and delaying gratification to pursue goals; recovering well from emotional distress.

Motivation
Using our deepest preferences to move and guide us toward our goals, to help us take the initiative and strive to improve, and to persevere in the face of setbacks and frustrations.

Empathy
Sensing what people are feeling, being able to take their perspective, and cultivating rapport and attunement with a broad diversity of people.

Social skill
Handling emotions in relationships well and accurately reading social situations and networks interacting smoothly; using these skills to persuade and lead, negotiate and settle disputes, for cooperation and teamwork.

Adapted from Goleman (1996).

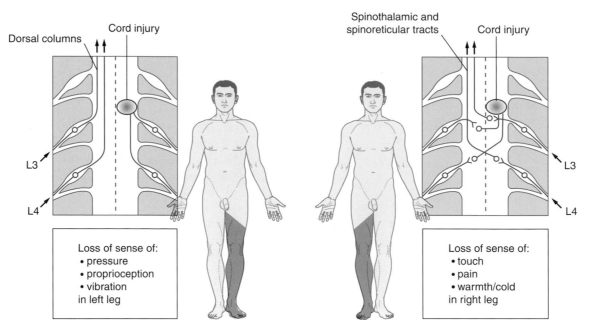

Fig. 4.17 Effects of an area of injury on one side of the spinal cord on sensation in the legs. Note that both legs are affected but in different ways (from Kindlen 2003, with permission).

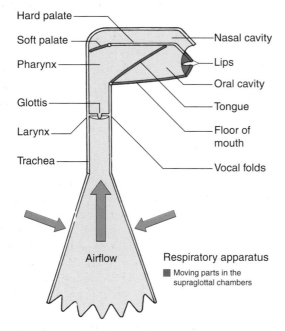

Fig. 4.18 The vocal instrument (from Kindlen 2003, with permission).

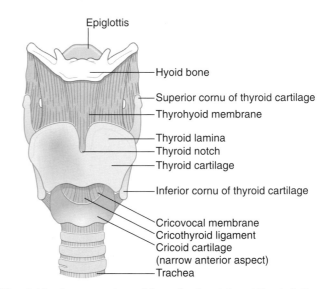

Fig. 4.19 Larynx – viewed from the front (from Waugh & Grant 2006, with permission).

and handles data in a variety of real-life situations, looking for problem-solving abilities of different kinds. This type of intelligence is built up through experience as well as through formal education and a bright mind 'discovers' new associations and comes up with original ideas and hypotheses. Intelligence in this sense also implies a rich and complex network of neuronal pools and circuits, with new synapses being developed all the time rather than staying static. There is, however, a strange exception to the idea of overall intelligence in a group of people rather insultingly called *idiots savants*. Defined as people with severe learning disabilities with a very low score in IQ tests, *idiots savants* have truly remarkable specific abilities such as in mental arithmetic, or in the ability to reproduce with startling accuracy ornate buildings seen only once, or a piece of music heard only once! Therefore, a single definition of 'intelligence' remains elusive and different kinds of intelligence need to be appreciated.

It was mentioned earlier in this chapter how integral self-awareness is to empathic and effective nursing. Communication is clearly dynamic, and it is important that a nurse has the skill to self-regulate, so that a negative attitude or mood does not adversely affect a patient's trust or confidence to communicate. The nature of nursing assessment across all the activities of living means that very personal and intimate questions can be asked and it must be clear that the motive for the question is that the information is needed to help plan effective care and not just for nosiness. Conveying this altruistic motivation presupposes empathy, self-regulation and social skill. It involves being self-aware to the point where little gestures of irritation, impatience or boredom are suppressed, since socially skilled people know that these are picked up unconsciously by others but can strongly influence the nature of the interaction.

Sociocultural factors

Crystal (1992, p. 37) states:

> *There is considerable overlap between the psychological, social and cultural aspects of our existence. People indicate psychological identity such as personality, intelligence, emotional state, and attitude through communication and interpersonal relations. Geographical identity comes from language, accent, and dialect and national, ethnic and cultural identity through language, dress, customs, beliefs, and values.*

In addition, social identity is indicated in terms of social stratification and social class, social role, and even gender through speech and language. From a growing body of sociolinguistic research, it is clear that we all make subtle, intricate and pervasive judgements about people based upon the way they speak (Trudghill 2001).

The 'languages' of health care clearly differentiate between different professions involved in health care. Nurses, doctors, occupational therapists, physiotherapists, speech and language therapists and other specialists develop their own professional language or 'jargon', often incomprehensible to others outside the profession. Medical terms, for example, are not so much professional jargon as ancient Greek or Roman. Most anatomical terms are taken directly from Latin and Greek and when translated into English are not at all mysterious.

It is possible to work out the meaning from the stems given: too many fats in the blood, too many red cells in the blood, study of cells and study of blood. If you learn the meanings of terms in this way, by trying as much as possible to get the meaning from roots, common beginnings and common endings they will be much easier to remember. There is a good section in Siviter (2005) on cracking the code of medical terminology. However, profession-specific terminology can continue to challenge interprofessional working, and the language used in interprofessional or collaborative care pathways needs to be very carefully agreed.

Terminology can also colour people's thinking, which is one of the reasons why there is regular debate and changes in terminology to try to ensure that it has no judgemental or pejorative overtones (Dumbleton 1998).

Nurses need to be able to use their understanding of medical terminology to liaise with the medical team and to be able to communicate with patients in a language that patients understand. If nurses are not able to do this, the principles of informed consent and ethical practice are breached and patients cannot be truly involved in care planning. Siviter (2005) warns against ever telling a patient something that you don't understand the meaning of yourself!

Sociocultural differences also operate nonverbally in the form of gesture, eye contact, facial expression, body posture, proximity and dress. There are other nonverbal differences in greeting, in leave taking, and in expressions of emotions such as love, liking, disliking and disgust. Culture, socialisation and the brain equip individuals with a perceptual filter, which can lead to different interpretations of the same event. For example, in Taiwan, blinking while another person is talking is regarded as impolite, but to North Americans it is hardly noticeable (Adler & Rodman 1991). In addition, a beckoning finger in most Middle and Far Eastern countries is an insulting gesture, but not in the Western world. Eye contact also differs in traditional Afro-Caribbean and Caucasian cultures. Caucasians tend to look away from a conversational partner when speaking and at the other person when listening. Black culture does the reverse, and misinterpretation may well occur (Adler & Rodman 1991).

Although there are many differences in body language in different cultures, according to Axtell (1991) the 'ultimate gesture' carries certain welcome characteristics unlike any other single gesture. This 'ultimate gesture' is known everywhere in the world, it is absolutely universal. It's a smile!

Environmental factors

Other environmental factors can influence communication. These include the auditory, visual and spatial features of the external physical environment as well as mental states of attention, concentration and distractibility. Health care settings have design difficulties in creating an environment that is public and private, sociable and peaceful and stimulating yet relaxed. The individual needs of patients with communication problems, and the different preferences people have in entertaining themselves have the potential to generate quite high noise pollution levels. Technology now makes the use of earphones, and networked radio and TV a welcome development in many hospitals. Different types of beds and equipment can also help. People can position themselves for conversation using four section-profiling beds or electronically operated beds. In the home, people can operate doors, switch on a television, radio or lights using POSSUM (an electronic, environmental control system). The system also enables people with paralysis, or much reduced mobility to communicate with others via an intercom system. An adaptation of the security system in shops can help keep people with orientation problems more safe. An armband, which the patient has agreed to wear, activates an alarm to alert staff and the patient that he or she has left the building. Consider the following brief case study.

Case study 4.2

Ethical issues in electronically 'tagging' a person

Sam is a 23-year-old man in a neurohabilitation ward, who is recovering from an assault 8 weeks ago when he sustained a brain injury. He is making a good recovery, can mobilise very well, and is making good progress. He is unaware of danger and has lost his sense of direction. The nurses are concerned for his safety because several times he has wandered outside to smoke a cigarette and then got lost.

1. What ethical and practical issues might be discussed with him about the possibility of using a 'tagging' system?

Electronic tagging is a form of surveillance, consisting of an electronic device, usually on a bracelet, pendant or lapel pin attached to a patient. A building or area of a building is fitted with receptors that sound an alarm when the individual has moved outside the area.

There are two main approaches to the ethical issues surrounding this form of restraint. One approach is the debate between safety and the infringement of civil liberties and the other approach is based on efficacy on tagging as a form of restraint compared with other alternatives. For example, some argue that on balance, electronic tagging allows more freedom of movement over a wider area and more 'personhood' than the alternatives of specialised and restrictive units. Others argue that if care was properly supported, adequately staffed and funded the use of these devices could be lessened if not eliminated and fear that they may be used as a cheap alternative to adequate staffing levels.

High-tech environments, such as Intensive Care Units, or Accident and Emergency Units can also make difficult and awkward communication environments. They often have very little daylight, windows are high, there is little to connect patients with the outside world, and high-tech equipment creates a disturbing background of hums, bleeps and sighs. This physical environment further compromises ease of conversation and the communication climate for example:

> 66 *The term communication climate refers to the emotional tone of a relationship as it is expressed in the messages that the partners send and receive. A climate does not involve specific activities as much as the way people feel about each other as they carry out those activities.* 99
> (Adler & Rodman 1991, p. 157)

Positive climates are characterised by value-affirming behaviour by the people in that environment such as praising and complimenting, showing appreciation, acknowledging by a wave or a smile, or listening attentively.

This is the sort of activity that could be carried out as part of your reflective practice, portfolio development and action planning to develop your communication skills in specific ways. It will be different on each ward, but by asking yourself these questions it may be possible to identify the common features in placements where the communication

Box 4.2	Communication behaviours
Confirming	**Disconfirming**
Sincere praise	Insults (even in fun)
Compliments	Humiliates
Acknowledging others, waving, smiling	Failing to return phone call, letter, greeting
Listening attentively	Interrupting, irrelevant, or ambiguous responses
Smiles	
Laughter	Frowns and scowls
Humour	

Adapted from Adler & Rodman (1991).

climate was good. For example in a ward or community setting where the team works well together you would probably identify that most of the behaviours fell on the side of confirming, and you might notice a positive correlation with this and the attitude towards patients and the patients' attitudes towards the staff. Good placement experiences of this type need to be analysed to try and 'unpack' the ingredients that make up the good communication climate.

Politicoeconomic factors

Political and economic factors influence health care and the quality of health care. These include government health policy such as the NHS Plan 2000, pay and spending decisions, health care reforms and auditing frameworks such as the Commission for Health Improvement. The UK Department of Health website (www.doh.gov.uk) gives comprehensive information on all of these aspects. However, health care is also influenced by nonspecific legislation relating to human rights. For examples see Box 4.3.

The Nursing and Midwifery Council (2007) also produces guidelines for records and record keeping, based on the principle that good record keeping is a mark of the skilled and safe practitioner, and that there are important features of content and style as well as legal aspects.

Confidentiality This is a legal requirement embedded in the above acts. The Nursing and Midwifery Council in the Code of Professional Conduct (2004) gives clear guidelines on the nature of confidentiality and how nurses can protect confidential information.

Consent to treatment There is some discussion on this aspect of care in the second part of this chapter, particularly focusing on the capacity to consent. There are also some further reading suggestions at the end of this chapter and the website address of the Department of Health which gives government guidelines on informed consent.

Other politicoeconomic influences are revealed through literacy levels in the community. Under *Skills for Life*, the current government's strategy for improving adult literacy, the following issue is addressed:

Box 4.3	Legislation relating to human rights

1976 Race Relations Act (amended 2000) which makes it unlawful to discriminate on racial grounds. The Act defines racial grounds as being colour, race, nationality, or ethnic or national origins. The Act also makes victimisation and harassment illegal. This would include verbal or physical bullying, jokes, or excluding people because of race or sex. (DoH 2000b)

1998 Human Rights Act which makes it unlawful for public bodies to act in a way that is incompatible with the Articles of the European Convention of Human Rights.

Article 2	Protection of life
Article 3	Freedom from inhuman treatment
Article 4	Freedom from servitude, slavery, or forced compulsory labour
Article 5	Right to liberty and security of person
Article 6	Right to a fair and public hearing
Article 7	Freedom from retrospective effects of penal legislation
Article 8	Right to respect for privacy
Article 9	Freedom of thought, conscience, and religion
Article 10	Freedom of expression
Article 11	Freedom of association and assembly
Article 12	Right to marry and found a family
Article 13	Right to an effective remedy before a national authority
Article 14	Prohibition of discrimination on the grounds of sex, race, colour, language, religion, political or other opinion, national or social origin, association with a national minority, property, birth or other status. (DoH 1998a)

1998 Data Protection Act which declares that all records about clients which are filed will be seen as data, whether electronic or paper. Individuals are given rights, which include:

- The right to know what information is held about them and to see and correct the information if necessary.
- The right to refuse to provide information.
- The right that data should be accurate and up to date.
- The right that information should not be kept longer than is necessary.
- The right to confidentiality – that the information should not be accessible to unauthorised people. (DoH 1998b)

The Department of Health (2002) has also produced guidelines for access to health records requests.

> *Seven million people have poor literacy and numeracy skills, including half a million or more who struggle with English because it is not their first language. People with poor literacy, numeracy and language skills tend to be on lower incomes or unemployed, and they are more prone to ill health and social exclusion.* (DfES 2001, p. 2)

Exercise

1. Why do you think people with literacy problems are more prone to ill health?
2. Find out how health education and health promotion material is made user friendly for people of all ages and ability levels.

People who have poor ability to read may not understand appointment slips, insurance forms, information leaflets, health education brochures, prescriptions and medicine bottles. They are less likely to understand informed consent forms. Often people are embarrassed about their poor reading or writing skills and will conceal the problem in various ways, sometimes by affecting lack of interest. Nurses need to find a tactful way to help their patients to understand written information if they suspect there might be a reading problem, possibly without asking them outright if they cannot read.

The NHS have produced a toolkit to help practitioners to develop user-friendly information leaflets. These can be downloaded at www.nhsidentity.nhs.uk/patientinformation toolkit/patientinfotoolkit.pdf.

THE MODEL FOR NURSING

USING THE MODEL TO INDIVIDUALISE NURSING FOR THE ACTIVITY OF LIVING: COMMUNICATING

This section uses case studies that illustrate a range of communication problems that may arise in clinical practice. The discussion links the components of the model of living (lifespan, dependence/independence and factors affecting communication) with the nursing process.

Assessment and collection of data when taking a nursing history

Taking into account the issues discussed, assessment needs to include the person's physical, psychological and sociocultural background, as well as the impact of environmental and politicoeconomic factors at work in the clinical setting, which affect communication. Nurses need to consider the relative advantages and disadvantages of the structured and unstructured means of gathering information and to differentiate between objectivity, subjectivity and interactivity in communication.

ASSESSMENT OF AL OF COMMUNICATING

The following guideline questions can help structure assessment.

Lifespan

- Are there any potentially relevant factors in relation to the person's age, development, or life experiences that may affect communication style?

Independence/dependence

- Does the person normally need any kind of help to communicate and interact with others in either one-to-one or group situations?
- Does the person have a preferred means of communication?
- What means does the care setting have to meet this person's normal communication needs?
- What sort of family/friend support network does the person normally have?
- How might the current health breakdown affect the person's normal communication style and abilities?

Factors affecting the AL of communicating

- *Biological:* What is the specific health problem and does it present an actual or potential problem?
- *Psychological:* What does the person currently understand about their health problem? How has this affected confidence, self-image, mood, relationships and emotional wellbeing? Does or will the person need help from specialists or other members of the health care team to meet their information, learning or counselling needs?
- *Sociocultural:* What is the person's normal communication style and are there any specific social or cultural factors to be taken into account?
- *Environmental:* How does the care setting affect the person's ability to communicate effectively and meet the needs for company and privacy?
- *Politicoeconomic:* Is the current health problem likely to have a detrimental effect on income and occupation in either the long or the short term? What legal and ethical issues need to be considered?

Consider these guidelines in the assessment of the patients in the following case studies. The first case study explores communication concerning an unconscious patient; the second is complex and concerns a patient who has aphasia following a stroke and whose first language is not English. The third study discusses a patient who has a chronic and progressive health problem affecting all areas of physical, psychological and social life. As you read the case studies, reflect on patients you have nursed with similar problems and relate the discussion of some of the more general points to that patient. This will help to consolidate your knowledge base and develop your clinical reasoning in practice.

Reflect on the data collection tools you use such as structured and unstructured interview, and structured observational assessment; include the less formal, conversational aspects of data collection. Finally, think about how you could use each of the tools to develop a care plan for the activity of communicating.

> ## Case study 4.3
>
> ### Paul
>
> Paul is an 18-year-old young man who has just started at university. It is Freshers' Week; when his friends found him lying on the ground and 'very groggy' outside the Student Union bar they called an ambulance. He is unconscious when the ambulance brings him to the Accident and Emergency Department. His friends arrive shortly after the ambulance.

Assessment of AL using guideline questions
Lifespan
Paul is in his late teens and in the first few weeks of a major life change in leaving home and attending university. However, we cannot draw any conclusions from this or make any inferences, since this may lead to stereotyping. There may be relevant factors unknown to us. For example, he may have a health problem, which has made him very familiar with a hospital setting, or he may never have set foot inside a hospital since childhood. He may have relatives or friends involved in health care which make him more familiar with the environment or service.

Dependence/independence
We do not know whether Paul's first language is English, or whether he has a hearing problem, a speech impediment or a sight problem. We do not know whether he is usually quiet and withdrawn or outgoing and gregarious. Neither do we know anything of his family whereabouts or his social network. The only means people in the care setting have to communicate with Paul on his immediate arrival is to talk to him, hoping he can hear and understand, to move and handle him carefully so that he is not afraid and to try to elicit a response using a neurological assessment.

Biological factors
Unconsciousness may develop from neurological, metabolic or vascular causes or from infection, intoxication or trauma. Whatever the reason, assessment of the conscious level is very important and there are specific guidelines to follow for certain conditions such as head trauma, stroke or diabetes. The full guidelines can be found at www.nice.org.uk. These guidelines are incorporated in the National Service Frameworks (DoH 2001, 2003a, 2005a) and many emergency units have already developed care pathways to ensure patients have access to the best possible care.

Neurological assessment
Although the best primary investigation to detect acute clinically important brain injuries is a CT scan, thorough neurological assessment and skull X-ray may be all that is available in settings that do not have scanners.

In Paul's case a CT scan would indicate if there is any brain trauma; blood results will indicate any toxic causes or other possible cause, as will ECG and other investigations. It may be that the results indicate a physiological problem such as diabetes, in which case the National Service Framework for Diabetes and the care pathway would be appropriate. Although these investigations and protocols will help establish the cause, the role of the nurse is to assess the way in which his altered conscious level has affected Paul in all his activities of living.

There are both structured tools and qualitative methods to help achieve a reasonable neurological assessment. This assessment can yield significant physical data about how the person's nervous system is functioning and what the level of consciousness is. From a nursing perspective it can:

- identify communication problems resulting from neurological damage
- detect life-threatening situations
- establish an initial database from which to develop a care plan, goal and nursing interventions
- compare data to previous assessments to determine change and trends, and to evaluate the effectiveness of the nursing interventions.

The Glasgow Coma Scale The initial tool to use in the emergency (after the Airway, Breathing and Circulatory protocol is carried out) in a patient with an altered conscious level is the Glasgow Coma Scale (GCS). This is a tool devised by two Glasgow neurosurgeons Jennet and Teasedale in 1974 (see Chapters 3 and 13). It is used all over the world and was welcomed because it is a reliable and valid objective measure of the level of consciousness, if carried out by those who are trained in its use. It allows nurses and medical staff to know over time whether the conscious level is lightening or worsening and whether further, possibly life-saving treatment needs to be initiated. The time factor is crucial and the GCS observations may need to be done several times in an hour if the situation is serious. CT scan is indicated if the GCS is less than 13 since injury.

Using the Glasgow Coma Scale This scale is divided into three subscales, eye opening, best motor response and best verbal response (see Chapters 3 and 13). For simple and easy-to-follow guidelines on how to carry this out read Fuller (2000).

Other neurological assessment A full neurological assessment supplements the coma score. Careful neurological assessment indicates his cognitive function, his cranial nerve function, his motor function and sensation. The role of nurses is usually to focus on pupil size, which reveals if there is damage to the nerve that controls pupil reaction. Nursing assessment of limb power can also help assess damage to motor nerves. Nurses record these findings, and an overall trend can emerge as all these things are taken into account.

Assessing the pupils of the eyes The findings of one pupil are always compared to the findings in the other pupil and the differences, if any, between the two are noted.

For an assessment you need a pen torch but before beginning follow these instructions.

- Watch the person and see if they open their eyes spontaneously.
- Introduce yourself and ask the person to open his or her eyes, explaining that you need to assess their pupils using a light.
- If the eyelids do not open to speech, explain that you are going to raise the eyelids and shine a light into his eyes to assess the pupils and that this will not hurt.
- Raise the eyelids with the one hand holding the torch in the other.
- Look at the pupils.
- Are they equal in size?
- Are they regular in outline?
- Are there any holes or foreign bodies in the iris?
- Shine the light in one eye.
- Look at the reaction of that eye (this is called the direct reflex) and then repeat and look at the reaction in the other eye (this is called the consensual reflex).
- The person should be looking into the distance rather than at the light if possible.
- Repeat for the other eye.

Recording the findings This depends somewhat on the type of recording sheets used, but most will ask you to indicate the size of the pupil and the type of reaction of each pupil. Normally the pupils are equal in size (about 2–6 mm)

and two methods are used to record pupil size: the millimetre scale, which is the most common, and verbal descriptors. These descriptors are:

- pinpoint
- small
- mid-sized
- large or dilated.

To record the information using the millimetre scale you need a diagrammatic gauge, usually illustrated on the recording sheet, which shows black circles ranging from 2 mm to 9 mm. Assessing and interpreting pupil size may take some experience before you feel confident. However, reliability always needs to be discussed as any changes can be very significant and must be the result of the change in the person rather than a change of observer. Most recording sheets will also ask you to record the rate of reaction to light in either words or symbols (see Glasgow Coma Scale chart on p. 84).

Assessing motor responses The next step in a neurological assessment is in evaluating motor function. Evans' (1995) explanation offers a good outline of what to look for (see Box 4.4).

Psychological/sociocultural factors

Other sources of information help identify actual, potential, temporary or long-standing problems with communication. Relatives and friends can give such information, and can tell the care team about people, places, activities and interests close to Paul's heart. These personal details can be used to stimulate a response at an emotional level, as these familiar things will have a more arousing effect. Nurses need

Box 4.4	Assessing limb power

Motor function

For a motor response to occur, nerve pathways from the brain to end organs and muscles must be intact. The upper motor neurones originate in the cerebral cortex and end at various levels in the spinal cord, where they synapse directly or via spinal neurones with lower motor neurones. Upper motor neurones are responsible for initiating voluntary movement. Lower motor neurones originate at various levels in the spinal cord and terminate on the muscle. They transmit upper motor neurone impulses or can be part of a motor reflex.

Evaluate motor nerve function by assessing muscle movement and strength.

Start by having the patient simultaneously squeeze both of your hands with his hands. Evaluate the strength of the grip in both hands; document his grip as equal or unequal, strong or weak. Evaluate subtle extremity weakness and problems with proprioception by checking for arm drift. Have the patient stand with his hands extended outward (perpendicular with the body with palms up) and with his eyes closed. An affected

arm slowly drifts down. In the comatose patient strength and grip cannot be tested voluntarily.

Ask the patient to move all his extremities. Record the presence or absence of movement or any unilateral or bilateral weakness. Determine whether movement is spontaneous or in response to command. Is spontaneous movement against gravity? Can the patient move an extremity against mild, moderate or forceful resistance? An entry might read 'Patient moves all Es in response to command, against gravity and against moderate resistance'.

Testing the patient's motor reflexes reveals the condition of sensory and motor pathways to and from muscle tendons and muscles to the spinal cord and brain. When the clinician taps on a muscle tendon (such as the one beneath the patella) with a reflex hammer, he is observing for an immediate, controlled jerk of the extremity in response to his action. A normal knee-jerk reflex indicates that the neural pathways to and from the spinal cord to the muscle and tendon are intact.

From Evans (1995, p. 10).

to note and pass on to others anything which appears to elicit a response, even if this is as little as an eyebrow flare or eyelid flickering.

Environmental factors

Emergency admissions departments are often busy and noisy and people with brain injury often have impaired concentration. When carrying out observations there should be minimal distractions in the immediate environment. This may mean simply excluding visual distractions by drawing the curtains round the bed or trolley, and ensuring that people are not talking around the bed.

Politicoeconomic factors

In this case, where Paul is unconscious, application of the principle of informed consent needs to be discussed. English law and codes of professional conduct require a nurse to obtain consent from the patient before treatment is given. If consent is not obtained, either verbally or in writing, civil or criminal proceedings could be instituted. In advanced and specialist practice, where the scope is extended, nurses can be involved in invasive procedures and take on extra accountability as a result. In addition, although a doctor may have obtained a patient's consent, communication studies have shown (Dickson et al 1997) that a patient may be confused or uncertain about their treatment choice and turn to the nurse for advice and clarification. This is linked with advocacy, where nurses act in the best interests of their clients (NMC 2004) and explain, in words patients and families can understand, the issues involved. Advocacy is concerned with promoting and safeguarding the wellbeing and interests of patients and clients. The advocacy function is still being developed and discussed and its boundaries are uncertain.

However, in Paul's case it is an emergency. Emergency treatment in the best interests of the patient is lawful without consent if the patient is unconscious or otherwise mentally incapable of valid consent. Emergency treatment may be taken to include all nursing care necessary to prevent significant deterioration.

Case study 4.4

Muhammed

Muhammed is a 72-year-old Asian man who has been admitted with a right-sided hemiplegia and aphasia. A CT scan shows that he has suffered a stroke and when his medical records arrive on the ward it becomes clear that he is also diabetic, and that this has unfortunately not been well controlled. He has lived in England since his early forties, working firstly in the local mill until it closed down 18 years ago, and then as a taxi driver. He speaks good English normally but his written skills in English are poor. His wife speaks very little English but his sons and two daughters are native English speakers. They also speak Urdu, which is Muhammed's first language.

Lifespan

Muhammed has learned to live his adult life using two languages and has been able to use English in his working and social life and Urdu with family and friends.

Dependence/independence

His spoken English is good in normal situations, but people who are suffering from illness or distress are more comfortable expressing themselves in their mother tongue (Robinson 1998).

His written English is less strong and his reading ability uncertain. We know so far that his sons and daughters can also speak both languages, but we do not yet know if the care setting has interpreters available.

Biological factors

The Royal College of Physicians (RCP 2004b) National Clinical Guidelines for Stroke make explicit recommendations for all disciplines involved in the care of stroke patients covering the whole care pathway from the acute event to longer-term management in the community. They can be downloaded at www.rcplondon.ac.uk/pubs/books/stroke/stroke_guidelines_2ed.pdf.

A 'stroke' is a cerebrovascular accident (CVA). The injury to the brain can be caused by a ruptured blood vessel, which is called a haemorrhagic stroke, or by gradual or sudden ischaemic damage caused by a clot or embolus lodging in a blood vessel. In either case some areas of the brain are deprived of oxygen and may make only a partial recovery. The neurological deficit will depend on individuals and which area of the brain has been affected. There may be common deficits in people who have suffered either a right-sided or a left-sided stroke and these are summarised in Box 4.5, but each person is unique and will have a unique combination of care needs.

Box 4.5	Functional differences in right-sided and left-sided hemiplegia	
Stroke syndrome on left side of brain (right-sided hemiplegia)	Stroke syndrome on right side of brain (left-sided hemiplegia)
Expressive aphasia, or Receptive aphasia, or	Spatial–perceptual deficits Denial and the deficits of the affected side require special safety considerations
Global aphasia Intellectual impairment	Tendency for distractability Impulsive behaviour; apparently unaware of deficits
Slow and cautious behaviour Defects in right visual fields	Poor judgement Deficits in left visual fields

From Hickey (1997, p. 552).

123

The World Health Organization (2002) uses an international classification system of impairments, activities (disabilities) and handicap (participation). These are:

- *Impairment:* Any loss or abnormality of psychological, physiological or anatomical structure or function.
- *Activities* (formerly disabilities): Any restriction or lack of ability to perform an activity as a result of an impairment in a manner or within a range which is considered normal for a human being.
- *Participation* (formerly handicap): A disadvantage for a given individual resulting from an impairment or a disability that limits or prevents the fulfilment of a role which is normal for that individual.

The social model of disability, which goes far beyond the physical impairment is discussed under environmental aspects.

Interdisciplinary care for Muhammed

The Royal College of Physicians strongly recommends that the World Health Organization terminology be used as a way of standardising the terminology used between different disciplines, since differences in the interpretation of commonly used words underlie many of the problems experienced in managing patients (RCP 2004a). The World Health Organization International Classification Framework introduces the concept of 'contextual factors' which impact on the manifestation of all diseases. These contextual factors are social, physical and personal, and emphasise that there is a dynamic between the person and the contextual factors. Although interdisciplinary teams may not use the Roper, Logan and Tierney model for nursing, if care is developed along the lines indicated by the RCP (2004a) there are clear compatibilities in the approaches, which should cross professional misunderstandings and promote good collaborative care.

Assessing Muhammed's communication abilities

Goodwin (1995) points out that a language disorder strikes at a fundamental 'taken for granted' ability to communicate. In Muhammed's situation, there are three components of communication to consider:

1. the kind of aphasia he has
2. other perceptual and motor problems which may affect his ability to communicate. He may, for example, have visual problems because of either his stroke or his diabetes and his right-sided weakness may further impair his ability to use written or visual communication aids
3. his normal sociocultural and family life.

Aphasia is the overall term used for a language disorder. Dysphasia is a classification of a type of language disorder, which may be described as receptive dysphasia or expressive dysphasia. Receptively the problem may be auditory (unable to process verbal information) or visual (unable to interpret written information) or both of these. Expressively the problem may be seen as difficulty in expressing thoughts in speech or writing. The different categories are summarised in Table 4.1 but it is important to remember that this rough guide is in no way a substitute for thorough, interdisciplinary, individualised assessment.

Aphasia (or dysphasia) may be accompanied by a perceptual problem called agnosia that makes it difficult to

Table 4.1 Difficulties experienced in different aphasias

Disorder	Clinical findings	Location of lesion
Broca's aphasia (motor expressive nonfluent)	Patient knows what he wants to say but has motor impairment and can't articulate spontaneously. Also patient understands written or verbal requests but can't repeat words or phrases	Frontal (posterior)
Wernick's aphasia (sensory receptive/ expressive fluent)	Patient articulates spontaneously and well but uses words inappropriately or uses neologisms. Also patient has difficulty understanding written or verbal requests and can't repeat words or phrases	Temporoparietal (anterior)
Global aphasia	Patient has profound expressive and receptive deficits and can barely communicate	Temporoparietal
Anomia	When given an object, patient can describe its characteristics (colour, size, purpose) but cannot name it	Parietal, subcortical or temporal
Apraxia	When asked to speak, patient can't coordinate movement of lips and tongue. When left alone he may be able to do so	Frontal
Dysarthria	Patient knows what he wants to say but has motor impairment and fails to speak clearly. Also patient has difficulty swallowing and chewing	Cerebellar or frontal (posterior)
Perseveration	Patient continually repeats one idea or response	Throughout the cerebrum (primarily anterior)

Source: Evans (1995).

recognise familiar objects, pictures or words. There may be some visual neglect, in which case the normal visual field is seriously distorted. There may also be apraxia, which means that the person has lost the ability to carry out planned purposeful movements. So for example, you may give Muhammed a pen to see if he is able to communicate that way. Inability to use the pen does not necessarily mean that the problem is with language. He may have other perceptual problems such as agnosia or apraxia that make it difficult for him to recognise or use the pen.

A speech and language therapist will carry out diagnostic aphasia assessment, using a range of test batteries and techniques. Nursing assessment aims to establish a therapeutic relationship, over 24 hours, meeting both information giving and receiving needs. The overall purpose of a nursing assessment in this situation is achieved through a sequence of more short-term purposes:

- to build a trusting relationship
- to identify positive communication attributes
- to identify effective modes of communication and how and when to use them
- to generate information about communication abilities occurring naturally over the 24-hour period which may help the family and other members of the team
- to build a relationship with the family
- to incorporate the recommendations of the speech and language specialists into the care interventions. (Iggulden 1994)

Benner (1984), through a series of patient vignettes identifies that at a very fundamental level people unable to communicate verbally have essential needs. These include:

- the need to understand
- the need to be reassured
- the need to learn trust
- the need to be involved.

Thus nurses are faced with situations in which the normal channels of communication are disrupted yet the nursing concern to meet the needs has to be resolved despite the inability to use language.

In Muhammed's case it might help to assess his needs when a family member or interpreter is available, making sure that:

- eye contact is made on the same level
- all are seated
- the curtains are drawn round the bed or the door to the room is closed to exclude visual and auditory distractions.

Explain to Muhammed, using facial expression, tone of voice and hand gestures where appropriate that his stroke has left him with some speaking problems and that it is important to establish a way of communicating with him. Note his nonverbal responses to you at this stage. It may be useful to ask a family member or interpreter to repeat your explanation and compare his responses. In order to establish an informal assessment of his verbal communication the next phase should be carried out using minimal nonverbal communication. The stages as outlined below can be helpful.

Assess understanding   Ask him simple questions.

- What is your name?
- What is/was your job?
- Where do you come from?

If he does not appear to understand repeat louder and use the translator.

Test his understanding   Ask questions with yes/no answers.

- Is this a pen? (Show something else such as a pair of scissors.)
- Check the consistency of yes/no responses as this is a vital and basic communication element.
- Give a one-step command: 'Open your mouth please' or 'Please point to the floor'.
- Give a two-step command such as: 'With your left hand touch your nose and with your right hand touch your tummy'.

If Muhammed appears to understand, but does not speak:

- Ask if he has difficulty finding the right word – this can elicit a good nonverbal response.
- Try to engage him in further, more natural conversation.
- Ask him about his job or his family using open questions so that he needs to reply in sentences and phrases.
- Take note of whether he speaks slowly, very indistinctly, or with difficulty or whether his voice lacks variable pitch and tone.

This may indicate that he has dysarthria rather than dysphasia. Dysarthria is a problem with the motor muscles of speech rather than a central problem of language in the cortex. This means that there is a strong possibility that other forms of graphical and symbolic language may be useful. For example, it may be possible to use eye pointing and gestures, as well as written communication and electronic communication aids.

If his speech is clear enough notice whether it is fluent, whether he uses words correctly, or whether he is unable to find just the word he is looking for. Asking him to name all the animals he can think of in a minute can further assess this word finding. The normal is 18–22 but Muhammed may not reach this anyway, as English is his second language. Then ask him to say all the words he can think of beginning with a particular letter, such as t or s. Word finding can also be assessed more practically by asking him to name objects in the room, items or components of clothing, or for washing or for eating.

Ability to repeat His ability to repeat can be assessed by:

- asking him to repeat a simple phrase, e.g. 'Today is Friday'
- asking him to repeat a more complicated phrase, e.g. 'There are 52 weeks in a calendar year'.

Reading and writing ability The final areas to check are his reading and writing ability, although in Muhammed's case his literacy skills were not good before his stroke.

- Use simple everyday tests such as a food menu or newspaper headline.
- Write down his name and ask him if that is his name.
- Ask him to write the names of the members of his family (be sure to repeat this in his native language).
- Document the nursing assessment in the activity of communicating, the aims, interventions and evaluation.

  A sample of such an assessment is shown in Table 4.2.

Interdisciplinary care for communication problems in people with stroke (RCP 2004b)

- Every patient with a dominant hemisphere stroke should be assessed for speech and language difficulties by a speech and language therapist using a reliable and valid method.

- If the patient has aphasia, the staff and relatives should be informed and trained by the speech and language therapist about communication techniques appropriate to the communication disability.
- Where achievable goals can be identified, and continuing progress demonstrated, patients with communication disabilities should be offered appropriate treatment with monitoring of progress.
- Patients with aphasia should have their suitability for intensive speech and language therapy assessed by a speech and language therapist. The trials suggest that the speech and language therapy should be for between 2 and 8 hours a week.
- For patients with long-term aphasia, a period of speech and language therapy intervention, including group communication treatment, should be considered.
- Any patient with severe communication disability but reasonable cognition and language should be assessed for and provided with appropriate alternative or augmentative communication aids.

Environmental factors

Pound et al (2000) suggest that a social model of disability shows that people are disabled not by their own disabilities,

Table 4.2 Suggested care plan for Muhammed

Assessment	Problem	Aim	Intervention	Evaluation
Muhammed attends to what is being said to him	Does not seem able to follow directions by language alone	Muhammed will understand and practise ways of overcoming language difficulty to make his needs known	Use gestures, clear simple speech, hand guided movements and aphasia boards	Record successful communication strategies in communication log-book
He is able to nod and shake his head appropriately and bows his head for thank you or waves his hand		Establish a consistent effective communication system with regard to meeting his elimination needs, nutritional needs and personal hygiene within the first 48 hours, negotiating with him and involving his family	Point to objects to increase his comprehension

Ask closed questions with yes/no response

Respond to his facial expressions by asking for confirmation, e.g. 'Did I frighten you?' | |
| His family say that his facial expressions are very similar to those he used before he had a stroke and that he clearly expresses puzzlement, surprise, annoyance and pleasure | | | | Evaluate his mood through his facial expression |
| He is able to recognise familiar objects such as a cup and a bar of soap and uses them appropriately when handed to him

He is not able to write his name or recognise his name written down | He does not yet recognise the male urinal or the call bell

He is not able to write his name or recognise his name written down | | Teach Muhammed how to use urinal and call bell

Record effective teaching strategies

Refer to speech and language therapist and liaise re interventions | Check continence levels using urinal

Evaluate perceptual function through his ability to recognise and use objects and equipment used in washing and dressing and eating and drinking |

but by the socially constructed barriers which spring up around them. Oliver (1996) identifies that these are:

- Environmental barriers, which in aphasia or dysphasia would include background noise that can make it more difficult for the person to process what is being said.
- In addition, spoken and written language can have a disabling effect if it is too fast, too complex or too vague.
- Structural barriers arise when resources, services and opportunities are not available.
- Informational barriers arise when the information is unavailable, irrelevant or incomprehensible.
- Attitudinal barriers occur when people with a language disorder are deemed to be 'persona non grata' and unable to think or function in any way – the 'Does he take sugar?' syndrome. This was the title of a BBC programme, demonstrating society's and individuals' attitudes towards disabled people as if they were totally incapable. The attitude fosters unwarranted assumptions about dependencies. Such an attitude, although it may be unconscious, and may stem from pity, fails to take into account an individual's abilities set against the disabling effects of society and the environment. Neither is the situation helped by the medicalisation of disability, such as discussing 'the deaf', or talking about people as 'bound' to wheelchairs. The language reflects a patronising attitude, an attitude being seriously challenged by social models of disability and disability rights activists.

The emphasis of the social model of disability can be compared with the other main 'individual' model as shown by Oliver (1996) in Table 4.3. Pound et al (2000) also discuss research evidence from sufferers themselves to support this view (see Box 4.6).

Box 4.6	Research evidence and aphasia

The subjective experience of people with language impairments has been relatively little explored. Reasons for the exclusion of people who are 'inarticulate' from social research seem complex and are not yet fully understood. Certainly, in terms of aphasia, personal stories have largely been used as material for 'expert' commentary, although this is now starting to change. The research project by Parr et al (1997) (cited in Pound et al (2000)) explored the consequences and significance of acquired language impairment from the perspective of the people who have it. The study set out to examine the personal perspectives on aphasia within a social, economic and political context. Fifty people with long-term aphasia took part in in-depth interviews in which they described the onset of aphasia; its consequences for employment, education, leisure and social life and personal relationships; their access to information; their experience and evaluation of health, welfare and social care services; their perceptions and understanding of disability. The findings from this qualitative study indicated that aphasia is experienced as a complex, dynamic process which influences every domain of social functioning, and affects the individual at a number of different levels – as someone who interacts with others, as a member of groups and communities and as a citizen.

From Pound et al (2000, pp. 11–12).

It becomes much clearer in the light of how disabling aphasia can be that a social model of disability really gets to the heart of the impact of aphasia on an individual and the family.

Sociocultural factors

Gerrish (2001) points out that a recurrent concern arising from examining the provision of health care to ethnic minority persons relates to the problems that develop when the health care practitioner and the patient do not speak the same language. Whilst it is true that Muhammed does normally speak English, he does have literacy problems and as Robinson (1998) suggests, when ill, people will tend to revert to their first language. Of the 6% of the population in the UK who are from an ethnic minority background, people from South Asia and African-Caribbean backgrounds form the largest communities (Office of Population Censuses and Surveys 1991). The level of ability to speak, read and write English varies considerably, but what is of greater significance perhaps is the extent to which stereotyping can influence our relationships with patients and their families. Robinson (1998, p. 137) explains that:

> 66 *A number of stereotypes operate in the encounter between black people and the state welfare agencies. These are stereotypes of African Caribbeans as aggressive,*

Table 4.3 A comparison of individual and social models of disability

Individual model	Social model
Personal tragedy	Social oppression
Personal problem	Social problem
Individual treatment	Social action
Medicalisation	Self-help
Professional dominance	Individual and collective responsibility
Expertise	Experience
Adjustment	Affirmation
Individual identity	Collective identity
Prejudice	Discrimination
Behaviour	Attitudes
Care	Rights
Control	Choice
Policy	Politics
Individual adaptation	Social change

From Oliver 1996 Understanding disability – from theory to practice. Macmillan, London, cited in Pound et al (2000, p. 9).

excitable and defiant, and images of Asian people as meek, passive and docile. One common stereotype assigned to Asians by whites is that Asian culture is dominated exclusively by men, women playing a dependent, submissive role ... although the wife of a family patriarch pays a formal, and often perfunctory deference to her husband, especially in front of strangers, she may exercise considerable domestic power, not merely among the other women of the household, but with her husband, and she often makes many of the vital decisions affecting the family's interests. 99

One stereotyped image which exists about Asian people is that 'they do not speak English'. However, a large proportion of the Asian community speaks English as a second language and many people speak two or three languages as well as English. Asian women who do not work outside the home and older Asians who migrated to Britain in their later years are more likely not to speak English. Muhammed does speak English, yet he may still need the help of an interpreter at this vulnerable time. Robinson (1998, p. 94) outlines some of the issues involved:

66 *In another study of social and health authority services 38 social services departments (SSDs) and 39 health authorities (DHAs) for elderly people from black and minority ethnic communities, ... half of both the SSDs and DHAs used no specifically funded interpreting services merely relying on families, phrase books or cards, or volunteers from their staff or community groups .... In an earlier survey of health authorities, all the respondents mentioned language as a major obstacle to health care.* 99

There are, however, general difficulties in using trained interpreters, untrained interpreters, and family members including:

- the possibility of bias as communication is dependent on a third party
- meanings can be changed in the process of translation.

The messages that leave both the practitioner and patient have the potential to be modified and changed by the interpreter.

- Interpreters are sometimes unfamiliar with the terminology used.
- Interpreters might wrongly reinterpret the patient's ideas, or abbreviate responses.
- An interpreter's presence may embarrass the patient when the problem is perceived as a taboo subject.
- Breach of confidentiality is a serious issue – some Asians reject interpreters who belong to the same community.

These last two will probably relate to Muhammed, particularly as it has been suggested that his family assist in helping to assess his communication needs (see Box 4.7).

Box 4.7	Family as interpreters

The role and practice of interpreters have become increasingly professionalised over the last decade or so. There is now a stress on codes or guidelines for standards of behaviour and practice. These include: maintaining impartiality and avoiding prejudice, fidelity to meaning in interpreting, intervention only for the purposes of clarification, maintaining confidentiality. These are not a complete match with the qualities that people who need interpreters value.

People with little English usually need to use a professional interpreter at some stage, when they cannot draw on their informal networks or in circumstances such as serious medical or legal matters. People recognise that knowledge of service procedures and specialist terms is beneficial, but they see the role of interpreter as involving more than the transfer of words across languages. In particular, they place an emphasis on the interpreter being proactive on their behalf, and especially on their personal character, attitude and trustworthiness. They want the advantages of familiarity and knowledge of the person who is acting as interpreter for them.

In sum, people want either a family member or friend who has professional skills and expertise, and who demonstrates some of the qualities evident in professional codes of good practice, or a professional interpreter who fulfils the obligations inherent in their role and is a proactive and familiar person.

From Alexander et al (2004).

Politicoeconomic factors

There are several issues here in relation to capacity to consent and ensuring privacy and dignity. The Mental Capacity Act (DoH 2005b) provides a statutory framework to empower and protect vulnerable people who are not able to make their own decisions. It makes it clear who can take decisions, in which situations, and how they should go about this.

The whole Act is underpinned by a set of five key principles:

- a presumption of capacity – every adult has the right to make his or her own decisions and must be assumed to have capacity to do so unless it is proved otherwise
- the right for individuals to be supported to make their own decisions – people must be given all appropriate help before anyone concludes that they cannot make their own decisions
- that individuals must retain the right to make what might be seen as eccentric or unwise decisions
- best interests – anything done for or on behalf of people without capacity must be in their best interests
- least restrictive intervention – anything done for or on behalf of people without capacity should be the least restrictive of their basic rights and freedoms.

Also, in assessing competence there are seven main aspects to consider:

- Is the environment conducive to decision making?
- What is the person's cognitive function and is it stable over time?
- How does the person cope with activities of daily living?
- Has the person been adequately informed and has the information been understood?
- Is the person's frame of mind conducive to decision making?
- What is the health professional's frame of mind?
- What family and social factors are at work?

In considering these questions Muhammed's initial nursing assessment shows some situations in which he would be able to indicate his wishes by nonverbal means, using gesture and facial expression. However, in other situations, particularly where there are no visual or concrete clues to offer him, such as when discussing his options for the future, the situation is more complex. The role of the nurse here is to work with Muhammed, his relatives and other members of the multidisciplinary team in reaching decisions which are in his best interests, i.e. in maintaining and furthering his health and welfare.

Privacy is also an area to consider for Muhammed. By virtue of the fact that he has aphasia or may need interpreters and the family to support his communication, he loses control over what people can know about him. For this reason, if at all possible, it is better to limit the number of people involved in assisting his communication, and to discuss with those who do, the confidentiality clause under which health care professionals work.

Finally in respect of both politicoeconomic factors and sociocultural factors, it is a sad fact that racism is widespread in the UK (Archibald 2000) and that racism is a major problem in the health service as a whole. Institutional racism, as Macpherson (1999) sees it, is the collective failure of an organisation to provide an appropriate and professional service to people because of their colour, culture or ethnic origin. He warns that it can be seen or detected in processes, attitudes and behaviour through unwitting prejudice, ignorance, thoughtlessness or racial stereotyping which disadvantage ethnic minority people.

A study undertaken by Tod et al (2001), although limited, found that in cardiac rehabilitation services there was poor access and use of interpreting services and that use of written material did not take into account patient literacy skills and concludes that 'the low uptake of cardiac rehabilitation education group may well be exacerbated by these communication problems identified' (p. 1031).

Communication standards for Essence of Care (DoH 2003b) and Muhammed

For Muhammed there are a number of factors that could make it challenging to achieve the standards set in the *Essence of Care* (DoH 2003b) document. These relate in particular

to the standards relating to his communication needs and his needs in relation to privacy and dignity. These standards do, however, promote holistic care for Muhammed and the use of the model in care planning with him and his family, and the interdisciplinary team takes into account specialist guidance on best practices as well as generic standards set by the *Essence of Care* (DoH 2003b).

Case study 4.5

Fiona

Fiona is a 38-year-old woman who developed multiple sclerosis (MS) 5 years ago. The progress of the disease has been very rapid in that time and she has needed help to support her in most of the Activities of Living. Every morning she has assistance from a carer to help her to wash, dress and prepare her and the children's breakfast. She is able to eat and drink independently as long as the shopping and food preparation is well thought out and of a suitable consistency and temperature. She is continent and uses self-catheterisation and a bowel management programme to maintain this. She can walk with the assistance of two sticks on good days, but can barely stand on bad days, on which occasions she uses a wheelchair.

Her relapse this time has brought her into hospital for further therapy and a review of her situation. She works two mornings a week teaching in the school at which she used to work full time before her illness. However, this current relapse has meant she has not been able to do this for the last 3 weeks. She separated from her husband 6 years ago and he has since remarried. Her two children are ten and eight; Fiona lives near her married sister and her mother who help her willingly. On this occasion Fiona is experiencing fatigue, she's very low in mood, tearful and feels that she is a nuisance to everyone. She fears that she won't be able to keep her job up much longer as the relapse has made it difficult to use the computer keyboard or control her handwriting. In addition, her speech is indistinct.

Lifespan

Up until 5 years ago Fiona had experienced a life of normal development of growth through babyhood, childhood, adolescence and young adulthood. She is well-educated and obviously intelligent and still works as a primary school teacher. However, Fiona has had very strong pressures on her coping mechanisms as she realises that her expectations and beliefs about her life and her future have been powerfully affected since the onset of her illness. As a mother she has not only the responsibilities of a single-parent family, she has the extra difficulties brought on by neurological diseases, which have affected her independence.

Dependence/independence

The Long-term (Neurological) Conditions National Service Framework (NSF) was launched in March 2005. The NSF aims to transform the way health and social care services support people to live with long-term neurological conditions.

Although Fiona has lost absolute independence over the last 5 years, with suitable support and equipment she has been able to maintain her independence in her home and working life and in her activities of daily living. This is a very positive aspect of her character and can be built on during this time when she is feeling very low. Even so, the fact that she has lost some motor control which interferes with her writing may mean she has lost the motor control for other ALs such as self-catheterisation, which she used to maintain her independence in elimination. Also the speech problem is a development and it is not yet known whether this will resolve or become an ongoing problem for her. Fiona is facing the reality of less physical independence in the present, and fears that she is moving towards a more dependent and lonelier future, as she physically weakens and loses touch because of her reduced communicative ability. The speech and language therapist needs to be involved. In the meantime, nurses caring for her need to understand the nature of dysarthria and the strategies that may be used to help her, which are discussed in the next section.

Biological factors

Multiple sclerosis is believed to be an autoimmune disease affecting the brain and spinal cord. It is the most common neurological condition, affecting approximately 85 000 people in the UK (Layward 1998). Although the exact cause remains uncertain, the effects on a neurone are that it damages the myelin sheath in which many neurones are encased. This slows down the nerve transmission, making it jerky and erratic. It affects both motor and sensory nerves in the central nervous system, but symptoms vary according to where the damaged nerve is situated. Common symptoms based on Graham (2001) include:

- blurring of vision, or double vision
- weakness or clumsiness or spasticity and lack of coordination of a limb
- altered feelings in the arms or legs such as tingling or numbness
- giddiness or lack of balance
- fatigue which is out of proportion to activity levels
- the need to pass water frequently and/or urgently.

Fiona is suffering from several of these symptoms and there is every possibility that they will resolve. There is a classification system, based on the course and duration of the symptoms, which shows that there is no single, inevitable pathway (Box 4.8). However, each individual suffering from MS will experience it differently and each individual will have a unique experience, although often fellow sufferers can provide support and understanding for each other. In meeting Fiona's needs therefore what is

Box 4.8	The four main types of multiple sclerosis

Benign
With this type the person may experience one attack and then nothing further for ten or more years.

Relapsing–remitting
This type affects 25% of people suffering from MS and goes through cycles of relapse when new symptoms appear, but which then may disappear as remission is achieved.

Secondary progressive
This is the most common type and affects nearly half of all sufferers. It usually develops from the relapsing–remitting stage, and people begin to notice deterioration progressing over time.

Primary progressive
This develops in mid-life and generally follows a progressively deteriorating course from the onset.

important is how she is experiencing her illness at this time and supporting her emotionally as well as physically.

Multiple sclerosis can be difficult to diagnose as there is no foolproof diagnostic test, and once diagnosed no one can predict how mild or severe, relapsing or progressive the course might be. Diagnosis is usually made following thorough neurological examination by a neurologist and other radiological and physiological investigations such as visual- and auditory-evoked potentials, lumbar puncture, myelogram and magnetic resonance imagery. Careful attention must be paid to feelings of fatigue and vague sensory disturbances, as it is these that may cause subtle deterioration in overall ability to function. It is clear at the moment that Fiona is suffering from fatigue. Although there is no 'cure' for MS the symptoms can often be successfully managed using a combination of drug therapy, complementary therapy, and the support of the multidisciplinary team and support groups. These are discussed below.

Drugs The commonest drugs used in the treatment of MS are:

- *Steroids.* These act by reducing the inflammation around the damaged nerve and are commonly used in relapse to assist recovery. They are usually given intravenously for a few days, when the effect is very rapid, or orally for a few weeks, with a gradually decreasing dose.
- *Baclofen.* This works in the central nervous system to calm down spasticity by reducing the neurotransmitters that cause such high tone in the muscles. Its use needs to be monitored carefully to ensure that weakness does not become a problem.
- *Oxybutinin.* This is commonly used because it relaxes smooth muscle and thus reduces the spasms that cause bladder difficulties. There may, however, also be

troublesome side-effects such as dry mouth, constipation, retention of urine and blurring of vision.

- *Amitriptyline*. This can be used in low doses to help alter the person's perception of pain. Pain may be a troublesome aspect of multiple sclerosis when sensory nerves are affected and cause neuropathic pain.
- *Carbamazepine*. This also helps to manage the neuropathic pain of MS and is thought to work by preventing excessive and spontaneous firing of sensory neurones.
- *Beta-interferon*. There are two types of beta-interferon, 1α and 1β. Interferons belong to a family of proteins that help to regulate the body's immune system. It is effective because it regulates the body's immune system against myelin and stops it from being destroyed. It comes in a prefilled syringe and can be conveniently self-administered at home once a patient or family member is taught how to do so. Although not a cure, beta-interferon can reduce the number and severity of attacks, and slow the progression of disability. The side-effects are mild to moderate and include flu-like symptoms such as fever, muscle aches and headache and there may be some irritation at the injection site.

Complementary therapies Complementary therapies treat 'the whole person' and for that reason have not been through the double-blind clinical trials used to assess the effectiveness of orthodox treatments. Also, what suits one person may not suit another, or it may take some time for the benefits or disadvantages of any treatment to become apparent. Acupuncture, acupressure, aromatherapy, cannabis (and the legal issues around this should make interesting reading), chiropractic and osteopathy, herbalism and homeopathy all have reputable organisations which can be consulted to find practitioners.

Support The most important factors in assessment are to establish how Fiona's symptoms are affecting her activities and to make sure that the interdisciplinary team are involved to ensure that treatment is timely and appropriate. The National Institute for Health and Clinical Excellence (NICE) has produced guidelines on several specific impairments.

For example, visual disturbances may interfere with Fiona's ability to read, watch television, or walk and she will need an assessment by an ophthalmologist. Each professional in contact with Fiona needs to assess the impact of her symptoms on her life and activities and implement good practice in relation to her pain, fatigue and dysarthria.

Dysarthria is the term used to describe the difficulty Fiona has in making her speech clear. The physiological processes of demyelination may affect the cranial nerves, particularly the motor nerves needed to produce speech. So it is a disorder of speech, caused by poorly innervated muscles of the lips, tongue, palate and throat. This means that pronouncing words is difficult, and sometimes the person may have slurred, drunken-sounding speech. In fact, the slurred speech of dysarthria is often mistaken for the speech of a person who is intoxicated. The rate of speech may be reduced and the slowed pace may lead listeners to infer that the thought processes are slow. This is not always so, and can lead to deeper problems if the person is treated as if they have cognitive impairment. Sometimes the speech may lack melody and the result can be a flattened speech that can make the person sound bored or depressed and lacking in emotion. The communication problem is therefore not just one of verbal information exchange, it also affects the communication of emotion and the whole interpersonal experience unless other means are developed to convey feelings and interpersonal communication.

In order to help with speech production nurses can:

- encourage Fiona to maintain a good posture whilst she speaks
- get her to use short sentences
- take appropriate breaths and break words up if necessary
- give her time
- phrasing questions that enable her to give short answers
- repeat what she has said to check your understanding
- use other assistive devices such as a lightwriter or communication board.

The important aim is to get the balance right between encouraging her to make herself understood verbally and yet not to allow this to make her feel fatigued.

Psychological factors

Fiona plays several roles in family, social and working life and in this respect it connects her with other women under the same stresses, strains and joys of these roles. However, there are additional psychosocial factors to be found amongst MS sufferers. In a study of 110 people at the National Hospital for Neurology, Ron & Logsdail (1989) found that irritability, poor concentration, low mood anxiety and elation were all seen significantly more frequently in people with MS than in the control group who were people with other physical disabilities. Depression is, however, by far the most common, although this does not seem to be correlated with brain pathology. It relates more to environmental factors such as social stress and lack of support (Ron & Logsdail 1989). Although cognitive impairment can be a feature of multiple sclerosis, it is by no means inevitable. Memory and attention impairments are usually the most commonly experienced problems, and these do tend to be correlated with brain pathology. We know that Fiona is tearful and low in mood, but it would be unreasonable to attribute this to a brain state caused by demyelination. Fiona needs immediate emotional support and it is important that nurses have the skills to offer that through what Burnard (1992) calls minimal counselling skills (see Box 4.9).

There are three main approaches to counselling, and some understanding of theoretical approaches is a valuable addition to basic skills.

Freud and his followers developed complex psychoanalytical theories, which, although they had such a profound influence on Western thinking were based on only

Box 4.9	Counselling skills

Formal counselling requires lengthy training but, says Burnard (1992), all nurses should be taught 'minimal' counselling skills to enable them to help clients with their problems in a positive, therapeutic way. He suggests:

- *Listening and attending:* giving the person one's full attention, and avoiding thinking about the 'rightness' or the 'wrongness' of what is being said – listening without being judgemental.
- *Using open-ended questions:* they usually begin with 'what', 'how' 'when' or 'where' enabling the person to expand on their problems, i.e. questions which avoid single word or yes, no answers.
- *Reflecting:* (a) reflection of thoughts, e.g. echoing the last few words the person has used; (b) reflection of feelings, i.e. echoing to the person, the feelings or unstated thoughts which underline a statement just made. Both need to be used judiciously, not over-used.
- *Summarising:* (a) to pull together disparate strands of conversation and help the person to organise their thoughts; (b) to end a therapeutic conversation while still focusing on the other person's concerns.
- *Checking for understanding*: seeking clarification by asking, e.g. 'Can I just check what you are saying?' or 'You seem to be saying that…'.

From Roper et al (1996, p. 125).

six published case histories that were, from the point of view of his patients, disasters (Dewdney 1997). Behaviour therapy approaches developed in complete contrast to this preoccupation with the unconscious workings of the mind.

Behaviour therapists felt that there was more to be gained by concentrating on behaviour rather than analysing underlying causes of behaviour. Therapists work with the person in a trusting and supportive relationship focusing very much on the here and now. They work with people through a range of techniques to help overcome problems, including anxiety and depression. It is, however, considered as being generally unsuitable in psychotic conditions.

Cognitive therapy, on the other hand, takes the view that behaviour is primarily determined by what a person thinks. This approach is particularly relevant in treating depression where thoughts of low self-worth and self-esteem are a common feature. Counselling challenges negative thoughts and explores the power of imagination, thought stopping and positive thinking to overcome problems.

Another approach emphasises the power of active listening, where the role of the therapist allows the person to talk about their problems, their feelings about their problems and feeds back their understanding of that problem.

In practice all these theories contribute to the helper's approach in finding ways to help the person to find solutions to their distress. Whatever the theoretical stance, therapeutic nursing helps a person to:

- feel accepted and understood and therefore able to talk openly
- develop an increased understanding of their situation
- discuss alternative understandings of their situation
- make a decision about what to do
- develop specific action plans
- carry out those plans with support if necessary
- adjust to a situation if that situation is unlikely to change.

In Fiona's present situation, apart from the possibility of mood changes caused by demyelination, she is experiencing feelings of loss, and apprehension about the future, which have at this time overwhelmed her coping strategies. Nurses can help in a number of different ways in developing a therapeutic relationship with her. Bowles et al (2001) found that this solution-focused brief therapy approach is relevant to nursing and offers a useful, cost-effective strategy towards training nurses in communication skills which is harmonious with nursing values. This approach may also be useful in determining whether Fiona may benefit from seeking the help of a qualified counsellor.

The NICE (2004) guidelines recognise the serious impact the emotional and psychological state can have on Fiona's wellbeing, and on people with similar problems:

- If depression is suspected, the person with MS should be assessed, and referred to a liaison psychiatrist if severe depression is present.
- In any person with MS who is depressed, a list of possible contributing factors (such as chronic pain and social isolation) should be drawn up.
- Assessment and interventions should be undertaken to ameliorate those contributing factors, where possible.
- Specific antidepressant medication, or psychological treatments such as cognitive behavioural therapy should be considered but only as part of an overall programme of depression management.
- Other concurrent psychological diagnoses, especially anxiety, should be considered.

Local implementation plans should include:

- which screening question or questionnaire is recommended locally
- which formal depression questionnaire is recommended locally
- which psychiatrist and/or clinical psychologist should be approached when more specialist advice or treatment is required
- what antidepressants are preferred locally.

Fiona also clearly has some anxieties in relation to her family and her future. NICE (2004) recommendations for good interdisciplinary practice advocate:

- Any person with MS whose function or happiness is being adversely affected by anxiety should be offered specialist assessment and management.
- In people with MS with marked anxiety, psychologically based treatment should be offered.
- Pharmacological treatment of anxiety should be through using antidepressants or benzodiazepines. The Committee on Safety of Medicines (CSM) guidelines on the use of benzodiazepines (reproduced in the British National Formulary) should be used.

Local implementation should indicate:

- how to access specialist psychological advice
- how to access specialist psychiatric advice.

Also as mentioned earlier, MS can affect cognition either because of physiological process or because of mood:

- Health care staff should always consider whether the person with MS has any impairment of attention, memory and executive functions sufficient to be a problem, or to be a contributing factor to their current clinical status.
- When a person with MS is being involved in making a complex medical decision, or is starting a course of complex treatment that requires their active participation, they should have their cognition sensitively assessed to ascertain their ability to understand and participate adequately, and to determine what support they may need.

Any person with MS experiencing problems due to cognitive impairment should:

- have their medication reviewed, to minimise iatrogenic cognitive losses
- be assessed for depression, and treated if appropriate
- be offered a formal cognitive assessment, coupled with specialist advice on the implications of the results advised, if necessary, about any vulnerability to financial or other abuse that may arise, advised how to reduce the risk and asked whether the results can be communicated to other people.

The local implementation plans need to:

- agree simple assessments of cognition for use by staff interacting with people with MS
- identify which specialist psychology service (usually that within the neurological rehabilitation service) should be approached for assessment and treatment, and how they are accessed.

Sociocultural factors

Fiona has a supportive family and clearly has coped well with help from some of the community services. It is unusual for her to be admitted to hospital in an acute relapse such as this. Arrangements will need to be made for the care of her children while she is in hospital and the care team will need to anticipate and discuss with her the level of help she will

need when she is discharged. It is the interface between the community and the interdisciplinary team and the effectiveness of the communication between them, which will go a long way towards helping Fiona. The people involved in the team may work in different care settings and different disciplines and because Fiona has an ongoing health problem that has made a big impact on her role and responsibilities, her care network is wide.

Interdisciplinary working Wilson & McLelland (1997, p. 8) highlight some of the problems of interdisciplinary working for both professionals and patients:

> 66 *There are many potential problems in working with people trained in different disciplines. Each discipline or profession has its own theoretical framework, traditions, sense of mission, priorities and rules. They run the risk however of reinforcing a reluctance to look for ideas from elsewhere, and they can also run the risk of competition and friction between professional groups, as well as between professions and patients.* 99

Fiona will probably come into contact with physicians, nurses, a specialist nurse, physiotherapists, occupational therapists, speech and language therapists, a social worker, and possibly a counsellor or clinical psychologist. Good teamwork not only across professions but also across care settings is essential if she is to experience continuity of care. Street & Blackford (2001) suggest a range of supporting strategies for effective formal modes of interdisciplinary communication across care settings in palliative care in Australia, although the communication problems they identify are universal:

- territoriality between professions
- lack of a common philosophy, language and style between professions and services
- restricted contact between busy professionals of one service and another.

Recent government initiatives in developing National Service Frameworks in the UK go some way towards helping to develop a framework which is more standardised, evidence-based and reliable in offering quality care. In the meantime, nursing practices in Britain continue to explore collaborative working practices such as Collaborative Care Plans, Integrated Care Pathways and patient-held records to try to improve continuity and communication in practice.

Environmental factors

Under this aspect for Fiona the social model of disability has a strong impact on her quality of life. Suitable adaptation of her home environment, provision of equipment and support to enable her to live as independently as possible, as well as help from a social worker can significantly improve her quality of life at home. Self-help organisations such as the Multiple Sclerosis Society can help Fiona overcome some of the wider environmental factors that may inhibit as full a social and communicative a life as possible. Wilson & McLelland (1997, p. 126) explain that:

> *Sometimes the natural history of a condition such as multiple sclerosis, arthritis, glaucoma, deafness or Parkinson's disease is known to be one of steady or periodic deterioration, but the levels of severe incapacity may not be obvious until well into retirement age. This means that in the early stages the threat of disability can be an anxiety affecting the individual much more than the actual physical problems that present. Work potential is certainly often affected, but this can result far more from worry about things that could be adapted than from the actual inability to continue to work. People with these problems may welcome regular long-term support and a review of adaptive measures or equipment.*

Politicoeconomic factors

For Fiona, a well-educated, professional, single parent with a chronic illness the economic implications are considerable because of her reduced ability to take on paid employment. Yet Wilson & McLelland (1997) point out that employment has significant wider functions (see Box 4.10).

The care team needs to be aware of these wider implications of the threat of the loss of the ability to work. Wilson & McLelland (1997) also warn that health care professionals may unwittingly make readjustment for patients more difficult by a preoccupation with clinical signs and pathologies (doctors), bowels and hygiene (nurses), painful physical jerks (physiotherapists) and the learning self-care tasks (occupational therapists). Patients with MS often find the service of an MS nurse specialist or the support of a self-help group such as the MS Society can help come to terms with the loss of social and economic status (p. 129).

Box 4.10	Work occupation and disability

Work gives human beings the opportunity to have certain basic needs met, and although most people complain about how busy and stressful and tiring work is, they would probably be much worse if forced into inactivity. This is true of both paid work and volunteer work.

Work has the following functions:

- *Income:* A job gives us the money to buy the goods and services others in society produce and provide. The 'poverty trap' is a term used to describe those who are not working (usually through disability) because its social benefits amount to more than could be earned.
- *Respect:* Social standards seem to favour those who are in work, and particularly those with high-status jobs. Individuals relying solely on benefits may feel low self-esteem and not respected by others.

Adapted from Wilson & McLelland (1997, p. 115).

CONCLUSION

This chapter has shown that good communication is at the heart of all interpersonal relationships, health care and teamwork. Nurses need excellent communication skills to assess patients' needs and negotiate holistic care, to interact and collaborate with other members of the interdisciplinary team, to implement nationally agreed standards of communication for health care personnel, ensure good record keeping wherever possible in collaborative care plans and to ensure patient privacy and dignity.

SUMMARY POINTS

1. Communicating can take many forms, including verbal and written. Nonverbal communication can have as important an impact as verbal.
2. As an AL communicating is central to effective assessment, underpins the therapeutic relationship and facilitates good collaborative care.
3. Nurses need to learn how to communicate with all age groups and take account of language and cultural differences in their care delivery.
4. Nurses need to take into account nationally set standards that affect the activity of communicating, and participate with the patient and interdisciplinary team to achieve the standards.

References

Adler RB, Rodman G 1991 Understanding human communication, 4th edn. Holt, Reinhart and Winston, London

Alexander C, Edwards R, Temple B 2004 Access to services with interpreters: user views. Joseph Rowntree Foundation, York

Archibald G 2000 The needs of South Asians with a terminal illness. Professional Nurse 15(5):316–319

Axtell RE 1991 The do's and taboos of body language around the world. John Wiley & Sons, New Jersey

Benner P 1984 From novice to expert. Addison-Wesley, London

Bowles N, Mackintosh C, Tom A 2001 Nurse communication skills: an evaluation of the impact of solution focused communication training. Journal of Advanced Nursing 36(3):347–354

Burnard P 1992 Counselling skills for health professionals, 2nd edn. Chapman and Hall, London

Crystal D 1992 The Cambridge encyclopaedia of language. Cambridge University Press, Cambridge

Department for Education and Skills 2001 Skills for life: A strategy for adult literacy and numeracy skills improving. HMSO, London

Department of Health 1997 The new NHS: Modern, dependable. The Stationery Office, London

Department of Health 1998a Data Protection Act 1998: protection and use of patient information. DoH, HMSO, London

Department of Health 1998b Human Rights Act 1998. DoH, HMSO, London (www.hmso.gov.uk/acts/acts1998/19980042.htm)

Department of Health 1998c A first class service: quality in the NHS (White Paper). The Stationery Office, London

Department of Health 1999 National service framework for mental health. The Stationery Office, London

Department of Health 2000a National service framework for coronary heart disease. The Stationery Office, London

Department of Health 2000b Race Relations Amendment Act. DoH, HMSO, London (www.homeoffice.gov.uk/raceact)

Department of Health 2001 National service framework for older people. The Stationery Office, London

Department of Health 2002 Guidance for access to health records requests under the Data Protection Act 1998 (www.doh.gov.uk/ipu/ahr/dpa1998.pdf accessed 30 Sept 2002)

Department of Health 2003a National service framework for diabetes. The Stationery Office, London

Department of Health 2003b Essence of care: patient focused benchmarking for health care practitioners. The Stationery Office, London

Department of Health 2004a National service framework for renal services. The Stationery Office, London

Department of Health 2004b National service framework for children, young people and maternity services. The Stationery Office, London

Department of Health 2005a National service framework for long term (neurological) conditions. The Stationery Office, London

Department of Health 2005b The Mental Capacity Act. The Stationery Office, London

Dewdney AK 1997 Yes we have no neutrons – a tour through the twists and turns of bad science. John Wiley & Sons, New York

Dickson D, Hargie O, Morrow N 1997 Communication skills training for health professionals, 2nd edn. Chapman and Hall, London

Dumbleton P 1998 Words and numbers … to describe people with learning disabilities. British Journal of Learning Disabilities 26(4):151–153

Evans MJ 1995 Neurologic neurosurgical nursing, 2nd edn. Springhouse Publications, Pennsylvania

Fromkin V, Rodman R 1983 An introduction to language, 3rd edn. CBS Publishing, London

Fuller G 2000 Neurological examination made easy, 2nd edn. Churchill Livingstone, Edinburgh

Gerrish K 2001 The nature and effect of communication difficulties arising from interactions between district nurse and South Asian patients. Journal of Advanced Nursing 33(5):566–574

Goleman D 1996 Emotional intelligence. Bloomsbury, London

Goodwin C 1995 Co-constructing meaning in conversations with an aphasic man. In: Jacoby S, Och E (eds) Research on language and social interaction (special issue on co-construction). Lawrence Erlbaum, NJ

Graham J 2001 What is MS? Multiple Sclerosis Society information booklet. Burnett Publications, London

Herz R 1997 Emotion experienced during encoding enhances odor retrieval cue effectiveness. American Journal of Psychology 110(4):489–505

Hickey JV 1997 Neurological and neurosurgical nursing, 4th edn. Lippincott, Philadelphia

Iggulden HM 1994 The nursing contribution in understanding and communicating with acute aphasia sufferers. Unpublished MSc Thesis, Manchester University

Kenny G 2002 Interprofessional working: opportunities and challenges (art and science multidisciplinary teams). Nursing Standard 17(6):33

Kindlen S 2003 Physiology for health care and nursing, 2nd edn. Churchill Livingstone, Edinburgh

Layward L 1998 Understanding MS research. Multiple Sclerosis Society information booklet. Burnett Publications, London

Leathard A 1994 Going interprofessional: Working together for health and welfare. Routledge, London

Macpherson W 1999 The Stephen Lawrence Inquiry: report of an enquiry by Sir William Macpherson of Cluny. HMSO, London

Masterson A 2002 Cross-boundary working: a macro-political analiysis of the impact on professional roles. Journal of Clinical Nursing 11(3):331

Millot J, Brand G 2001 Effects of pleasant and unpleasant ambient odors on human voice pitch. Neuroscience Letters 297:61–63

Moonie N 2000 Advanced health and social care, 3rd edn. Heineman, Oxford

NHS Executive 1999 Clinical governance: quality in the new NHS. NHSE, London

NICE 2004 Multiple sclerosis national clinical guideline for diagnosis and management in primary and secondary care. NICE, London

Nursing and Midwifery Council 2004 Code of professional conduct. NMC, London

Nursing and Midwifery Council 2007 Record keeping guidance. NMC, London

Office of Population Censuses and Surveys 1991 Census, local base statistics. HMSO, London

Oliver M 1996 Understanding disability: From theory to practice. Macmillan, London

Ovreteit J, Mathias P, Thompson P 1997 Interprofessional working for health and social care. Macmillan, Basingstoke

Pound C, Parr S, Lindsay J, Woolf C 2000 Beyond aphasia. Winslow Press, Bicester

Robinson L 1998 'Race,' communication and the caring professions. Open University Press, Buckingham

Ron MA, Logsdail SJ 1989 Psychiatric morbidity in multiple sclerosis: A clinical and MRI study. Psychological Medicine 19:887–895

Roper N, Logan WW, Tierney AJ 1996 The elements of nursing, 4th edn. Churchill Livingstone, Edinburgh

Royal College of Physicians 2004a Multiple sclerosis: national clinical guidelines for diagnosis and management in national and clinical care. RCP, London

Royal College of Physicians 2004b National clinical guidelines for stroke, 2nd edn. RCP, London

Rutishauser S 1994 Physiology and anatomy: A basis for nursing and health care. Churchill Livingstone, Edinburgh

Sharples N 2002 Communicating with patients who are prelingually profoundly deaf. Personal communication, University of Salford

Siviter B 2005 The student nurse handbook. Elsevier, Edinburgh

Street A, Blackford J 2001 Communication issues for the interdisciplinary community palliative care team. Journal of Clinical Nursing 10:643–650

Sully P, Dallas J 2005 Essential communication skills for nurses, Elsevier Mosby, Edinburgh

Tod AM, Wadsworth E, Asif S, Gerrish K 2001 Cardiac rehabilitation: the needs of South Asian cardiac patients. British Journal of Nursing 10(16):1028–1035

Trudghill P 2001 Sociolinguistic variation and change. Edinburgh University Press, Edinburgh

Waugh M, Grant A 2006 Ross and Wilson anatomy and physiology in health and illness, 10th edn. Churchill Livingstone, Edinburgh

WHO International classifications of functions, disability and health (www3.who.int/icF2002 accessed 3.12.02)

Wilson BA, McLelland DL 1997 Rehabilitation studies handbook, Cambridge University Press, Cambridge

Further reading

Aveyard H 2003 The patient who is unable to consent to nursing care. International Journal of Nursing Studies 40:697–705

Barnes MP, Ward AB 2000 Textbook of rehabilitation medicine. Oxford University Press, Oxford

Barret D Sellman G Thomas J 2005 Interprofessional working in health and social care. Palgrave, Macmillan, London

Darley M 2002 Managing communication in health care. Baillière Tindall, London

Day J 2006 Expanding nursing and health care practice interprofessional working. Nelson Thornes, Cheltenham

Griffin J, Tyrell I 1999 Psychotherapy and the human givens. Monograph. The European Therapy Studies Institute, London

Mann E, Carr E 2006 Pain management. Blackwell Publishing, Oxford

Parr S 2005 The stroke and aphasia handbook. Connect Press, London

Parr S, Byng S, Gilpin S, Ireland C 1997 Talking about aphasia; living with loss of language after stroke. Open University Press, Buckingham

Piteroni M, Vaspe A 2000 Understanding counselling in primary care – voices from the inner city. Churchill Livingstone, Edinburgh

Robb M, Barrett S, Komaromy C 2003 Communication, relationships and care: a reader. Routledge, Oxford

Sundin K, Jansson L 2003 Understanding and being understood as a creative caring phenomenon in care of patients with stroke and aphasia. Journal of Clinical Nursing 12(1):107–116

Useful websites

www.aphasia.org (National Aphasia Association)

www.bac.co.uk (British Association of Counselling and Psychotherapy)

www.connectuk.org (communication disability site)

www.cultsock.ndirect.co.uk (communication, cultural and media studies)

www.doh.gov.uk (Department of Health)

www.ethnicityonline.net (Ethnicity Online – addresses the need for a better understanding of ethnic differences in health care)

www.freedomtocare.org (ethics in health care)

www.headway.org.uk (Brain Injury Association)

www.mssociety.org.uk (Multiple Sclerosis Society)

www.nmc-uk.org (Nursing and Midwifery Council, UK)

www.pals.hns.uk (PALS Online: website of the national network of NHS Patient Advice and Liaison Services)

Breathing

Jane Jenkins

INTRODUCTION

Roper et al (2000, p. 22) highlight the fact that breathing appears to be 'effortless and people are not usually consciously aware of the AL of breathing until some abnormal circumstances force it to their attention'. Being able to breathe normally ensures that we can attempt other activities without any difficulty, for example walking, running and swimming. However, breathing can be affected by health problems which relate to other Activities of Living (ALs), such as being overweight through unhealthy eating causing the individual breathing difficulties when running, walking or even talking. It is important to remember that we are all individuals with life activities that are interlinked and when illness causes one or more activity to be affected then most of the activities can become compromised. This may then result in physical, emotional or social problems.

This chapter will focus on the following:

1. **The model of living**
   - breathing activity in health and illness across the lifespan
   - dependence and independence in relation to the activity of breathing
   - factors which influence the activity of breathing.

2. **The model for nursing**
   - nursing care of individuals with health problems which affect their activity of breathing.

THE MODEL OF LIVING

Initially, you will need to be able to answer the question 'How do we breathe?' It may be necessary for you to review your knowledge of the normal anatomy and physiology of the respiratory and circulatory systems before you continue with the chapter. (See Further reading at the end of this chapter and the section entitled Biological Factors.)

BREATHING ACTIVITY IN HEALTH AND ILLNESS ACROSS THE LIFESPAN

At birth

Breathing is usually an independent activity immediately following birth. A mother's initial question, following the joys of labour, is to ask if the baby is alright. Whatever response is given, the first cry that is uttered from the baby signifies to the mother that all is well. From a health care professional's point of view that cry signifies that the baby is able to breathe on their own, albeit that suction may have been required to remove secretions from the upper respiratory tract which collect during the birth process. Observations of the baby's respiratory function will take place unobtrusively to ensure that this vital AL is not compromised in any way. It is important that the rate, depth and pattern of respiration is monitored along with the colour of the baby's skin.

Childhood

Children expend an enormous amount of energy and need a respiratory system that can meet these demands. The activity of breathing is performed effortlessly and children will be totally unaware of breathing unless they experience childhood illnesses, such as whooping cough and asthma.

Adulthood/older person

As in childhood, the activity of breathing continues to take place without conscious thought and is very much taken for granted. However, problems with the respiratory and cardiovascular system occur more commonly in adults and older people and breathing can then become a major factor in their lifestyle.

You may have noticed that the baby's or child's rate of breathing was much faster than that of an adult and older person. The normal range for a baby is about 30 or more breaths per minute, 22–28 per minute for a child, 18–22 per minute for an adolescent, 14–20 per minute for an adult and slightly higher in an older person. In healthy people, there is a relationship between their pulse rate and their respiratory rate. This is fairly constant and one breath occurs to every four or five heart beats. Where there are more than the usual number of respirations (above 24) then this is known as tachypnoea and bradypnoea if below 12. The depth of their respiration is again fairly constant and is often described as 'normal', 'shallow' or 'deep', but in an older person then the depth may become more shallow. Normal relaxed breathing is usually effortless, automatic, regular and almost silent according to Richards & Edwards (2003). If any of the people you observed had any health problems which affected breathing, such as the common cold, you may have noticed that their breathing rate was faster than normal and the pattern may have been altered and their breathing required effort and was possibly noisy.

DEPENDENCE AND INDEPENDENCE IN RELATION TO THE ACTIVITY OF BREATHING

The degree of independence is closely related to the position on the lifespan with most of the activities. However, breathing is probably the exception to the rule as, already discussed, most individuals breathe unaided and independently from birth throughout their lifespan until the moment of death. In fact, it is the cessation of breathing that signifies death for most people.

Roper et al (1996) identified that, even in health, individuals can become dependent upon certain aspects in relation to breathing, such as organising outdoor pursuits when the pollen count is low as they suffer from hayfever, or by ensuring that they take their respiratory or cardiovascular medications so that they can carry out their normal ALs.

However, some individuals are not able to breathe on their own and are totally dependent upon specialised equipment and constant care. This may range from the need to

have a constant supply of oxygen in their own home, to the person needing to be intubated and attached to mechanical ventilation. This latter level of dependency may be as a result of an accident which has caused paralysis of the nerves which affect breathing, infection such as poliomyelitis which causes paralysis of the muscles of the chest or many other clinical problems such as respiratory failure, pneumonia or congenital problems. Although care for these patients requires specialist knowledge and skills, it is important that you have an awareness of mechanical ventilation as emergency situations may arise.

In relation to how mechanical ventilators work you may have discovered that there are different types of mechanical ventilators, e.g. the most common type being either positive pressure ventilators, or negative pressure ventilators which were commonly used for patients with poliomyelitis. Dickson & Martindale (2002) describe positive pressure ventilators as those which deliver gases directly into the lungs through a tube and an artificial airway, such as an endotracheal or tracheostomy tube, whereas negative pressure ventilators do not require an artificial airway as they work on the principle of removing air from within a closed container by generating negative pressure. This negative pressure causes the lungs to expand and air to flow into them as in the 'iron lungs' that were used for patients suffering from poliomyelitis; however, these are rarely used now.

Negative pressure ventilators may be used by individuals in their own homes but in Intensive Care Units it is usually the positive pressure ventilators that are used. There are also different modes of ventilating such as negative intermittent positive pressure ventilation (NIPPV) and continuous positive airway pressure (CPAP).

Mechanical ventilation provides artificial support for breathing, maintains vital functions and optimum gaseous exchange and ensures adequate tissue perfusion, therefore allowing physiological functions to continue.

A bellows action within the ventilator acts as the diaphragm and the thoracic cage, thereby delivering oxygen to the lungs so that gaseous exchange can take place. The positive pressure ventilators allow oxygen to be delivered at a preset pressure at a concentration of 21–100%. This may be via either 'controlled ventilation' where the individual makes no respiratory effort and is totally dependent on the ventilator or via 'assisted ventilation' where the individual is able to make some respiratory effort but they are partially dependent on the ventilator to assist them to breathe adequately (Dickson & Martindale 2002).

You may have watched medical programmes where patients are (or appear to be) ventilated or you may have been able to observe patients being nursed on a ventilator in an Intensive Care Unit or in an Operating Theatre. These patients are critically ill and require specialised care.

However, there are principles of care which you may be able to recognise, such as airway maintenance by appropriate endotracheal suctioning, delivery of warmed, humidified, filtered oxygen, observations of patient's vital signs (colour, oxygen saturation levels, consciousness, temperature, pulse, blood pressure, fluid balance), amount of sedation required and its effect on respiration, correct positioning for lung function, and physiotherapy; whilst doing all of this technical activity it is vital to communicate with the patient. Care of the patient's skin is essential and the nurse must ensure that the patient is adequately hydrated and well nourished and that hygiene needs are maintained. Patients requiring this level of care are totally dependent on the health care professionals for the maintenance of all of their ALs.

Specific monitoring devices for the measurement of arterial pressure, central venous pressure and pulmonary artery pressure will be utilised. Observation of the ventilator tubing and endotracheal cuff pressures will take place in addition to the other observations noted. (Further details of caring for the critically ill and ventilated patient can be found in Smith 2006, Sheppard 2003.)

Your response to how you may feel about being dependent on a ventilator will be affected by many aspects, e.g. 'Are you aware of the problem?', 'Is it long term?', 'Have you any previous knowledge of this type of care?'. However, you may well have thought that you would be frightened knowing that you could not breathe on your own, or angry at not being able to breathe or talk, or perhaps frustrated as you are not able to communicate with other people or become depressed and withdrawn because of lack of ability to communicate and worrying over the potential outcome. Responding to patients' mental, social and spiritual needs are as important as attending to their physical needs and technical equipment.

Another area of dependency to consider is in relation to smoking and this form of addiction. Because smoking is highly addictive, smokers find it difficult to give up smoking and therefore become dependent upon it for a variety of reasons.

The World Health Organization (WHO) (2006) has now classified tobacco and nicotine dependency as a 'Mental and behavioral disorder' in the *International Classification of Diseases; ICD-10* (Classification F17.2). The WHO (2006) identifies that various behavioural, cognitive and physiological changes develop after repeated use of tobacco, and this includes a strong desire to smoke, difficulties in controlling its use, persisting in its use despite harmful consequences, a higher priority given to smoking than to other activities, increased tolerance and sometimes a physical withdrawal state.

The WHO (1980) has defined three types of dependency:

1. *Social dependency* – the person depends on a chemical in order to conform to the behaviour patterns of his particular community.
2. *Psychological dependency* – the person depends on a chemical to provide enjoyment and/or suppress or come to terms with mental or emotional conflicts.
3. *Physical dependency* – the person depends on a chemical for normal functioning.

Exercise
1. Find out why people start smoking and try to find different age groups to see if reasons have changed.
2. Identify their smoking habits, i.e. number smoked, type, how soon after waking do they smoke.
3. Find out if any of them have tried to stop and if so how successful they have been.
4. Discuss with them how smoking affects their breathing and their day-to-day living activities.

You will probably have found many reasons why individuals start smoking. Children may start smoking to show their independence, because their friends or siblings do, because adults tell them not to, or to follow their role models. Advertising in sporting events or on billboards is also a reason why children start to smoke, as identified by the Department of Health (DoH 1998a). The Tobacco Advertising and Promotion Act (DoH 2002a) now prohibits advertising and promotion of tobacco products in the UK and the Department of Health estimates that this will lead to 2.5% reduction in smoking levels of the population. Smoking may initially start as an experiment but unfortunately they are unable to give up. Older people, especially men, may say they started smoking during the war periods where tobacco was given to troops. Now, older people may start smoking due to pressures at work or home and use it as a stress reliever (DoH 1998a).

A survey on smoking-related behaviour and attitudes by Taylor et al (2005) identified that people in routine or manual occupations are more likely to smoke than those in managerial or professional occupations (32% compared to 16%). The number of cigarettes smoked daily has remained fairly static, with 42% smoking 10–19 a day, 30% smoking 10 a day and 28% smoking 20 or over a day.

Social dependency may have been the originator of smoking for most people but this then slowly moves into psychological and physical dependency later on. The time after waking before the first cigarette is smoked is indicative of the person's level of dependency. Taylor et al (2005) reported that 14% of smokers did so within 5 minutes of waking up and this was significant in those classed as heavy smokers (20 and over a day). At the physical dependency stage, it is more difficult to quit than at the previous levels of dependency. As the smoker has become dependent on the chemical, i.e. nicotine, unpleasant symptoms result from the withdrawal of this chemical, such as depression, irritability, anxiety, restlessness and lack of concentration as Roper et al (1996) identify.

You may have found out that smokers find it extremely difficult to stop, some may not wish to and some may have restarted after stopping smoking for a period of time. Taylor et al (2005) identified that smoking has decreased since 1996 when 28% of the adult population smoked whereas in 2005, 24% of the adult population smoked with minimal differences between the number of men and women. This equates to over 1 million fewer smokers. The statistics relating to smoking as found in *Smoking Kills* (DoH 1998a) and *Statistics on Smoking* (DoH 2003a) provides sober reading and demonstrates not only the dependency but also the cost in health.

Exercise

Read or show the statistics in Box 5.1 to:

1. smokers – young and older persons.
2. a parent of a teenager.

Discuss with them their views on the facts raised by the Department of Health statistics.

You may find that a smoker may read them and pass no comment, or confirm that they already know the risks but still wish to smoke, or they may believe them and express a wish to quit. A parent who is a smoker or a non-smoker may be horrified at these statistics and want to know how they can help to prevent their child from starting smoking.

As smoking is known to be the key avoidable cause of premature death in the UK, the government has built on the *Smoking Kills* White Paper (DoH 1998a) and produced a further White Paper, *Choosing Health* (DoH 2004a). This promises new action on tackling tobacco issues and reducing the 106 000 deaths caused by smoking in the UK each year. It aims to do this by reducing the numbers of people who smoke, by using media and education campaigns; reducing exposure to secondhand smoke or passive smoking; reducing the availability of tobacco products and regulating their supply; continuing with NHS Stop Smoking Services and nicotine replacement therapy; restricting tobacco advertising, and providing support to local authority enforcement of underage tobacco sales. Also, all enclosed public places and workplaces have been smoke-free since 2007. (See Department of Health website www.dh.gov.uk for further information.)

Box 5.1	Statistics relating to smoking

- 13 million adults smoke in UK.
- More than 120 000 deaths were caused by smoking in the UK in 1995; that is, one in five of all deaths.
- 13 people will die each hour, in the UK, due to illnesses directly related to smoking.
- UK citizens smoke more cigarettes per person than in Europe.
- Smoking is the principal avoidable cause of premature deaths in the UK.
- Smoking is the major cause of cancer (46 500 deaths per year in UK).
- Smoking is the major cause of heart disease (40 300 deaths per year in UK).
- Smoking is the major cause of 30 600 deaths from lung cancer.
- Smoking is high in people with severe mental illness.
- Increasing numbers of young people smoke.
- Smokers who take up the habit as teenagers generally go on to smoke all of their lives.
- Half of those (life-time smokers) die of the habit.
- A quarter die before the age of 69.
- Smokers lose 16 years from their life expectancy compared to non-smokers.
- Someone starting smoking at 15 is three times more likely to die of cancer than someone who starts smoking at 25.
- UK death rates due to smoking are high compared to EU countries except Denmark.
- Higher rate of smoking in manual workers is matched with higher rates of disease.
- In 2001, the prevalence of cigarette smoking continued to be higher for people in manual than non-manual socioeconomic groups (32% compared with 21%).
- In 2001, 66% of smokers in England wanted to give up smoking.
- In 2002, 10% of children aged 11–15 smoked cigarettes regularly; 9% of boys and 11% of girls.

Department of Health (1998a, 2003a).

FACTORS INFLUENCING THE ACTIVITY OF BREATHING

As identified by Roper et al (1996, 2000) speaking, laughing and eating alter breathing patterns even though individuals are rarely aware of this. Even in the healthy person a number of factors can and do influence the rate, depth and rhythm of breathing and other vital signs of pulse and blood pressure. These factors will be explored individually but include:

1. Anatomy and physiology related to breathing (biological factors).
2. Emotional issues related to breathing (psychological factors).

3. Practices, associated health beliefs and habits in different cultures related to breathing (sociocultural factors).
4. Pollutants in the air and how these are related to breathing (environmental factors).
5. Policies, laws and economics related to breathing (politicoeconomic factors).

Anatomy and physiology related to breathing (biological factors)

In order to promote health and be able to care for individuals who have breathing problems it is necessary for you to understand the normal structure and function of all systems in the body. In relation to breathing, the anatomy and physiology of the respiratory system and the cardiovascular system need to be considered.

The function of the respiratory system is twofold:

- to provide an adequate supply of oxygen to the cells, so that they can function properly
- to provide a means of removing the carbon dioxide, which is produced by the cells, as a waste product, following their activity.

The organs of the respiratory system allow the oxygen, present in the atmosphere, to enter the body and ultimately the cells, and for carbon dioxide to exit the body from the cells. It is vital that the cells receive this supply of oxygen as without it, even for a few minutes, major problems can result and death can occur. Breathing is effortless or laboured depending on how 'stiff' the respiratory system is and how narrow the airways are.

Respiration, according to Kindlen (2003), is the term used to describe the processes which ensure that oxygen is transported to, and used by, the cells and that when carbon dioxide is produced it is taken away from the cells (see Fig. 5.1). For this process to work, it is necessary for the cardiovascular system to be utilised. The blood is the fluid medium used to transport oxygen and carbon dioxide, the blood vessels are the means by which the gases are transported to and from the cells in the blood and the heart provides the pump to ensure that the blood flows around the body in the blood vessels to deliver the oxygen and pick up the carbon dioxide.

These two systems (respiratory and cardiovascular) interlink to provide three processes, according to Kindlen (2003), ventilation of the lungs with air, gaseous exchange between air and blood and perfusion of the lungs with blood. These processes will be briefly discussed in relation to the activity of breathing but you may need to refer to anatomy and physiology books noted in the Further Reading list at the end of this chapter for further details.

Ventilation process involving the respiratory system

Various organs make up the respiratory system (nose, pharynx, larynx, trachea, bronchi, bronchioles, lungs, alveoli,

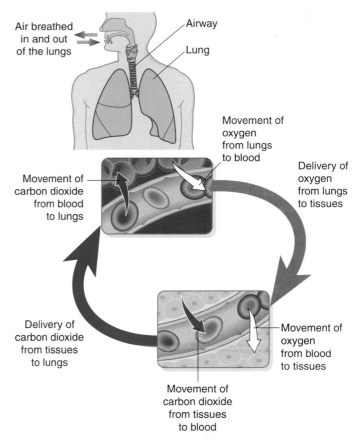

Fig. 5.1 Processes involved in the delivery of oxygen to the tissues and the elimination of carbon dioxide (from Kindlen 2003, with permission).

pleura and thoracic cage) and you need to be aware of the position, structure and function of each organ (Waugh & Grant 2006). The positions of these organs are shown in Figure 5.2.

The initial activity of the respiratory system is that of ventilation, moving air in and out of the lungs. Initially, air breathed in through the nose is warmed, moistened and filtered by the vascular, moist mucosal layer of the nose and the hairs in the nose. The mucus traps any inhaled particles and the cilia (hairs) help to drive this mucus with the particles up and out of the airway. As the air passes down the pharynx and larynx, the air continues to be warmed and moistened and is at body temperature when it reaches the trachea, although warming can still take place in the bronchi and bronchioles. The alveoli are at the end of the respiratory tract and it is here that gaseous exchange takes place between the air and the blood (Waugh & Grant 2006). The lower respiratory tract can be seen in Figure 5.3.

For gaseous exchange to occur, the lungs need to inflate and this is achieved by increasing the size of the thoracic cavity due to the muscular activity of the external intercostal muscles (which are stimulated by the nervous system) and the diaphragm and this is known as inspiration. The diaphragm contracts and pushes the abdominal organs down,

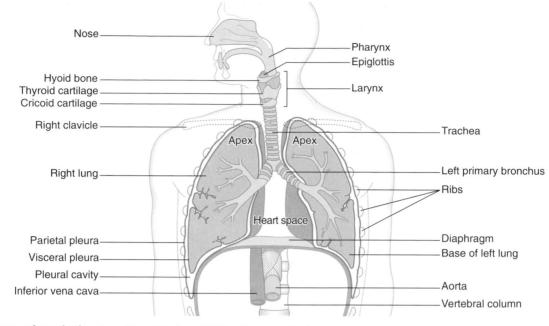

Fig. 5.2 Organs of respiration (from Waugh & Grant 2006, with permission).

whilst the lower ribs swing outwards so increasing the size of the thoracic cavity to allow the air into the lungs. When the external intercostal muscles and the diaphragm relax, air is pushed out of the lungs and this is known as expiration. No effort is normally needed for expiration to occur.

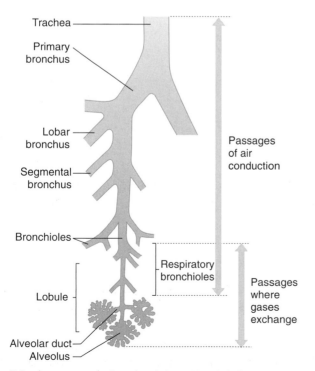

Fig. 5.3 Lower respiratory tract (from Waugh & Grant 2006, with permission).

The changes in the capacity of the thoracic cavity during ventilation are shown in Figure 5.4 (Waugh & Grant 2006).

You can also feel these changes if you place your hands on the sides of your rib cage and breathe in and breathe out. You will be able to realise that with extra effort (for example, lifting up shoulders) you can increase the size of the thoracic cavity and therefore breathe in more air; however, breathing out just happens. These changes occur because of the links with the nervous system. The intercostal muscles are stimulated by the involuntary system which includes the respiratory centre in the brain stem. The respiratory centre receives information from the respiratory system itself on the state of the lungs and also from special receptors on the oxygen and carbon dioxide levels in the bloodstream as described by Kindlen (2003) and is shown in Figure 5.5.

According to Kindlen (2003), the amount of air breathed in and out varies between individuals, but in quiet breathing this should be about 500 ml and is known as the tidal volume (TV). However, the total lung capacity (TLC) is far greater than this and could be up to 6 litres of air. The total lung capacity includes the total amount of air that can be breathed in and out and also that which remains in the respiratory tract as not all air can be expelled. Extra air which can be breathed in, with maximum effort, could be up to 2 litres and is called the inspiratory reserve volume (IRV). The largest amount of air that can be breathed out, with maximum effort, is about 1 litre and is known as the expiratory reserve volume (ERV). The amount of air that cannot be expelled is known as the residual volume (RV) and is approximately 1500 ml. The last two volumes (ERV + RV) give the functional residual capacity (FRC), which is the amount of air left in the system at the end of normal

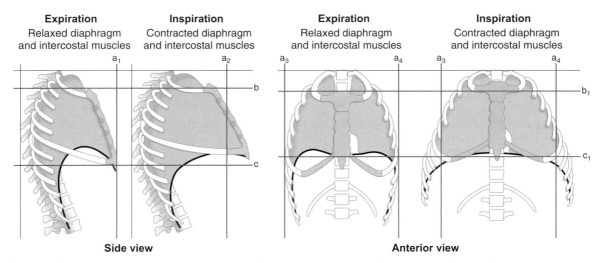

Fig. 5.4 Changes in the capacity of the thoracic cavity during breathing (from Waugh & Grant 2006, with permission).

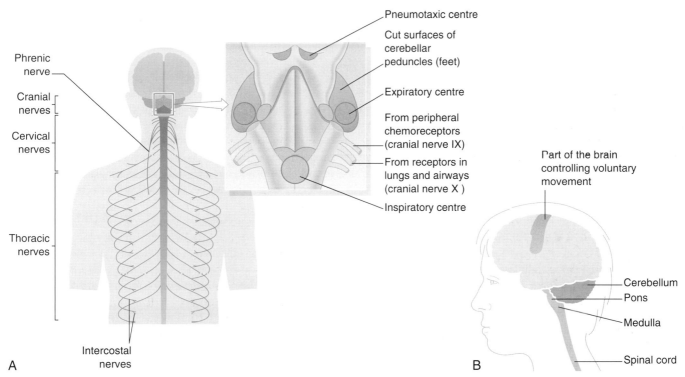

Fig. 5.5 Parts of the nervous system involved in controlling breathing, (A) brain, brain stem, spinal cord and nerves with enlarged inset showing respiratory centres in medulla and pons, (B) position of medulla and pons (from Kindlen 2003, with permission).

expiration and should be between 2 and 3 litres. The maximum amount of air that can be moved in and out of the lungs (TV + IRV + ERV) is the vital capacity (VC) and is normally between 3500 and 4800 ml (Kindlen 2003). The pattern of breathing and measurements of lung volumes can be recorded by spirometry as shown in Figure 5.6.

Respiratory function is assessed using these lung volumes and therefore it is important to be aware of their meanings in health and illness.

Exercise

1. Investigate what alterations are found in lung volumes with individuals who have respiratory problems.

You may have been able to observe spirometry being carried out at the bedside, in a clinic, GP's surgery or at the patient's home. You may have visited a pulmonary function laboratory or discussed this with a Respiratory Specialist

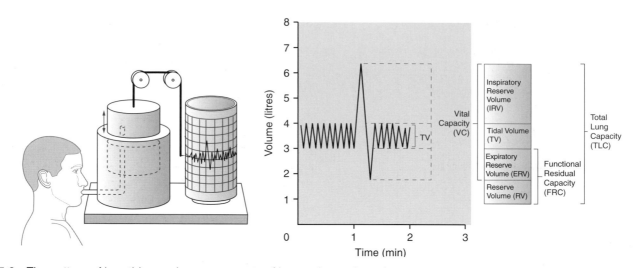

Fig. 5.6 The pattern of breathing and measurements of lung volumes by spirometry (from Kindlen 2003, with permission).

Nurse. The British Thoracic Society (1997) recommend using spirometry as opposed to peak expiratory flow for diagnosing patients with chronic obstructive pulmonary disease and Sayer (1999) comments on the increasing use of spirometers in GP surgeries. However, Jackson & Hubbard (2003) concluded that peak expiratory flow rate is as good as spirometry at detecting chronic obstructive pulmonary disease in the community. Although spirometry can provide extra information, it is time consuming and complex and they question its value in primary care.

Patients who have obstructive airway disease (e.g. asthma) may have a normal or slightly reduced vital capacity (VC) as air is trapped in the lungs because individuals have difficulty in breathing out. Both the residual volume (RV) and functional residual capacity (FRC) are increased as more air remains in the lungs after each expiration.

You may have experienced difficulties in observing or finding out information in relation to lung volumes but you may have observed peak flow rate measurements (peak expiratory flow rate or PEFR) possibly using a Wright peak flow or mini-Wright peak flow meter (Esmond 2003, Brooker 2005). There are other peak flow meters but Nazir et al (2005) does caution users as significant differences in values can be obtained from different types; therefore it is important to always use only one type with each person to limit inaccuracies. Higgins (2005a) outlines the procedure. This can be undertaken at home, in a clinic, GP's surgery or at the bedside to assess respiratory function by an individual breathing in fully and then breathing out as fast and fully as possible into a peak flow meter. Therefore, it tests the maximum rate at which an individual can breathe out or exhale in litres per minute. As the rate at which the air flows through the airways is measured by the PEFR, it gives an indication of the size of the airways. If they are wider then the air flows easier through them and the PEFR will be higher but if the airways are narrowed then it will be harder for the air

to flow through and the PEFR will be lower and problems will be experienced.

The normal range, in health, is 400–600 litres per minute but individuals with asthma, for example, will have a lower peak flow rate when their airway is narrowed. Many asthma sufferers monitor their own peak flow rate measurements to ascertain the effect of medication and act as a warning mechanism before they experience obvious alterations in their breathing. Sayer (1999) assesses the use and reliability of peak flow meters. Although there may be some discrepancies in readings due to product variations, user error or falsification of results, Sayer (1999) considers that the benefits are numerous as trends in respiratory function can be monitored, compliance with treatments may be improved and response to changes in therapies can be noted.

Gaseous exchange involving the respiratory and cardiovascular systems

Air has now reached the lungs and, in particular, the alveoli, and oxygen needs to be transferred from the air in the alveoli to the blood and carbon dioxide needs to be transferred from the blood to the alveoli (Waugh & Grant 2006). The oxygen moves from the alveolar air to the blood by diffusion and stops when the partial pressure of oxygen in the blood is the same as that in the alveoli. The carbon dioxide moves from the blood to the alveolar air again by diffusion and stops when the partial pressure of carbon dioxide in the alveoli is the same as that in the blood, as illustrated in Figure 5.7.

To understand how these gases exchange by diffusion, it is necessary to consider the differences in the partial pressures of the gases in the atmosphere and the alveolar air. According to Kindlen (2003), the composition of air can be described in two ways, namely by the amount of each gas which is present in atmospheric air and alveolar air in terms of the percentage and the partial pressures or concentration of these gases (kPa). The atmospheric pressure, at sea level,

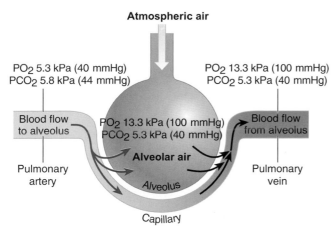

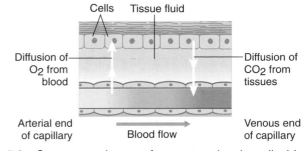

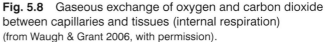

Fig. 5.8 Gaseous exchange of oxygen and carbon dioxide between capillaries and tissues (internal respiration) (from Waugh & Grant 2006, with permission).

Fig. 5.7 Gaseous exchange of oxygen and carbon dioxide between alveolar air and blood (external respiration) (from Waugh & Grant 2006, with permission).

is 100 kPa or 760 mmHg, and the percentage composition of oxygen is 21%, i.e. oxygen forms 21% of air. So the part of the atmospheric pressure due to oxygen is called the partial pressure of oxygen and is 21% × 100 kPa. This gives a partial pressure of oxygen which is 21 kPa. Carbon dioxide, on the other hand, is measured at only 0.04% of the atmospheric air, so the partial pressure of carbon dioxide is 0.04% × 100 kPa, giving a partial pressure of carbon dioxide of 0.04 kPa. In alveolar air, the percentage composition changes as the gases move through the respiratory tract to the alveoli. The percentage composition of oxygen, in the alveolar air, falls to 13.2%, so the partial pressure of oxygen is 13.2 kPa (13.2% × 100 kPa). The carbon dioxide level in the alveolar air is higher, 5.3%, giving a partial pressure of 5.3 kPa (5.3% × 100 kPa). The partial pressure of gases or concentration in the blood stream is denoted as pO_2 or pCO_2 kPa.

Oxygen moves from the alveolar air, which has a partial pressure of oxygen of pO_2 13.2 kPa, into the bloodstream, as the partial pressure of oxygen in the bloodstream only measures pO_2 5.3 kPa. This movement continues until the pO_2 is the same in the alveoli and the blood. Carbon dioxide leaves the alveolar air in the same way. The partial pressure of carbon dioxide (pCO_2) in the bloodstream is 6 kPa and as this is higher than in the alveolar air (pCO_2 5.3 kPa), the carbon dioxide moves from the blood into the alveoli and is eventually breathed out. Again the movement of the gases continues until the partial pressure of carbon dioxide is the same in the alveoli and the blood. Kindlen (2003) explains that this process occurs very quickly.

It is useful to identify and differentiate between the terms external and internal respiration (Waugh & Grant 2006). External respiration is the term used to explain the process by which the blood is oxygenated and the subsequent elimination of carbon dioxide from the body, i.e. gaseous exchange as explained above. The use of the oxygen at cell level and the production of carbon dioxide is known as internal respiration and is illustrated in Figure 5.8.

Before birth, gaseous exchange is performed by the placenta and the exchange is between the mother's blood and that of the fetus. Immediately after birth, the gaseous exchange is taken over by the newborn baby's lungs.

> **Exercise**
> 1. Identify what effects there may be on the fetus if the mother smokes and give the reasons why these problems may occur.
> 2. What information would you give a pregnant mother who smokes?

It is recognised that smoking is addictive and is therefore difficult to give up but there are serious health risks, not only to the mother, but to the unborn child and the baby as serious illnesses and cot deaths are more prevalent in houses where the mother smokes. There is evidence to support the fact that smoking during pregnancy harms the unborn child and leads to lower birth weights and increased risk of miscarriage. These problems arise possibly because of a decrease in the blood flow to the placenta. There is also evidence that the mother can pass on harmful carcinogens to the baby. Some nicotine will also pass into the baby's bloodstream if the mother smokes when breast feeding (DoH 1998a).

The Department of Health (1998a) states that 24% of women smoke during pregnancy and only 33% give up during pregnancy. It is vital that mothers quit smoking during pregnancy because of the problems noted and the target is to reduce the proportion of pregnant women who smoke to 15% by 2010.

Helping mothers to give up smoking during pregnancy has many benefits. Not only should the health of the mother and baby be better but the NHS will save money also. This is because low-weight babies need intensive care which is extremely costly. Therefore, members of the primary health care team (midwives and health visitors in particular) have an important role to play in helping pregnant women to give up smoking.

NHS Stop Smoking Services (previously known as smoking cessation services) are prominent at present as the risk of illness and death decrease with each year after stopping smoking. Therefore, it is vital that during pregnancy, health education is given, not only for the health of the fetus but for the pregnant mother's own health. Support groups, acupuncture and hypnosis are being used to assist smokers to quit (DoH 1998a).

The National Institute for Health and Clinical Excellence (NICE 2002) has produced guidelines on the use of nicotine replacement therapy (NRT) and bupropion for smoking cessation. These treatments are cost effective in helping people stop smoking without experiencing withdrawal symptoms. Unfortunately, neither NRT nor bupropion are advocated in the UK at present with pregnant women without consultation. A UK quitline was launched in 1997 and is run by the charity 'Quit'. There is a section on their website (www.quit.org.uk) with advice for pregnant mothers who wish to quit smoking. In the first year, it answered 3000 calls and agreed individual smoking cessation programmes and has now helped over 2 million smokers quit the habit. There is evidence that prenatal counselling involving at least 10 minutes person-to-person contact and the use of written materials can double the quit rates (DoH 1998a). Support needs to continue after the birth to ensure that the mother doesn't start smoking again.

Perfusion involving the respiratory and cardiovascular system

The amount of oxygen and carbon dioxide that can be diffused and therefore exchanged is dependent on the amount of blood passing through the lungs (Kindlen 2003). For this to occur we must have a pulmonary circulation (Fig. 5.9).

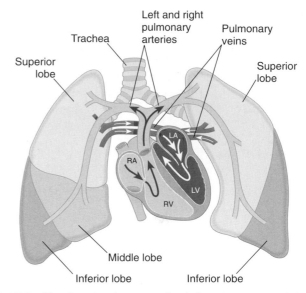

Fig. 5.9 Heart and pulmonary circulation (from Waugh & Grant 2006, with permission).

Oxygen is transported mainly by the red blood cells and is linked to haemoglobin; it is then called oxyhaemoglobin and gives blood its bright red colour when oxygen levels are high. However, when the oxygen leaves the red blood cell rendering the oxygen levels low, the deoxyhaemoglobin (deoxygenated haemoglobin) gives blood a purplish colour (Kindlen 2003). Carbon dioxide is transported by reacting with several constituents of blood. At rest, the cells in the body use 250 ml of oxygen per minute and during exercise this can rise to 7500 ml. Two hundred ml of carbon dioxide are made when the body is at rest (Casey 2001).

Exercise
1. Identify how the blood gets from the right side of the heart to the lungs.
2. Identify how the blood gets from the lungs to the left side of the heart.

Exercise
1. Using your knowledge of the physiology of breathing, work out what happens to the breathing activities (short and long term) of the following individuals:

   a. A woman, aged 20, of average height, weighing 15 stones (95 kg), who decides to jog for 15 minutes a day as part of her new keep fit regime.
   b. A man, aged 50, who already undertakes regular aerobic exercise, three times a week by swimming, decides to start running 3 miles a day.

You should have identified that the blood leaves the right side of the heart by the pulmonary artery (so named as, although carrying deoxygenated blood, it is taking blood to somewhere) to go to the lungs and then returns to the left side of the heart via four pulmonary veins (so called as they are taking blood away from somewhere, even though oxygenated now); check this in Figure 5.9. This results in a massive blood flow through the two systems at any time, as all the blood in the right ventricle goes to the lungs and all the blood in the lungs is returned to the left atrium. At rest, this is approximately 5 litres per minute and up to 25 litres per minute with maximum exertion (Kindlen 2003).

You may have decided that their breathing would be influenced by their age, weight and fitness levels. As muscles require more oxygen during physical exercise then, in a healthy adult, the respiratory rate will increase to provide this. According to Law & Watson (2005), there is a sudden increase in respiratory rates at the very onset of exercise and an equally rapid, although larger, decrease in respiratory rates immediately exercise ceases. Equally, as respiratory rates and pulse rates are linked then the pulse rate will also rise. The young woman is overweight and is new to exercise and therefore you would expect that her respiratory rate and pulse rate will increase quicker than the older man who is more used to exercise. When the body rests, then the respiratory and pulse rates will decrease. It may be that the older man's respiratory and pulse rates return to normal quicker than the younger woman's.

Other factors need to be considered, such as the amount and effectiveness of the delivery of oxygen to the tissues, as this will also affect individuals' responses to lifestyle changes. Three factors determine the delivery of oxygen to the tissues: oxygen saturation, amount of haemoglobin in the bloodstream and how well it is transported around the body (Casey 2001).

Oxygen binds to haemoglobin molecules depending on the concentration of oxygen in the plasma and this is noted as PO_2. This figure is measured when taking arterial blood gases as a pressure in millimetres of mercury (mmHg). The amount of oxygen in the arterial blood depends on the amount entering the plasma as the blood passes through the lungs.

According to Casey (2001), at sea level, during inspiration, air is drawn in at a pressure of about 760 mmHg and this atmospheric air contains 21% oxygen. Through its passage to the alveoli, the air is warmed and humidified (water vapour pressure 47 mmHg) and this lowers the pressure of oxygen available to about 150 mmHg, i.e. PO_2 of 150 mmHg (760 mmHg – 47 mmHg × 21%). This pressure is lowered further because of the dead space in the lungs where gaseous exchange doesn't take place (nose, trachea and bronchi). As blood entering the lungs has a PO_2 of 40 mmHg, diffusion occurs, thereby allowing oxygen to move from the air to the blood.

Changes occur when an individual experiences a change in altitude, for example athletes competing in other countries or climbers attempting to climb Mount Everest. For people who live in such places their breathing, lungs and red cells adapt to having less oxygen but for people who only visit for a short time problems can occur.

Exercise

1. Calculate the inspired air pressure for climbers in Mount Everest (about 8000 m above sea level) where the air pressure is 250 mmHg, using the formula: air pressure = water vapour pressure of 47 mmHg × oxygen % of 21%.
2. Consider the effect this would have on the body.

The inspired air pressure, i.e. PO_2 at the top of Mount Everest is 42 mmHg (250 mmHg – 47 mmHg × 21%), with the PO_2 being 40 mmHg in the blood entering the lungs. Consequently, diffusion doesn't occur as the difference in the two pressures is not enough. The body would not be able to function properly as oxygen would not be entering the bloodstream and therefore would not be transported to the tissues. It is for this reason that individuals who climb at altitude may use oxygen (Casey 2001).

Oxygen can be used at different pressures: 24%, 28% or 40%. Using the same formula as above, it can be seen that any increase in oxygen pressures will increase the inspired air pressure, i.e. PO_2 and therefore aid diffusion (Casey 2001). For 24% oxygen the inspired air pressure, i.e. PO_2 is 171 mmHg, for 28% it is 200 mmHg and for 40% it is 285 mmHg. As these are all considerably higher than the blood PO_2 of 40 mmHg, then oxygen will be diffused into the bloodstream far more easily.

Arterial blood gas (ABG) samples are used to evaluate the partial pressures of oxygen and carbon dioxide in the blood and according to Coombs (2001), are commonly taken from acutely ill patients with respiratory and cardiac disease to assess their disorders. It is important to appreciate the physiological underpinnings of blood gas analysis and relate to changes that can occur in health as well as illness.

Normally the arterial partial pressure of carbon dioxide (P_aCO_2) is 4.5–6 kPa (35–45 mmHg). Changes in people's breathing or ventilation affects the carbon dioxide levels, so by measuring the P_aCO_2 levels this will give an indication of the person's breathing and ventilation function. For example, in patients who are hyperventilating (breathing very fast and deep) large amounts of air are breathed in and out of the lungs. This lowers the amount of carbon dioxide and the P_aCO_2 level falls to below 4.5 kPa and causes respiratory alkalosis, which occurs when there is a fall in oxygen levels associated with high altitude (Coombs 2001). Anxiety may also cause people to hyperventilate and this can be treated by placing a paper bag over their nose and mouth and encouraging them to breathe in and out of the bag. This recycles the expired carbon dioxide so lowering the rate and depth of the respirations (Cornock 1996).

Respiratory acidosis arises when the person is hypoventilating (slow or shallow breathing) and so small amounts of air are breathed in and out of the lungs. This raises the amount of carbon dioxide and the P_aCO_2 level rises to above 6 kPa and causes respiratory acidosis, which can occur when there is an obstruction to the airways following inhalation of a foreign body (Coombs 2001). In this instance the obstruction needs to be removed to return respirations and blood gases to normal.

Normally, the arterial partial pressure of oxygen (P_aO_2) is 8–12 kPa (60–90 mmHg) and measures the amount of oxygen dissolved in the blood. This level indicates the amount of oxygen which is potentially available to oxygenate the tissues. If the P_aO_2 levels fall below 8 kPa (hypoxaemia) then the cells are deprived of oxygen (hypoxia) and this can lead to cell damage and cell death. Hypoxaemia occurs following hypoventilation, obstructed airway and sometimes in older people. Lynes (2003) and Allen (2005) offer stepped approaches designed to enable nurses to interpret blood gas analysis quickly and accurately. These involve reviewing P_aO_2, pH, P_aCO_2 and bicarbonate ion concentration (HCO_3^-) readings to identify possible acid–base imbalances.

Arterial blood gases can form part of an acutely ill patient's assessment alongside oxygen saturation levels. The oxygen saturation level (S_aO_2) can be measured by a pulse oximeter, using a finger probe, and is a useful monitoring device for evaluating the oxygen status of patients in a variety of clinical areas. It is important to remember that S_aO_2 measures the amount of oxygen being carried by haemoglobin in the arterial (oxygenated) blood but not the amount of oxygen that is delivered to the tissues. The oxygen saturation level should be 95–98% in a healthy adult (Casey 2001, Brooker 2005) and provides useful information when assessing a patient. Higgins (2005b) provides information relating to this procedure. However, there are a variety of nonclinical factors which can affect the accuracy of pulse oximetry, such as nail polish, movement as in shivering or fits, and dark skin, and it may not be reliable in severe respiratory disease, so care must be taken when interpreting the readings. Clark (2002) raises concerns that readings are being used without full knowledge of aspects which could affect their interpretation. Howell (2002) concurs with this after finding a knowledge deficit of pulse oximetry in nurses and medical staff when completing a small-scale audit in a large general hospital. However, Giuiliano & Liu (2006) found an increased level of pulse oximetry knowledge in critical care nurses than previously reported but recommends that further research is conducted to assess whether this knowledge is applied in clinical practice.

Other less invasive measurements can give useful information relating to respiratory function. Observing for cyanosis (blue–purple colour visible in nail beds, skin and mucous membranes, such as lips) is vital and this occurs when oxygen saturation levels fall below 70% and indicates that there is a large volume of haemoglobin which is poorly saturated and the oxygen levels are therefore low. Esmond (2003) notes that the oral mucosa and tongue should be examined in people with dark skin as lip colour changes may be difficult to see.

First-aiders may be involved in situations where individuals have collapsed due to shock, circulatory and respiratory failure; Brooker (2005) describes basic life support (BLS) using the mnemonic ABC: Airway (open and clear the airway), Breathing (give mouth-to-mouth resuscitation), and Circulation (carry out external cardiac compression). Finding individuals in a collapsed state, such as this, can be a frightening experience for onlookers; however, there have been publicity and road shows to teach the general public how to resuscitate people.

Another problem that individuals may experience in their everyday lives is that called the 'flight or fight' response which can help survival at times of extreme danger. The response to danger is to raise the respiration rate and depth, heart rate, blood pressure and blood flow to the muscles. This response prepares the body for physical action so that the individual can either run away from danger or stand and fight (Brooker 2005).

Emotional issues related to breathing (psychological factors)

Emotional events in life can affect breathing (Roper et al 1996). Consider the following exercise.

> ### Exercise
> 1. Observe individuals, when watching different programmes on TV, and identify the effect emotions have on their respirations, e.g. when happy, sad, grieving, anxious or frightened.
> 2. Ask a friend or colleague to observe your breathing whilst watching television programmes, a visit to the cinema or a sports event (making sure they do not make you aware of when they are doing this). Discuss your findings and theirs.

The actor's ability may have affected what you observed, but within your own family you may be able to confirm the associated changes in respiration. Roper et al (1996) identified that sadness and grieving can affect the rate and depth of breathing resulting in audible and visible activities such as sobbing and sighing. Also when individuals are frightened their respirations change and this can be noted by an initial indrawing and gasping respiration followed by an increase in breathing and pulse rates. Equally, pleasure and excitement result in raised breathing and respiratory rates. For some people, anxiety and panic attacks can result in marked changes in respiration.

West & Popkess-Vawter (1994) discuss classic literature from the 1960s which reports on the psychosocial aspects of breathlessness. For example, Dudley et al (1964), in West & Popkess-Vawter (1994), studied the effects of life stress on pulmonary function of individuals with normal and diseased lungs and concluded that psychological orientation was a major factor in the person's respiratory response to life events as changes in respiration rates during anger or anxiety were similar to respiratory changes during exercise.

Equally, Burns & Howell (1969), also cited in West & Popkess-Vawter (1994), studied chronic bronchitis patients who reported disproportionately severe breathlessness when compared with their lung function tests. Their level of breathlessness was found to be unrelated to the amount of exertion or their environment, but was related to their emotional status, where hyperventilation was associated with an emotionally distressing event.

West & Popkess-Vawter (1994) propose a holistic breathlessness model linking current life experiences (biological, psychological and social triggers) with antecedent conditions (perceived threat, past negative experiences, stress response, disease changes, fatigue and pulmonary congestion) which can then present with varying degrees of breathlessness, according to the individual's response.

Relaxation techniques and biofeedback can help individuals during periods of high anxiety or panic attacks and they should be encouraged to plan relaxation periods into their daily life. Biofeedback can also be used for individuals who suffer from migraine headaches, high or low blood pressure, epilepsy or even with paralysis. Kaushar et al (2005) found that biofeedback-assisted diaphragmatic breathing and relaxation was useful in migraine and had better long-term effect than using propranolol. Biofeedback systems use electronic systems to measure stress and feed back the results in the form of a movement of a pen on graph paper or by the pitch of sound through earphones. Individuals can then practise using different techniques and compare the effects, such as being taught how to identify factors which trigger their problems, how to cope with these problems, how to change their lifestyles and how to gain self-control. These techniques are a reminder that behaviour, thoughts and feelings can influence physical health and although they cannot cure disease they can help an individual. However, for this to occur the individual must accept responsibility for their own health.

Practices, associated health beliefs and habits in different cultures related to breathing (sociocultural factors)

According to the British Thoracic Society (2006a), the link between social inequality and lung disease is highlighted and the report states that social inequality causes a higher proportion of deaths in respiratory diseases than in any other disease area. Almost half the deaths (44%) are associated with social class inequalities compared to 28% of deaths from ischaemic heart disease. Men aged 20–64 employed in unskilled manual occupations are 14 times more likely to die from chronic obstructive pulmonary disease (COPD) and nine times more likely from tuberculosis (TB) than men in professional roles. The burden in the community is also noted: 24 million GP consultations are linked to respiratory diseases and 1 million hospital admissions were respiratory related (www.brit-thoracic.org.uk/BurdenofLungDisease2).

It is important that you consider the practices of individuals in relation to breathing. Most of the time, individuals are not aware of breathing until they have a problem, e.g. cough, choke, spit or sneeze. Coughing can be a sign of ill health (particularly cancer) if it is a nagging cough with hoarseness. The spread of disease through coughing, spitting and sneezing is well known, yet some individuals exhibit antisocial behaviour with regard to this, such as spitting on the pavement whilst walking along the street. It is obvious by observing onlookers, that this behaviour is perceived to be in poor taste. Tolerance to individuals polluting the air in social places warrants consideration, as does occupational practices and their effect on breathing and ill health.

> **Exercise**
> 1. Identify links between various occupations and lung disease.
> 2. How is smoking tolerated in social places such as restaurants, public houses, workplaces, theatres or on public transport?
> 3. Identify if there are any differences in cultural attitudes to breathing habits.

There are numerous occupations linked to lung diseases. For example, long-term exposure to coal dust or cotton dust predisposes workers to lung disorders, such as pneumoconiosis and silicosis.

Another industrial disease, malignant mesothelioma, is linked to asbestos, which was used in the building industry in the 1960s and 1970s. Millar (2000) reports that experts estimate that between the years 2000 and 2035 more than 250 000 people will die from this disease in Western Europe. The UK death rate is expected to be higher than any other European country, except The Netherlands with some 1750 dying from this disease. Men born between 1945 and 1950 and who worked as plumbers, gas fitters, carpenters and electricians, are at greatest risk. However, their family members are also at risk from secondary exposure via the asbestos fibres on their clothing. Millar (2000) reports on the development of a nurse-led project aimed at improving access to services and providing information on mesothelioma. The National Institute for Health and Clinical Excellence (NICE 2007) is in the process of finalising guidelines in relation to recommending the use of pemetrexed disodium as part of the treatment for mesothelioma. According to NICE there were 1700 cases of mesothelioma diagnosed in UK in 2004 and a further 2000 cases per year are expected between the years 2011 and 2015, culminating in over 65 000 cases between the years 2002 and 2050.

The general attitude to cigarette smoking in the early 20th century was that it relieved tension and produced no ill effects. However, it was noticed that lung cancer, rare before the 20th century, had dramatically increased and the link to lung cancer was made. Various measures have taken place since the 1960s in an attempt to limit smoking and the resultant diseases. Warnings on cigarette packets were introduced and all cigarette advertising was banned on television and radio.

The Hospital In-Patient Enquiry (OPCS 1985) reported that in a one in ten sample, 46 023 patients in England and Wales were suffering from respiratory illnesses and a further 5499 had lung cancer. The mortality rate, in 1986, for England and Wales for respiratory illness was found to be over 63 000 and a further 35 000 from lung cancer (OPCS 1986). Although the death rate in men from lung cancer was halved from 1971 to 1992, the death rate for women increased by 16% (Central Statistical Office 1995). Cancer trends in England and Wales in the second half of the century (1950–1999) demonstrate that mortality from cancer

To help reduce problems, smog levels, particularly ozone levels, are included in weather forecasts to alert the general public of this risk and individuals who are sensitive to ozone should limit outdoor exercise during the latter part of the day. Prevention of smog is also done by controlling smoke from chimneys, furnaces, industrial plants and noxious emissions from cars. Recent changes in the internal combustion engines and the use of catalytic converters have made these emissions lower in an attempt to lower the risk of smog (DoH 1991, 1995). Fine dust particles, suspended in the air, contain pollen, silica, animal fibres, bacteria and moulds. In cities these dust particles also contain smoke from industry and can cause a serious pollution problem and may cause silicosis. There is a need to use filters to obtain dust-free air. Public transport issues such as park and ride, car sharing, congestion charges in cities, predestination of town areas all help to limit the air pollution. (See www.defra.gov.ukl/ environment/airquality for further information.)

Furthermore, COMEAP produced a report in February 2006 with regards to the link of air pollution and cardiovascular disease for the Department of Health (2006). It concluded, from a larger number of studies, that there was convincing evidence between air pollutants and cardiovascular disease reflected in risk of death, hospital admissions and. reduction in life expectancy. This supports earlier work by Poloniecki et al (1997) who reported that there was a significant relationship between the incidence of myocardial infarction and air pollutants (Department of Health 1999b). This relationship was identified by analysing the number of hospital admissions with myocardial infarctions in London and the previous day's air pollution levels. Poloniecki et al (1997) suggest that exposure to air pollutants may be linked to 6000 patients per year who suffer myocardial infarctions.

Another hazard, first noted in 1976, is that of *Legionella pneumonophila,* a bacterium which causes infection and inflammation of the lung tissue. The bacteria are found in stagnant water in water tanks, shower heads and air conditioning systems so the source of the bacteria has often been linked to hotels and hospitals. It is known to transmit Legionnaires' disease which produces symptoms of bronchopneumonia, complicated by gastrointestinal problems, headache, confusion and renal failure (Waugh & Grant 2006). The figures for 2003 identified that 315 people (239 men, 76 women) had contracted Legionnaires' disease with 175 associated with travel, resulting in 35 deaths compared with 182 cases with 23 deaths in 1980. Due to the link with travel, a working group has set out European Guidelines for Control and Prevention of Travel Associated Legionnaires' Disease available on www.ewgli.org/data/ europoean_guidelines. However, an increase in this disease was noted in England and Wales in 2006 with some 273 cases being reported up to August 2006, an increase of 68 cases from the 2005 figures, but only a small proportion of these cases are related to foreign travel (Health Protection Agency 2006a) and it is therefore important for nurses to be alert to this disease.

Severe acute respiratory syndrome (SARS) is another severe respiratory disease caused by SARS coronavirus which was first recognised in China in 2002 and spread worldwide before being contained in July 2003 (Health Protection Agency 2006b). Over 8000 cases were reported in 30 countries and symptoms include a fever of over 38°C with a cough, or difficulty breathing or shortness of breath. Pneumonia or respiratory distress syndrome is noted on X-ray along with a recent travel history to China and Hong Kong. Hospitalisation is required and strict infection control practices are required to prevent spread. (Further details can be found on www. hpa.org.uk/infections/topics/a-z/SARS.)

According to the Health Protection Agency (2007), avian influenza A (H5N1) (bird flu) in humans is a rare but severe disease and must be closely watched because of the potential of this virus to evolve in ways that could start a global outbreak (pandemic). H5N1 affects poultry flocks and other birds but people who come into contact with infected birds can contract the disease. There is no firm evidence to support that H5N1 is able to pass from person to person as yet. The disease follows an unusually aggressive pathway; initially symptoms include a high fever over 38°C and influenza-like symptoms but a rapid deterioration occurs with high fatality as viral pneumonia and multi-organ failure are common. The first cases were found in Hong Kong where 18 cases were reported in 1997 and 6 of these patients died. Up to December 2006, 261 people caught the infection and 157 of these died. They are mainly from China, Cambodia, Indonesia, Thailand and Vietnam, and most cases occurred in previously healthy children and young adults. No human cases of bird flu have been reported in the UK but a swan was found in Scotland in 2006 which had died from the disease. Hospitalisation, strict infection control practices and specific antiviral drug therapy can be used, e.g. oseltamivir. (See www.who.int and dh.gov.uk for further details.)

Policies, laws and economics related to breathing (politicoeconomic factors)

Roper et al (2000, p. 119) clearly identify that political, economic and social issues are 'major determinants of health' and that health is not solely the concern of the National Health Service (NHS) but relates to public policies. The economic state of a country affects the living conditions, which in turn affect the health and illness of that population.

The Public Health Act of 1875 heralded major reforms in the UK, with emphasis on sanitation and water supplies. Combined with this, as Roper et al (2000) discuss, there was a general improvement in the country's economy and as a result, living conditions improved. The general health of the population improved and diseases that in those days were killers were seen to decline prior to the implementation of preventative and curative care.

Today, preventative health measures are needed to promote health and prevent illness. As health care costs increase then the need for preventative health care is increased. For example, immunisation is now used to prevent respiratory diseases such as tuberculosis and influenza (flu). Every autumn, a national campaign is run in the UK, offering influenza (flu) vaccinations to protect people who are at risk of serious illness should they catch the flu. This includes everyone who is 65 years old and above and those who already suffer from chronic diseases, such as asthma, diabetes and heart disease. The vaccinations are given in GPs' surgeries usually, but NHS Trusts also provide this service to their workers. Guidance has been produced by NICE in 2003 for the prevention and treatment of flu. Amantadine is not recommended for the treatment of flu but oseltamivir or zanamivir can be used in certain circumstances (NICE 2003a, 2003b).

Environmental issues link to this factor also in relation to air pollutants as previously discussed, e.g. policies in relation to the purity of air, lessening the emissions from cars and industry and the banning of certain substances, e.g. asbestos. Poorer industrial towns have a higher than expected death rate compared to more affluent areas linking the effects of social factors and illness. For example, Harding & Reid (2000) identified that mortality levels were lower in the South and the death rate of men aged 26–64 was the highest in the North and West Midlands and in women aged 26–59, the lowest mortality rate was in the South East and West and East Anglia. The North–South divide was shown in all age ranges with urban and industrial areas having the highest mortality according to Fitzpatrick et al (2000).

Exercise

1. Look on the Department of Health website (www. dh.gov.uk).
2. Identify the current health policies relating to breathing and smoking.

You should have found numerous links to breathing, smoking and related health problems on this website. Within health and social care topics there are at least four areas that relate to breathing, e.g. air pollution, pertussis (whooping cough), tobacco, and tuberculosis. The National Service Framework for COPD has been advocated and is due to be completed in 2008. Information about various advisory committees is also included, such as SCOTH (Scientific Committee on Tobacco and Health) and COMEAP (Committee on the Medical Effects of Air Pollutants).

The first ever White Paper on smoking and tobacco published in 1998 entitled *Smoking Kills* set out three targets in relation to smoking:

1. Reduce smoking amongst children from 13% to 11% or less by the year 2005 and to 9% by 2010.
2. Reduce smoking amongst adults in all social classes from 28% to 26% or less by the year 2005 and to 24% by 2010.
3. Reduce smoking amongst pregnant women from 23% to 18% or less by the year 2005 and to 15% by 2010.

Following this, the NHS Plan was published in 2000 by the Department of Health (2000a), and this identified the need for a major expansion in smoking cessation programmes. As a result, 26 Health Action Zones (HAZ) were established in England in areas of deprivation and poor health to tackle inequalities and provide services. Smoking cessation services consisting of specialist support sessions were launched in 1999/2000, with £53 million being made available for these services plus extra for nicotine replacement therapy. A range of different services ensued until April 2001 when a minimum standard was set to include weekly support for 4 weeks after quit attempt.

The initial results for 1999/2000 published by the Department of Health (2001b) (www.doh.gov.uk/public/sb0105.htm) showed that 14 600 people had set a quit date through these services in HAZs and 5800 (39%) had successfully quit smoking at the 4-week follow up.

Further action was deemed necessary and the 'Stop Smoking Service' is one arm of the Department of Health's strategy to combat smoking and reduce the preventable deaths from this addiction. Stop Smoking Services have now replaced Smoking Cessation Services and are one part of a comprehensive tobacco control strategy. The Department of Health's (2002c) Priorities and Planning Framework 2003–2006 was published in October 2002 and included new targets for smoking cessation services for Primary Care Trusts to achieve over the period. These targets were as follows:

1. 50 000 smokers successfully quitting at the 4-week stage for 2001–02
2. 100 000 smokers successfully quitting at the 4-week stage for 2002–03
3. 800 000 smokers successfully quitting at the 4-week stage by 2006.

All of these targets were met and exceeded with 832 900 smokers having successfully quitted by March 2006. Although, according to the figures published in the Department of Health's (2003a) *Statistics on Smoking: England, 2003*, the original Smoking Kills targets were not fully achieved, progress is being made on all aspects of smoking cessation.

Exercise

1. Review these targets and consider what action will be needed to meet these from the political perspective.
2. Discuss with colleagues the implications of these targets for health education initiatives and service providers.

You may have read the government's strategy in relation to these targets in which a need for a wide and integrated range of measures is identified by the Department of Health

(1998a) or later work by West et al (2003) or McNeill et al (2005). This includes tobacco education campaigns, reducing the availability of tobacco, regulating supply of the actual products and reducing advertising. Policies on tobacco and smoking are wide ranging and a new campaign designed to target young adults commenced in September 2006. A major issue is to help protect young people by helping them to quit and to prevent them from starting smoking. As a result, £138 million was made available to the NHS Stop Smoking Services between 2003 and 2006 with a further £112 million for PCTs in 2006 and 2007.

NICE (2006b) produced guidelines in relation to brief interventions and referrals for smoking cessation in primary care and other settings. Silagy & Stead (2001) reviewed 34 trials, conducted between 1972 and 1999, involving 27000 smokers and concluded that simple advice from physicians had a small effect on smoking cessation rates. Potential benefits were also found by Rice & Stead (2001), when 15 studies were reviewed to assess the effectiveness of nursing interventions in relation to smoking cessation. The odds of quitting were significantly increased when smoking cessation advice and counselling were given by nurses.

Anthonisen et al (2005) completed a randomised controlled trial of a 10-week-long smoking cessation intervention with 5887 smokers with asymptomatic airway obstruction. Fourteen-year mortality rates were found to be lower in the smoking cessation group even when only a minority stopped smoking. Telephone counselling was found to increase smoking cessation rates amongst young adult smokers according to a randomised control trial completed by Rabius et al (2004) and a systematic review by Stead et al (2006) concluded that telephone counselling can help as part of a programme to help people stop smoking. Etter & Perneger (2004) tested the effect of a computer-tailored smoking cessation programme and found that this doubled the odds of quitting smoking but the effect was only maintained whilst the programme was active. Further research is needed to follow individuals who have ceased smoking and whether this has reduced their risk of developing lung cancer.

Initially, 1 week's nicotine replacement therapy (NRT) was made available free to those who were less able to purchase them, but in 2001 NRT was made available on NHS prescription. NICE (2002) guidelines considered the use of NRT and bupropion to be cost effective for smoking cessation. NRT is currently available in the form of gum, patches, lozenges, inhalators, sublingual tablets and nasal sprays with gum, lozenges and patches being available on open sale. Statistics for the NHS Stop Smoking Services in England (Information Centre 2006) identified that in April 2005–March 2006 some 603174 people had set a quit date through the NHS Smoking Services and at the 4-week follow-up 329854 had successfully quit with the majority in receipt of NRT (Information Centre 2006). The cost of the prescription items in England was £43.5 million for NRT and £4.6 million for bupropion and the expenditure on

NHS Stop Smoking Services was £52 million. However, the annual cost to the NHS of treating patients with smoking-related disorders is around £1500 million according to NICE (2002).

A European ban on all tobacco advertising and sponsorship has been in place since 2006. Smoking is to be reduced in public places and a new Charter for Smoking in the licensed trade and a new Approved Code of Practice on smoking at work has been agreed. The tax increase on tobacco products will remain above inflation in an attempt to deter people from smoking due to the cost and stricter measures will be used to cut tobacco smuggling.

Health care professionals have an important role to play in ensuring that these targets are met in relation to health promotion activities, being non-smoking role models and supporting individuals through smoking cessation programmes. It is recognised that some health care professionals smoke but these individuals can still play a role in ensuring that these targets are met and maybe take some personal responsibility in this and work with smokers through a Stop Smoking Service.

An example of how legislation impacts upon health in breathing is in relation to the Health and Safety at Work Act (DoH 1974) which is directed at protecting the public. Within this Act the employer has a duty to provide a safe working environment and to inform and instruct employees about health risks and the precautions to be taken. Economic factors are a major influence in relation to breathing from the politicians' and individuals' perspective. Smoking costs the NHS £1.7 billion pounds per year. But how much does it cost the individual in monetary terms.

Exercise

1. Working on the basis of cigarettes costing £4 for a packet of 20, work out how much it will cost an individual who smokes:

   a. 10 cigarettes a day for 1 week, 1 month, 1 year, 15 years, 30 years and 50 years.
   b. 20 cigarettes a day for 1 week, 1 month, 1 year, 15 years, 30 years and 50 years.

You may be shocked at the cost of this activity. At 10 cigarettes a day, the cost in monetary terms is £14 a week, £60 a month, £730 a year, £10950 for 15 years, £21900 for 30 years and £36500 for 50 years. For someone smoking 20 cigarettes a day, then these figures are obviously doubled, giving £28 a week, £120 a month, £1460 a year, £21900 in 15 years, £43800 in 30 years and £73000 in 50 years.

The cost of nicotine replacement therapy is between £10 to £20 a week and with a course lasting about 10 weeks, it amounts to costing between £100 and £200 to quit smoking. Surely an incentive of monetary gains is worthy of advertising.

CONCLUSION

The framework of the model of living has been used to demonstrate how the model can be used to guide your understanding of health and everyday life in relation to the activity of breathing (Fig. 5.10). From this it is hoped that you have been able to engage in the exercises and can appreciate the complexity of the model and the interrelativeness of the other Activities of Living. The final two exercises will concentrate on the interrelativeness with other activities and the factors which affect breathing specifically through the use of mini case studies to demonstrate how individuality in living occurs.

> **Exercise**
> 1. Read through the family scenario in Case study 5.1 and consider how their activity of breathing may affect each other and the other Activities of Living.

> **Case study 5.1**
>
> ### Effect of smoking on ALs
> John is 60 years old and has smoked 20 cigarettes a day for 40 years and has worked in the building trade for most of his life. His wife does not smoke now but she has done in the past. They have two children, aged 35 and 28. The elder son has two children and they visit their grandparents regularly, as well as going abroad on holiday as a family. Their youngest daughter, who also smokes, is expecting her first child.

You may have considered the following points:

- *Maintaining a safe environment* – safety issues relating to fire hazards in the home
  – effects of stress in relation to smoking and quitting
  – air pollution and passive smoking
  – immunisation of grandchildren
- *Communicating* – smell of cigarettes on breath and teeth affected
- *Eating and drinking* – food and taste affected by smoking
- *Eliminating* – predisposition to cancers
- *Mobilising* – difficulty with walking, running etc., if suffer from shortness of breath
- *Expressing sexuality* – fetal damage possible
- *Maintaining body temperature* – predisposition to chest infections as noted by pyrexia
- *Working and playing* – social activities curtailed by nonsmoking areas
  – cost of smoking
  – building work itself with dust and possible asbestos exposure
  – holidays abroad and risk of respiratory diseases
- *Sleep and rest* – coughing may affect sleep patterns
- *Dying* – predisposition to lung cancer for all the family.

> **Exercise**
> 1. Read through the scenario in Case study 5.2 and consider how the activity of breathing is affected by biological, psychological, sociocultural, environmental and politicoeconomic factors.

> **Case study 5.2**
>
> ### Breathing and factors affecting health
> A 20-year-old young man, who suffers from asthma, is taken ill at a disco. He takes his inhaler but unfortunately because he panics he is unable to control his breathing.

You may have considered the following:

- *Biological factors* – effect of asthma on lung tissue, effect on breathing, effects of smoke on lungs
- *Psychological factors* – anxiety, not using inhaler properly leading to panic state and hyperventilation
- *Sociocultural factors* – peer pressure to smoke and visit discos, macho male image
- *Environmental factors* – possible smoky environment
- *Politicoeconomic factors* – cost of smoking for a student.

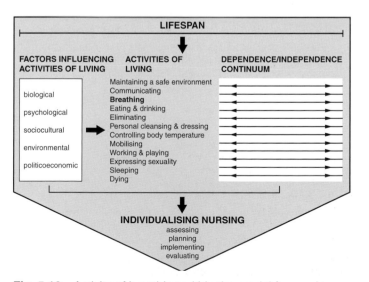

Fig. 5.10 Activity of breathing within the model for nursing (from Roper et al 1996, with permission).

SUMMARY POINTS

1. Breathing is affected by all the factors.
2. Breathing can affect all of the other ALs.
3. Smoking is one of the major contributors to breathing problems.
4. Pollutants are a major problem worldwide which can cause respiratory problems.

THE MODEL FOR NURSING

USING THE MODEL FOR NURSING TO INDIVIDUALISE NURSING FOR THE ACTIVITY OF BREATHING

Introduction

This part of the chapter will link the components of the model of living (lifespan, dependency/independency and factors affecting breathing) with the model for nursing in states of health and ill health in relation to breathing. Exercises, mini case scenarios and one major case scenario will be used to allow you to apply the knowledge gained from the model of living section. The application of the model for nursing is based upon the integration of the model of living components and the four stages of the nursing process, according to Roper et al (1996), as shown in Figure 5.10. (See Chapter 1 for further details relating to the nursing process, i.e. assessing the individual, planning nursing activities, implementation of care and evaluation of care planned and given.) The initial stage of this process, i.e. assessment, begins with the point of contact of the nurse and the patient and is the start of the nurse–patient relationship. The aim of the assessment stage in relation to breathing is to collect information about how the individual relates to this Activity of Living when they are well and when they are ill.

Breathing in health

In order to do this assessment, all the other aspects of the model should be integrated into the breathing Activity of Living as shown in Box 5.2.

This Activity of Living in health is complex and the nurse needs to be aware of the normal health states of individuals before considering the activity of breathing in ill health. You will need to be able to integrate this information in each stage of the nursing process to identify individual patient needs and problems.

Breathing in ill health

The components of the model will be used to show you how a variety of ill-health issues affect the activity of breathing.

Box 5.2	Summary of the model for nursing with the activity of breathing – in health

Lifespan
- Consider effect of age on breathing, pulse rate, blood pressure.

Dependence
- Dependency is linked to lifespan and ill health, e.g. infection, congenital, trauma, paralysis.

Independence
- Independence linked to health.

Factors affecting breathing
Biological
- Degree of physical activity.
- Body's physiological responses to stressors.
- Intact respiratory system to enable effective internal and external respiration.
- Intact circulatory, lymphatic and nervous system to ensure that bodily systems benefit from the actions of the respiratory system.
- Noted by observations of normal breathing: rate, depth, rhythm, sound, patterns.
- Note any abnormal breathing: cough, wheeze, sputum produced, exposure to pollutants.

Psychological
- Effects of emotional state on breathing such as crying, laughing, anxiety, panic, fear.

Sociocultural
- Religious practices related to bathing/meditation/breathing control.
- Expectoration of sputum and coughing habits.

Environmental
- Exposure to microorganisms.
- Exposure to air pollutants at home, work, travelling.

Politicoeconomic
- Mechanisms to limit smoking-related diseases and air pollutant diseases.

Exercise
1. Using the components of the model (lifespan, dependency–independency continuum, factors affecting health – physical/biological, psychological, sociocultural, environmental, politicoeconomic) and your clinical experience to date, consider what illnesses patients may have in relation to breathing.
2. Check Box 5.3 for some examples.

| Box 5.3 | Summary of the model for nursing with the activity of breathing – ill health |

Lifespan
- Congenital abnormalities.
- Childhood, e.g. asthma, bronchiolitis.
- Adult, e.g. chest trauma, tumours.
- Older person, e.g. range of illnesses as below.

Dependence/independence
- Breathing difficulties will affect many of the other Activities of Living and therefore the individual may become dependent on others, e.g. difficulties with mobilising due to dyspnoea.

Factors affecting breathing
1. *Biological*
   a. *Damage to respiratory tract*
      - Airway obstruction, e.g. chronic obstructive pulmonary/airways disease, emphysema, asthma, chronic bronchitis.
      - Allergic reaction, e.g. bronchial asthma.
      - Infection, e.g. pneumonia, pleurisy, SARS.
      - Trauma, e.g. chest injuries, flail chest, fractured ribs, haemothorax.
      - Tumours, e.g. benign, primary bronchogenic carcinomas, metastatic tumours.
      - Blood flow obstruction, e.g. pulmonary embolism in pulmonary capillaries.
   b. *Damage to cardiovascular tract*
      - Congestion, e.g. cor pulmonale, congestive cardiac failure, pulmonary oedema.
      - Blood flow obstruction to myocardium, e.g. myocardial infarction.
      - Lack of oxygen in blood, e.g. iron deficiency anaemia.
   c. *Damage to nervous tract*
      - Respiratory muscle paralysis, e.g. poliomyelitis, Guillain–Barré syndrome.
      - Brain/spinal cord damage, e.g. coma/head injuries.

2. *Psychological*
   - Link with stress and anxiety, e.g. asthma.

3. *Sociocultural*
   - Cultural differences, e.g. pulmonary tuberculosis.
   - Smoking habits (active/passive), e.g. lung cancer.

4. *Environmental*
   - Pollens/irritants, e.g. hayfever, asthma.
   - Smoking, e.g. lung cancer.
   - Inhalation of dust, e.g. silicosis, asbestosis.
   - Damp/overcrowding poor living conditions, e.g. bronchial asthma, pulmonary tuberculosis.

Reflect on these conditions and identify your learning needs following this exercise. It may be useful for you to discuss your learning needs with a qualified nurse and formulate action plans to address them.

ASSESSING THE INDIVIDUAL

The aim of this section, related to assessing an individual in relation to breathing, is to demonstrate how you can utilise the components of the model of living to carry out the following three phases involved in assessment:

1. Collection of data when taking a nursing history in relation to the activity of breathing and other related activities.
2. Interpretation of data collected to assess the degree of alteration in the activity of breathing and the effect on other Activities of Living.
3. Identification of individuals' actual and potential problems related to the activity of breathing and other related activities.

It is noted that assessment is a continuous activity but a thorough initial assessment is vital and this chapter will describe how the components of the model can be integrated to support the assessment process. (For further details relating to assessment refer to Chapter 1.)

Collection of data when taking a nursing history in relation to the activity of breathing and other related activities

The assessment stage is vital, as all the other stages of individualising nursing are dependent upon it. Therefore, it is important to plan this activity and consider what may affect the collection of data, their interpretation and the identification of patients' problems.

Exercise
1. Consider that you have been asked to assess a patient who has been admitted to your clinical area with severe breathlessness.
2. Identify what physical, psychological, sociocultural, environmental and politicoeconomic factors may influence the collection of the data required.

You may wish to refer to Box 5.4 to check these factors and consider how you can minimise the influence these factors may have.

Reflect on how you can ensure that the collection of data is accurate and how these factors can be minimised so as not to influence the information collected. As noted, there are many factors that may affect the collection of the data and therefore you will need to use a variety of skills when collecting data. The following exercise will enable you to consider the skills needed.

Box 5.4	Factors influencing activity of breathing

Physical
- Actual physical state of breathing as they may be unable to talk due to severe breathlessness, coughing or wheezing.
- May be in pain which will affect their ability to communicate.

Psychological
- Actual mental state due to oxygen transport being affected so may be hypoxic.
- Actual emotional state due to fear and anxiety relating to dying, may feel sense of shame.
- Actual knowledge of disease and past experiences.

Sociocultural
- Different social/cultural backgrounds of patient and nurse which may affect their ability to communicate.
- Level of interpersonal skills of the patient and the nurse.
- Presence, attitudes and reactions of others.

Environmental
- Ward environment noisy and not very private causing distractions and repetition of answers.

Politicoeconomic
- Time to conduct the interview.

Exercise
1. What skills will you need to develop to enable you to obtain a comprehensive nursing history from a breathless patient?
2. Check Box 5.5 with regard to these skills.
3. Reflect on your abilities in these skills. Consider which of these skills you believe you have mastered. Then identify the skills which you may need to improve upon and consider how you can do this.
4. Discuss this with your mentor or preceptor in practice and write an action plan for this learning need.

Having identified that various factors may affect your ability to collect information and that a variety of skills are equally required, it may be useful to consider what data you need to collect specifically and what purpose these data will be used for.

Exercise
1. Reflect upon a recent admission you have been involved with and identify potential questions that would help you collect specific data.
2. You may wish to check Box 5.6 for possible questions.

Box 5.5	Assessment skills – AL breathing

Interviewing skills
- Asking open and closed questions as appropriate so as not to tire the individual.
- Explain issues in lay terms and check understanding.
- Use of silence to allow individual to rest or think.
- Prioritise questions.
- Involve relatives.

Observation skills
- Verbal and nonverbal cues.
- Physical signs, e.g. pulse rate, respiratory rate, peak flow, pulse oximetry.
- Psychological cues, e.g. anxiety.

Listening skills
- Therapeutic relationship skills.
- Use own body language appropriately.

Box 5.6	Assessment questions – AL breathing

Lifespan and independence
- Does the individual breathe normally in relation to the expectations of the time of the lifespan?

Dependence
- Has the individual experienced any difficulties with breathing in the past or do they have a long-standing breathing difficulty?
- How has the individual coped with these difficulties experienced with breathing?
- How is the individual coping with these breathing difficulties?
- Could the individual experience difficulties with breathing in the future?

Factors affecting breathing
Physical
- What specific difficulties is the individual experiencing and what are the causes?
- What specific abnormalities are noted in the person's breathing pattern or habit?
- What other Activities of Living affect the individual's breathing difficulties?
- What effect does the individual's breathing difficulties have on the other Activities of Living?

Psychological
- What emotional responses affect breathing?
- What information or advice is required now or in the future to aid breathing and promote independence?

Sociocultural
- What are the individual's beliefs and attitudes to coughing, spitting and smoking?

| Box 5.6 | Assessment questions *(continued)* |

Environmental
- What factors may alter/affect the individual's breathing at home, work and hospital?

Politicoeconomic
- What information and resources does the individual have or need, to assist in coping with any breathing difficulties to aid independence?

You may need to reflect on how you feel about asking these questions and how you would ask these questions in a conversational manner. You then need to consider specific questions which would be needed for patients with specific ill-health issues related to breathing. The following exercise will allow you to consider additional questions relevant to three different ill-health breathing problems. You are required to read the mini case studies in Box 5.7 to complete this exercise.

Exercise
1. Identify specific questions relating to the mini case studies in Box 5.7 with specific ill-health breathing problems.

Here are some potential specific questions.

Scenario A questions
- When did the fall occur?
- Where is the pain specifically?
- What is the type of pain?
- When is the pain worse – on breathing in or out?
- What helps the pain?
- Have the problems/difficulties got worse?

Scenario B questions
- When did all the problems start?
- What type of cough does the individual have?

| Box 5.7 | Mini case studies |

A. A 45-year-old builder, who has fallen at work, is complaining of severe right-sided chest pain. A fractured rib is suspected. The patient has been admitted to the Accident and Emergency Department.

B. A 70-year-old Asian man, with suspected pulmonary tuberculosis (TB), complains of feeling tired, night sweats, loss of weight and is coughing and expectorating sputum throughout the interview, following admission to a medical admissions unit.

C. An 18-year-old female, new university student, who has asthma is reporting to a practice nurse for a review of her medications and life style.

- Is there any sputum being expectorated?
- What colour and consistency is it?
- How difficult is it to expectorate?
- When is the cough the worst – day, night, with exercise?
- How long do you normally sleep for and how long do you sleep now?
- How much weight have you lost?
- What is your appetite like?
- Why are you not eating as well as before?
- What effect does coughing have on you?

Scenario C questions
- How effective is your present medication?
- When and how do you use your inhalers?
- Have you experienced any changes in breathing habits?
- Have you noticed any increase in wheezing, choking and coughing?
- How has your lifestyle changed now you are at university?
- Have you experienced problems with smoky atmospheres, stress, etc?
- How do you cope with your breathing problem in public?

It is impossible to cover all adult health problems and their associated breathing difficulties in this chapter but it is important for you to consider that the objective is to collect information to identify:

- the individual's normal habits when they are well
- whether there are any difficulties now in relation to their independence in breathing
- previous coping strategies with breathing and associated AL-specific problems now.

However, there are common difficulties experienced by individuals with breathing problems such as:

- changes in rate, depth, rhythm of breathing
- marked changes in breathing habit (dyspnoea and wheezing)
- coughing
- production of abnormal secretions (sputum and haemoptysis)
- respiratory pain.

It is useful for you to consider how each of these difficulties can be assessed and what observations would be required.

Changes in rate, depth and rhythm of breathing

Mallik et al (2004, p. 145) state that it is 'relatively simple for a nurse to assess breathing by observing the rate, depth and rhythm of respiration' and these will give a basic indicator of respiratory function. Observations should be taken on admission, pre- and postoperatively, monitoring the patient's condition following invasive procedures and with patients who have respiratory, cardiovascular and neurological problems. Ferns & Chojnacka (2006) consider that, as respiratory rates are sensitive predictors of impending deterioration, it is vital that nurses assess, monitor, chart and act upon changes in the rate, depth or rhythm of patients' respiratory effort.

As noted previously the normal respiratory rate is 12–18 times per minute in usually fit adults and is called eupnoea. A rapid rate (tachypnoea) may indicate increased activity, anxiety, pain, pyrexia, sepsis, shock or obstructed airway. Slow breathing (bradypnoea) may indicate sleep, head injury, brain tumours, hypothermia or depression of respiratory centre by drugs, e.g. opioids or pre cardiac arrest. Apnoea is the absence of breathing for at least 10 seconds and can occur in 'sleep apnoea' and causes snoring by a brief obstruction of the upper airways or can be the reason for 'cot deaths' (Mallik et al 2004).

The depth of respiration depends on the amount of air inhaled and can be observed by noting the movement of the chest wall during inspiration and is described as normal, shallow or deep. Observation of the chest movements is important as the thorax is usually symmetrical and breathing should be effortless. However, abnormal chest movements can be seen when an injury results in a flail chest. A flail chest occurs when several successive ribs are fractured in two places and become dissociated from the rest of the rib cage which presents with breathing which is known as paradoxical. On inhalation, the rib cage expands and air is sucked in and the flail segment collapses in on the lung thus preventing proper expansion and ventilation and is forced out on exhalation (Dickson & Martindale 2002). A peak flow meter or spirometer will give a more objective measurement of the depth of respirations (see Fig. 5.11).

Normally, adults have a regular breathing rhythm or pattern and their breathing is effortless, even, regular and automatic, but it can become irregular when the respiratory centre is affected or the person has respiratory problems. Some of these are noted in the next section.

Marked changes in breathing habit (dyspnoea and wheezing)

It is, according to Dickson & Martindale (2002), important to identify when the person becomes breathless and the effect this has on their normal activities including their sleep patterns. It is useful to listen to the person talking and assess whether it is jerky, with short phrases being used with an apparent effort or audible, effortless and clear. Another useful area to assess is the coping strategies they use to minimise their problems, such as pursed lips respirations. Francis (2006) discusses various tools to aid the assessment of individuals' experience of breathlessness, such as one by Gift (1990) which is based on a visual analogue scale of 0 = 'No breathlessness' to

1. Fit disposable mouthpiece to peak flow meter

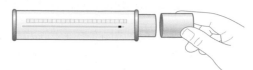

2. Ensure patient stands up or sits upright and holds peak flow meter horizontally without restricting movement of the marker. Ensure the marker is at the bottom of the scale

3. Ask patient to breathe in deeply, seal lips around mouthpiece and breathe out as quickly as possible

4. Repeat steps 2 and 3 twice more. Choose and record the highest of the three readings

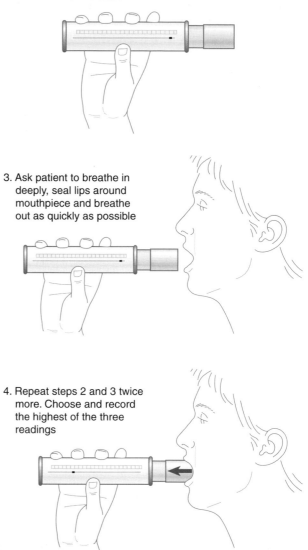

Fig. 5.11 Measuring Peak Expiratory Flow Rate (PEFR) using a peak flow meter (from Brooker 2005, with permission).

10 = 'Worst breathlessness imaginable' and the patient marks on the scale to indicate their perception of their dyspnoea. Kendrick et al (2000) modified a previously produced breathlessness assessment scale by Borg which is perhaps easier for patients and clinical staff to use. This

uses descriptive words linked to a scale of 0 to 10, for example 2 = 'Slight breathlessness' and 7 = 'Very severe breathlessness'.

Dyspnoea or shortness of breath or difficulty with breathing is accompanied by the use of accessory muscles of respiration, e.g. nostrils flaring and shoulder girdle raised, anxiety, restlessness and perspiring. This is a very distressing symptom but does indicate that the body is attempting to compensate by conveying more oxygen to the tissues. Orthopnoea is when the person experiences dyspnoea when lying down but is relieved when sitting up and is often found in patients who have heart failure. Another form of dyspnoea is that called paroxysmal nocturnal dyspnoea which occurs in patients with heart failure and pulmonary oedema and is characterised by sudden breathlessness at night.

Cheyne–Stokes respirations can occur as death approaches and are characterised by a cyclical pattern of a few seconds of apnoea (up to 20 seconds), followed by increase in rate and depth to a peak intensity followed by a period of apnoea again. Kussmaul's respirations, associated with diabetic ketoacidosis and pneumonia, involve an increase in the rate and depth with panting and grunting expirations (Dougherty & Lister 2004).

Breathing is usually silent so it is important to listen for breath sounds as discussed by Dickson & Martindale (2002) and Mallik et al (2004). Wheezing or rhonci occurs when whistling or musical sounds are heard which are associated with spasm of the bronchi and occur on expiration and are common in people with asthma and chronic bronchitis. Wheezing may also occur in response to exercise and inhalation of toxic substances. Severe bronchospasm is life threatening as the size of the bronchi is reduced and secretions are retained which become infected. Another distinctive noise is a harsh, high-pitched sound on inspiration, known as a stridor and is caused by an obstruction in the larynx, this again is life threatening.

Coughing

According to Francis (2006), coughing is a reflex action directed towards the removal of foreign bodies, such as bacteria trapped in mucus and is a frequently encountered problem. The nurse needs to note the presence, frequency, depth, nature and sound of a cough. Coughs may be described as strong/weak, dry, hard, racking, croupy, hacking, shallow, deep, rattling, with a whooping sound. It may be worse in the morning or associated with exercise. It should be noted what effect the coughing has on the person, e.g. tired, not able to talk, sleepless nights or not able to carry out normal Activities of Living. It may be accompanied by sputum and this should be expectorated (coughed out) to prevent its accumulation within the lungs. A 'dry' cough has little sputum whereas a 'loose' cough is associated with sputum production.

The British Thoracic Society (2006b) has published recommendations for the management of cough in adults. The report differentiates between acute and chronic coughs, and provides recommendations relating to specific respiratory diseases, investigations, drug therapy and the provision of specialist cough clinics.

Production of abnormal secretions (sputum and haemoptysis)

Adults usually produce 100 ml of mucus a day; however, this is increased when the air passages are irritated and is then known as sputum and according to Esmond (2003) and Francis (2006) should be observed to note any change in colour, consistency and quantity. The colour must be noted as this may indicate an infection if purulent and green or if blood stained (called haemoptysis) which is found in inflammatory conditions (tuberculosis or pneumonia) that cause erosion of tissues and blood vessels, or lung cancer. Haemoptysis is very frightening for the patient and anyone else in the vicinity. It is also necessary to observe the consistency of the sputum as it may be watery or frothy (long-term respiratory conditions and/or cardiac problems as well), purulent (infections) or tenacious or thick (acute respiratory problems). The amount may need to be measured to show the effect of the disease or treatments. Specimens of sputum can be collected and laboratory analysis of bacteriological culture of microorganisms can aid the diagnosis of respiratory and cardiovascular problems. As pathogens may be present in sputum, meticulous handwashing is needed to limit the cross-infection risk.

Respiratory pain

Pain in any part of the body can, as Roper et al (1996) point out, cause alterations in breathing. In relation to breathing, it can indicate infection, inflammation or trauma (Mallik et al 2004). The pain may be poststernal and is associated with coughing (usually inflamed trachea) or sharp, stabbing pain worsened by deep breathing and coughing (usually inflammation of the pleura or trauma). Therefore it is important to note if pain is associated with breathing activities or coughing, the nature, type, duration, severity of the pain and the strategies used to minimise the pain.

Interpretation of data collected

Once the data have been collected you need to utilise your knowledge and decision-making skills to interpret the information prior to the identification of the individual's actual and potential problems. Using the assessment questions outlined in Box 5.6 you need to consider the information that you may gather from Case study 5.3 by considering the components of the model.

Case study 5.3

Tom Jackson

Tom Jackson, a 78-year-old widower, has been admitted to the elderly assessment ward following an episode of severe breathlessness. He is a retired mill worker and has been treated by his GP for a chronic chest condition with inhalers and tablets. He says that he is a bit confused with the inhalers and tablets. He lives alone in a terraced house since the death of his wife some 12 months ago. The house is rather damp and is in need of some repairs and modernisation as he only has coal fires in the downstairs rooms. His only daughter lives a few miles away and visits once or twice a week with his two grandchildren. He smokes some 10–15 cigarettes a day even though he is rather wheezy and his coughing keeps him awake at night. He used to enjoy a visit to the local pub but finds the walking too troublesome now as even going from room to room is difficult at times. He says that he has lost some weight since his wife died as he cannot shop or cook very well. His daughter does bring prepared meals with her when she visits but he prefers plain food so doesn't always eat them.

Over the last few days, he has felt too tired to shave himself or wash his hair. He has to stop many times during the interview to rest and cough. You note that his respirations are rapid and that he has a loose cough and is expectorating some sputum.

Exercise

1. Using the assessment questions found in Box 5.6 consider the possible responses in relation to Tom Jackson.
2. Consider the factors which may have led to Tom's health breakdown.
3. Identify the effect on other Activities of Living with the main case scenario.
4. Check your answers with those in Box 5.8.

From this exercise it can be seen that Mr Jackson has:

- an acute breathing problem affecting other Activities of Living
- a long-standing chronic breathing problem
- a knowledge deficit in relation to smoking
- an environmental problem regarding a damp and cold house
- alterations in social factors since bereavement and acute illness.

Following this interpretation of the data, it is then necessary to complete the final stage of the assessment process and identify actual and potential problems.

Identification of actual and potential problems

Actual breathing problems will be specific to the actual health problems but common problems have already been identified in relation to:

| **Box 5.8** | **Factors contributing to health breakdown** |

1. Factors leading to this health breakdown
- Age possibly may be a factor.
- Dependency continuum altering now as dependent on daughter for some meals and company.
- Physical – long-standing chronic chest condition/smoking/mill worker.
- Psychological – bereavement.
- Sociocultural – losing social contact as not able to walk too far.
- Environmental – damp terraced house, no heating in bedroom, fumes from coal fires, previous exposure to dust in mills.
- Politicoeconomic – pension rates affected by death of wife, cost of food/heating.

2. Other activities being affected
- Maintaining safe environment – due to not taking his medication properly.
- Communicating – having to rest during interview as breathless, wheezing and tired.
- Eating and drinking – following bereavement and not being able to walk far, affecting shopping and cooking abilities which were already reducing.
- Mobilising – due to breathlessness and coughing.
- Expressing sexuality – self-esteem affected by appearance.
- Working and playing – not able to walk to the pub. Lacks company since wife died.
- Sleep and rest – coughing during the night.

- changes in rate, depth, rhythm of breathing (see p. 159–160)
- marked changes in breathing habit – dyspnoea and wheezing (see pp. 160–161)
- coughing (see p. 161)
- production of abnormal secretions – sputum and haemoptysis (see p. 161)
- respiratory pain (see p. 161).

Potential breathing problems

There are many potential problems which may be identified; some will relate to the individual's breathing condition, some specific to the factors which affect the individual. There are, however, two potential problems which may affect any individual with a breathing difficulty, namely being at risk of obstructed air passages and cardiac/respiratory arrest. It is important that you are able to recognise these potential problems so that prompt action can follow as both problems are potentially fatal. For example:

1. *At risk of obstructed air passages.* Airway obstruction may be due to a variety of causes, e.g. trauma, tumours, oedema, foreign bodies, blood, vomit or tongue falling backwards and occluding the airway. It may occur in the nasal passages, pharynx, larynx, trachea or bronchus. Hoarseness,

dyspnoea, stridor, cyanosis and increased but ineffective respiratory effort can be seen (see pp. 171–175 for further care).

2. *At risk of cardiac/respiratory arrest.* Dougherty & Lister (2004, p.159) define the term cardiac arrest as implying 'a sudden interruption of cardiac output (which) may be reversible with appropriate treatment'. Events leading up to an arrest may be varied, e.g. surgery, asphyxia, accidents such as drowning, cardiac arrhythmias or respiratory failure. The diagnosis of an arrest is, according to Webster & Thompson (2006), an abrupt loss of consciousness, absent respirations, absence of carotid and femoral pulses. Jevon (2006) considers that it is not straightforward to confirm cardiorespiratory arrest, but advocates that the nurse should look, listen and feel for signs of breathing for up to 10 seconds and if experienced may check for the carotid pulse for up to 10 seconds if the person is not breathing. Although there are similarities in how you can recognise this event, there is one important difference between cardiac and respiratory arrest. In cardiac arrest there is an absence of an arterial pulse, whereas in a respiratory arrest the arterial pulses are present, although they may be difficult to locate and time should not be lost in trying to palpate these, just for a differential diagnosis. It is vitally important that these signs are noted early as cerebral damage can be caused by anoxia, i.e. no oxygen getting to the brain, if breathing and circulation are not restored effectively within 4 minutes. Basic life support measures are needed to restore breathing and circulation (see pp. 175–178 for further care).

Exercise

Re-read the case scenario in Case study 5.3 (Tom Jackson).

1. Using the 12 Activities of Living as a framework, identify Tom's actual and potential problems.
2. Check your identified actual and potential problems with those in Box 5.9.

By working through this section you will have considered how to collect data when taking a nursing history in relation to the activity of breathing and other related activities; interpret the data collected to assess the degree of alteration in the activity of breathing and the effect on other Activities of Living and to identify individuals' actual and potential problems related to the activity of breathing and other related activities.

PLANNING NURSING ACTIVITIES

Planning nursing activities involves the following:

- identifying priorities
- establishing short- and/or long-term goals
- determining nursing actions/interventions required
- documenting the plan (refer to Chapter 1 for further information).

To ensure that the nursing activities are planned appropriately, you must review the individual's actual and potential problems and then consider the level to which the activity of breathing can be helped. There are different levels of helping, such as:

1. to solve or alleviate actual problems
2. to prevent potential problems becoming actual ones
3. to prevent solved problems from re-occurring
4. to develop positive strategies for any problems which cannot be solved.

Exercise

1. Re-read the three mini case studies in Box 5.7.
2. Consider these three case studies and identify the levels of helping within them.

Box 5.9	Actual and potential problems – Case study 5.3 (Tom Jackson)	
Activity of Living	**Actual problems**	**Potential problems**
Maintaining safe environment	Tom has difficulty complying with the correct medication due to his stated confusion over his medication.	
Breathing	Tom has difficulty with breathing due to the exacerbation of his breathing disorder as shown by a loose cough, a raised respiratory rate and an audible wheeze.	
Communicating	Tom has difficulty communicating due to breathlessness and cough.	
Eating and drinking	Tom has difficulty cooking food so his dietary intake has decreased due to breathlessness affecting mobility and his ability to cook and shop.	
Eliminating		Tom may have difficulty getting to the toilet due to breathlessness.
Personal cleansing and dressing	Tom has difficulty maintaining his hygiene needs due to his breathless state.	*(continued)*

Box 5.9	Actual and potential problems *(continued)*	
Activity of Living	**Actual problems**	**Potential problems**
Mobilising	Tom has difficulty mobilising due to his breathlessness.	Tom may develop pressure sores, deep vein thrombosis, pulmonary embolism, and constipation due to limited activity.
Sleep and rest	Tom is experiencing difficulty sleeping due to coughing at night.	
Work and play	Tom is becoming isolated as he cannot socialise as he did previously due to breathlessness affecting his mobility.	
Expressing sexuality		Tom has difficulty maintaining his body image due to his breathing and mobility problems.
Maintaining body temperature	Tom may have difficulties maintaining body temperature due to his lack of mobility and because his house is in need of modernisation having only coal fires downstairs.	
Dying		Tom may be worried about the severity of his condition and he is still coming to terms with the death of his wife.

You may have considered the following levels of care were appropriate:

Scenario A
- To alleviate severe right-sided chest pain.
- To prevent potential problems following rib fracture such as chest infection due to poor breathing and coughing habits.

Scenario B
- To alleviate congestion, tiredness, night sweats, weight loss and promote expectoration.
- To prevent possible spread of infection to others.

Scenario C
- To develop positive coping strategies for lifestyle changes so that potential problems don't become actual problems.

The focus must be on the individual's problems and what they want as opposed to the nurse's ideas. Therefore, involvement of the patient is crucial at this stage. However, this may be affected by the problems that the patient may have, e.g. pain, difficulty with communicating verbally as noted previously.

Many factors may influence the nurse and the patient in the planning stage of nursing activities with a patient with breathing difficulties. Consider this in relation to a patient you have nursed with breathing difficulties and check these in Box 5.10.

Identifying priorities
Following the assessment the next stage is to plan the care. You will need to determine priorities of care and this skill is a vital component of any nurse's repertoire. You need to be able to determine which problem is the most important and you could grade it as follows:

Box 5.10	Factors which influence planning care for a patient with breathing difficulties

Nurse's perspective
- Knowledge of normal physiology and specific pathophysiological processes in relation to breathing disorders.
- Knowledge of normal living and dependency across the lifespan in various cultures in relation to breathing.
- Knowledge of breathing difficulties specific to the patient's problem.
- Knowledge of nursing interventions available and research-based evidence.
- Accuracy of assessment.
- Skills in relation to observing, assessment, interpreting and prioritizing.
- Staffing levels and skill mix on individual shifts.

Patient's perspective
- Ability and degree of involvement of patient in the decisions related to care to be planned.
- Knowledge of breathing difficulties specific to their problem.
- Personal beliefs, attitudes, experiences and coping strategies.
- Enactment of the sick role.

- life threatening – totally dependent
- urgent – mainly dependent but some ability to be independent
- semi-urgent – some dependency but mainly independent
- non-urgent – totally independent.

This priority status may change day by day, shift by shift or hour by hour and therefore assessment must be a continuous activity to ensure that you remain alert to possible changes.

Exercise

Re-read the actual and potential problems that have been identified for Tom Jackson in Case study 5.3.

1. Identify which problems are life threatening, urgent, semi-urgent and non-urgent.
2. Decide which would be the first three problems that need to be addressed, giving a rationale for this choice.
3. Check your decisions with those found in Box 5.11.

It can be seen that Tom's problems are varied in relation to their priorities and are complex in nature. A suggested priority order is:

1. has difficulty with breathing due to exacerbation of breathing disorder as shown by loose cough, raised respiratory rate and audible wheeze
2. has difficulty with mobilising because of breathlessness and may develop pressure sores, deep vein thrombosis, pulmonary embolism and constipation due to limited activity
3. has difficulty sleeping due to coughing at night.

The rationale for the priority order is that difficulties with breathing are the main problem that Tom has which is affecting many of his other Activities of Living. If nursing actions are not planned then the breathing difficulties will worsen. If, however, nursing actions are planned and implemented, then not only will the breathing difficulty be alleviated but also the difficulties with the other Activities of Living will be eased.

Mobilising difficulty will be eased once Tom's breathing difficulty is alleviated. In the meantime, however, potential problems which may become life threatening, e.g. deep vein thrombosis leading to pulmonary embolism, could occur and therefore it is important to address this problem with preventative care.

Box 5.11	Priority status of actual problems – Case study 5.3 (Tom Jackson)	
Activity of Living	**Actual problems**	**Problem status**
Maintaining safe environment	Tom has difficulty complying with the correct medication due to his stated confusion over his medication.	Urgent
Breathing	Tom has difficulty with breathing due to the exacerbation of his breathing disorder as shown by a loose cough, a raised respiratory rate and an audible wheeze.	Urgent
Communicating	Tom has difficulty communicating due to breathlessness and cough.	Semi-urgent
Eating and drinking	Tom has difficulty cooking food so his dietary intake has decreased due to breathlessness, affecting mobility and his ability to cook and shop.	Non-urgent
Personal cleansing and dressing	Tom has difficulty maintaining his hygiene needs due to his breathless state.	Semi-urgent
Mobilising	Tom has difficulty mobilising due to his breathlessness.	Urgent
Sleep and rest	Tom is experiencing difficulty sleeping due to coughing at night.	Semi-urgent
Work and play	Tom is becoming isolated as he cannot socialise as he did previously due to breathlessness affecting his mobility.	Non-urgent
Expressing sexuality	Tom has difficulty maintaining his body image due to his breathing and mobility problems.	Non-urgent
Eliminating	Tom may have difficulty getting to the toilet due to breathlessness.	Non-urgent
Mobilising	Tom may develop pressure sores, deep vein thrombosis, pulmonary embolism, and constipation due to limited activity.	Semi-urgent
Maintaining body temperature	Tom may have difficulties maintaining body temperature due to his lack of mobility and because his house is in need of modernisation having only coal fires downstairs.	Non-urgent
Dying	Tom may be worried about the severity of his condition and is still coming to terms with the death of his wife.	Semi-urgent

Difficulty with sleeping is important to alleviate quickly as Tom's wellbeing is affected by lack of sleep.

Goal setting

Goal setting is based upon sound assessment and the identification of problems and priorities. Goals can be short term (hourly to generally less than a week) or long term (for a longer period). Many short-term goals may be needed to achieve long-term goals.

The goal statement is essential so that the process of evaluation can take place. It is therefore important that the goal is written in the terms of what the patient ought to be able to, or has agreed to, achieve. The goals should be written in observable, realistic and measurable behavioural terms so that it is easier to monitor and evaluate the patient's progress. (Refer to Chapter 1 for further details on goal setting.) This may be a skill that you need to develop and practise. One example is shown in Box 5.12 for you to reflect upon.

Exercise
Re-read Tom Jackson's problems related to the main scenario, listed in Case study 5.3.

1. Choose three of these problems and set short- and long-term goals using one of the frameworks noted in Chapter 1.
2. Check the example given in Box 5.12.

Once the short-term and long-term goals have been set you will need to determine the appropriate nursing actions which will aid the alleviation of problems and the achievement of the short- and long-term goals.

Determining nursing actions

It is vital that the appropriate nursing actions are chosen to alleviate patients' problems. It is vital that each nurse constantly updates their knowledge and skills to ensure that care given is evidence based and delivered in a safe, competent and professional manner. Nursing actions will be considered in relation to dependency, comforting and preventative care with patients who have 'difficulty with breathing'.

Roper et al (1985) used these three aspects, in their second edition of *Elements of Nursing* to discuss care and it may be useful to consider their use in this activity.

Nursing actions associated with dependency care

The purpose of nursing actions associated with dependency care, related to breathing difficulties, is that you, the carer, provide specific care to the individual who is not able to provide care for themselves. The place on the lifespan, the level of dependency and biological factors identified in the model of living will need to be considered when the nursing actions are planned. There are many nursing actions, related to dependency care, which affect breathing but some of the main actions include:

- nursing observations of vital signs – temperature, pulse and respiration (TPR), BP, peak flow, O_2 saturation levels, tissue perfusion
- administration of prescribed oxygen therapy
- administration of non-invasive and invasive ventilation
- administration of prescribed drug therapies/ inhalers/nebulisers
- localised airway passage obstruction
- postural drainage and chest physiotherapy
- artificial airway maintenance
- cardiopulmonary resuscitation
- underwater seal chest drain.

Let us consider these.

Nursing observations of vital signs

These actual observations have already been noted earlier in this chapter (see p. 159–160). However, it is important that you consider when these observations are done and how often. This will depend on the severity of the patient's condition and whether the problems are acute or chronic. The initial assessment of vital signs will be used as a baseline for future evaluations. It may be that these observations are carried out continuously as the patient is in a critical care environment and is monitored, or that they are carried out 4-hourly or daily. You may need to refer to Chapters 3 and 9 in relation to the activities of maintaining a safe environment and maintaining body temperature for further information.

Box 5.12	Short- and long-term breathing goals set for Tom Jackson	
Problem	Short-term goal	Long-term goal
Tom has difficulty with breathing due to exacerbation of his breathing disorder as shown by a loose cough, raised respiratory rate and audible wheeze.	Tom will be able to breathe more easily and more quietly with the aid of oxygen with a lower respiratory rate than on admission and is able to expectorate secretions.	Tom will be able to breathe normally, unaided before discharge, with no audible wheeze, no cough or sputum produced and have a respiratory rate of within 18–24 respirations per minute at rest for a minimum of 4 hours.

It is the nurse who usually decides on the site for temperature recordings to be taken and the device to be used. Oral temperature recordings would be difficult for someone who is dyspnoeic and therefore the axilla or tympanic membrane would be the preferred site. Safety aspects, cost and ease of use may be the influencing factors and Tempadot and tympanic membrane thermometers should be used rather than glass or mercury thermometers.

The temperature observation could be completed when the pulse and respiration rates are being counted. The pulse rate and respiratory rate need to be counted for a full minute each as sufficient time is needed to detect irregularities or abnormalities and these may not be identified if a full minute is not used (Jamieson et al 2002, Mallik et al 2004, Docherty & Coote 2006). The blood pressure would normally be completed after the other vital signs have been recorded, as the patient will be at rest and factors which may affect their blood pressure, such as exercise, will have been minimised.

The use of automatic blood pressure machines, e.g. 'Dinamap', have speeded up the process of taking measurements of vital signs. These machines can also provide a recording of pulse rates and oxygen saturation levels. You must, however, remember to observe and touch the patient as pulse recordings and oxygen saturation levels on the 'Dinamap' machine only produce a reading; it does not give any indication to the fullness of the beat, the irregularity of the beat or the texture and colour of the skin. Peak flow recordings may be used as a general indicator of respiratory activity and are recorded 4-hourly or daily or they may be used to assess the effectiveness of medication and therefore the recordings may be done before and after medication has been taken.

As breathing is affected by mobilising, eating and communicating, you would need to take these issues into account and record the vital signs prior to these activities. It is important for nurses to rationalise why such observations are being undertaken for each individual patient and in particular the frequency of these measurements. Ritualistic practices, particularly in relation to observations, have been identified and the recording of 4-hourly observations may well be an established practice but may not be necessary. As Walsh & Ford (1989, p. ix) identify, 'Ritual action implies carrying out a task without thinking it through in a problem solving, logical way'.

When the observations have been taken, you must ensure that the recordings are accurately recorded on the appropriate chart and the significance of the observations identified and reported to senior members of the health care team. For example, if the recordings taken were as follows: pulse and blood pressure rising, pulse weaker, respirations initially increased, with sighing, yawning and dyspnoea being present, this combined with restlessness, confusion and decreasing conscious level may indicate hypoxia (insufficient oxygen for cells to work) and oxygen therapy may be required.

Administration of oxygen therapy

Oxygen therapy can be used for a variety of patients, e.g. acute and chronic respiratory problems, in an emergency situation, as a short- or long-term measure, but it must be remembered that it is a drug and therefore has regulations as to its administration. Serious consequences can develop if oxygen is administered inappropriately or incorrectly. Usually, as noted by Kindlen (2003) and Law & Watson (2005), breathing is stimulated when the carbon dioxide levels are high. However, for people with chronic respiratory disease, their stimulus to breathe is due to an oxygen lack and not a build up of carbon dioxide. If these people are given above 24% of oxygen, then their stimulus to breathe is removed with potential fatal consequences. Oxygen should therefore, as noted by Jevon & Ewens (2001), always be prescribed and the flow rate, delivery system, duration and monitoring of treatment should be specified. This should be guided by arterial blood gas levels, for high concentrations of oxygen over a long period of time may cause severe lung damage, and so it is important that its use is monitored carefully. Local protocols, relating to its emergency use, should be available in every health care environment.

There are numerous delivery systems available and you need to be able to rationalise the choice to the patient and the other health care professionals. All of the systems include an oxygen supply (portable black cylinder with a white top clearly marked oxygen or piped oxygen), flow meter to regulate rate of oxygen per minute, oxygen tubing (usually green) and a delivery device with humidifier. The delivery device used may be low-flow, which provides variable oxygen concentration, or high-flow, which provides fixed or controlled oxygen concentrations, and the choice depends on the amount and concentration of oxygen needed, compliance with the therapy and the condition.

Low-flow devices, e.g. nasal cannulae or simple face mask, allow the patient to inhale room air and mix it with the oxygen being administered so giving a variable amount of oxygen. Both nasal cannulae and face masks are for single patient use only and should be disposed of after use with one patient. Care must be taken when disposing of the devices if the patient is expectorating sputum because of any contamination. The respiratory rate and depth will affect the concentration of oxygen received. High-flow devices, usually Venturi masks or non-rebreathing masks, deliver a precise concentration of oxygen to the patient irrespective of their respiratory effort (Francis 2006, Esmond & Mikelsons 2001, Esmond 2003, Dougherty & Lister 2004). See Figure 5.12 for these devices.

Nasal cannulae deliver oxygen via a length of tubing with two prongs which fit into the nostrils. They can deliver oxygen concentrations of 24–44% at a flow rate of 1–6 litres per minute, although patients may experience difficulties above 4 litres per minute. If a patient breathes through the mouth then the efficiency of this method is lessened and masks may be necessary.

air from outside the mask plus oxygen delivered through the system (Francis 2006, Esmond & Mikelsons 2001, Esmond 2003, Dougherty & Lister 2004).

High-flow, fixed-performance or Venturi masks deliver accurate concentrations of oxygen as they are not affected by the patient's breathing pattern. The concentration of oxygen tends to be lower, but levels of 24–40% can be given. There are a number of holes in the side of the mask and this allows the expired air to escape and therefore eliminate the chance of rebreathing carbon dioxide. Hence, they can be used for people who retain carbon dioxide and use the lack of oxygen as their stimulus to breathe. Non-rebreathing masks can be used to deliver oxygen concentrations of 90–100%, at a flow rate of 12–15 litres per minute, as no outside air or expired air is allowed in through the mask (Francis 2006, Esmond & Mikelsons 2001, Esmond 2003, Dougherty & Lister 2004).

Irrespective of the type of delivery device used, patients will require frequent mouth and nasal care because humidification of the inspired air will be lessened and breathing dry gas dries and irritates the mucous membranes. Specific measures to humidify the oxygen delivered may be necessary also, especially when oxygen concentration levels of 35% and above are prescribed, but not with nasal cannulae or Venturi masks (see Figure 5.12). As all masks must fit closely over the nose and around the chin, these areas must be inspected and pressure relieved on the underlying tissues (Francis 2006, Esmond 2003).

You would need to ensure that the patient and their relatives received explanations, in relation to the need for oxygen therapy and the safety issues relating to this combustible gas, e.g. no smoking (Francis 2006, Esmond 2003). A calm approach is needed and once the oxygen delivery system is in place the nurse needs to stay with them to ensure that the patient is able to tolerate the oxygen flow. They would need to be nursed in an observable position in the care environment and be nursed in an upright position in bed or a chair. Jamieson et al (2002) point out that the administration of oxygen does not require aseptic technique but that adequate cleanliness should be maintained to prevent cross-infection. The inside of the oxygen mask may become wet with condensation and can be dried to increase the patient's comfort and tolerance of the oxygen administration. Sheppard & Davis (2000) state that oxygen masks should be cleaned regularly, particularly if the patient has a productive cough and that the nurse must wash their hands after disposing of the oxygen equipment, to prevent cross-infection.

Long-term oxygen therapy (LTOT), i.e. oxygen delivered for over 15 hours per day, according to Francis (2006), is often prescribed for patients with progressive lung disease (COPD) and can be administered in the home. If patients are able to comply and use LTOT for more than 15 hours per day their life expectancy is improved. An oxygen concentrator, as opposed to a cylinder, is used to deliver low-flow oxygen in the home. Oxygen can be delivered at up

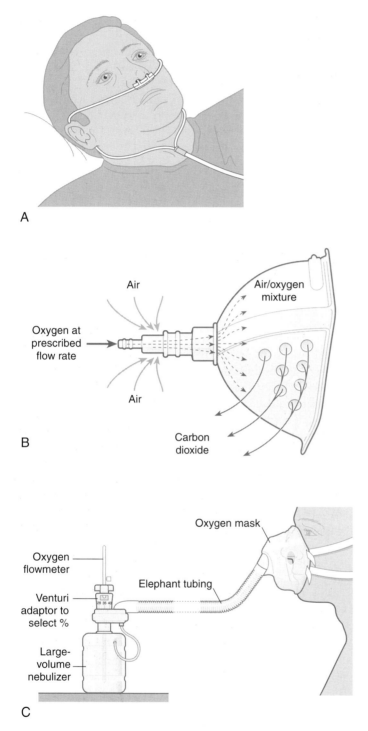

Fig. 5.12 Oxygen delivery devices, (A) low-flow device – nasal cannulae, (B) high-flow device, Venturi mask, (C) humidification of oxygen (from Brooker 2005, with permission).

Masks can be used to deliver various concentrations of oxygen and are designed to fit over the patient's nose and mouth or trachea. Simple low-flow masks can deliver oxygen concentrations of 21–60% but the amount of oxygen received will vary according to the patient's respirations as the patient rebreathes their own expired air, combined with

to a flow rate of 4 litres per minute and is usually via nasal cannulae. NICE (2004) guidelines for COPD are available and include advice on the selection of patients for LTOT; this assessment must be overseen by a suitably experienced respiratory physician. Education, support and follow-up are also supported by respiratory nurse specialists (Esmond 2003). Portable oxygen is also available for home use and Esmond & Mikelsons (2001) discuss the indications and assessment of its use and also issues related to travel in the UK and abroad for individuals who require oxygen therapy. The British Thoracic Society (2002a) has issued recommendations with regard to air travel and respiratory disease.

Administration of non-invasive and invasive ventilation

In patients with severe respiratory failure it is sometimes necessary to use either non-invasive or invasive ventilation according to Francis (2006). Non-invasive ventilation (NIV) or non-invasive positive pressure ventilation (NIPPV) uses a nasal mask or full face mask along with a pressure or volume preset ventilator machine. Careful assessment of the patient and a full explanation of the treatment are required. It can provide adequate oxygen levels and carbon dioxide clearance, improves quality of sleep, and allows the patient to communicate and eat and drink when off the machine. The patient may need to use the machine for the first 24–48 hours and then decrease its use as they become more stable. The machine can be used in the home but the patient will need education and support to ensure they can cope independently. Therefore the nurse needs to be skilled in the use of the machine and be able to problem-solve as difficulties with mask leaks, skin trauma, nutrition etc. can occur (Mikelsons & Esmond 2001, British Thoracic Society 2002b, Esmond 2003).

Continuous positive airway pressure (CPAP, see Fig. 5.13), can also be used as a non-invasive ventilation method where positive airway pressure is maintained throughout inspiration and expiration by using a tight-fitting full face mask or nasal mask, or can become invasive ventilation when it is used through an endotracheal or tracheostomy tube. Either mode requires a skilled team to care for the patient as there are problems with this method, such as vomiting and aspiration of gastric contents, and damage to skin integrity (Esmond 2003, Dougherty & Lister 2004, Francis 2006).

Invasive ventilation occurs when an artificial airway is used, e.g. endotracheal tube or tracheostomy to allow the commencement of mechanical ventilation via negative or positive pressure ventilators. This decision should not be taken lightly as the patient would be unconscious for the treatment to be effective and this brings along other problems (Francis 2006, British Thoracic Society 2002b).

Administration of drug therapies/inhalers/nebulisers

Moist inhalations may be used to loosen secretions in the upper respiratory tract and promote expectoration, especially when infection is present. Tincture of benzoin or menthol

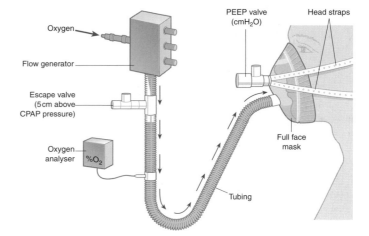

Fig. 5.13 Continuous positive airway pressure (CPAP) (from Esmond 2003, with permission).

crystals can be used with a jug and bowl or a Nelson's inhaler. Care must be taken to prevent scalding when handling the hot water and when in contact with the hot vapour. The vapour is breathed in through the mouth and out through the nose using a jug and bowl of hot water.

Bronchodilators are used to prevent or treat bronchoconstriction, e.g. salbutomol (Ventolin). Metered-dose inhalers (MDI) with or without spacers are commonly used so that each time an inhaler is used the same amount of drug is delivered into the respiratory tract. The dose is usually two puffs three times a day. There are other types of inhalers, e.g. dry powder or breath-actuated devices, and it is important to choose the right type of inhaler for the patient to ensure compliance with the therapy and effectiveness of the treatment (Esmond 2003, Francis 2006) (see Fig. 5.14). Corticosteroids, e.g. beclomethasone (Becotide), can be used with bronchodilators to reduce bronchial reactivity and broad-spectrum antibiotics, e.g. amoxycillin (Amoxil), may be used at the earliest signs of infection (Murphy 2001, Hateley 2001). Specific treatments for respiratory diseases are guided by British Thoracic Society and NICE guidelines (see further reading section).

Exercise

1. Identify the drugs (bronchodilators and corticosteroids) that have been prescribed for a person you have nursed with asthma or COPD.
2. Look in a copy of the BNF or the online BNF at www. bnf.org.
3. Identify the doses, routes, actions, side-effects etc.
4. Discuss your findings with your patient to assess their knowledge of their drug therapy.
5. Discuss your findings with your mentor, preceptor, clinical supervisor or respiratory nurse specialist.

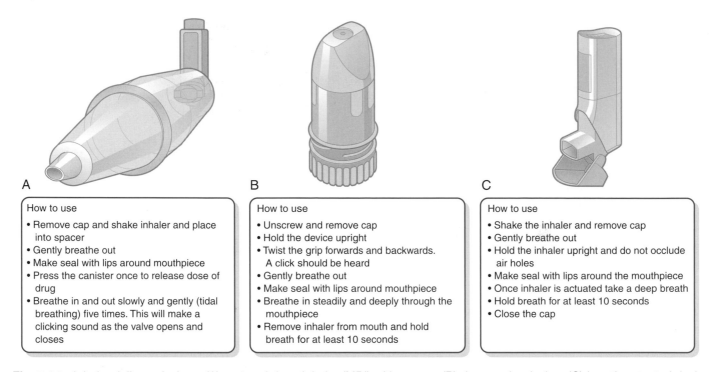

A

How to use
- Remove cap and shake inhaler and place into spacer
- Gently breathe out
- Make seal with lips around mouthpiece
- Press the canister once to release dose of drug
- Breathe in and out slowly and gently (tidal breathing) five times. This will make a clicking sound as the valve opens and closes

B

How to use
- Unscrew and remove cap
- Hold the device upright
- Twist the grip forwards and backwards. A click should be heard
- Gently breathe out
- Make seal with lips around mouthpiece
- Breathe in steadily and deeply through the mouthpiece
- Remove inhaler from mouth and hold breath for at least 10 seconds

C

How to use
- Shake the inhaler and remove cap
- Gently breathe out
- Hold the inhaler upright and do not occlude air holes
- Make seal with lips around the mouthpiece
- Once inhaler is actuated take a deep breath
- Hold breath for at least 10 seconds
- Close the cap

Fig. 5.14 Inhaler delivery devices, (A) metered dose inhaler (MDI) with spacer, (B) dry powder device, (C) breath-actuated device (from Esmond 2003, with permission).

It is important for you to be aware of the doses, effects and side-effects of any drug therapy given. You will have found that bronchodilators can be either short acting or long acting (e.g. Salbutamol or Serevent). Short-acting medications are best for treating relief from acute bronchospasam as they provide quick, temporary relief from asthma symptoms and usually take effect within 20 minutes or less, and can last from 4 to 6 hours. If taken 15–20 minutes prior to exercise or exposure to cold air, they can also prevent asthma symptoms being triggered. Long-acting bronchodilators help to control and prevent symptoms and are taken routinely in order to control and prevent bronchoconstriction. They are not intended for fast relief. These medications take longer to begin working, but relieve airway constriction for up to 12 hours.

Corticosteroids such as beclometasone (Becotide) is a potent glucocorticoid steroid drug and used in an inhaler for the prophylaxis of asthma. Occasionally it may cause a cough when inhaled and deposits of a white coating on the tongue and throat which may be oral thrush. This can usually be prevented by rinsing the mouth with water after using the inhaler.

Teaching of inhaler techniques is vital and awareness of the different types of inhalers is needed so that patient's treatment can be tailored to their abilities. See Jordan & White (2001) and Francis (2006) for further information concerning bronchodilators and the implications for nursing practice in relation to the education of patients and in particular inhaler techniques.

Nebulisation is a method of converting a drug or liquid into an aerosol mist which can be used as a therapeutic inhalation, according to Jamieson et al (2002) (see Fig. 5.15). Nebulisers may be indicated when bronchodilators need to be administered or when mucolytic medication is required to lower the viscosity of sputum to aid expectoration. The medication and the air (oxygen is rarely used and only with selected clients because of the dangers) must be prescribed and the procedure should be coordinated with physiotherapy and peak flow readings taken before and afterwards to evaluate the prescribed therapy. Usually all the solution is administered in 10 minutes and it is important that you discourage the patient from speaking at this time and to breathe normally. There is emerging a body of evidence discussed by Francis (2006) to suggest that there is no benefit in the use of nebulisers over MDIs combined with large volume spacers but further research is needed and nebuliser therapy is still a feature of hospital and community care.

Nebulisers are for single patient use but must be cleaned after every use, and changed every 24 hours to prevent infection (Jamieson et al 2002). As the procedure doesn't sterilise the nebuliser, it must be discarded if the patient has an infectious illness. Guidelines for the cleansing of nebulisers will be found on the information leaflet that is provided with the equipment. However, it is usual that the residual drug is emptied from the nebuliser and water run through the nebuliser for 1 minute. The individual components of the nebuliser are washed in hot soapy water, rinsed in clean

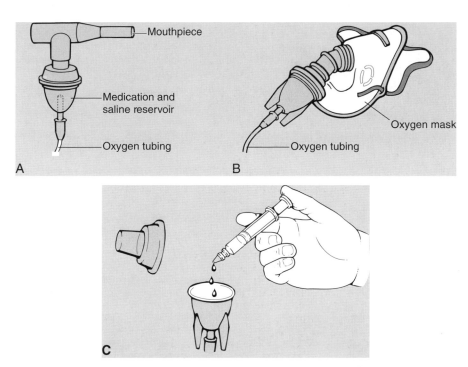

Fig. 5.15 Nebulisers, (A) attached to a mouthpiece, (B) attached to an oxygen mask, (C) taken apart to introduce a prepared medication (from Jamieson et al 2002, with permission).

water to remove any residue and dried thoroughly. The nebuliser is reassembled, run on the compressor to remove any excess water and stored in a dry, clean place (plastic bag), ready for the next administration. (See further reading section for nebuliser treatment from British Thoracic Society 1997a.)

Localised airway passage obstruction

Where the airway is obstructed by a foreign body or the tongue, the positioning of the individual is important to ensure that the airway is patent and it may be necessary to insert an airway. This may be done by lying the patient flat on their back and then lifting up the jaw before inserting the airway, followed by placing them in the recovery position (see Fig. 5.16). Suction may be required to remove foreign material, blood or vomit. Prompt emergency measures are needed if the obstruction is at the larynx or trachea level as death may ensue as a result of asphyxia (Dickson & Martindale 2002).

The Resuscitation Council (UK) 2005 has produced guidelines for choking and recommends that if it is a severe airway obstruction in a conscious person, then five sharp back blows between the shoulder blades may move the obstruction or if this fails then abdominal thrusts (Heimlich manoeuvre) may be used. If the individual cannot stand, then the Heimlich manoeuvre is performed by placing crossed hands just below the ribcage and exerting a firm thrust upwards. If they are able to stand then this manoeuvre is carried out differently. Someone stands behind the individ-

ual and places their arms around the individual's trunk, just below the diaphragm, clasping the hands in front. Pressure is then applied with the arms and the hands which forces air out through the airway and may dislodge the obstruction. This is repeated five times and if unsuccessful, then alternate with five back thrusts with five abdominal thrusts. If this is not successful, then an emergency tracheostomy may need to be performed to maintain the airway prior to the obstruction being cleared. When a foreign body enters a child's airway, they will usually cough to expel it; however, if the cough is ineffective and the child is conscious then five back blows followed by five chest thrusts for infants or abdominal thrusts for children over the age of 1 year is recommended by the Resuscitation Council UK (2005). See Figure 5.17 for the Heimlich manoeuvre; the algorithms produced by the Resuscitation Council UK (2005) addressing adult choking treatment and paediatric foreign body airway obstruction (FBAO) treatment are shown in Figures 5.18 and 5.19.

Postural drainage and chest physiotherapy

Roper et al (1996) identified that certain lung disorders produce an excessive amount of sputum which can obstruct the airways and must be removed or the oxygenation of the blood will be affected. Postural drainage, along with chest physiotherapy, can be used to remove these excessive secretions (Hateley 2001). Repositioning of patients allows gravity to assist in the clearance of each lung segment and is particularly used for patients with cystic fibrosis, where they have persistent recurrent lower respiratory tract infections

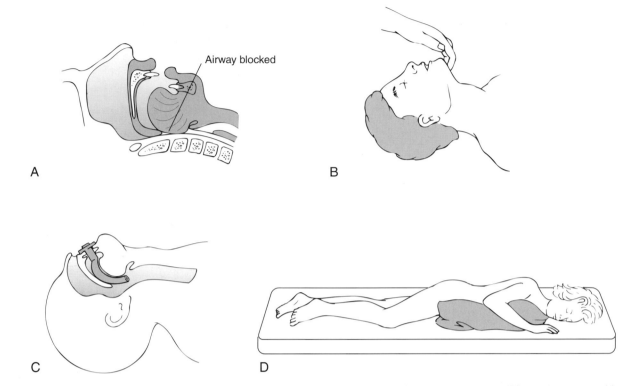

Fig. 5.16 Maintenance of airway, (A) airway blocked by tongue, (B) jaw lifted, (C) airway inserted, (D) semiprone position (from Roper et al 1996, with permission).

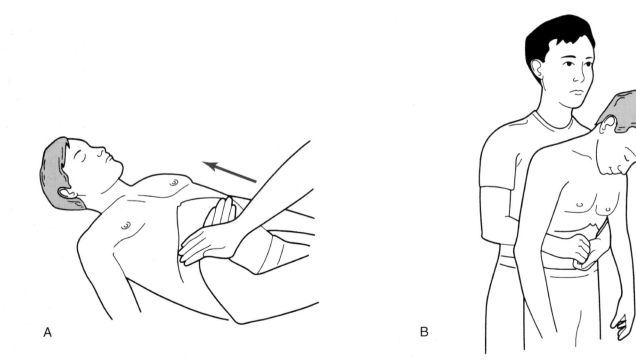

Fig. 5.17 Heimlich manoeuvre, (A) lying down, (B) standing up (from Dickson & Martindale 2002, with permission).

which result in lung damage. Figure 5.20 illustrates the positions used to enable postural drainage to take place.

Time needs to be spent teaching the patient and their relatives how to perform postural drainage along with specific breathing and coughing exercises. Patients may be

exhausted following this exacting form of physiotherapy and the nurse may need to plan a rest period afterwards. Privacy is required as the expectoration of large volumes of sputum may be unpleasant for all concerned but the relief is great, especially in the morning after secretions have gath-

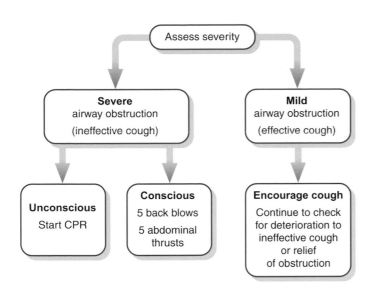

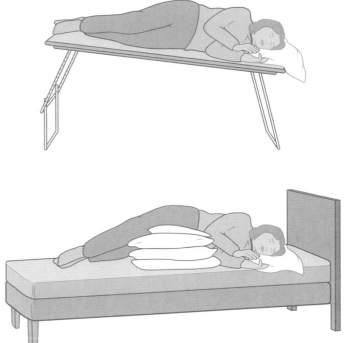

Fig. 5.18 Adult choking treatment algorithm (from Resuscitation Council (UK) 2005, with permission).

Fig. 5.20 Postural drainage for physiotherapy (from Esmond 2001, with permission).

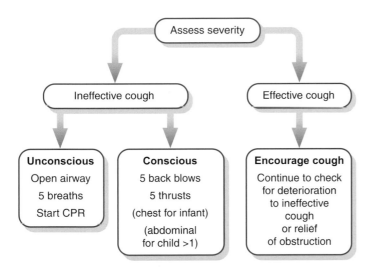

Fig. 5.19 Paediatric foreign body airway obstruction (FBAO) treatment algorithm (from Resuscitation Council (UK) 2005, with permission).

ered overnight where movement is minimal. Airway clearance techniques appear to be effective in the short term with regard to mucus clearance in cystic fibrosis patients according to a systematic review conducted by van de Schans et al (2006). Guidelines on physiotherapy and respiratory care are available from the British Thoracic Society.

Artificial airway maintenance

It may not be possible to clear the airway by physiotherapy, postural drainage, deep breathing and coughing exercises and suctioning, if there are excessive secretions and sputum retention. It is imperative that the airway is maintained and this may be achieved by the insertion of

an endotracheal tube (through the mouth into the trachea) or by performing a tracheostomy (surgical opening in the trachea).

An endotracheal tube is held in situ by inflating a cuff with a specified volume of air (see Fig. 5.21), whereas the tracheostomy tube is inserted into the trachea and held in place by inflating a cuff and by tapes being tied at the back of the neck (see Fig. 5.22). These measures may be temporary or permanent and can be carried out as a planned or emergency procedure (Dickson & Martindale 2002).

You would need to plan a variety of nursing actions once an endotracheal tube has been inserted or a tracheostomy has been performed. Humidified oxygen will be required to ensure that an adequate intake of moist oxygen is delivered. Secretions will need to be removed by the use of sterile catheters and an appropriate suctioning technique which is not harmful to the sensitive mucosa. Explanations are needed prior to suction being used, as it can be a frightening procedure for the patient. Jamieson et al (2002) and Dougherty & Lister (2004) provide a description of the procedure for this. Figure 5.23 illustrates the position of a tracheostomy tube and aspiration of secretions from a tracheostomy tube.

Care of the skin around the tracheostomy tube needs to be considered as the secretions and the tape used to hold the tube in place can irritate the skin, so keyhole dressings can be placed underneath the tracheostomy tube and replaced twice a day. Mouth care and mouthwashes should be given

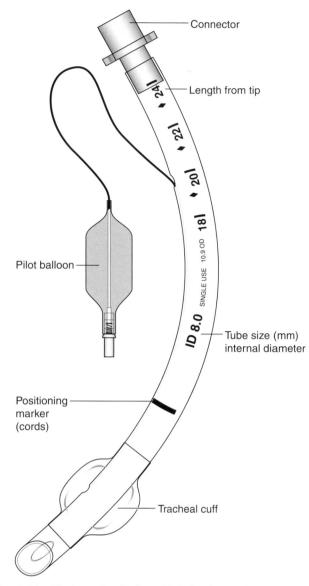

Connector

Length from tip

Pilot balloon

ID 8.0 SINGLE USE 10.9 OD 18 20 22 24

Tube size (mm) internal diameter

Positioning marker (cords)

Tracheal cuff

Fig. 5.21 Endotracheal tube with inflatable cuff (from Dickson & Martindale 2002, with permission).

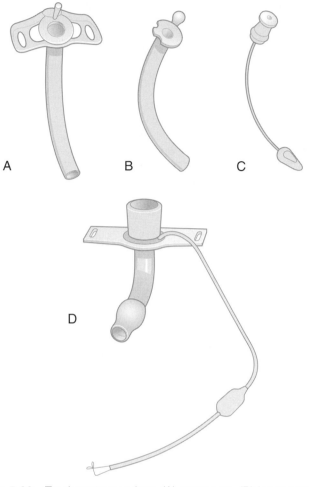

Fig. 5.22 Tracheostomy tubes, (A) outer part, (B) inner part, (C) introducer, (D) cuffed tube (from Dickson & Martindale 2002, with permission).

with care. The tracheostomy tube does need changing at various intervals and the nurse needs the appropriate knowledge and skill to do this. There are many different types of tracheostomy tubes, and Jamieson et al (2002), Dickson & Martindale (2002) and Dougherty & Lister (2004) discuss their specific care and the general care of patients requiring artificial airway maintenance. The patient will not be able to talk, initially, with an endotracheal or tracheostomy tube in position so the nurse must plan activities and use other communication methods such as a call bell and pen and paper to ensure that the patient can express their feelings and wishes to others. It may be useful for you to read the article by Serra (2000) for further information on tracheostomy care.

Mechanical ventilation will be required for patients who cannot breathe spontaneously and therefore maintain their own oxygen and carbon dioxide levels. Mechanical ventilators

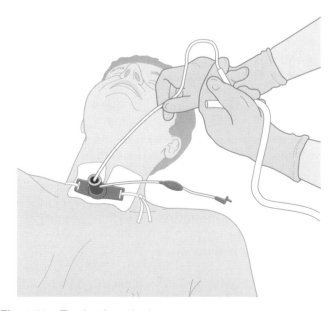

Fig. 5.23 Tracheal suctioning (from Nicol et al 2004, with permission).

(negative or positive pressure) automatically expand the chest, and oxygen is delivered into the lungs. Further details can be found earlier in this chapter and in Esmond (2001), Dickson & Martindale (2002) and Francis (2006).

Cardiopulmonary resuscitation in adults

Many writers discuss this action (Jamieson et al 2002, Nicol et al 2004, Mallik et al 2004, Dougherty & Lister 2004, Webster & Thompson 2006, Jevon 2006) and there is consensus that it involves three procedures. However, it is important to note that the guidelines produced by the Resuscitation Council (UK) in 2000 were revised in 2005 (www.resus.org.uk). The main difference for basic life support is the need to increase the number of chest compressions to optimise performance and minimise interruptions. The algorithms addressing adult basic life support (out of hospital and in hospital) are shown in Figures 5.24 and 5.25.

The revised recommendations are:

1. *Airway* – providing and maintaining a clear airway by removing any visible obstruction is the initial consideration. The head is then tilted backwards and the mandible pulled forward. This will open the airway and an oral

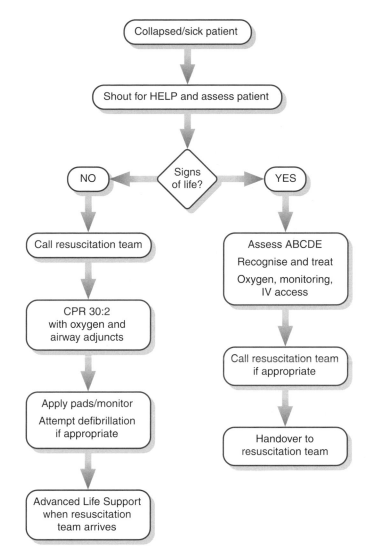

Fig. 5.25 Adult basic life support – in-hospital resuscitation algorithm (from Resuscitation Council (UK) 2005, with permission).

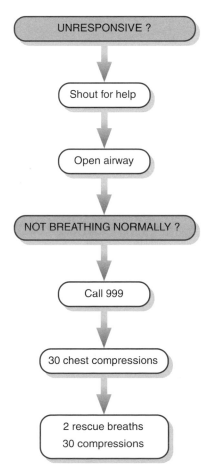

Fig. 5.24 Adult basic life support – out of hospital resuscitation algorithm (from Resuscitation Council (UK) 2005, with permission).

airway may be inserted at this time. Care must be taken if a neck injury is suspected.

2. *Breathing* – It is then important to check for normal breathing. If they are not breathing normally, then resuscitation is required but no initial ventilations are recommended until chest compressions have commenced as the blood oxygen level remains high for the first few minutes. The only exception to this is in the case of a near drowning situation where two initial ventilations are recommended. Supplying oxygen to the blood by means of artificial ventilation is vital after initial 30 chest compressions. Mouth-to-mouth ventilation can be used, and a chest compression ratio of 30 to a ventilation ratio of 2 is recommended in adults. The rise and fall of the chest should be noted to confirm that air is entering the respiratory tract. However, this method can only deliver 16% oxygen to the individual and there may a risk from contact with body fluids. If at all possible, an airway should be used and ventilation continued with a Ambubag or a

mask. Up to 90% oxygen can be delivered by this route but it needs practice to do this.

3. *Circulation* – forcing the blood out of the heart into the arterial system by means of cardiac compressions is needed if no carotid pulse can be found within 10 seconds. If the arrest is witnessed, then commence with 30 chest compressions. The correct position for chest compressions is vital and the Resuscitation Council UK (2005) and Jevon (2006) advocate placing the heel of one hand in the centre of the person's chest and placing the heel of the other hand on top of the first hand. The fingers should then be interlocked with no pressure being applied to the person's ribs, upper abdomen or lower end of the sternum. The arms are kept straight and the elbows locked and the sternum is then compressed by 4–5 cm towards the spine. After each compression, all the pressure should be released on the chest without losing contact with the sternum. The chest compression then needs to be repeated at a rate of 100 times per minute. After the first 30 compressions then two effective rescuer breaths should be administered. Chest compressions and rescue breaths should continue in a ratio of 30:2 and should not be interrupted unless the person starts to breath normally. If there is more than one rescuer present, another should take over CPR about every 2 min to prevent fatigue. It is necessary to ensure that there is a minimum delay during the changeover of rescuers (see Fig. 5.26).

The use of a precordial thump (blow to the lower half of a person's sternum using the lateral aspect of a closed fist) should be considered according to the Resuscitation Council UK (2006) only if the arrest is witnessed, where ventricular fibrillation (VF) or ventricular tachycardia (VT) is shown on ECG monitoring and where there is no defibrillator at hand. However, training is required before this procedure can be carried out. Advanced life support for adults and paediatrics is not covered in this chapter but recommendations can be found in the Resuscitation Council UK (2005) guidelines.

Paediatric life support was also revised by the Resuscitation Council (UK) in 2005. After opening the airway and confirming that the child is not breathing normally, five rescue breaths are given as the priority is oxygenation. If the child remains unresponsive, then this is followed by 15 chest compressions followed by two rescue breaths, and this 15:2 ratio continues. The Resuscitation Council (UK) 2005 algorithm addressing paediatric basic life support is shown in Figure 5.27.

Exercise

If you are able to observe a person being resuscitated then consider:

1. Were these recommendations followed?
2. What drugs were used during the resuscitation attempt? Check in a copy of the BNF or online (www. bnf.org).
3. How did you feel after the attempt (successful or not) and how did you deal with this?

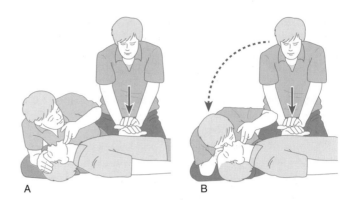

Fig. 5.26 Cardiopulmonary resuscitation, (A) two resuscitators – ratio of 30:2, (B) one resuscitator – ratio of 30:2 (from Jamieson et al 2002, with permission).

If you have not been able to observe a resuscitation then discuss this with your mentor, preceptor, clinical supervisor or resuscitation officer.

You may have found some differences depending on the updating of staff with the revised guidelines issued by

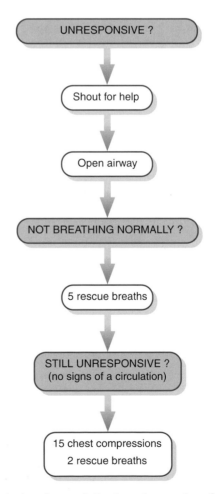

UNRESPONSIVE ?

↓

Shout for help

↓

Open airway

↓

NOT BREATHING NORMALLY ?

↓

5 rescue breaths

↓

STILL UNRESPONSIVE ? (no signs of a circulation)

↓

15 chest compressions
2 rescue breaths

After 1 minute call resuscitation team then continue CPR

Fig. 5.27 Paediatric basic life support resuscitation algorithm (from Resuscitation Council (UK) 2005, with permission).

Resuscitation Council UK (2005). It is essential that all health care professionals are trained in cardiopulmonary resuscitation techniques. Although a literature review conducted by Hamilton (2005) identified various studies, over some 20 years, that have demonstrated poor knowledge and skills retention following cardiopulmonary resuscitation training for health care professionals, training programmes for the general public have been promoted and well attended. The Resuscitation Council (UK) commenced basic life support and advanced life support courses in 1993 and there is some evidence that there has been an increase in the number of successful resuscitations since this time (Handley & Swain 1996).

You may have noted drugs being used during CPR such as adrenaline, amiodarone, lidocaine (only used if amiodarone is not available) and atropine. Other less commonly used drugs that you may have seen used during CPR are magnesium sulphate, sodium bicarbonate, or calcium chloride. The Resuscitation Council UK (2005) and Gallimore (2006) give more details about these drugs, their routes, actions, doses and side-effects.

There are legal, ethical and professional issues relating to resuscitation and you may need to consider these issues as well as the skills that are needed. According to Mallik et al (2004), there is no legal duty of care in the UK to a neighbour. So a nurse need not legally stop to give first aid to help someone in the streets but there is a moral issue of whether this is right. However, if the first-aider has presented themselves as a nurse, then they do have a professional duty of care to help and would be responsible and liable for their acts and omissions in relation to the care given. It is, therefore, important that nurses have some form of personal indemnity insurance.

Policies about decisions relating to CPR have been reviewed following the implementation of the Human Rights Act 1998 (DoH 1998b) (see www.opsi.gov.uk/ACTS/acts1998/19980042.htm).

Exercise

1. Locate a copy of the Human Rights Act 1998 on the internet.
2. Identify the section noted as 'Articles'.
3. Identify which Articles relate to resuscitation and discuss these with your mentor, preceptor or clinical supervisor.

Health care professionals must be able to demonstrate that their decisions are compatible with the human rights set out in the Articles contained within the Act. Those Articles particularly relevant to decisions about attempted CPR include the right to life (Article 2), to be free from inhuman or degrading treatment (Article 3), to respect for privacy and family life (Article 8), to freedom of expression, which includes the right to hold opinions and to receive information (Article 10) and to be free from discriminatory practices in respect of these rights (Article 14). If there is any doubt about the legality of an advance decision about attempting resuscitation, legal advice should be sought.

However, when the nurse is an employee and the arrest occurs in the context of employment, then the nurse would be classed as the designated first-aider as defined in the Health and Safety at Work Act (1974). In this situation, it would probably be the employer who would be sued for negligence and not the individual nurse.

The Nursing and Midwifery Council (NMC) Code of Professional Conduct (2004a) however, complicates the matter as it states that 'As a registered nurse, midwife or specialist community public health nurse, you must: protect and support the health of individuals and clients, protect and support the health of the wider community, act in such a way that justifies the trust and confidence the public have in you and uphold and enhance the good reputation of the professions' (p. 4, Section 1.2). This appears to override the legal issues and indicates that all nurses and midwives must render first aid to all people, whether they are in a health care setting or not.

Resuscitating individuals also raises ethical dilemmas and the issues of 'Do not resuscitate' policies and 'Living Wills' complicate this already 'grey area'. A joint statement was set out by the British Medical Association, the Resuscitation Council (UK) and the Royal College of Nursing in 2002 stating that all establishments that face decisions about attempting resuscitation should have in place local policies for decision making. The purpose of these guidelines is to outline legal and ethical standards for planning patient care and decision making in relation to cardiopulmonary resuscitation. (See Box 5.13 for the summary of these guidelines, and new BMA, Resuscitation Council (UK) and RCN guidelines (2007).)

Another issue is that of whether relatives have the right to witness the resuscitation of their loved ones. Even though, according to Resuscitation Council UK (1996), approximately 30 000 resuscitation attempts take place each year in the UK, there is still much discussion and debate regarding whether relatives should be allowed to stay. Most resuscitation attempts take place in the Accident and Emergency Department or Intensive Care Units, where relatives are often present. Walker (1999) concludes that the relative's right to witness resuscitation is dependent on the health care professional's beliefs and attitudes.

There are, therefore, many issues for you to consider when the decision to resuscitate someone is taken. Following a resuscitation event, debriefing is advocated by Gamble (2001) and the Resuscitation Council (UK) (2004) as the unpredictability of the event can result in unique feelings in the carer. The initial resuscitation call activates the stress response system known as the 'general adaptation syndrome'. If the effect of this stress response system is not discussed then the carer may be left with physical and psychological issues unresolved.

Box 5.13	Summary of the decisions relating to cardiopulmonary resuscitation

Principles
- Timely support for patients and people close to them, and effective, sensitive communication are essential.
- Decisions must be based on the individual patient's circumstances and reviewed regularly.
- Sensitive advance discussion should always be encouraged, but not forced.
- Information about CPR and the chances of a successful outcome needs to be realistic.

Practical matters
- Information about CPR policies should be displayed for patients and staff.
- Leaflets should be available for patients and people close to them explaining about CPR, how decisions are made and their involvement in decisions.
- Decisions about attempting CPR must be communicated effectively to relevant health professionals.
- *In emergencies,* if no advance decision has been made or is known, CPR should be attempted unless:
  – the patient has refused CPR
  – the patient is clearly in the terminal phase of illness or
  – the burdens of the treatment outweigh the benefits.

Advance decision making
- Competent patients should be involved in discussions about attempting CPR, unless they indicate that they do not want to be.
- Where patients lack competence to participate, people close to them can be helpful in reflecting their views.

Legal issues
- Patients' rights under the Human Rights Act must be taken into account in decision making.
- Neither patients nor relatives can demand treatment which the health care team judges to be inappropriate, but all efforts will be made to accommodate wishes and preferences.
- In England, Wales and Northern Ireland relatives and people close to the patient are not entitled in law to take health care decisions for the patient.
- In Scotland, adults may appoint a health care proxy to give consent to medical treatment.
- Health professionals need to be aware of the law in relation to decision making for children and young people.

British Medical Association, Resuscitation Council (UK) and Royal College of Nursing (2002).

Underwater seal chest drain

A chest drain or intrapleural drain, according to Dougherty & Lister (2004) is used to remove a collection of air, fluid, pus or blood from the pleural space into a collecting bottle in order to restore normal respiratory expansion and function. Many different clinical situations may require the insertion of a chest drain, such as following a pneumothorax, postoperative cardiac surgery and pleural effusions. The British Thoracic Society (BTS) produced guidelines for the insertion, management and removal of chest drains in 2003 and advocates that patients with chest drains should be managed on specialist wards by staff trained in chest drain management.

The insertion of the chest drain is not a nurse's role but it is explained in Jamieson et al (2002) and Dougherty & Lister (2004) (see Fig. 5.28). Francis (2006) discusses the nurse's role when the tube is being inserted as one of providing explanations, correct positioning and observation of the patient. Once the drain has been inserted the nurse must ensure that the tube is sutured securely and it is connected to a closed drainage system which is always kept below the patient's chest. The nurse then needs to: check that the apparatus is functioning; apply a sterile dressing; observe for swinging and bubbling of the fluid in the bottle on inspiration and expiration; note the type and amount of drainage; and provide adequate analgesia. The position of the tube should be checked by a chest X-ray. The British Thoracic Society (2003) guidelines discuss the clamping of chest drains and there are specific times when the tube should not be clamped, e.g. when the chest drain is still bubbling or prior to its removal. The chest tube can be removed either while the patient performs the Valsalva manoeuvre or during expiration. Two health care professionals are required, one to remove the drain and one to tie the suture in place and apply a dressing.

Nursing actions associated with comforting care

You will need to consider what the best position for the patient is so that they can increase lung inflation, aid emptying of the lungs and decrease respiratory effort. The patient may breathe more easily sitting up and leaning forward, resting arms and shoulders on a bed table in a well-ventilated area near a window. They may choose to sit in a chair as opposed to being in a bed. The nurse needs to adopt a calm approach to care, talking to the patient using closed questions and allaying their fears of dying. Deep breathing, coughing exercises and relaxation techniques need to be taught appropriately (see Fig. 5.29).

Nursing actions associated with preventative care

The nurse's role in health promotion and the prevention of disease is noted within the Department of Health's (1999c) document *Saving Lives*, and within the activity of breathing

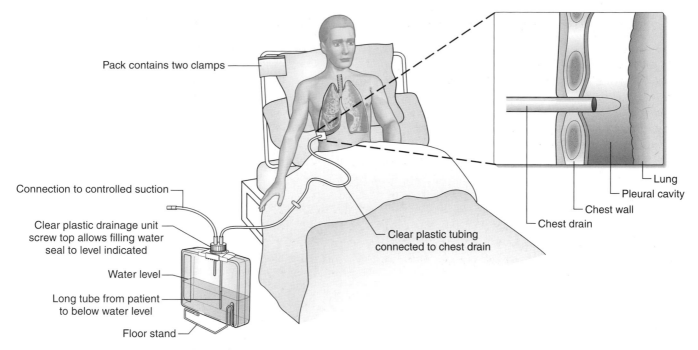

Pack contains two clamps

Connection to controlled suction

Clear plastic drainage unit screw top allows filling water seal to level indicated

Water level

Long tube from patient to below water level

Floor stand

Clear plastic tubing connected to chest drain

Lung
Pleural cavity
Chest wall
Chest drain

Fig. 5.28 Underwater seal chest drainage (from Edmond et al 2006, with permission).

there are many areas where this role is paramount to the patient's wellbeing. Their role in smoking cessation programmes has already been discussed in this chapter.

Self-management is the mainstay of acute and chronic respiratory problems. So patients, and therefore nurses, need to have knowledge and skill in administering drugs via inhalers and/or nebulisers and need to be able to recognise when their regime may need altering and when medical assistance is needed. They need to know about the actions, side-effects and method of administration of drug therapies. In particular, you will need to support patients with their inhaler technique as this is vital to the effectiveness of this therapy. Patients need to be able to identify allergens that precipitate an attack and consider what actions can be taken to try and minimise problems. Patient compliance with their medication is vital and the nurse needs to use appropriate strategies as outlined by Murphy (2001) to aid compliance.

In hospital, it is important to recognise 'at risk' or critically ill patients as common signs are displayed when patient's condition deteriorates, according to the Resuscitation Council (UK) (2005). Many hospitals have adopted Early Warning Scores (EWS) where points are allocated to routine vital sign measurements on the basis of their deviation from normal ranges. The score is then used to alert ward staff and/or an outreach service (usually clinical nursing teams or a medical emergency team (MET) which is able to respond to acute crises and is available 24 hours a day) to the deterioration of the patient. Naeem & Montenegro (2005) consider that there is insufficient evidence to support the benefit of EWS to prevent in-hospital cardiopulmonary arrest. However, more recent studies of the medical emergency teams have shown a significant decrease in cardiac arrests and overall mortality rates with this intervention. The Resuscitation Council UK (2005) has recommended various strategies for the prevention of avoidable in-hospital cardiac arrests and these can be found in Box 5.14. It would be useful to discuss these with your mentor, preceptor, clinical supervisor or Resuscitation Officer to ascertain if these are in place within your organisation.

It can be seen that there are numerous nursing actions and these vary between emergency procedures and health promotion measures. You, therefore, may need to develop your knowledge and skills to ensure that you are able to give competent professional care to all patients alike.

Documenting the care plan

Once the nursing actions have been identified then the care plan needs to be written. Care plans should abide by the NMC (2007) *Record Keeping Guidance* and identify individualised actions and specify:

- who should be involved in the care planned
- what care should be given
- why that care should be given
- when the care should be given
- where the care should be given
- how the care should be given.

Exercise

1. Write the care plan for Tom Jackson (Case study 5.3) to address the three problems identified on p. 165.
2. Check your answers with the care plan in Box 5.15.

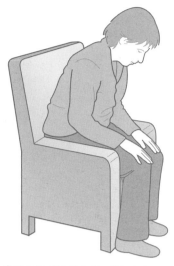

Sitting in chair leaning forward

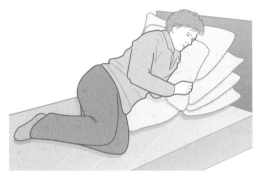

High side lying

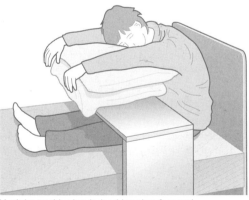

Upright positioning in bed leaning forward
onto pillows or bedside table with pillows

Fig. 5.29 Positioning the breathless patient (from Brooker 2005, with permission).

It may also be useful for you to consider the five factors (physical, psychological, sociocultural, environmental and politicoeconomic) when writing the nursing care plan. Re-read the nursing care plans and decide if all the factors are utilised.

Once the nursing care plan has been written then you must communicate this to other health care professionals by verbal handover ready for the next stage – implementation.

| Box 5.14 | Recommended strategies for the prevention of avoidable in-hospital cardiac arrests |

1. Place critically ill patients, or those at risk of clinical deterioration, in areas where the level of care is matched to the level of patient sickness.
2. Regularly monitor such patients using simple vital sign observations (e.g. pulse, blood pressure, respiratory rate). Match the frequency and type of observations to the severity of illness of the patient.
3. Use a EWS system to identify patients who are critically ill, at risk of clinical deterioration or cardiopulmonary arrest, or both.
4. Use a patient vital signs chart that encourages and permits the regular measurement and recording of early warning scores.
5. Ensure that the hospital has a clear policy that requires a clinical response to deterioration in the patient's clinical condition. Provide advice on the further clinical management of the patient and the specific responsibilities of medical and nursing staff.
6. Introduce into each hospital a clearly identified response to critical illness. This will vary between sites, but may include an outreach service or clinical team (e.g. MET) capable of responding to acute clinical crises. This team should be alerted, using an early warning system, and the service must be available 24 hours a day.
7. Ensure that all clinical staff are trained in the recognition, monitoring, and management of the critically ill patient.
8. Agree a hospital 'Do Not Attempt Resuscitation' (DNAR) policy, based on national guidelines, and ensure that it is understood by all clinical staff. Identify patients who do not wish to receive CPR and those for whom cardiopulmonary arrest is an anticipated terminal event for whom CPR would be inappropriate.
9. Audit all cardiac arrests, 'false arrests', unexpected deaths, and unanticipated Intensive Care Unit admissions, using a common dataset. Audit the antecedents and clinical responses to these events.

Resuscitation Council (UK) (2005).

IMPLEMENTING NURSING ACTIVITIES

Implementation of nursing activities involves three stages:

1. Preparatory stage of reading the care plan, receiving handover report and ensuring that staff know what is required to accomplish the goals and decide on the skill mix needed.
2. Implementation where safe, competent practice is the key to successful care. The plan is then put into action and shows the artistic and scientific side of nursing.
3. Post-implementation stage when nursing activities are communicated to health care professionals (written and verbally) via progress notes.

Box 5.15	**Nursing care plan – Tom Jackson**

PROBLEM 1

Tom has difficulty with breathing due to exacerbation of his breathing disorder as shown by a loose cough, raised respiratory rate and audible wheeze.

Short-term goal

Tom will be able to breathe more easily and more quietly with the aid of oxygen with a lower respiratory rate than on admission and is able to expectorate secretions.

Long-term goal

Tom will be able to breathe normally, unaided before discharge with no audible wheeze, no cough or sputum produced and have a respiratory rate of 18–24 respirations per minute at rest for a minimum of 4 hours.

Nursing care plan

- Observe respiratory rate, rhythm and character of breathing 4-hourly.
- Observe sputum production for quantity, consistency and colour, ability to expectorate.
- Observe the duration and frequency of Tom's coughing and when his coughing is worse and the effect coughing has on Tom.
- Observe colour of skin, lips and nail beds.
- Observe temperature and peak flow recordings 4-hourly.
- Report changes in any of the observations immediately.
- Send a specimen of sputum for culture and sensitivity.
- Give oxygen, 2 litres per minute, via humidified MC mask as prescribed and note effect.
- Assist in the investigations ordered by the medical staff, e.g. chest X-ray, blood gases.
- Assist the physiotherapist in teaching and supervising deep breathing exercises and encourage Tom to expectorate sputum.
- Give oral care and nasal care 4-hourly.
- Ensure adequate hydration is maintained with 2 litres of oral fluids encouraged per day.
- Explain the need to expectorate sputum.
- Ensure a call bell is at hand and stay calm when with the patient.
- Ensure that Tom has a balance between company and rest.
- When talking to Tom allow him time to reply and if needed use closed questions so that Tom doesn't get overexerted trying to answer questions.
- Ensure the room is well ventilated and that Tom is sat up in bed or in an armchair, well supported by pillows.
- Ensure a bed table is at hand with pillows on it if this aids Tom's breathing.
- Ensure sputum pots are to hand and tissues available.

PROBLEM 2

Tom has difficulty with mobilising because of his breathlessness and may develop pressure sores, deep vein thrombosis, pulmonary embolism, constipation due to limited activity.

Long-term goal

Tom will be able to mobilise unaided, without dyspnoea and will not experience complications of bed rest as shown by intact skin, calf soft, pain-free and normal size, no chest pain, bowels opened normally for him.

Nursing care plan

- Observe Tom's ability to mobilise and his breathing rate.
- Rest in bed initially, sitting up in bed supported well by pillows.
- Ensure that Tom is comfortable.
- When able to mobilise with minimal dyspnoea then encourage Tom to do so.
- Complete risk assessments for pressure sores and plan accordingly.
- Observe pressure areas 4-hourly, report redness and any breaks in the skin.
- Reposition 2–4 hourly.
- Move and handle appropriately.
- Ensure skin is clean and dry.
- Observe calf size for changes. *(continued)*

References

Allen K 2005 Four-step method of interpreting arterial blood gas analysis. Nursing Times 101(1):42–45

Anthonisen N, Skeans M, Wise R et al 2005 The effects of a smoking cessation intervention on 14.5-year mortality. Annals of Internal Medicine 142(4):233–239

British Medical Association, Resuscitation Council (UK), Royal College of Nursing 2002 Decisions relating to cardiopulmonary resuscitation: a joint statement from the British Medical Association, the Resuscitation Council (UK) and the Royal College of Nursing. British Medical Association, London (www.bma.org.uk/ap.nsf/Content/cardioresus)

British Medical Association, Resuscitation Council (UK), Royal College of Nursing 2007 Decisions relating to cardiopulmonary resuscitation: a joint statement from the British Medical Association, the Resuscitation Council (UK) and the Royal College of Nursing. British Medical Association, London (www.bma.org.uk/ap.nsf/)

British Thoracic Society 1997 Guidelines for the management of chronic obstructive pulmonary disease. Thorax 52(Suppl): S1–28 (www.brit-thoracic.org)

British Thoracic Society 2002a Managing passengers with respiratory disease planning air travel: British Thoracic Society recommendations. Thorax 57:289–304 (www.brit-thoracic.org)

British Thoracic Society 2002b Non-invasive ventilation in acute respiratory failure. Thorax 57:192–211 (www.brit-thoracic.org)

British Thoracic Society 2003 Guidelines for the insertion of a chest drain. Thorax 58(Suppl 11): ii53–ii59 (www.brit-thoracic.org)

British Thoracic Society 2006a Burden of lung disease, 2nd edn (www.brit-thoracic.org.uk/BurdenofLungDisease2)

British Thoracic Society 2006b Recommendations for the management of cough in adults. Thorax 61(Suppl I): i1–i24 (www.brit-thoracic.org)

Brooker C 2005 Mini encyclopaedia of nursing. Churchill Livingstone, Edinburgh

Burns BH, Howell J 1969 Disproportionately severe breathlessness in chronic bronchitis. Quarterly Journal of Medicine 38:277–294

Casey G 2001 Oxygen transport and the use of pulse oximetry. Nursing Standard 15(47):46–53

Clark A 2002 Legal lessons: 'But his O$_2$ Sat was normal!' Clinical Nurse Specialist 16(3):162–163

Castle F 1999 The breath of life. Nursing Standard 13(33):20

Central Statistical Office 1995 Annual abstract of statistics. HMSO, London

Clothier C, MacDonald C, Shaw D 1994 Independent enquiry into deaths and injuries on the Children's ward at Grantham and Kestevan General Hospital during the period February to April 1991 (Allitt Inquiry). HMSO, London

Coombs M 2001 Making sense of arterial blood gases. Nursing Times 97(27):36–38

Cornock MA 1996 Making sense of arterial blood gases and their interpretation. Nursing Times 92(6):30–31

Department of Health 1974 Health and Safety at Work Act. HMSO, London

Department of Health 1991 Advisory group on the medical aspects of air pollution episodes first report: ozone. HMSO, London

Department of Health 1995 Advisory group on the medical aspects of air pollution episodes. Report: health effects of exposure to mixtures of air pollutants: fourth report of the advisory group on the medical aspects of air pollution episodes. HMSO, London

Department of Health 1998a Smoking kills. A white paper on tobacco. HMSO, London

Department of Health 1998b Human Rights Act 1998. HMSO, London

Department of Health 1999a Committee on the medical effects of air pollutants. Statement on the health effects of indoor exposure to carbon monoxide in the UK. HMSO, London

Department of Health 1999b COMEAP statement on the study by Poloniecki et al: Daily time-series for cardiovascular hospital admissions and previous day's air pollution in UK. HMSO, London

Department of Health 1999c Saving lives. HMSO, London

Department of Health 2000a NHS plan. HMSO, London

Department of Health 2000b COMEAP advice: The health effects of air pollutants July 2000 (www.advisorybodies.dh.gov.uk/comeap/statementsreports/healtheffects)

Department of Health 2001a Committee on the medical effects of air pollutants report on long-term effects of particles on mortality. HMSO, London

Department of Health 2001b Statistical bulletin, HMSO, London (www.doh.gov.uk/public/sb0105.htm)

Department of Health 2002a Tobacco Advertising and Promotion Act. HMSO, London (www.dh.gov.uk)

Department of Health 2002b Carbon monoxide: The forgotten killer. HMSO, London (www.dh.gov.uk)

Department of Health 2002c Priorities and planning framework 2003–2006. Improvement, expansion and reform. HMSO, London (www.dh.gov.uk)

Department of Health 2003a Statistical Bulletin 2003/21 Statistics on smoking: England, 2003. HMSO, London (www.dh.gov.uk)

Department of Health 2003b Ozone – effects on respiratory symptoms in panel studies – summary. Addendum to COMEAP/2003/9a. (www.advisorybodies.dh.gov.uk/comeap/issues)

Department of Health 2004a Choosing health: Making healthier choices easier. (www.dh.gov.uk)

Department of Health 2004b Scientific Committee on Tobacco and Health (SCOTH). Secondhand smoke: review of evidence since 1998. Update of evidence on health effects of secondhand smoke. (www.dh.gov.uk)

Department of Health 2005 Indoor air pollution – carbon monoxide. (www.dh.gov.uk/airpollution)

Department of Health 2006 Cardiovascular disease and air pollution A report by the Committee on the Medical Effects of Air Pollutants. (www.advisorybodies.dh.gov.uk/comeap/issues)

Dickson A, Martindale G 2002 Caring for the patient with a respiratory disorder. In: Walsh M (ed) Watson's clinical nursing and related sciences, 6th edn. Chapter 13. Baillière Tindall, London.

Docherty B, Coote S 2006 Respiratory assessment as part of track and trigger. Nursing Times 102(44):28–29

Dougherty L, Lister S 2004 The Royal Marsden Hospital manual of clinical nursing procedures, 6th edn. Blackwell Publishing, Oxford

Dudley DL, Martin CJ, Holmes TH 1964 Psychophysiologic studies of pulmonary ventilation. Psychosomatic Medicine 26:645–659

Durmaz E, Laurence S, Roden P et al 1999 Carbon monoxide poisoning and hyperbaric oxygen therapy. British Journal of Nursing 8(16):1067–1072

Edmond CB, McLean J, McGlone J et al 2006 The respiratory system. In: Alexander MF, Fawcett JN, Runciman PJ (eds) Nursing practice hospital and home 3rd edn, Chapter 3. Churchill Livingstone, Edinburgh

Esmond G 2001 Respiratory nursing. Baillière Tindall, Edinburgh

Esmond G 2003 Nursing patients with respiratory disorders. In: Brooker C, Nicol M (eds) Nursing adults: the practice of caring, Chapter 20. Mosby, Edinburgh

Esmond G, Mikelsons C 2001 Oxygen therapy. In: Esmond G (ed) Respiratory nursing, Chapter 7. Baillière Tindall, Edinburgh

Etter J-F, Perneger TV 2004 Post-intervention effect of a computer tailored smoking cessation programme. Journal of Epidemiology and Community Health 58:849–851

European guidelines for control and prevention of travel associated legionnaires' disease 2005 (www.ewgli. org/data/europoean_guidelines)

Ferns T, Chojnacka I 2006 Conducting respiratory assessments in acute care. Nursing Times 102(7):53–55

Fitzpatrick J, Griffiths C, Kelleher M 2000 Geographic inequalities in mortality in the United Kingdom during the 1990s. Examines inequalities in mortality by country, region and local authority within the United Kingdom between 1991 and 1997. Health Statistics Quarterly 7:18–31

Francis C 2006 Respiratory care. Blackwell Publishing, Oxford

Gallimore D 2006 Understanding the drugs used during cardiac arrest. Nursing Times 102(23):24–26

Gamble M 2001 A debriefing approach to dealing with the stress of CPR attempts. Professional Nurse 17(3):157–160

Gift A 1990 Dyspnea. Nursing Clinics of North America 25(4): 955–956. In: Francis C. 2006 Respiratory care. Blackwell Publishing, Oxford

Giuliano K, Liu L 2006 Knowledge of pulse oximetry among critical care nurses. Dimensions of Critical Care Nursing 25(1):44–49

Hamilton R 2005 Nurses' knowledge and skill retention following cardiopulmonary resuscitation training: a review of the literature. Journal of Advanced Nursing 51(3):288–297

Handley AJ, Swain A (eds) 1996 Ethics and legal aspects. In: Advanced life support manual. Resuscitation Council, London,

Harding S, Reid A 2000 Trends in regional deprivation and mortality using the longitudinal study. Examines trends in regional mortality using a deprivation index based on individual characteristics. Health Statistics Quarterly 5:17–25

Hateley P 2001 Respiratory infections. In: Esmond G (ed) Respiratory nursing, Chapter 9. Baillière Tindall, Edinburgh

He J, Vupputuri S, Allen K et al 1999 Passive smoking and the risk of coronary heart disease – a meta analysis of epidemiologic studies. New England Journal of Medicine 340:920–926 (www.jr2.ox.ac.uk/bandolier/booth/hliving/Passive.htlm)

Health Protection Agency 2006a Legionnaires' disease (www.hpa.org.uk/infections/topics_az/legionella/menu.htm)

Health Protection Agency 2006b Severe acute respiratory syndrome (SARS) disease (www.hpa.org.uk/infections/topics/a-z/SARS)

Health Protection Agency 2007 Avian flu (www.hpa.org.uk/infections/topics_az/influenza/avian/)

Higgins D 2005a Measuring PEFR. Nursing Times 101(10):32–33

Higgins D 2005b Pulse oximetry. Nursing Times 101(6):34–35

Howell M 2002 Pulse oximetry: an audit of nursing and medical staff understanding. British Journal of Nursing 11(3):191–197

Information Centre 2006 Statistics on NHS Stop Smoking Services in England, April 2005 to March 2006. Q4–quarterly report (www.ic.nhs.uk/pubs/nhsstopsmokingstats2005to2006q4)

Jackson H, Hubbard H 2003 Detecting chronic obstructive pulmonary disease using peak flow rate: cross sectional survey. British Medical Journal 327:653–654

Jamieson EM, McCall JM, Whyte LA 2002 Guidelines for clinical nursing practices, 4th edn. Churchill Livingstone, Edinburgh

Jevon P 2006 An overview of the new resuscitation guidelines. Nursing Times 102(3):25–27

Jevon P, Ewens B 2001 Assessment of a breathless patient. Nursing Standard 15(16):48–53

Jordan S, White J 2001 Bronchodilators: implications for nursing practice. Nursing Standard 15(27):45–52

Juurlink DN, Buckley NA, Stanbrook MB et al 2006 Hyperbaric oxygen therapy for carbon monoxide poisoning. Cochrane Database of Systematic Reviews Issue 3

Kaushar R, Kaushik RM, Mahajan SK et al 2005 Biofeedback assisted diaphragmatic breathing and systematic relaxation versus propranolol in long term prophylaxis of migraine. Complementary Therapies in Medicine 13(3):165–174

Kendrick K, Baxi S, Smith R 2000 Usefulness of the modified 0–10 Borg scale in assessing the degree of dyspnoea inpatients with COPD and asthma. Professional Nurse 7(11):748–754

Kindlen S 2003 Physiology for health care and nursing, 2nd edn. Churchill Livingstone, Edinburgh

Law C, Watson R 2005 Respiration. In: Montague SE, Watson R, Herbert RA (eds) Physiology for nursing practice, 3rd edn. Chapter 5.3. Elsevier, Edinburgh

Lynes D 2003 An introduction to blood gas analysis. Nursing Times 99(11):54–55

Mallik M, Hall C, Howard D 2004 Nursing knowledge and practice: Foundations for decision making, 2nd edn. Baillière Tindall, Edinburgh

McNeill A, Raw M, Whybrow J, Bailey P 2005 A national strategy for smoking cessation treatment in England. Addiction 100(Suppl 2):1–11

Millar B 2000 A cruel and nasty disease. Nursing Times 96(21):32–33

Mikelsons C, Esmond G 2001 Respiratory support techniques. In: Esmond G (ed) Respiratory nursing, Chapter 8. Baillière Tindall, Edinburgh

Murphy S 2001 Respiratory medication. In: Esmond G (ed) Respiratory nursing, Chapter 5. Baillière Tindall, Edinburgh

Naeem N, Montenegro H 2005 Beyond the intensive care unit: a review of interventions aimed at anticipating and preventing in-hospital cardiopulmonary arrest. Resuscitation 67(1):13–23

Nazir Z, Razaq S, Mir S et al 2005 Revisiting the accuracy of peak flow meters: a double-blind study using formal methods of agreement. Respiratory Medicine 99(5):592–595

NICE 2002 Guidance on the use of nicotine replacement therapy (NRT) and bupropion for smoking cessation. Technology Appraisal Guideline No 38. NICE, London

NICE 2003a Flu treatment – zanamivir (review), amantadine and oseltamivir. Technology Appraisal Guideline No 58. NICE, London

Eating and drinking

Jackie Solomon

INTRODUCTION

Eating and drinking are essential to existence (Roper et al 1996, 2000) and nutritional status is influenced by general health, chronic disorders, mobility and psychological or socio-economic factors as well as age (McLaren et al 1997). The ability or inability to eat and drink can impact on many of the other ALs, if not all, for example overeating resulting in obesity may impact on the ability to mobilise or lack of adequate fluids may lead to dehydration and imbalance of homeostasis thus impacting on the activity of maintaining a safe environment. It is important to remember that ALs are closely related to each other and when illness compromises one activity then this will undoubtedly impact on the other ALs. The Roper, Logan and Tierney model for nursing provides nurses with a framework through which they are able to recognise and take account of the interrelatedness of the Activities of Living when assessing, planning, implementing and evaluating patient care. The nurse has a primary role, within the multidisciplinary team, in ensuring that patients receive food, fluids and adequate nutrition whilst they are in their care and health education regarding a healthy diet. Sadly, numerous reports and public concern have highlighted the poor nutritional status of patients in hospital and care homes, the lack of nurses' knowledge of nutrition and involvement in the nutritional care of patients, poor staffing levels, and the need for medical and nursing staff to assess patient's nutritional status (Lennard-Jones 1992, McWhirter & Pennington 1994, Kowanko et al 1999, Corish et al 2004, Woo et al 2005, Leslie et al 2006, Age Concern 2006). To maintain a healthy diet we all need to ensure that we have an adequate supply of nutrients and in the right proportions for our need. Throughout this chapter the term malnutrition is used to include undernutrition due to inadequate food intake; overnutrition due to overconsumption of food; deficiencies in nutrients; and dietary imbalance (Bond 1997).

This chapter will focus on the following:

1. **The model of living**
   - eating and drinking in health and illness (across the lifespan)
   - dependence/independence in eating and drinking
   - factors influencing the AL of eating and drinking.

2. **The model for nursing**
   - nursing care of individuals with health problems affecting the AL of eating and drinking.

THE MODEL OF LIVING

Eating and drinking are essential to our survival as human beings (Roper et al 1996, 2000). Food, water and essential nutrients are necessary to provide energy, growth and repair of body tissue, and to maintain physiological functioning (Green & Jackson 2006). Eating and drinking form part of our social activities and psychological wellbeing, and a certain level of intelligence is required to understand the requirements of a well-balanced diet. The availability of food and drink is subject to social, economic and political influences, and within well-developed countries is often taken for granted, unlike in less-developed countries where the access to food and drink is a daily struggle. Food safety and access to uncontaminated water sources is of vital importance. Eating and drinking is also a feature of cultural and religious rituals and ceremonies, for example the service of communion within a Christian community and fasting during Ramadan, as well as formal meals to celebrate birthdays and weddings.

The nurse has a vital role in ensuring patients' nutritional needs are met as well as being involved in health education programmes. Working within a multidisciplinary team, nurses are responsible for assessing the nutritional needs of patients, ensuring that patients receive the right food, encouraging patients to eat and drink or managing artificial feeding regimes. They are also ideally placed to ensure a pleasant environment at mealtimes, minimise interruptions and advise on menu choices. In today's health care environment there are often times when it may be necessary for the nurse to delegate the nutritional care of patients to unregistered staff. In such circumstances the registered nurse is responsible for ensuring that the member of staff has the knowledge and skill required to undertake the required task (Nursing and Midwifery Council (NMC) 2004).

EATING AND DRINKING IN HEALTH AND ILLNESS (ACROSS THE LIFESPAN)

Before birth

Before birth the fetus obtains its essential nutrients for growth and development from the mother via the placenta and amniotic fluid. Therefore it is important that the mother during her pregnancy maintains a healthy diet to provide nourishment for the growing fetus and successful lactation, and if she drinks alcohol that she reduces her intake to avoid the risk of birth defects (Roper et al 1996).

After birth

After birth the action of suckling stimulates the formation of milk and the mother produces a substance known as colostrum from her breasts in the first instance followed by breast milk, which begins to flow on or around the third day after delivery. Both colostrum and breast milk contain all the nutrients that a baby needs in the right proportions. The 'fore milk' which is full of lactose and quenches the baby's thirst is followed by a richer food known as the 'hind milk' that contains the calories that the baby requires. It is easily digested and absorbed and contains antibodies that help to protect the baby against infection and disease (Quigley et al 2006). For further information see Kindlen (2003) or Montague et al (2005).

> **Exercise**
> 1. Discuss with your colleagues or family your views (and theirs) about breastfeeding.
> 2. Access the Baby Friendly Initiative website (www.babyfriendly.org.uk or www.breastfeeding.nhs.uk) to find more information about breastfeeding and find out what advantages breastfeeding has for the mother and the baby.
> 3. Find out about the UNICEF Baby Friendly Initiative standards and accreditation. How are these being applied in your local area?

Breastfeeding has been shown to be advantageous for both the baby and the mother in preventing certain diseases. You may have found that there is some evidence to indicate that breastfeeding can protect the baby against gastroenteritis, otitis media, respiratory infections, urinary infections and diabetes mellitus. Breast milk also provides the baby with added immunity and enhances the benefits from immunisation. There is a belief that there are some situations in which breastfeeding might not be in the best interest of the baby, including some maternal medications and specific viral infections such as HIV, hepatitis and T-cell leukaemia. Since breastfeeding protects against infant deaths from infectious diseases an overwhelming majority of babies will benefit from breastfeeding, even those born to HIV-infected women (Dobson 2002).

> **Exercise**
> 1. Find out it if there is any information available on the number of women who started to breastfeed within your local area over a period of time.
> 2. What initiatives are available to support and encourage mothers to breastfeed their babies?
> 3. What advice is given to expectant and breastfeeding mothers about their own nutrition?

UNICEF estimates that 1.5 million babies worldwide die each year because they are not breastfed. Infant feeding surveys are conducted on behalf of the Department of Health every 3 years and have shown a significant increase in breastfeeding rates within the four countries of the UK between 2000 and 2005 (Bolling et al 2007). In England 78% of mothers breastfed their babies and of those 48% were still breastfeeding at 6 weeks. Factors which influence breastfeeding are social demographic characteristics, e.g. social class, age and education. The survey showed that mothers in managerial and professional occupations, first-time mothers and those aged 30 years or over were more likely to breastfeed. However, around 22% of mothers in England do not breastfeed. Factors that influence uptake include an acceptance that artificial feeding is the cultural norm, the father or partner's commitment to breastfeeding and the provision of facilities in public places where women can breastfeed their baby. Breastfeeding a baby can be difficult for some women and it is important that they receive instruction and support in how to breastfeed successfully. In some areas mothers who have breastfed act as peers to help and support new mothers to breastfeed.

You may have also found out about a number of initiatives designed to increase the prevalence of breastfeeding within your local health community including:

- breastfeeding targets set by the Department of Health
- breastfeeding policy
- media campaigns
- health education activities
- support groups
- peer support
- training for both mothers and health professionals.

> **Exercise**
> 1. If you or your partner has had children, how did you feed your baby? If you breastfed your baby reflect on why you chose to do so and who or what helped you.
> 2. If you or your partner has not had children, discuss with a relative or colleague who has breastfed their child or children. Why did they choose to do so and who or what helped them?

Despite an increase in breastfeeding rates only 25% of mothers chose to breastfeed their baby as the sole form of

the recommended maximum daily levels of alcohol and are at risk of developing alcoholic liver disease, cancer and cardiovascular disease. Significant numbers of admissions to hospitals are linked to alcohol and cost the health service in the region of £1.7bn per annum (Cabinet Office 2004).

The decline of oestrogen levels in women approaching the menopause and increased bone reabsorption can lead to osteoporosis. Whilst osteoporosis is usually seen in the older person, increasing the level of calcium and vitamin D supplements in the diet alongside medication can help to slow down the disease in those at risk of other calcium-deficient diseases in adulthood, including osteomalacia and Paget's disease. Calcium also has a role in controlling blood pressure and reducing the likelihood of kidney stones. Some foods which contain phyto-oestrogens, are thought to be especially beneficial to menopausal women (Sutcliffe 2001). These are believed to control excess oestrogens in the body and prevent excess excretion of calcium from our bones. Phyto-oestrogens are found in fruit and vegetables and the soya bean. Soya milk contains more protein than cow's milk; it is high in fatty acids and also contributes to reducing cholesterol levels. Some women prefer to use phyto-oestrogens as an alternative to hormone replacement therapy.

Older people

By 2040 a quarter of the population of the UK (16 million) is expected to be over the age of 65 (NAO 2003). The largest increase is predicted in those older people over the age of 85, who are the greatest users of public and health services, from 1.1 million to 4 million by 2051. A healthy diet in later life is essential to optimum health. With advancing age an older person becomes less active and may lead a more sedentary lifestyle than younger people. They tend to have less muscle leading to a fall in their basal metabolic rate. Older people follow the same recommended nutritional guidelines as those for adults in enough quantities to meet their energy requirements. Older people are more likely to suffer from debilitating factors associated with ill health, psychological, physiological and biological changes, social isolation, reduced income and environmental issues that impact on their ability to take an adequate diet and maintain an appropriate nutritional status (Bond 1997). They are also likely to be receiving medication that may cause side-effects (e.g. nausea, constipation), and alter their appetite, absorption of nutrients and their sense of taste, and/or influence their nutritional status. If an older person has a problem with incontinence or urine they may be reluctant to drink enough fluids, resulting in dehydration and electrolyte imbalance. (For further information on fluid and electrolyte balance see Alexander et al 2006, Ch. 20.)

A decrease in the ability to handle food and cutlery, perhaps due to arthritic hands or reduced mental capacity, difficulty with shopping and cooking, declining oral health and ill-fitting dentures, as well as loss of senses such as taste and smell, can contribute to malnutrition in the older person. Malnutrition in the older person is a frequent and serious problem (Chen et al 2001) and often goes unnoticed, mistaken instead for signs of ageing or symptoms of underlying disease (Furman 2006). Untreated it will lead to increased mortality and morbidity, and influence the length of admission to hospital (Lennard-Jones 1992). In the UK around 10–40% of all people admitted to hospital are thought to be undernourished, and one in seven people over the age of 65 are at risk of malnutrition, although this can vary according to where one lives (Elia 2003). Whilst many older people will continue to live a normal active life, others will require some form of care either in sheltered accommodation, or a residential care setting. Malnutrition in nursing or care homes often goes unrecognised and untreated despite adequate food being available (Leslie et al 2006). A Swedish study found that a high proportion of older people in long-term care were reported as having lower energy and nutrient levels than was recommended and a higher mortality rate (Elmståhl et al 1997). With a rapidly increasing elderly population the issue of malnutrition is gaining the interest of policymakers and professional bodies (DoH 2001c,d).

Exercise

1. Talk to a teenager, an adult and an older person and find out:
   - What do they eat and drink and when?
   - Are there any foods that they avoid and if so why?
   - Do they shop for their food?
   - Do they cook for themselves or others?
2. Compare what they say they eat against the Balance of Good Health plate model (see Fig. 6.1). What differences are there?
3. Monitor your diet for a week. Do you need to make any changes to your diet?

You may have discovered differences in response to your questions. A teenager living at home will more likely still be reliant on their parents to provide their food. Their lifestyle may mean that they rely on convenience or fast foods. Because they are still growing and need high energy levels, they are likely to eat bigger portions and have snacks between meals. There may be some foods that they dislike and therefore avoid.

The adult's choice and variety of food may be constrained or enabled by their socioeconomic status and access to healthy foods. The times and frequency with which they eat may depend on working patterns, and if a parent, children's routines and choice of food. Their view of what constitutes a healthy diet may be influenced by their knowledge and health beliefs and this in conjunction with their financial circumstances will have a bearing on their purchase of food. Environmental factors relating to facilities for the safe storage and cooking food may also be a factor.

The older person is more likely to suffer from health problems, have limited mobility, live alone and have a reduced income. Cooking for one person and eating alone reduces the pleasure associated with mealtimes and perhaps after a lifetime of preparing food for others they see no purpose in the preparation of food (Gustafsson & Sidenvall 2002). They may find it hard to adapt recipes for one person and choose ready-prepared meals instead. If the older person is housebound they are reliant on others to shop thus limiting their choice. They may also adapt their diet to help control health problems, for example diabetes or heart complaints. Older people with few teeth or dentures are likely to avoid fruit, raw vegetables and salads. The older person is likely to have lower activity levels and a more sedentary lifestyle than younger people and therefore may believe that they do not need to eat as much as a younger person. Dietary beliefs based on childhood and lifetime experiences, access to food, the cost and quality of the food can influence what people eat (McKie et al 2000).

> **Exercise**
> 1. List the essentials of a healthy diet.
> 2. How does the activity of eating and drinking change over a person's lifespan?

The Nursing and Midwifery Practice Development Unit (2002) in Scotland has produced a best practice statement which provides a useful tool to guide practice in the clinical area for physically frail older people.

DEPENDENCE/INDEPENDENCE

Dependence/independence in the ALs is closely related to an individual's lifespan and the other Activities of Living (Roper et al 1996, 2000). Viewed as a continuum it is central to the concept of the model (see Fig. 6.2).

Whilst in the uterus the fetus is dependent on the mother for its nutrients via the umbilical cord. After birth, babies and young children are very dependent on adults to provide them with food and drink. By the age of 18 months a baby will be making attempts to feed itself and by the age of 2 years most children are able to undertake this activity

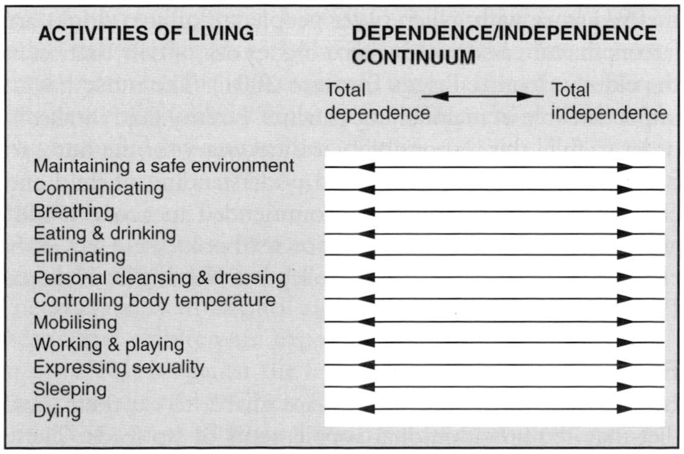

independently. However, children will continue to depend on adults to make informed choices about the purchase, provision and safe preparation of food and drink for some considerable time and those who are physically disabled or suffer from learning difficulties may be dependent on others to assist them to eat and drink for even longer. Ill health, physical or psychological disability in all ages may impact on an individual's ability to be independent in the activity of eating and drinking (Roper et al 1996).

> **Exercise**
> Consider the following brief case studies.

> **Case study 6.1**
>
> ## Temporary disability
> Mark is a 22-year-old university student. He has recently been involved in a road traffic accident and injured both his arms. He lives in student accommodation with two other students. He is reluctant to move back home as he needs to attend lectures in preparation for his exams later in the year.

> **Exercise**
> 1. How will Mark's temporary disability impact on his independence in the activity of eating and drinking?

Mark will need help from his friends and colleagues, if they are willing, to buy in and prepare the food. He may require help to feed himself and to attend to his personal hygiene, washing and dressing and elimination. He may be unable to clean his teeth, resulting in altered sense of taste and lack of appetite. However, his dependence is temporary and he should return to independence within a short timescale.

> **Case study 6.2**
>
> ## Dependence on others
> Agnes is a 48-year-old lady who suffers from multiple sclerosis. She lives with her husband, who is the main wage earner, and two teenage children. She is wheelchair dependent and needs assistance with most ALs.

> **Exercise**
> 1. In what way is Agnes dependent on others in relation to the activity of eating and drinking?
> 2. What help does she need to maintain her independence?

ACTIVITIES OF LIVING	DEPENDENCE/INDEPENDENCE CONTINUUM	
	Total dependence	Total independence
Maintaining a safe environment	←	→
Communicating	←	→
Breathing	←	→
Eating & drinking	←	→
Eliminating	←	→
Personal cleansing & dressing	←	→
Controlling body temperature	←	→
Mobilising	←	→
Working & playing	←	→
Expressing sexuality	←	→
Sleeping	←	→
Dying	←	→

Fig. 6.2 Dependence/independence continuum (from Roper et al 1996, with permission).

Multiple sclerosis is a chronic degenerative disease and its effects vary from person to person. Recurring relapses will increase Agnes's dependency on others for assistance with

pressure or a tachycardia, or be in a state of shock. In cases of mild dehydration it may be possible to replace fluids orally but in more severe cases intravenous fluids may be needed. The administration and monitoring of intravenous fluids is an important task that the nurse working in acute care will undertake regularly. It is important that the nurse has a firm understanding of the physiology of fluid replacement when administering and monitoring fluid intake and output and managing complex fluid regimes (Gobbi et al 2006). Safe administration of intravenous fluids also requires knowledge of professional and legal responsibilities, an understanding of the fluids being administered and the reasons why they are being administered (Hand 2001).

Exercise

1. Access a physiology textbook and update your knowledge of fluid and electrolyte balance.
2. What skills and knowledge do you need to be a safe and competent practitioner when administering an intravenous infusion to a patient?
3. If you are a student nurse on a clinical placement find out how fluid balance is documented.
4. Are there any factors that limit the accuracy of this process?
5. Include these responses in your development plan and arrange to discuss these with your mentor and personal tutor.

Nutrients   A person needs a constant supply of nutrients to maintain health. Nutrients fall into two main categories.

Macronutrients

- *Carbohydrates* are the main source of heat and energy for the body and should supply the majority of calories needed. There are three main groups of carbohydrates: sugars, starches and complex polysaccharides. These can be found in bread, potatoes, cereals, fruit and vegetables. During digestion carbohydrates are broken down into glucose before being absorbed.
- *Protein* is required for repair and growth. Whilst protein is found in most foods, the extent to which the body can absorb proteins, in the form of amino acids, from some foods differs considerably. Protein from animal products, for example meat, fish and eggs, and from legumes, has a higher absorption rate than that of plants or cereals.
- *Fats* also provide a source of energy and insulation. Fat is an essential component of the body composition and of the diet but taken in excess it can contribute to a number of health problems including obesity. Saturated fats found in foods from animals may contribute to an increase in blood cholesterol levels and likelihood of coronary heart disease. However, not all fats are unhealthy; polyunsaturated fatty acids, such as omega-3 fatty acids found in oily fish, have been shown to reduce the risk of coronary thrombosis.

Micronutrients

- *Vitamins* are found in fruit and vegetables, dairy products and meat and oily fish. There are two main types of vitamins, fat-soluble (A, D, E, K) which we can store in our body and water-soluble (B, C) which we need to get from our daily food but are easily lost. A deficiency in one or more of the vitamins may result in specific diseases such as scurvy (vitamin C). Five portions of fruit and vegetables per day are recommended.
- *Minerals* are found in many different foods and are essential for health. They have many different roles including hormonal, enzymatic, transportation of molecules and electrolyte balance. A major trace element, iron, is necessary for the transportation of haemoglobin around the body, whereas sodium, a mineral, is essential in maintaining the electrolyte balance within the cells. Other minerals include calcium, phosphorus, potassium, chlorine, magnesium and sulphur.

For a more comprehensive description of both these groups of nutrients and to gain a greater understanding of their function in the body and risks associated with deficiency refer to a physiology textbook such as Kindlen (2003) or Montague et al (2005).

Sociocultural factors

The AL of eating and drinking extends to more than just providing nutrients for the body, it forms an important part of our personal, religious, sociocultural and ethical aspects of living (Roper et al 1996, 2000). In many cultures eating and drinking are given a great deal of attention and provide much pleasure. For example, Henley & Schott (1999, p. 104) state that:

> 66 *Food is not simply a matter of nutrition; it often has deep personal significance, symbolising, for example, security, love, moral and religious values and identity.* 99

Exercise

1. Think about your own mealtimes.
2. Do you eat together as a family or group?
3. Do you observe any rituals?
4. Discuss your observations with a colleague. Are there any differences or similarities in eating behaviours and customs?

Some families make a point of sitting down at a table as a family for a meal at least once a day, others may never eat at a table. Others may only eat as a family at special occasions, family birthdays or holidays and have special foods. In some cases adults may eat separately from the children. Some people may pray before a meal. Other rituals may be considered to be polite or respectful, like waiting until everyone has sat down and has been served food before eating. Some cultures and religions observe different rituals.

In some family structures the male and female roles are clearly distinguished. For example in the Jewish orthodox faith the mother is responsible for the home and children and the father for religious education. Only food that is kosher (permitted by the Torah) is allowed and dairy products are not eaten at the same time or following a meal containing meat unless several hours have elapsed (Collins 2002). On the Sabbath (Saturday) Jewish families celebrate with a special family supper and lighting of candles. There are many religious groups that follow dietary restrictions and observe rituals. There are also strong beliefs in some cultures about what one should eat to keep healthy and what to avoid.

Chan (1995) discusses the influence of the Chinese philosophy of yin and yang on dietary beliefs and customs. The Chinese believe that harmony and health can only exist when these two competing forces are balanced. Yin is linked to cold energy and to infections, gastric upsets and anxiety. Foods that are said to be yin are vegetables, milk, water and dairy products. Yang, on the other hand, is related to hot energy and dehydration, fever and irritability; these are foods such are red meat, alcohol, wheat and fatty foods. Dietary remedies are an important part of the Chinese culture and relatives may bring in food and herbal remedies to redress the balance of yin and yang.

Not all people use a knife and fork to eat a meal. The Chinese use chopsticks, and people living in South Asia and Muslim countries use only their right hand and often their fingers to eat their food. Their left hand is reserved for washing and using the lavatory (Henley & Schott 1999, Akhtar 2002).

Fasting from food and drink is expected in some religions. Fasting is one of the five pillars of Islam and it teaches Muslims self-discipline and self-restraint and reminds Muslims of those in poverty and hunger. During the month of Ramadan Muslims will avoid food and drink from sunrise to sunset. Strict Buddhists may decline food after midday (Northcot 2002).

Exercise
1. From the following list of different religious cultures choose one or two different to your own and find out what dietary restrictions and rituals are observed.
   - Chinese community
   - Islam
   - Hinduism
   - Sikhism
   - Christianity.
2. Visit the catering department in a hospital and find out about the diets available for these groups of people.

When visiting the sick, relatives and carers will often bring food. Taking time to provide food for a person who is ill is a sign of caring or love (Henley & Schott 1999). If a patient is unable to eat or drink this can be very stressful for the relatives or carers. The wish to preserve life at all costs is, in some cultures, very intense. Some people will insist on artificial feeding, even in patients in the final stages of death. They may see the reluctance of medical and nursing staff to feed a patient artificially as failing in their duty of care. A decision to commence artificial feeding is a clinical decision with of course the informed consent of the patient. The British Medical Association's guidance for decision-making *Withholding and Withdrawing Life* recognises legal and ethical dilemmas and the emotional and psychological burden on staff involved with withdrawing or withholding treatment (BMA 1999). Every mentally competent adult has the right to refuse treatment; there are, however, situations and circumstances where a patient is unable to consent or refuse treatment, for example mental incapacity, illness or unconsciousness. In these circumstances and in the absence of an advanced directive the law permits doctors to treat patients under the principle of necessity. The law, however, requires the approval of the court to discontinue artificial feeding for patients in a persistent vegetative state (Lennard-Jones 2000). Nurses will need to be aware of the implications of the Mental Capacity Act 2005 and their legal responsibilities with regard to commencing and withdrawing artificial feeding, should a patient be incapacitated.

Exercise
1. Explore your views of the legal and ethical implications of commencing and withdrawing artificial feeding in critically ill patients with a group of your peers.
2. Compare your views with the NMC Code of Professional Conduct and Ethics (NMC 2007).
3. What is meant by informed consent?
4. Discuss this activity with your tutor and mentor.

Environmental factors

Environmental factors have an important role to play in the AL of eating and drinking. The quality and availability of food and water depends on a stable and safe environment. Many people in the world depend on local produce and on access to good soil and amenable weather conditions (Roper et al 1996). Climate changes can mean the difference between a good harvest and starvation for many thousands of people in some countries. The World Health Organization website (www.who.int) has up-to-date information on the number of people affected by famine in the world. In countries with access to good road and rail networks, people have access to a wide variety of foods, which are imported to and exported from many different parts of the world. Easier access to package holidays and foreign travel has also increased the demand for different foods.

Access to a safe supply of drinking water is a fundamental health requirement. Approximately 20% of the world's population lack access to safe drinking water. Contamination of the water supplies is of grave concern to the more affluent countries. Within the UK the Department for Environment, Food and Rural Affairs is responsible for all aspects of water policy, supply and research.

> **Exercise**
> 1. Access the Department for Environment, Food and Rural Affairs website (www.defra.gov.uk). Increase your knowledge about maintaining safe water supplies.

Where, when and with whom we eat and drink can determine how we enjoy our food. An environment that promotes a relaxing atmosphere contributes to both the physiological and psychological enjoyment of eating and drinking. If we are rushed we are less likely to enjoy our food.

> **Exercise**
> 1. Think about a meal you have enjoyed in the restaurant with friends or family.
> 2. Now think about a meal you have taken whilst at work or in a snack bar.
> 3. Did the environments differ and how did they contribute to your enjoyment?

You may have enjoyed the ambience of the restaurant, being able to choose your food from a menu and being served your food by others. The comfort of the restaurant and company of others may have added to your enjoyment of your meal. However, if the restaurant was dirty, noisy or the service slow and the food poor quality then this may have affected your enjoyment of your meal. On the other hand, you may have found that the meal at work was rushed because of lack of time and you did not have time to enjoy your food and the choice of food on offer may have been limited and of poor quality. Once again this may not always be the case and a chance to sit down with colleagues and enjoy a meal may prove an enjoyable experience. Ensuring a pleasant environment and patient experience at mealtimes is an important role of the nurse.

> **Exercise**
> 1. If you are a student nurse on a clinical placement, observe the patient environment at mealtimes.
> 2. Speak to patients and ask them how they enjoyed their meal.
> 3. How did the environment contribute to the patient's experience?
> 4. Compare this to your own experiences.
> 5. Are there any changes you would make to improve the patient's experience?

Food hygiene and the provision of a safe and clean environment for food storage, preparation and cooking are essential to health and wellbeing. Hospitals, restaurants, cafes, bars, in fact anywhere food is sold, prepared, cooked and served to the public are required to comply with stringent standards to ensure the general public is not put at risk.

> **Exercise**
> 1. Increase your knowledge about food hygiene and food safety.
> 2. Access the Food Standards website (www.foodstandards.gov.uk).
> 3. Look in your own refrigerator. How do you store your foods?
> 4. Find out about any guidelines within the clinical area regarding the serving of food and storage of food within the clinical area.

You will have found out about the importance of strict handwashing and the separation of cooked meats from uncooked meats both within the refrigerator and in retail outlets, ensuring foods are cooked thoroughly and at the correct temperature, and ensuring food is not used after its sell-by date.

Psychological factors

As Roper et al (1996) point out, individuals require a certain level of intelligence to be able to select, prepare and cook a healthy diet. They need to understand the role of the major nutrients and to be able to prepare foods safely.

The amount of food one eats depends on a number of factors, not only on the degree of hunger but also on appetite and the function of the hypothalamus. Appetite can be affected by emotional state, mood and behaviour, for example overeating or undereating due to stress or loss of self-esteem.

> **Exercise**
> Think about a time when you have felt stressed. This may have been before an examination or interview for a new job.
>
> 1. How did you feel?
> 2. Did you use food to help you cope with the stress?
> 3. If so what foods did you eat?
> 4. Did you increase your intake of alcohol?

Some people when stressed might eat more cakes, sweets and chocolates than when less stressed. Research has shown that some people crave carbohydrates when depressed (Rinomhota & Rollins 2001).

Eating disorders

People who experience symptoms of depression are likely to report loss of appetite and eating disorders. A number of well-known people have admitted to suffering from eating disorders. Most notably Princess Diana admitted that she had suffered from bulimia, as did the actors Jane Fonda and Joan Rivers.

Eating disorders, whilst usually associated with young women, can affect both men and women of any age and background (Cremin & Halek 1997). Anorexia nervosa usually presents during adolescence and can persist throughout life. Individuals present with severe loss of weight due to strict dieting, they are preoccupied with their weight and have a distorted image of their body. Bulimia, on the other hand, usually manifests itself in later life. Those who suffer bulimia crave food and binge on food before vomiting the food up. They are reluctant to seek help as they see this as giving up the control they have over their food intake. Depression and suicidal thoughts and behaviours are not uncommon and require psychological treatment.

Obesity

Within the Western culture a slim body shape is preferred. People who are overweight are often stigmatised and suffer discrimination. If intake of food exceeds activity levels over a period of time then there is a risk that this will result in weight gain. Obesity is defined as where someone puts on weight to the point that it damages health. In the UK the number of people who are obese or overweight continues to grow. It is estimated that by 2010, 12 million adults and 1 million children will be obese (NICE 2006a).

The reasons for this are believed to be a gradually more sedentary lifestyle, a change in eating patterns and genetic factors.

In 1998, the direct costs of obesity in England were £2.6 billion. This will increase to £3.6 billion in 2010 if the prevalence continues to rise at the present rate (NAO 2001). Obesity increases the risk of many common diseases (see Fig. 6.10 and Box 6.6) and is an important public health problem. Specifically there is a strong association between obesity and heart failure as shown in the Framington Heart Study (Kenchaiach et al 2002).

The National Service Framework for Coronary Heart Disease (DoH 2001a) and Diabetes (DoH 2001b) have highlighted the need for health promotion, promotion of a healthy diet and weight reduction. A body mass index of $>30\,kg/m^2$ increases the risk of cardiovascular disease. Any approach to reducing weight needs to induce a negative energy balance, by reducing calorie intake and/or increasing energy expenditure. Whilst there are several diets and weight-loss products on the market there is no evidence to demonstrate their effectiveness and indeed some products may be deficient in essential nutrients. Dietary and behavioural interventions combined with exercise have been found to be successful for individuals but have had no impact on reducing the rise in obesity (NICE 2006b). The National Institute for Health and Clinical Excellence have produced guidelines which recognise the need for agencies to work together to address the problem of obesity.

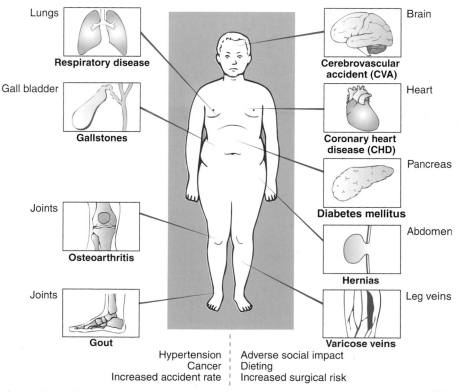

Fig. 6.10 The effects of obesity on the body (from Alexander et al 2000).

| Box 6.6 | Impact of being overweight on the body |

Being overweight can affect most parts of the body:

- coronary heart disease
- breathlessness
- cancer
- osteoarthritis
- back pain
- sleep difficulties
- infertility
- sweating
- difficulties in walking
- low self-esteem, poor body image.

Adapted from Brooker & Nichol (2003).

Weight alone is not an accurate indicator of whether a person is over- or underweight. The body mass index (BMI) is an indicator and estimation of total body fat (see Box 6.7). However, this is a general guide as very muscular people may have a high BMI without being overweight and some people may be underweight without being thin.

Exercise

1. Using the calculations outlined in Box 6.7 calculate your BMI.

The shape of a person's body is also an important indicator of risk of heart disease and diabetes. A person who carries a lot of weight around the middle of his or her body ('apple shaped') has a greater health risk than someone who is 'pear shaped' (see Box 6.6 for impact of being overweight). Waist measurement is an indicator of the risk of coronary heart disease and should be taken into account along with BMI and any accompanying risk factors (NICE 2006a).

Politicoeconomic factors

Malnutrition is a global problem and contributes to nearly 5.25 million deaths each year. The World Health Organization has

| Box 6.7 | Body mass index |

The BMI is calculated by dividing a person's weight (in kilograms) by the square of their height (in metres). For example, someone with a body weight of 57 kg and a height of 1.62 m has a BMI of $57/1.62^2 = 22.3\,\text{kg/m}^2$. The ideal range is 18.5–24.9; 25–29 indicates overweight; 30.0–34.9 is obese (class 1) and 35.0–39.9 obese (class 2) and greater than 40 is obese (class 3).
Care should be take when using BMI as a predictor of risk in a very old person (British Dietetic Association 2003).

From Green & Jackson (2006).

sought the help of all sectors of society to help tackle malnutrition in infants and young children, which is causing grave concern. Global communications bring pictures of the crop failures in Africa into our homes. These serve to remind us of the plight and fight for human survival of these people who are undernourished and live in extreme poverty. Roper et al (1996) highlight the complex reasons for the misdistribution of food throughout the world including poor soil and crop rotation, lack of irrigation, social unrest, natural disasters, and lack of funding, poor education and food regulation.

Within the UK, the NHS Improvement Plan (DoH 2004a) set out the government's plans to focus on health and wellbeing, not just illness. From 2005 the performance of the NHS and independent healthcare organisations has been monitored by the Healthcare Commission (www.healthcarecommission.org.uk) to ensure they meet the requirements of the National Service Frameworks and national plans with particular regard to reducing obesity through action on nutrition. The Government's White Paper *Choosing Health: Making Healthy Choices Easier* (DoH 2004b) sets out principles for supporting the public to make healthier and informed choices with regard to reducing obesity and improving health. The need to ensure a healthy diet by working in partnership with business, voluntary agencies, communities, media, local government and faith organisations, is a core theme flowing throughout the document.

There are also economic reasons why it is important that people eat a healthy diet. Coronary heart disease is the main cause of premature death in the UK and the most costly disease in the UK (www.bhf.org.uk). The cost of heart disease, including the cost of informal care, is in the region of £7 billion including around £3 billion in lost earnings to the economy, and £1.73 billion for the NHS (Liu et al 2002). The cost of treating patients with malnutrition is higher than in other patients as they require more tests and take longer to recover, resulting in a longer stay in hospital (Royal College of Physicians 2002).

Exercise

1. Visit the Department of Health and Health Development Agency websites (www.dh.gov.uk and www.hda.nhs.uk) and update yourself on recent developments and progress on health policy strategies.
2. Find out about initiatives and interventions aimed at encouraging people to adopt a healthier diet and lifestyle.

You may have found out that the UK government is working with industry to increase the provision of fruit and vegetables by encouraging the establishment of food cooperatives that allow people to increase the availability of fresh fruit and vegetables at affordable prices. Other interventions may be aimed at increasing the knowledge of a healthy diet within schools, for example the 'Cooking for Kids' initiative, which reinforces food hygiene and nutrition. Initiatives such as breakfast clubs are aimed at encouraging children to have a breakfast and those from low-income families to have at least one nutritious meal a day. Food suppliers, supermarkets and retailers also support healthy eating campaigns by providing nutritional information on foods and food packaging.

On an individual basis there are resource implications in ensuring a healthy diet, including enough money to buy or grow food, access to the right sort of food, access to food storage facilities, cooking utensils and equipment, and access to health and social services support if necessary.

Malnutrition in hospital

Brooker (2005) defines malnutrition as 'the state of being poorly nourished' resulting from inadequate intake of nutrients either from malabsorption, disease or obesity. Protein-energy malnutrition results from an inadequate intake of protein associated with anorexia, starvation, and is also seen in hospital patients and older people in care homes. The incidence of malnutrition in older people is high and often goes unnoticed (Holmes 2006). The seminal King's Fund Centre report by Lennard-Jones (1992) raised awareness of the nutritional status of patients admitted to hospital as a consequence of illness. The report indicated that as many as half of certain patient groups (surgical and medical) were malnourished on admission to hospital and during prolonged hospital stay, malnutrition often becomes worse or develops for the first time (Table 6.2).

The report recommended a multidisciplinary team approach to recognising and dealing with malnutrition and acknowledged the nurse's role as essential within that team. McWhirter & Pennington (1994) undertook a prospective study of the nutritional status of patients admitted to a Scottish hospital and found that 40% (200) of patients were undernourished and had a body mass index of less than 20; of these, only 96 patients had any information on nutrition documented in their case notes. This problem is not unique to the UK. Kowanko et al (2001) undertook a similar study in Australia and found that the nutritional intake of many patients was poor. Lennard-Jones et al (1995) found that most nurses and doctors in 70 hospitals failed to recognise the importance of asking patients questions about nutrition and height and weight. Attempting to raise awareness of the importance of assessing nutritional needs, Reilly et al (1995) developed a simple assessment tool to be used on admission to encourage staff to assess nutritional needs.

As a result of the recommendations of the King's Fund report (Lennard-Jones 1992), the British Association for Parenteral and Enteral Nutrition (BAPEN) was formed. BAPEN subsequently published two reports: the first 'Organisation of Nutritional Support in Hospitals' (Silk 1994) recommended that nutrition support teams responsible for organising the diagnosis and treatment should be established; the second report set standards of clinical practice in nutritional support (Sizer 1996). Both reports highlighted the general lack of awareness of both medical and nursing staff of nutrition and the importance of nutritional assessment. A number of different assessment or

Table 6.2 Malnutrition

Causes	Effects
Causes	**Effects**
• Reduced appetite	• Impaired growth and development of children
• Difficulties with eating	• Weight loss
• Nausea and vomiting	• Loss of muscle strength
• Depresssion/anxiety	• Delayed wound healing
• Environment	• Increased risk of pressure ulcer development
• Pain	• Impaired immune response leading to increased risk of infection
• Starving for tests	• Impaired psychological wellbeing
• Difficulties with shopping and cooking	• Depression of appetite
• Side-effects of medication	• Prolonged recovery and rehabilitation
Increased Nutritional Requirements	• Increased morbidity and mortality
• Liver disease	• Increased dependence
• Renal disease	
• Respiratory disease	
• Abdominal losses (e.g. through stoma)	
• Major surgery/trauma	
• Increase in involuntary movements secondary to neurological condition	
Impaired Ability to Utilise, Absorb Metabolic Nutrients	
• Crohn's disease	
• Untreated coeliac disease	
• Untreated diabetes	
• Laxative abuse	

Lennard-Jones (1992).

screening tools have been developed for use in hospital or community settings to guide care planning. However, many have not been subject to evaluation and may not demonstrate reliability, validity or sensitivity and specificity (Green & Watson 2006). The British Association for Parenteral and Enteral Nutrition (BAPEN) have published a Malnutrition Screening Tool (MUST) that has been validated for use in adults in a range of care settings both in hospital and community. Obtaining a dietary history and assessing dietary intake, undertaking a physical examination, measuring body weight and height, and biochemical tests are all important ways of assessing a patient's nutritional status (McLaren & Green 1998).

In response to a report by the Association of Community Health Councils (1997) and concern about the dietary care in hospitals in the UK, the Department of Health through the Chief Nursing Officer supported the development of a resource pack 'Eating Matters' (Bond 1997). The pack was designed to assist nurses and organisations to improve the nutritional needs of patients.

The UK government through the NHS Plan (DoH 2000) sought to redress the unacceptable variations in standards of catering and nutrition in hospitals across the country. Initiatives such as the Department of Health 'Better Food for Hospitals' scheme have resulted in nurses, modern matrons, dietitians, hospital managers and catering staff looking at ways in which the patient's experience of food could be improved by introducing new menus and ward housekeepers or ward hostesses, and ensuring that patients are not disturbed during mealtimes by closing wards and refraining from consultant ward rounds. Sadly it would still appear that nutrition continues to receive less priority than other nursing activities and is an international concern (Xia & McCutcheon 2006, Watson 2006).

The Essence of Care patient-focused benchmarks for clinical practice include a toolkit for practitioners (DoH 2003b). Food and nutrition is one of nine essential aspects of care. Benchmarking is seen as a process through which best practice is identified and continuous improvement pursued through comparison and sharing. Nutrition and hydration are important aspects of nursing care and are just as important as monitoring vital signs. Assessing and meeting the needs of patients at risk is a fundamental part of a nursing assessment and planning care to ensure that 'patients get the right sort of food and drink, in the right place at the right time, with the right

help' (Mullally 2000, p.1). Nurses are well placed to identify poor nutritional status of patients. However, they do not work in isolation and meeting the nutritional needs of patients requires a multidisciplinary approach.

During your allocation you may have met with the following health care professionals and providers:

- *Ward or community nurse* – who has overall responsibility for ensuring that the patient's nutrition and hydration needs are identified, that there is a plan of care designed to meet individual needs and subject to ongoing evaluation. The nurse will work in collaboration with other health care professionals and coordinate their input.
- *Health care assistant or home care worker* – who is responsible for ensuring that patients receive the right food at the right time and receive any assistance that they need. Some hospitals may have introduced ward housekeepers whose role is to support ward staff by serving meals and preparing snacks.
- *Occupational therapist* – who will assess the patient's ability to feed themselves and provide specialised equipment where necessary.
- *Dietitian* - who will assess nutritional status, calculate dietary requirements, monitor patients on nutritional support and provide specialist dietary advice and support to patients.
- *Catering manager or community meals provider* – who is responsible for the catering arrangements, menus and nutritional content of meals.
- *Doctor* – who has overall responsibility for the nutritional regimes and the suitable route of nutritional support.
- *Pharmacist* – who will supply intravenous foods and advise on how drug regimes may impact on appetite, nutrition, parenteral, enteral and intravenous regimes.
- *Gastroenterologist* – who is increasingly becoming involved in artificial nutrition support.
- *Chemical pathologist* – who will monitor the biochemical activity.
- *Microbiologist and infection control nurse* – who together will provide support and monitoring of possible catheter-related sepsis.
- *Speech and language therapist* – who will assess the patient's muscular control and swallowing reflex and work with patients to improve swallowing.
- *Social worker* – who will advise on eligibility for financial and community care support, for example meals on wheels, luncheon clubs, home care etc.

SUMMARY POINTS

1. Food and water are essential for our survival.
2. Access to sufficient food and water for survival, however, is affected by many different politicoeconomic as well as sociocultural factors.
3. What we eat and drink is very much affected by the culture we live in as well as our health status, e.g. whether we are ill or not.

Exercise

1. If you are a student nurse on a clinical placement in a hospital or in primary care find out which health professionals have a role in ensuring that patients' nutritional and hydration needs are met.
2. Arrange to meet with one or two of these professionals and find out more about their role and how you can refer for specialist advice and support.
3. How might a patient's care in the hospital influence their care in primary care and vice versa? What information needs to be shared between the two organisations?

THE MODEL FOR NURSING

INTRODUCTION

Within this chapter, in addition to the following main case study, you will be encouraged to transfer your understanding of eating and drinking to other individual patients and consider its relationship to other ALs. Using the model for nursing you will consider what information you would obtain from a main case scenario, identify patient problems and develop a plan of care. You may choose to record the information on the Patient Assessment Sheets provided in Appendix 3.

Assessing individual needs and problems

If patients' expectations are to be understood and their problems (whether actual or potential) with this AL are to be addressed then an assessment must be undertaken. Assessment involves the following three phases:

- collecting information from the patient and nursing history
- interpreting the information collected
- identifying the patient's actual and potential health problems.

However, if the nurse is to undertake a comprehensive and holistic nursing history it is essential that all the Activities of Living as seen in Chapter 1 are taken into account. This is not only undertaken at the beginning of the patient's episode of care or admission to hospital but is an ongoing and dynamic process. Before assessing the AL of eating and drinking in ill health the nurse must first of all understand and have knowledge of the AL of eating and drinking in health.

Assessing the individual

Assessment is the cornerstone on which the patient's care is planned, implemented and evaluated. In most cases the nurse undertakes an initial nursing assessment within the first few hours of admission to hospital by gathering information that informs the nursing assessment without overburdening the patient and duplicating assessments. However, we must remember that nursing assessment is continuous and patients must be reassessed as their condition changes or in response to the outcome of evaluation.

Using the model of living as a framework to collect information on the patient's normal habits and routines and any factors that might cause the activity to be altered is the first step in applying the Roper et al (1996, 2000) model of nursing in practice. Box 6.8 provides a summary of the key factors, which you may consider in assessing the activity of eating and drinking.

When assessing the patient you will need to use interviewing, observational and listening skills (see Chapter 4). In addition you will also need to understand the biological, sociological, psychological and environmental issues associated with eating and drinking. Poor or incomplete assessment subsequently leads to poor care planning and

| Box 6.8 | Assessment framework for the activity of eating and drinking |

Lifespan
- Consider the effect of age on the activity of eating and drinking.

Dependence/independence
- Dependence is linked to lifespan and age, e.g. childhood/old age.
- Dependence is linked to specific needs, e.g. disability, communication, certain foods and drink.
- Ill health affects the dependence/independence balance, e.g. dehydration, neurological problems.

Factors affecting eating and drinking
Biological
- Ingestion
- Vomiting
- Digestion
- Absorption
- Neurological impairment
- Metabolism
- Nutrients
- Exercise
- Medication.

Psychological
- Attitudes to eating and drinking, health behaviour and beliefs
- Intellectual capacity
- Emotional state
- Cognitive state
- Social class
- Body image.

Sociocultural
- Recognition of individual attitudes, beliefs and values
- Sociocultural similarities/differences
- Religion.

Environmental
- Access to food and drink
- Food storage and food hygiene
- Cooking facilities
- Environment.

Politicoeconomic
- Finance
- Access to feeding aids
- Access to health and social services support.

implementation of the care plan (Sutcliffe 1990). The care plan should identify the nursing interventions required to meet patient needs related to eating and drinking. These interventions may include promoting health, preventing ill health, providing nutritional support, helping patients to eat and drink and maintaining a safe environment.

Exercise

1. Consider the activities in Box 6.9 and identify which skills you have already and the ones you need to develop when undertaking an assessment of eating and drinking.

A thorough patient assessment is the basis on which a relevant and realistic individualised nursing care plan is founded. The nursing care plan should aim to:

- solve actual problems
- prevent potential problems becoming actual problems
- prevent solved problems from recurring
- alleviate problems which cannot be solved
- help the person cope with temporary or permanent altered states
- provide information to others to enable the delivery of individualised care
- provide information on the effectiveness of nursing care through evaluation.

PATIENT ASSESSMENT

When assessing the Activities of Living you may consider the following questions which can be adapted to fit the nursing context either within primary care or in hospital.

Lifespan

- How old is the person?
- Do they have a life history of health problems?
- Is there anything in their life history that may affect the way in which they view their present health problems?

Box 6.9	Skills and behaviours necessary for undertaking assessment

Interviewing
- Asking open and closed questions relevant to the health status of the patient
- Use of appropriate language
- Determining the priority of the questions to be asked
- Giving information, relating and checking understanding
- Involving relatives and carers.

Observation
- Verbal and nonverbal responses
- Body language
- Appearance
- Vital signs
- Height and weight
- Skin condition
- Oral health and dentures
- Dexterity
- Swallowing reflex
- Anxiety and stress.

Listening
- Verbal and nonverbal cues
- Checking out understanding and giving explanation.

Dependence/independence

- Has the individual experienced any difficulties in relation to independent living?
- Are they able to prepare food and drink or are they dependent on others?
- Are they able to shop for food and drink or are they dependent on others?
- Will they experience difficulties in the future as a result of their current health problems?
- Are they dependent on particular types of substances, food or drink?
- Do they have any support in the community to enable them to maintain their independence?

Factors affecting health
Biological

- What specific health problem are they suffering from?
- What do they understand about their present health status?
- Are there any disabilities?
- What is their BMI?
- What is their waist measurement?
- Is there evidence of loss of weight recently?
- Are there any allergies to food and/or drink?
- What is their nutritional status? You may choose to use one of the recognised nutritional assessment tools to assess their nutritional status as discussed previously in this chapter.
- Is there any pain?
- Is there any vomiting?
- What medication do they take?

Psychological

- Is there any intellectual deficit?
- What effect is their health problem having on their emotional wellbeing?
- Are there any emotional problems?
- Is the patient suffering from stress?
- Are there any memory problems?
- What is their motivation?

Socioeconomic

- Are there any specific spiritual or religious practices or needs?
- Do they have any religious or cultural beliefs about food and diet?
- What support do they have in the home and from whom?
- Do they have any contact with others?
- Is there any indication of poverty or lack of financial support?

Environmental

- What type of housing does the individual live in?
- What facilities are there for the storage and preparation of food and are these suitable and safe?

- Does the individual have any environmental needs which affect nutritional care?
- Are they exposed to any environmental hazards or risks of infection?

Politicoeconomic

- What resources could be required to help the individual manage their health problems in hospital or in the home?
- Is the patient aware of the resources or benefits that are available?
- Are there any financial constraints compromising recovery or maintenance?
- What effect is this having on their nutritional status?

Whilst helping patients maintain an adequate nutritional intake is everyone's responsibility, as a nurse you will have the most contact with patients. Working in partnership with other health professionals, you are in a unique position to ensure that that patient's nutritional needs are met and not compromised (Bond 1997, Norton 1996, Roper et al 1996, Wood & Creamer 1996).

Case study 6.3

Admission to hospital

Mavis, an 83-year-old woman, is admitted to your ward after being found on the floor at home by a neighbour. She has a history of arthritis and hypertension. She lives alone in her own home. Her husband died 4 years ago and she has a son and a daughter and three grandchildren. Her daughter lives 50 miles away and visits at weekends. Until recently she has been fiercely independent and refused any form of support other than help with her cleaning and assistance with shopping from her son. On admission or visiting she is dehydrated and disorientated and her son has noticed that she has lost weight recently.

Exercise

1. Using your knowledge of the Roper et al model for nursing and the questions listed on this and the previous page, reflect on how you will include these in your assessment of the patient in Case study 6.3.

Using the Roper et al (1996) model for nursing, you may have decided to devise a number of questions that will enable you to identify the patient's normal habits and routines in relation to the ALs, dependency, and identify actual and potential problems associated with the AL of eating and drinking and how this might impact on the other ALs. Even if the patient is able to communicate effectively, it is usually helpful with the permission of the patient to make arrangements to speak to the patient's relatives or carers to elicit any extra information and opinions.

Having considered your questions and likely responses check these out against the following.

Lifespan

In later life nutritional status is influenced by physiological changes as a result of normal ageing, disease, chronic disorders and reduced mobility. Mavis, an 83-year-old widow, may not fully understand the importance of nutrition in later life. Her medical records reveal that she has a history of osteoarthritis in her knees and hip and hypertension. Osteoarthritis is more likely to occur in older women and is a noninflammatory degenerative condition which affects the hyaline cartilage of the synovial joints (Lucas 2006).

Physically frail older patients are more likely to have problems associated with eating and drinking and suffer from malnutrition. This should alert you to the importance of ensuring adequate nutrition whilst in hospital and also when she returns home, thus highlighting the nurse's role and responsibility for health education.

Dependence/independence

Mavis has been fiercely independent and has refused any help other than help from her son with shopping and her neighbour's help to do the cleaning. You may have questioned Mavis about how she manages to do the cooking, who helps her with the cooking and whether there are there any constraints. You will need to consider how her chronic health problems, in particular her osteoarthritis, is affecting her independence. The answers to these questions will provide information on Mavis's normal functioning. Admission to hospital and a change in health status will impact on Mavis's current level of dependence/independence. Therefore you will need to assess any change from the normal functioning.

An older person can find admission to a hospital ward disorientating. You will need to take account of whether the patient has been in hospital before and how they coped. You will need to assess what the impact of hospital admission will have on Mavis's independence and if necessary what help she will need to regain her independence. Taking account of her current situation, is she able to eat by herself? Does she need help to feed and if so what help does she need? How will she respond to changes to her independence as a result of her admission?

You will have also considered the impact of dehydration and that Mavis will be dependent on the medical and nursing staff to restore hydration and rectify her electrolyte balance by intravenous fluid replacement.

Exercise

1. Reflect back on your discussions with your mentor and tutor following the previous exercise.
2. Is there anything else you need to know, see and do in relation to meeting the hydration needs of patients?

Biological

It is important to understand Mavis's normal health situation. When was she diagnosed with osteoarthritis and hypertension and how did this impact on her ALs? You would want to understand what Mavis could remember about the incident and any symptoms or events leading up to her fall. You would need to know if she had any physical difficulties or disabilities, including any sensory loss (sight, hearing, smell, taste) or pain. Whilst people don't normally feel ill with osteoarthritis they are likely to suffer dull nagging pain or periods of acute pain, which will require medication for pain relief. You will need to know if the presence of pain has had any effect on Mavis's appetite.

You would want to understand how her raised blood pressure is affecting her health status. Hypertension can be defined as primary, where no cause is found, or secondary, due to underlying medical conditions for example renal disease. If the rise in blood pressure is only moderate and occurs over a long period of time it is said to be mild, whereas a sudden increase in blood pressure is referred to as malignant (Webster & Thompson 2006). A number of dietary factors are associated with hypertension, including obesity, sodium intake and alcohol, and so you would need to take these factors into account when assessing Mavis's normal Activities of Living.

To understand Mavis's current health status you would monitor her vital signs and in discussion with medical staff determine the frequency of future monitoring. You would record her temperature, pulse, respiration and blood pressure and observe for any signs of infection. Mavis's son thinks she has lost weight over the last 6 months. You should also check for any altered skin integrity particularly for bruising, dry skin or presence of petechiae and any signs of fatigue and lethargy (Holmes 2006). A record of her weight and height should be made and her BMI calculated (see Box 6.7). A patient with a BMI of less than 19 is said to be 'at risk' and associated with higher mortality (Bond 1997). You should assess for any signs of weight loss. It is important to record this in her medical and nursing notes against which any future weight gain or loss can be monitored.

Observation of Mavis's physical condition will also aid your assessment in relation to the activity of eating and drinking. You would want to observe whether there is evidence of recent loss of weight. Do her clothes or rings look too big? Is there any evidence of oedema in her lower limbs? Can she grip your hands? Is there any evidence of loss of muscle power?

You will need to know what medication Mavis is taking and if this has the potential to affect her appetite, for example non-steroidal anti-inflammatory medication and some cardiovascular medicines are associated with gastrointestinal side-effects. You should refer to the British National Formulary for further information or seek advice from the ward or local pharmacist.

Psychological

As psychological factors can affect people's attitude to food and drink, you would need to understand Mavis's attitude towards her diet and if this has changed recently. Your questions and observations would be aimed at establishing her understanding and knowledge of her current situation. Does she give any indication that she might be suffering from depression? Does she understand the importance of a healthy diet? Has she any problems with her memory? Does she have any abnormal attitudes about her weight or body image?

Sociocultural

We know that Mavis was bereaved 4 years ago and that her son and a neighbour support her. Her daughter lives some 50 miles away and visits whenever she can. You would need to determine her normal social situation and how her current health problems impact, or have the potential to impact, on this. You might have considered the following:

- What social contacts and support does she have?
- Does she get out of the house?
- Does she meet up with friends?
- Is she isolated?

The older person living alone can become isolated and this can influence their motivation and interest in eating and drinking. Gathering this information will assist you to discuss with Mavis any support she might wish to access on her discharge from hospital to help her maintain a healthy living style.

Whilst she is in hospital you would also need to understand any food preferences that Mavis has in relation to any religious beliefs or cultural upbringing. Does Mavis avoid any foods, e.g. spicy foods? Does she have any beliefs about particular foods? What time of day does she have her main meal? Does she eat breakfast? Beginning to understand our patients' food habits will enable us to know if a patient is eating appropriately or not and inform future health education needs and any support the patient needs to maintain the AL.

Environmental

When taking environmental factors into account you would need to consider both the home and hospital environment. In the home you would need to understand the design of the home and facilities. Does she have hot and cold running water? What cooking and food storage facilities does she have? Can she use these safely? What about toilet facilities? If Mavis's only toilet facilities are upstairs, and she is unable to negotiate the stairs without feeling pain, she might be reluctant to drink. Have there been any adaptations made to her accommodation?

As previously discussed there have been several studies that have highlighted the prevalence of malnutrition in patients in hospital (Lennard-Jones 1992, McWhirter & Pennington 1994). You will also need to consider the impact being in the hospital environment might have on Mavis's nutritional status. She is unlikely to be able to find her way around the ward or understand the routines. Depending on the type of ward she has been admitted into, she will be in contact with other ill patients who might have feeding difficulties, and exposed to different sights and smells that might affect her appetite and ability to eat and drink. She might not be familiar with the type and standard of food served in hospital. You should also have taken into account the impact the environment has on her ability to reach her food and drink.

Politicoeconomic

Sensitive questioning and observation may reveal any concerns or issues relating to lack of financial support that may influence Mavis's access to adequate nutrition. You may enquire if she is accessing any resources to which she is entitled and if she requires any advice or support from a social worker.

> **Exercise**
> 1. Find out how to access a social worker.
> 2. What is their role?
> 3. What resources and agencies do they have access to?
> 4. What support would be available to someone like Mavis?

By using the components of the model we are able to identify how lifespan, dependency, psychological, sociocultural and economic factors have contributed to health breakdown. We are also able to discover normal coping mechanisms and identify which of the other ALs may also be affected. In addition we are able to begin to recognise actual and potential problems associated with the activity of eating and drinking.

However, Roper et al (2000) point out that each Activity of Living does not stand alone and it is the interaction between each of these that contributes to the individualisation of nursing. Hence we need to assess the patient's other Activities of Living to obtain a holistic view.

> **Exercise**
> 1. Consider how you might assess each of the other ALs in order to provide a holistic assessment of the patient.

You may have considered and observed the following:

1. **Breathing**
   - Does she have any problems breathing?
   - Does she smoke and if so how many and how often?

2. **Eating and drinking**
   - How much fluid is she drinking?
   - Is her appetite affected? If yes, what has she eaten in the last 5 days?
   - Is she able to eat and drink? If not, why not?
   - Does she need help to eat and drink?
   - When does she eat and drink?
   - What does she eat and drink?
   - Does she take any food supplements?
   - Is she taking any medication that may affect her appetite?
   - Does she avoid or have allergies to any foods or drink?
   - Does she have any problems with oral hygiene, e.g. loose-fitting dentures, crowns, gum disease?

   - Is there any nausea, vomiting or swallowing difficulties?
   - Can she prepare a meal?

3. **Eliminating**
   - Is she continent?
   - How often is she able to open her bowels?
   - Has she any gut problems?
   - What does her urinalysis tell you?
   - Can she get to the toilet?

4. **Mobilising**
   - Has she any disability that restricts her mobility or ability to eat and drink?
   - If so how does this impact on her ability to eat and drink, obtain and/or prepare food?

5. **Expressing sexuality**
   - What is her appearance?
   - Do her clothes or jewellery fit or are they loose?
   - What does she like to wear?
   - Is she in a relationship?

6. **Personal cleansing and dressing**
   - Is she able to shower or bathe?
   - How frequently does she bathe or shower?
   - Does she require any assistance to get dressed?

7. **Working and playing**
   - How does she spend her day?
   - Does she have any visitors?
   - Is she able to get out of the house?
   - Does her health problem impact on her home and social life?

8. **Communicating**
   - Is she able to express her needs?
   - Does she require glasses or hearing aid?

9. **Maintaining a safe environment**
   - Is she safe in the kitchen?
   - Does she have any pain?
   - Does she have any visual or auditory impairment?
   - Are there any risks, e.g. infection, pressure sore development, falls, and moving and handling?
   - Does she understand her medication regime?

10. **Sleeping**
    - How does she sleep?
    - Does anything disturb her sleep?
    - What helps her to sleep?

11. **Controlling body temperature**
    - Does she feel cold?
    - How does her diet influence her body temperature?
    - How does she keep warm at home?
    - What heating system does she have?
    - Is she able to maintain this?

12. Dying
- Does she express any beliefs about dying?
- Does she have any spiritual or religious beliefs?

PLANNING NURSING ACTIVITIES AND CARE

Maintaining an accurate nursing record of a patient's assessment and plan of care is a fundamental part of professional nursing practice and the care process. Nursing records provide a valuable tool for communication with patients and other members of the health care team and good record keeping is seen as an indication of quality of patient care (NMC 2007).

Within the UK, nursing records may be called and used in evidence in a court of law by the Health Service Commissioner; the Nursing and Midwifery Council Fitness to Practice Committee may also use them when investigating complaints about professional conduct, or they may be used to investigate a local complaint.

Key principles that underpin good nursing records include:

- a full account of your assessment and the care you have planned and provided
- relevant information about the condition of the patient or client and the measures you have taken to respond to their needs
- evidence that you have understood and honoured your duty of care for the patient and that any acts or omissions on your part have not compromised their safety in any way
- a record of any arrangements you have made for the continuing care of a patient or client.

The Nursing and Midwifery Council provide regular advice and guidance on record keeping and practitioners are advised to keep up to date with changes at regular intervals via the NMC website.

By using the Roper et al (1996) model for nursing to assess, plan and implement care we will be able to demonstrate a holistic patient assessment, develop an individualised plan of care and take account of the input of other health care professionals in the patient's care. This involves the following activities:

- identifying the problems or needs
- identifying priorities
- establishing short- and long-term goals
- determining the nursing actions and interventions required
- documenting the care plan.

Identifying problems or needs

Roper et al (2000, p. 80) state that:

> *The specific function of nursing is to assist the individual to prevent, alleviate or solve, or cope positively with problems (actual or potential) related to the ALs.*

Whilst undertaking the nursing assessment the nurse should be able to detect potential problems, which the patient may not be aware of. This is where the nurse's knowledge of the factors relating to ill health, socioeconomic, biological, psychological and environmental is important.

During the initial nursing assessment the nurse may obtain a considerable amount of information from the patient, their relatives or carers, other health care professionals and the patient's medical records. Roper et al (2000) seek to clarify the use of the word assessment in relation to their model for nursing as follows:

- collecting information from or about the person
- reviewing the collected information
- identifying a person's problems with Activities of Living
- identifying priorities amongst the problems.

It must be remembered that assessment is an ongoing and interactive process. Having undertaken a thorough assessment you should be able to identify any problems or patient needs and determine the nursing interventions required in order to meet those needs. It is important to stress that such problems and needs must be patient-focused and must relate to the nursing assessment and what is needed to aid recovery in the immediate, short and long term. They may be actual or potential problems or needs and should be prioritised to take account of life-threatening situations.

Prioritising problems

Prioritising problems is an important component of care planning. By using the independence/dependence continuum of the model of living it is possible to identify and prioritise patients' problems that require nursing care and assistance to regain or maintain their independence, or those where the patient is totally dependent on the nurse (Roper et al 2000).

There are different ways by which dependency scoring can be used and you should discuss with your mentor or preceptor local systems of prioritisation or dependency scoring systems. Alternatively you may wish to use the following example as suggested by Whittam in Chapters 3 and 11.

Dependency/independency priority criteria
- *Priority 1:* Completely independent in the AL/independency maintained.
- *Priority 2:* Potential problems in the AL/remains mostly independent.
- *Priority 3:* Actual problems identified within more than one AL/some dependency noted but remains mainly independent.
- *Priority 4:* Existence of actual and potential problems in a number of other ALs with associated increasing dependency.
- *Priority 5:* Life-threatening actual and potential problems/total dependency.

Once the patient's problems or needs have been identified and prioritised the nurse can review these and plan the nursing interventions required to:

- solve actual problems
- prevent potential problems occurring
- prevent solved problems from re-occurring
- develop positive coping strategies for any problem that cannot be solved.

Exercise
1. Reflect on what skills and knowledge you consider a nurse will need to plan care for a patient.
2. Check your knowledge and skills against your list and those listed below.
3. Identify any areas for further learning and/or skills development.
4. Discuss these with your personal tutor and mentor.

Knowledge and skills required to plan care:

- analytical skills
- problem-solving skills
- knowledge of the illness
- knowledge of anatomy and physiology
- decision-making skills
- negotiating skills
- priority setting.

Identifying actual and potential problems

Having undertaken a nursing assessment let us consider what actual and potential problems have been identified and how these might be prioritised. Within the context of this chapter we will focus on those problems, actual and potential in relation to the activity of eating and drinking that might be relevant to Mavis's admission to hospital. We will also demonstrate how using the Roper et al (1996, 2000) model for nursing can contribute to provide a holistic nutritional assessment and inform care planning and nursing interventions.

Nutritional risk assessment screening

As previously discussed there are a number of nutritional assessment tools available that are designed to help nurses to identify patients who may be malnourished or at risk of malnutrition. Some tools include guidelines on when to refer to dietitians and advice on nutritional interventions according to a given score. However, nurses need to ensure that assessment tools are based on evidence rather than rhetoric and are validated in practice.

Exercise
1. Locate literature on a nutritional risk assessment tool and the evidence to support its use in practice. Discuss the value and/or limitations of the tool with your personal tutor and mentor.
2. If you are a student nurse undertaking a clinical placement, find out if a nutritional risk assessment tool is used and find out how it is used in practice.
3. If so, establish how this is used, what information is collected and what guidelines are in place to support its use.
4. What evidence base is there to support its use?
5. If a tool is not used find out why and if any plans are underway to introduce one.
6. You may wish to discuss your findings with your mentor or personal tutor.

The Malnutrition Universal Screening Tool (MUST) (BAPEN 2006) includes the following:

- body mass index (BMI)
- percentage weight loss in the last 3–6 months
- ability to eat and drink/absorb food for 5 days or more.

If a patient is assessed at risk then the nurse should follow local policies to develop a plan of care.

Having undertaken a thorough nursing assessment using the Roper et al (1996, 2000) model for nursing you should have sufficient information to complete a nutritional screening tool, and identify actual and potential problems associated with the activity of eating and drinking and maintaining adequate nutrition.

Now let us return to the main case study. Using the Roper et al (1996, 2000) model for nursing has enabled us to undertake a thorough nursing assessment, which may look something like the following hypothetical example for Mavis.

1. Breathing
- Mavis has never smoked and has no problems with her breathing.

2. Eating and drinking
- She has reduced her fluid intake because her toilet is upstairs and she is unable to negotiate the stairs without pain in her hip.
- Her appetite has been poor and she has not felt like cooking for herself: 'What's the use of cooking for one?'
- Mavis is able to feed herself but with IV therapy in place she finds this difficult.

- She has toast for breakfast, a sandwich at lunchtime and soup for her evening meal. Mavis used to like to cook for her husband. Her BMI is 16.
- She doesn't like fish or tomatoes.
- She likes a small whisky at night before going to bed.
- Her mouth is dry and her dentures are too big.
- She has a sore mouth.

3. Eliminating
- Mavis has recently had some incontinence of urine and is complaining of constipation.

4. Mobilising
- Mavis is experiencing pain in her hip and has found it increasingly difficult to move around recently. There is one step down into her kitchen. She used to like to go out to Age Concern to meet up with her friends for lunch but her mobility problems have made this increasingly difficult recently.

5. Expressing sexuality
- Mavis was always very proud about her appearance but her recent weight loss has made her clothes look untidy and she feels she is not smart. She likes to wear smart clothes and used to visit the hairdresser each week.

6. Personal cleansing and dressing
- Until recently Mavis has been able to get into her shower but because of mobility problems she is finding it increasingly difficult. Under normal circumstances she does not need any assistance to dress herself.

7. Working and playing
- Before she retired Mavis was a schoolteacher. Until recently she was able to do most of her own housework, shopping and cleaning. She had a circle of friends whom she would meet in Age Concern and at church social events. Since she has been unable to get out of the house her friends have been visiting her at home. Mavis is a Christian and regularly attended church on a Sunday. She spends most of her day watching the television or listening to the radio.

8. Communicating
- Mavis is able to communicate; she wears a hearing aid and glasses. Mavis has a telephone and frequently phones her daughter and speaks to her grandchildren. Her eyesight has begun to deteriorate recently and she is unable to read the newspaper.

9. Maintaining a safe environment
- Mavis has pain in her hip when mobilising. She has had a couple of falls at home and walks with a stick. Her eyesight is poor and there is a risk of further falls.
- Because Mavis is undernourished she is at risk of developing pressure ulcers.
- Mavis understands her medication although she does not understand that because she is hypertensive she needs to reduce her salt intake.

10. Sleeping
- Normally Mavis sleeps well for 7½ hours but recently she has had difficulty in getting off to sleep.
- She likes to have a small drink of whisky before retiring.

11. Controlling body temperature
- Her house is centrally heated but she is unwilling to keep it on because of the high cost of fuel bills.

12. Dying
- Mavis does not express any beliefs openly about dying but she was very upset when her husband died. Her Christian beliefs have helped her to cope.

Exercise
1. Having undertaken a thorough nursing assessment you will have already begun to identify a number of potential and actual problems in relation to the activity of eating and drinking (see Table 6.3).
2. Make a list of what you think these might be and check your list against those identified below. This list might not be exhaustive but will give some indication to those that you might consider in relation to eating and drinking. You should remember to take account of the factors which influence the Activities of Living, i.e. physical, psychological, sociocultural, environmental and politicoeconomic.

Whilst undertaking this exercise you will begin to appreciate the interrelatedness of the actual and potential problems relating to the other Activities of Living. For further information and reading on these Activities of Living you are referred to the relevant chapters in this book. You may like to return to the brief case studies and consider the actual and potential problems that might arise and discuss these with your personal tutor.

Discharge planning
It is at this point you should be starting to plan for her discharge back home. Every patient wants to know how long they are likely to remain in hospital and more importantly when they are able to go home. A successful discharge is part of patients' experience of care in hospital (DoH 2004c). Discharging a person back safely into the community requires a multidisciplinary and multi-agency approach. The discharge process is governed by legislation (Community Care (Delayed Discharge) Act 2003) and NHS policy (NHS Plan 2000).

Exercise
1. Whilst on a clinical placement familiarise yourself with the discharge policy.
2. Arrange, with your mentor and/or discharge coordinator, involvement in planning the discharge of a patient.
3. Revisit the case study and identify actions that need to be taken to secure a successful discharge.
4. Discuss these with your mentor or tutor.

Table 6.3 Potential problems – Case study 6.3 (Mavis)

Activity of Living	Actual problem	Potential problem
Eating and drinking	Mavis is dehydrated and reluctant to drink	Fluid and electrolyte imbalance
	IVI in place, which may hamper Mavis's ability to reach her food and to feed herself	Mavis may not eat her meals and receive adequate nutrition
	Mavis's BMI is 16	Further weight loss and protein energy malnutrition whilst in hospital
	Mavis's appetite has been poor and she has not felt like cooking for herself	Mavis may not receive adequate nutrition
	Mavis is disorientated due to dehydration and hospital admission	Mavis may not understand how to choose her meals from the menu or how to call for help
Eliminating	Occasionally incontinent of urine	Reluctance to drink fluids thus increasing symptoms and effects of dehydration
	Constipation due to reduced fluid intake	Impacted faeces
Mobilising	Pain on mobilising	Depression due to pain and inability to get out and socialise
Personal cleansing and dressing	Unable to wash and dress due to IVI in situ	Mavis will become unkempt
Communicating	Poor eyesight and hearing	Inability to see menus due to poor eyesight
		Inability to hear dietary instructions and advice
Maintaining a safe environment	Risk of further falls	Risk of fractured femur due to falls
	Risk of pressure ulcer development due to loss of subcutaneous fat	

When discharging a patient from hospital the nurse will need to take account of a patient's physical, cultural, social, economic and environmental needs. Using the Roper, Logan and Tierney model as a framework for assessment will provide a baseline on which to build a comprehensive discharge plan. It is important to involve carers, with the patient's consent, at all stages of discharge planning. Poor discharge planning can have a detrimental effect on patients, their families and carers. For further information on discharge planning see Dougherty & Lister (2004).

Setting goals

Having identified the actual and potential problems, it is now necessary to agree, ideally with the patient, short- and long-term goals or outcomes for nursing care and nursing interventions. This will enable you to evaluate whether the expected outcome has been achieved.

Goals should be realistic, achievable and measurable. It is advisable to include dates and times to indicate when the goal is to be achieved. This enables the nurse to evaluate progress and achievement and demonstrate how nursing has benefited the patient (Roper et al 1996). In some cases it may be necessary to agree long-term goals. Roper et al (1996, 2000) liken goals to signposts on a journey indicating when you have arrived at your destination.

Table 6.4 shows examples of how goals might be set in the case of Mavis in relation to her activity of eating and drinking.

You may have considered other goals in relation to her psychological, sociocultural and environmental needs that have been identified in the case study. For example you may have considered the need for a home assessment in relation to her ability to negotiate the kitchen and prepare meals or referral to a social worker to assess if she is eligible for financial support and how she might access services to enable her to get out more. You may wish to include these in your nursing care plan.

Determining nursing actions and interventions

Having undertaken a nursing assessment and identified actual and potential problems, the nurse is now ready to develop the nursing care plan. Roper et al (1996) point out that 'the nursing care plan is just that – a plan'. The nursing care plan, in addition to the direct observation of the patient, monitoring of vital signs and verbal report, should guide professional and ethical practice, care delivery, care management and personal and professional development (see Box 6.10).

Availability of resources

When planning the care and determining nursing actions and interventions the nurse must take account of the resources available, including staffing levels, knowledge and skills, the environment and equipment and any evidence-based guidelines, protocols or policies. They will also need to take account of any interventions and care prescribed by other members of the health care team and incorporate these in to the nursing care plan where necessary. A registered nurse remains at all times accountable for the appropriate delegation to unregistered staff and making sure that the person is competent to undertake the task or duty (NMC 2004).

Table 6.4 Eating and drinking goals

Actual problem	Potential problem	Goal
1. Mavis is dehydrated and reluctant to drink	Fluid and electrolyte imbalance	Mavis will receive IV fluids as prescribed Mavis will drink 1.5 litres of water a day
2. IVI in place, which may hamper her ability to reach her food and to feed herself	Mavis may not eat her meals and receive adequate nutrition	Mavis will receive assistance to reach her food and drink
3. Mavis's BMI is 16	Further weight loss and protein energy malnutrition whilst in hospital	Further weight loss whilst in hospital will be prevented
4. Mavis's appetite has been poor	Mavis may not receive adequate nutrition	Mavis's dietary intake will be monitored Mavis will state that her appetite has improved
5. Mavis is disorientated due to dehydration and hospital admission She also has poor sight and hearing	Mavis may not understand how to choose her meals from the menu or how to call for help	Mavis will receive assistance and explanation on how to choose nourishing meals
6. Sore mouth due to loose dentures	Mavis may be reluctant to eat because of pain	Mavis's painful mouth will be relieved
7. Mavis is constipated	Faecal impaction	Mavis will receive dietary advice and increase amount of fibre in her diet and fluid intake Mavis will report normal bowel movements

---

Box 6.10	**Objective of the plan**

- To prevent identified problems with any of the ALs from becoming actual ones
- To solve actual problems
- Where possible to alleviate those that cannot be solved
- To help the person cope positively with those problems that cannot be alleviated or solved
- To solve identified actual problems
- To prevent recurrence of a treated problem
- To help the person to be as comfortable and pain free as possible when death is inevitable.

From Roper et al (1996, p. 57).

Care pathways

The introduction of clinical governance into the NHS in the UK (DoH 1998) has placed greater emphasis on ensuring quality care to patients and effective outcomes. A care pathway is a tool that sets out the evidence-based care a patient should receive for an episode of care (Ellis & Johnson 1999). When planning the nursing care of a patient it is necessary to consider where care pathways have been developed and take account of these when determining the nursing interventions and individualising care. (Further information on care pathways can be found at www.library.nhs.uk/pathways.)

Collaboration

As we have already discussed, nurses do not work in isolation; they work in teams and in collaboration with others. In hospital nurses are with the patients for 24 hours a day

and in many cases they may take the lead role in coordinating the care of the patient, referring if necessary to specialist nurses and health care professionals.

> **Exercise**
> 1. Revisit Mavis's assessment and identify other health care professionals who may be involved in her care.
> 2. What would be their role?

You may have considered the following:

- dietitian
- medical staff
- junior medical staff
- pharmacist
- physiotherapist
- health care assistant
- ward hostess.

Other professionals who may input indirectly or at a later date include:

- social worker
- dentist
- occupational therapist
- discharge liaison coordinator.

When preparing a nursing care plan and discharge plan you will need to take account of the input and assessments undertaken by these professionals.

Return to the brief case studies and consider which other professionals are likely to be involved.

Nursing interventions

The nursing care plan details the nursing interventions required to achieve the stated goals. The plan should enable other staff including other health care professionals to provide continuity of care for the patient (Roper et al 2000). The nursing care plan may be paper-based or computerised.

When determining the nursing interventions you will need to consider where the patient is on the independency/dependency continuum as identified in the model of living (Roper et al 1996). The nurse provides nursing interventions for a dependent patient, whereas nursing interventions in an independent patient aim to encourage and maintain independence. As discussed in the first part of this chapter, dependency may be influenced by the factors associated with living across the lifespan.

Problem 1: Mavis is dehydrated and is reluctant to drink

The nurse has an important role in ensuring that the patient's hydration needs are met. In Mavis's case the nursing actions would involve ensuring that the intravenous fluids are administered safely and according to the medical prescription. You would need to ensure the integrity and patency of the cannula site and that it does not pose a problem with washing, dressing or feeding. The nurse must observe the cannula site for any signs of phlebitis or extravasation, the most common complications of intravenous therapy. The intake and output of fluids must be accurately monitored, measured and charted. The reasons for intravenous therapy should be explained to Mavis.

You would need to agree with Mavis how often she would take oral fluids and what she preferred to drink. It is sometimes useful to agree with the patient that they would keep a record of what they drink and when. You would ensure that fluids are made available and within reach or that Mavis understands how to call for assistance to drink if necessary.

Problem 2: Mavis has an IVI in place, which may hamper her ability to reach her food, and feed herself, she may therefore not eat her meals or receive adequate nutrition

Intravenous access is more likely to be made through one of the lower extremities, such as the arm or hand. When determining which arm or hand, consideration should be given to using the arm other than the one she uses to feed herself. Consideration should be given to her positioning for meals and whether she can reach her food. Whilst wishing to promote independence, Mavis may require nursing assistance according to her dependency to drink or feed herself. Food should never be left out of the reach of the patient.

Problem 3: Mavis is underweight with a BMI of 16

A person with a BMI of 16 is regarded as underweight. Mavis should be referred to the dietitian who will undertake a more detailed nutritional history and determine if Mavis requires a therapeutic diet. Some hospitals will have guidelines or procedures on when to refer to a dietitian and provide nutritional food supplements, based on a patient's nutritional assessment score. Nutritional food supplements contain nutrients and are used in the short term to complement the normal hospital diet (Bond 1997). A doctor or dietitian must prescribe some food supplements unless there is a locally agreed protocol.

You may consider recording Mavis's food intake for a period of 3 days to enable a more detailed assessment of Mavis's nutritional intake whilst in hospital. Nurses, health care assistants and ward hostesses should be alerted to the need to monitor and observe Mavis's dietary intake, especially any food supplements. Mavis will also need assistance with choosing food from the menu.

In order to monitor any improvement you would need to check Mavis's weight at least once a week. You should try to do this using the same machine each time and ensuring that Mavis wears the same clothes each time.

Problem 4: Mavis's appetite is poor

As in the previous problems you would discuss Mavis's likes and dislikes and help her to choose nourishing meals from the hospital menu. The hospital environment including smells and other patients' behaviours can have an influence on a person's appetite. You should attempt to ensure the environment is as conducive as possible at mealtimes and there are no interruptions so that they are as pleasurable as possible (Tolson et al 2002). Attention to the presentation, amount and serving of meals can help to encourage patients to eat. You will need to discuss with Mavis reasons why she believes her appetite is poor and try to identify any underlying reasons for this. You should aim to discuss strategies for improving her appetite and monitor and record her food intake, especially when removing her food tray at the end of a meal. You should also check with the pharmacist and doctor that her medication is not contributing to her lack of appetite.

Problem 5: Mavis is disorientated due to hospital admission. She also has poor eyesight and hearing

It is not uncommon for older patients to be disorientated on admission to hospital. Mental state is affected by malnutrition and Mavis may well have little motivation, energy or will to help herself. Mavis will need to be orientated to her surroundings and any procedures and routines explained. It should be explained to her that by eating a better diet she might begin to feel better. She will need instructions and assistance in completing any relevant forms for her menus. She might be unused to the type of food on the menu and will need to be helped to choose nourishing high-calorie food. This may provide an opportunity to promote healthy eating and offer patient information leaflets to support your advice in readiness for her discharge.

Problem 6: Mavis has a sore mouth due to loose dentures

Because Mavis is dehydrated her mouth is dry, and as she has also lost weight her dentures are too big, resulting in a sore mouth and a reluctance to eat and drink. Older people have specific oral care needs and it is essential that nurses understand and are able to meet these needs (Fitzpatrick 2000). You may choose to use one of a number of oral hygiene assessment tools developed to assist nurses in assessing patient's needs to identify any nursing actions or interventions (Holmes & Mountain 1993). Nursing interventions should include inspection of her oral cavity, noting any ulceration or abnormality. The plan should include the frequency of oral hygiene, cleansing of dentures, advice on removal of debris and any prescribed use of topical anaesthetic mouthwash or lozenges and possible referral for dental advice. It is important to consider Mavis's dignity and self-esteem when attending to her oral hygiene.

Problem 7: Mavis is constipated

Constipation may be caused by low fluid intake, therefore an increase in fluid intake should assist in returning to normal defecation. Mavis's problems with mouth pain and her inability to cope with foods that need to be chewed can also contribute to constipation. In addition, unfamiliarity with her surroundings and access to toilet facilities will also compound the problem. Therefore nursing interventions and actions should aim to increase fluid intake, administer any prescribed medication or laxatives, reduce mouth pain and familiarise Mavis with her surroundings. Her bowel movements should be monitored and recorded daily.

IMPLEMENTING THE PLAN

When implementing the plan of care, nurses need to take account of the resources available, including staff and skill mix, knowledge, the skills required to deliver care and systems of organising nursing care delivery.

Exercise
1. Arrange to spend some time observing how nursing care is organised on the ward or within a team.
2. How does the system of organising care delivery contribute to individualising patient care?

You may have observed one of the following methods:

- Task allocation is a system where nurses are assigned to tasks such as taking temperatures for a group of patients or a whole ward. This method leads to fragmentation of care and lack of continuity. Patient care is not individualised and no one nurse will have an overall view of an individual patient.
- Team nursing is where nurses work in teams to deliver the care to a group of patients, sometimes in a defined area of the ward. Nurses could be allocated to a team for a whole shift or allocated to a team permanently. This system of care delivery can provide continuity of patient care but there is always a danger that the team can revert to task-centred nursing within a team.
- In primary nursing a nurse is responsible for the care of a patient for the whole period of care from admission to discharge. Because they are unable to be present 24 hours a day they work with an associate nurse who will assume delegated responsibility in his or her absence. This method provides continuity for the patient and the nurse.

Alternatively, you may have observed hybrid systems of care delivery being used depending on the number of nurses and their level knowledge and skills available to meet the individual needs of patients.

Exercise
1. What factors would you need to take into account when implementing the plan of nursing care for Mavis?
2. Organising the nursing care of patients in their own homes will need different approaches. How might this differ from in a hospital?

You may have considered the following:

Factors influencing implementation
- the philosophy of care on the ward, department or team (beliefs and values, advocacy)
- the nursing model used
- the care delivery system (primary nursing, team nursing, case management or task allocation)
- resources available (skill mix of staff available, equipment, support staff and other health care professionals).

Knowledge required when implementing nursing activities
- anatomy and physiology of digestive system and nutrition
- psychological effects associated with eating and drinking
- sociocultural issues relating to eating and drinking
- environmental issues and concerns
- political and economic concerns.

Skills required when implementing nursing activities
- caring skills (listening, comforting, reassuring, helping)
- clinical psychomotor skills (catheterisation, intravenous infusions)
- management skills (organisational, supervision, delegation)
- counselling skills (listening, problem solving, advising)
- teaching skills
- research skills (literature searching, critical appraisal, synthesis)
- problem-solving skills (problem identification, goal setting, priority setting)
- leadership skills (advocacy, teamwork, transformational leadership skills, networking).

Exercise
1. Reflect on these and assess your current knowledge and skills in relation to the activity of eating and drinking.
2. Record your reflections in your diary.
3. Identify those areas in which you need further development.
4. Take these to your next tutorial or clinical supervision session. Discuss with your mentor or preceptor how you plan to develop these further.

EVALUATION OF NURSING ACTIONS AND INTERVENTIONS

Evaluation of nursing care is an important part of professional practice and provides feedback on the patient's progress. It is an ongoing process, which should be undertaken by the nurse in conjunction with the patient and his or her relatives or carers and other health care professionals (for further information refer to Chapter 1).

Evaluation consists of checking the patient's progress against the identified goals and timescales to determine whether these have been fully or partially met or indeed not been met at all.

When evaluating the care plan you will need to establish if the goals have been completely met, partially met or not met at all. If the goal has not been met or partially met then the nurse must consider if the agreed timescale was realistic. If not then you may decide to extend the timescale. Alternatively you may need to reassess the problem and modify the plan. In some cases the problem may have changed or the goal may have been inappropriate. Not all goals will be achievable during a hospital stay, in which case you might need more information on the problem. Is it worse or has it changed?

You might also reconsider the appropriateness of the prescribed nursing actions and interventions – do these need to be changed or modified? By involving patients in their nursing care planning it is possible to identify and agree realistic goals and meaningful evaluation of outcomes.

SUMMARY POINTS

1. This chapter introduced the fourth Activity of Living, eating and drinking as described by Roper, Logan and Tierney in their model of nursing (Roper et al 1996, 2000). It systematically explored the framework of the model and its application in clinical practice, the use of a case scenario, exercises, and reflection and directed reading. It has been impossible within this chapter to cover every aspect in relation to the activity of eating and drinking and it is important that you keep up to date with new information and evidence-based practice in order to be able to meet the changing needs of patients and health care delivery.

2. The activity of eating and drinking is essential to existence and nurses have a very important role in ensuring the quality of the patient experience and that patient needs are met. There is a significant amount of evidence that patients' nutritional needs in hospital are not being met. Throughout this chapter it has been shown how the ability or inability to eat and drink can impact on many of the other Activities of Living and how, by using the Roper, Logan and Tierney model for nursing as a framework, nurses are able to recognise and take account of the patient's nutritional needs when assessing, planning, implementing and evaluating holistic patient care.

References

Age Concern 2006 Hungry to be heard. The scandal of malnourished older people in hospital. Age Concern, England

Akhtar S 2002 Nursing with dignity: Part 8: Islam. Nursing Times 98(16):40–42

Alexander MF, Fawcett JN, Runciman PJ (eds) 2000 Nursing practice: hospital and home, the adult, 2nd edn. Churchill Livingstone, Edinburgh

Alexander MF, Fawcett J (Tonks) N, Runciman PJ (eds) 2006 Nursing practice: hospital and home (the adult), 3nd edn. Churchill Livingstone, Edinburgh

Anderson C, Nathan A 1991 Promoting oral health (3). Pharmaceutical Journal 15:734–736

Association of Community Health Councils for England and Wales 1997 Hungry in hospital. ACHEW, London

Bolling K, Grant C, Hamlyn B et al 2007 Infant feeding survey 2005. Information Centre for Health and Social Care. Part of the Government Statistical Service (www.ic.nhs.uk)

Bond S (ed) 1997 Eating matters: A resource for improving dietary care in hospitals. Centre for Health Services Research, University of Newcastle, Newcastle

British Association for Parenteral and Enteral Nutrition (BAPEN) 2006 Malnutrition Universal Screening Tool (MUST) (www.bapen.org.uk/must-tool.html)

British Medical Association 1999 Withholding and withdrawing life: prolonging medical treatment. Guidance for decision making. BMA, Buckingham

British Nutrition Foundation 2004 Balance of good health plate model (www.nutrition.org.uk)

Brooker C, 2005 Churchill Livingstone's mini encyclopaedia of nursing. Elsevier, Edinburgh

Brooker C, Nichol M, 2003 Nursing adults. The practice of caring. Mosby, London

Butterworth ACE 1974 The skeleton in the hospital closet. Nutrition Today March/April:4–5

Cabinet Office 2004 Alcohol harm reduction strategy for England. Prime Minister's Strategy Unit, London (www.strategy.gov.uk)

Chan JYK 1995 Dietary beliefs of Chinese patients. Nursing Standard 9(27):30–34

Chen CG, Schilling LS, Lyder CH 2001 A concept analysis of malnutrition in the elderly. Journal of Advanced Nursing 36(1):131–142

Collins A 2002 Nursing with dignity. Nursing Times Series Part 1, Judaism. Nursing Times 98(9):33–35

Cooper DB 2006 Substance abuse. In: Alexander MF, Fawcett J (Tonks) N, Runciman PJ (eds) Nursing practice hospital and home (the adult), 3rd edn. Churchill Livingstone, Edinburgh

Corish CA, Flood P, Kennedy NP 2004 Comparison of nutritional risk screening tools in patients on admission to hospital. Journal of Human Nutrition & Dietetics 17(2):133–139

Covington CY, Cybulski MJ, Davis TL et al 2001 Kids on the move: Preventing obesity of urban children. American Journal of Nursing 101(3):73–75, 77, 79, 81–82

Cremin D, Halek C 1997 Eating disorders: Knowledge for practice. Nursing Times Learning Curve 451(5):5–8

Crowther R, Dinsdale H, Rutter H et al 2007 Analysis of the National Childhood Obesity Database 2005–06. A report for the Department of Health South East Public Health Observatory on behalf of the Association of Public Health Observatories. (www.dh.gov.uk)

Department of Health 1992 Health of the nation report. HMSO, London

Department of Health 1998 A first class service: Quality in the new NHS. The Stationery Office, London

Department of Health 2000 The NHS plan: a plan for investment – a plan for reform. The Stationery Office, London

Department of Health 2001a National service framework for coronary heart disease. The Stationery Office, London

Department of Health 2001b National service framework for diabetes. The Stationery Office, London

Department of Health 2001c Modern standards and service models of older people: National Service framework for older people. The Stationery Office, London

Department of Health 2001d Caring for older people: Nursing priority integrating knowledge, practice and values. Report by the Nursing & Midwifery Advisory Committee, HMSO, London

Department of Health 2003a Five a day. DoH. Leeds

Department of Health 2003b The essence of care: patient-focused benchmarking for health care professionals. The Stationery Office, London

Department of Health 2004a NHS Improvement Plan. Putting people at the heart of public services. The Stationery Office, London

Department of Health 2004b Choosing health: making healthy choices easier. The Stationery Office, London

Department of Health 2004c Achieving timely simple discharge from hospital. A toolkit for the multidisciplinary team. Downloaded from www.dh.gov.uk

Diabetes: State of the Nation 2006 Progress made in delivering the national diabetes framework. A report from Diabetes UK. Downloaded from www.diabetes.org.uk, December 2006

Dobson R 2002 Breast is still best even when HIV prevalence is high, experts say. British Medical Journal 324:1474

Dougherty L, Lister S 2004 The Royal Marsden Hospital manual of clinical nursing procedures, 6th edn. Blackwell Publishing, Oxford

Drummond C, Oyefeso A, Phillips T et al 2005 The alcohol needs assessment research project (ANARP). The 2004 national alcohol needs assessment for England. Department of Health, London (www.gov.uk/publications)

Elia M. 2003 The MUST report. Malnutrition Advisory Group British Association for Parenteral and Enteral Nutrition, Redditch

Ellis BW, Johnson S 1999 The care pathway: a tool to enhance clinical governance. British Journal of Clinical Governance 4(2):61–71

Elmståhl S, Person M, Andren V et al 1997 Malnutrition in geriatric patients: a neglected problem? Journal of Advanced Nursing 26:851–855

Fitzpatrick J 2000 Oral health care needs of dependent older people: responsibilities of nurses and care staff. Journal of Advanced Nursing 32(6):1325–1332

Food Standards Agency 2003 The balance of good health. Food Standards Agency, Middlesex

Frobisher C, Maxwell SM 2001 The attitudes and nutritional knowledge of a group of 11–12 year olds in Merseyside. International Journal of Health Promotion and Education 39(4):121–127

Furman EF 2006 Undernutrition in older adults across the continuum of care: nutritional assessment, barriers and interventions. Journal of Gerontological Nursing 32(1):22–27

Gobbi M, Cowen, M. Ugboma, D 2006 Fluid and electrolyte balance. In: Alexander MF, Fawcett J (Tonks) N, Runciman PJ (eds) Nursing practice hospital and home (the adult), 3rd edn. Chapter 20. Churchill Livingstone, Edinburgh

Green S, Jackson, P 2006 Nutrition. In: Alexander MF, Fawcett J, (Tonks) N, Runciman PJ (eds) Nursing practice hospital and home (the adult), 3rd edn. Churchill Livingstone, Edinburgh,

Green SM, Watson R 2006 Nutritional screening and assessment tools for older adults: literature review. Journal of Advanced Nursing 54(4):477–490

Gustafsson K, Sidenvall B 2002 Food-related health perceptions and food habits among older women. Journal of Advanced Nursing 39(2):164–173

Hamilton-Smith S 1972 Nil by mouth? Royal College of Nursing, London

Hand H 2001 The use of intravenous therapy. Nursing Standard 15(43):47–55

Henley A, Schott J 1999 Culture, religion and patient care in a multi-ethnic society. A handbook for professionals. Age Concern Books, Glasgow

Hill AJ 2006 Motivation for eating behaviour in adolescent girls: the body beautiful. Proceedings of the Nutrition Society 65(4):376–384

Holmes S 2006 Barriers to effective nutritional care for older adults. Nursing Standards 21(3):50–54

Holmes S, Mountain E 1993 Assessment of oral status: Evaluation of three oral assessment guides. Journal of Clinical Nursing 2:35–40

Iggulden H 2006 Care of the neurological patient. Blackwell Publishing, Oxford

Joanna Briggs Institute 2001 Best practice: maintaining oral hydration in older people. Evidence Based Practice Information Sheets for Health Professionals, vol 5, issue 1

Joint FAO/WHO/UNU Expert Consultation 1985 Energy and protein requirements. WHO Technical Report Series 724. WHO, Geneva

Kelly R 2006 Disorders of the mouth. In: Alexander MF, Fawcett J (Tonks) N, Runciman PJ (eds) Nursing practice hospital and home (the adult), 3rd edn. Chapter 15. Churchill Livingstone, Edinburgh

Kenchaiach SK, Evans JC, Levy O et al 2002 Obesity and the risk of heart failure. New England Journal of Medicine 347(5):305–313

Kindlen S 2003 Physiology for health care and nursing. Churchill Livingstone, Edinburgh

Kowanko I, Simon S, Wood J 1999 Nutritional care of the patient: nurses knowledge and attitudes in an acute setting. Journal of Clinical Nursing 8:217–224

Kowanko I, Simon S, Wood J 2001 Energy and nutrient intake of patients in acute care. Journal of Clinical Nursing 10:51–57

Lennard-Jones J 1992 A positive approach to nutrition as treatment. The Kings Fund Centre, London

Lennard-Jones J 2000 Ethical and legal aspects of clinical hydration and nutritional support. British Journal of Urology 85:398–403

Lennard-Jones J, Arrowsmith H, Davison C et al 1995 Screening by nurses and junior doctors to detect malnutrition when patients are first assessed in hospital. Clinical Nutrition 14:336–340

Leslie WS, Lean MEJ, Woodward M et al 2006 Unidentified under-nutrition: dietary intake and anthropometric indices in a residential care home population. Journal of Human Nutrition and Dietetics 19(5):343–347

Liu JLY, Maniadakis N, Gray A et al 2002 The economic burden of coronary heart disease in the UK. Heart 88:597–603

Lucas B 2006 Disorders of the musculoskeletal system. In: Alexander MF, Fawcett J (Tonks) N, Runciman PJ (eds) 2006 Nursing practice hospital and home (the adult), 3rd edn. Churchill Livingstone, Edinburgh

McKevieth B 2004 The nation's diet: promoting healthy eating. Nursing Standard 18(48):45–52

McKie L, MacInnes A, Hendry J et al 2000 The food consumption patterns and perceptions of dietary advice of older people. Journal of Human Nutrition and Dietetics 13(3):173–183

McLaren S, Green S 1998 Nutritional screening and assessment. Nursing Standard 12(48):26–29

McLaren S, Holmes S, Green S et al 1997 An overview of nutritional issues relating to the care of older people. In: Bond S (ed) Eating matters: A resource for improving dietary care in hospitals, pp 15–21. Centre for Health Services Research, University of Newcastle, Newcastle

McWhirter JP, Pennington CR 1994 Incidence and recognition of malnutrition in hospital. British Medical Journal 308:945–948

Madden C 2000 Nutritional benefits of drinks. Nursing Standard 15(13–15):47–52

Martyn K 2003 Nutrition. In: Brooker C, Nichol M (eds) Nursing adults. The practice of caring. Chapter 11. Mosby, London

Metcalf C 2002 Crohn's disease: an overview. Nursing Standard 16(31):45–52

Montague SE, Watson R, Herbert RA 2005 Physiology for nursing practice, 3rd edn. Elsevier, Edinburgh

Mullaly S 2000 The chief nurse's view. Nursing Times Plus 96(8):1

NAO 2001 National audit report: Tackling obesity in England, report by the Comptroller and Auditor General. The Stationery Office, London

NAO 2003 Developing effective services for older people. The Stationery Office, London (www.nao.gov.uk)

National Patients Safety Agency 2005 Safety advice to NHS on reducing harm caused by the misplacement of nasogastric feeding tubes. (www.npsa.nhs.uk)

NICE 2004 Eating disorders: core interventions in the treatment and management of anorexia nervosa, bulimia nervosa and related eating disorders. Clinical Guideline 9. NICE, London

NICE 2006a Obesity: the prevention, identification, assessment and management of overweight and obesity in adults and children. NICE, London

NICE 2006b Nutrition support in adults: oral nutrition support, enteral tube feeding and parenteral nutrition. Clinical Guideline 32. NICE, London

Northcot N 2002 Nursing with dignity. Part 2: Buddhism. Nursing Times 98(10):36–38

Norton B 1996 Malnutrition in hospitals: The nurse's role and prevention. Nursing Times 92(26):Suppl 1(1)

Nursing and Midwifery Council 2004 Code of professional conduct: standards for performance and ethics. NMC, London (www.nmc-uk.org)

Nursing and Midwifery Council 2007 NMC Record keeping guidance (www.nmc_uk.org)

Nursing and Midwifery Practice Development Unit 2002 Nutrition for frail older people. Best practice statement, available at www.nhshealthquality.org

Parliamentary Office of Science and Technology 2003a Childhood obesity. Online publication (www.parliament.uk/post)

Parliamentary Office of Science and Technology 2003b Improving children's diet. Online publication (www.parliament.uk/post)

Pearson C 2004 Inflammatory bowel disease. Nursing Times 100(9):86–90

Prior, F 2003 Water and electrolyte balance. In: Kindlen S (ed) Physiology for health care and nursing, Chapter 14. Churchill Livingstone, Edinburgh

Quigley MA, Cumberland P, Cowden JM et al 2006 How protective is breast feeding against diarrhoeal disease in infants in 1990's England? A case-castrol study. Archives of Disease in Childhood 91(3):245–250

Reilly HM, Martineau JK, Moran A et al 1995 Nutritional screening - evaluation and implementation of a simple nutrition risk score. Clinical Nutrition 14:269–273

Rinomhota S, Rollins H 2001 Energy, mood and behaviour: part 2. NT Plus Nursing Times 97(44):50, 52

Roper N, Logan WW, Tierney AJ 1996 The elements of nursing: A model for nursing based on a model for living, 4th edn. Churchill Livingstone, London

Roper N, Logan WW, Tierney AJ 2000 The Roper–Logan–Tierney model of nursing based on activities of living. Churchill Livingstone, Edinburgh

Royal College of Nursing 2005 Perioperative fasting in adults and children. RCN Guideline for the Multidisciplinary Team. RCN, London

Royal College of Nursing, National Patient Safety Agency 2007 Water for health. Hydration best practice tool kit for hospitals and health care. Online publication (www2.rcn.org.uk.)

Royal College of Physicians 2001 Alcohol: can the NHS afford it? Online publication (www.rcplondon.ac.uk/pubs/wp-actnhsai-summary.htm)

Royal College of Physicians 2002 Nutrition and patients: A doctor's responsibility. RCP, London

Rutishauser S 1994 Physiology and anatomy: A basis for nursing and health care. Churchill Livingstone, Edinburgh

Scottish Intercollegiate Guidelines Network 2004 Management of patients with stroke. Identification and management of dysphagia. Publication 78. SIGN, Edinburgh

Shireff A 1990 Pre-operative nutritional assessment. Nursing Times 86(8):68–72

Silk D (ed) 1994 Organisation of nutritional support in hospitals: A report by a working party of BAPEN. The British Association for Parenteral and Enteral Nutrition, Maidenhead, Berks

Silverman K, Evans SM, Stragin EC et al 1992 Withdrawal syndrome after the double-blind cessation of caffeine consumption. New England Journal of Medicine 327(16):1109–1114

Sizer T (ed) 1996 Working Party of the British Association for Parenteral and Enteral Nutrition. Standards and guidelines for nutritional support of patients in hospital. BAPEN, Maidenhead

Smith GD 2005 The acquisition of nutrients. In: Montague SE, Watson R, Herbert RA (eds) Physiology for nursing practice 3rd edn. Elsevier, Edinburgh

Sutcliffe A 2001 Osteoporosis: prevention and treatment. Nursing Times 97(3):53–55

Sutcliffe E 1990 Reviewing the process progress. A critical review of the literature on the nursing process. Senior Nurse 10(a):9–13

Thomas AE 1987 Pre-operative fasting, a question of routine. Nursing Times 83(49):46–47

Tolson DT, Schofield J, Booth R et al 2002 Best practice statements. Part 2: Nutrition for the physically frail older people. Nursing Times 98(28):38–40

Watson R 2006 Editorial. Mealtimes in hospital: When will we ever learn? Journal of Clinical Nursing 15(10):1212

Waugh A, Grant A 2006 Ross and Wilson anatomy and physiology in health and illness, 10th edn. Churchill Livingstone, Edinburgh

Webster RA, Thompson DR 2006 Disorders of the cardiovascular system. In: Alexander MF, Fawcett J (Tonks) N, Runciman PJ (eds) Nursing practice: hospital and home, the adult, 3rd edn. Chapter 2. Churchill Livingstone, Edinburgh

Westergren A, Karlsson S, Andersson P et al 2001 Eating difficulties, need for assisted eating, nutritional status and pressure ulcers in patients admitted for stroke rehabilitation. Journal of Clinical Nursing 10:257–269

Woo J, Chi I, Hui E et al 2005 Low staffing level is associated with malnutrition in long-term residential care homes. European Journal of Clinical Nutrition 59(4):474–479

Wood S, Creamer M 1996 Malnutrition in hospitals. Nursing Times 92(26):67–68

Xia C, McCutcheon H 2006 Mealtimes in hospital – who does what? Journal of Clinical Nursing 15(10):1221–1227

Further reading

Holland K, Hogg C 2001 Cultural awareness in nursing and health care. Arnold, London

NHS Scotland 2003 Food fluid and nutritional care in hospitals. Nursing and Midwifery Practice Development Unit, Edinburgh (www.nhshealthquality.org)

Useful websites

www.ageconcern.org.uk (Age Concern)

www.bapen.co.uk (British Association for Parenteral and Enteral Nutrition (BAPEN))

www.bda.uk.com (British Dietetic Association)

www.bnf.org (British National Formulary)

www.nutrition.org.uk (British Nutrition Foundation)

www.defra.gov.uk (Department for Environment, Food and Rural Affairs)

www.dh.gov.uk (Department of Health)

www.foodstandardsagency.gov.uk (Food Standards Agency)

www.joannabriggs.edu.au (Joanna Briggs Institute)

www.breastfeeding.nhs.uk (NHS Breastfeeding)

www.hda.nhs.uk (Health Development Agency)

www.nelh.nhs.uk/maternity (MIDIRS informed choice)

www.nhlbi.nih.gov/aboutframington (National Heart, Lung and Blood Institute)

www.npsa.nhs.uk (National Patients Safety Agency)

www.nmc-uk.org (Nursing and Midwifery Council)

www.nhshealthquality.org (Nursing and Midwifery Practice Development Unit (NMPDU))

www.rcpsych.ac.uk (Royal College of Psychiatrists)

www.rcplondon.ac.uk (Royal College of Physicians)

www.sign.ac.uk/guidelines (Scottish Intercollegiate Clinical Guidelines)

Eliminating

Jackie Solomon

INTRODUCTION

Elimination is an activity that individuals undertake several times throughout each day and is necessary to rid the body of the waste products (urine and faeces) associated with metabolism. It is an activity that is undertaken in private. Influenced by societal and cultural norms, the inability of individuals to control elimination is often frowned upon in all but the very young child. The ability to control elimination is referred to as being 'continent' and relies on mature physiological systems. Illness or disability may impact on the ability to remain continent. Problems associated with elimination may impact and compromise many of the other Activities of Living (ALs), such as mobilising, eating and drinking, expressing sexuality, personal cleansing and dressing, working and playing, and maintaining a safe environment. Each AL is closely related to the others (Roper et al 2000) and it is important that the nurse takes these into consideration when assessing, planning, implementing and evaluating care of patients.

This chapter will therefore focus on the following:

- elimination in health and illness
- dependence/independence in the AL of elimination
- factors influencing the AL of elimination
- nursing care of individuals with health problems affecting the AL of elimination.

THE MODEL OF LIVING

ELIMINATION IN HEALTH AND ILLNESS (ACROSS THE LIFESPAN)

Childhood and adolescence

At birth babies have no control of their bladder or bowels and depend solely on their parents to keep them dry and clean. Most children will gain control around the age of 18 months and many children will be dry during the daytime by the time they reach 3 years with boys taking longer than girls to do so. As soon as the child is able to recognise the need to pass urine or faeces and is able to understand simple instructions and pull his/her clothes up and down, parents will begin potty training. Later when the child progresses to using the toilet they may require a low stool and toddler seat to make it less daunting and easier to sit on. A boy will learn that it is acceptable to stand to pass urine and in front of other children. In the early days a child is likely to have 'accidents' when they lose control and are incontinent, especially if they are upset, excited, distracted or engrossed in something.

> **Exercise**
> 1. Reflect on your own childhood. Can you recall an event or situation in which you were unable to control your bladder or bowel? What were you doing at the time? How did you feel?
> 2. How does society view the young child who is unable to control his bladder? Would this attitude change if this were an older person?

Environmental and psychological factors can have an influence on a child's toileting regime. During a period of excitement, activity or fear, a child may become incontinent. Some children may suppress the need to go to the toilet in a different environment, for example at school, preferring instead to use their own toilet at home. It is important to be sympathetic and provide reassurance about any accidents. If the child gets worried then the problem may become worse. Whilst society understands that a young child is unable to control their bladder, it is much less tolerant of the older child or adult who is incontinent.

Enuresis

If a child is unable to control his or her bladder either during the day or night this is known as enuresis. Daytime wetting can be either due to delaying the need to go to the toilet, giggling, or urge incontinence due to detrusor instability (Rogers 2002). Being dry at night takes a little longer and there are the inevitable bedwetting accidents. Bedwetting or nocturnal enuresis is the most common type of incontinence in childhood and affects 15% of 5 year olds;

7% of 8 year olds; 5% of 10 year olds; and 2% of 15 year olds. Around 15% of children per annum are cured spontaneously. Less than 50% of parents who have a child who wets the bed seek medical advice and children from socially deprived areas are less likely to be brought to the attention of medical staff (Hjalmas et al 2004). Usually the reason is unknown; although it may be caused by urinary tract infection or congenital abnormalities, and it can run in families.

Most children are able to control their bladder by the age of five; however, boys may take a little longer. If a child continues to wet the bed and has no other urinary symptoms or disease this is known as nocturnal enuresis (Glazener et al 2003). Some children who have been dry for some time may begin to wet the bed again. This is known as secondary enuresis and may occur if a child is upset or feeling insecure, for example if a new baby has arrived in the family. During the foot and mouth outbreak in 2001, a number of children living in Cumbria were reported as suffering from secondary enuresis (Beaton 2001). It is important to give encouragement and support and identify those children who require physiological and psychological help at an early stage.

> **Exercise**
> 1. What do you think are the consequences of bedwetting (a) for the child, (b) for the parents?
> 2. What practical advice might be offered to a parent whose child suffers from nocturnal enuresis?

You may have found out about local and national support groups and organisations that provide written information to parents such as the Enuresis Resource and Information Centre (ERIC) (www.enuresis.org.uk) or the Continence Foundation (www.continence-foundation.org.uk). These organisations provide information and practical help to parents and professionals. They may be able to put parents in contact with other parents with children with similar problems. The general practitioner will be able to undertake a physical examination to determine if there are any physical or congenital abnormalities and to exclude a urinary infection. Local health services may have a team of health professionals including specialist nurses, physiotherapists and psychologists to provide expert advice and therapy.

There are a number of treatments or interventions for children of school age with nocturnal enuresis. These include: enuresis alarms, dry bed training, the use of star charts, and medication, e.g. antimuscarinic medicines, tricyclic antidepressants or hormones. Enuresis alarms are pads with sensors, which are placed on the bed or worn on the body and an alarm sounds when the child begins to pass water. The use of alarms for nocturnal enuresis is an effective treatment for nocturnal bedwetting in children. Alternatively parents may choose to wake their child every 2 hours to go to the toilet. Both these require a high level of parental intervention. Hormonal or tricyclic antidepres-

sant treatment has been shown to be effective but was not sustained in the long term (Glazener et al 2004).

It may be difficult for parents to cope with continual wet beds and they may become stressed and impatient due to lack of sleep. They may also suffer a financial burden if they need to buy pads and extra bed linen to cope with the wet beds. The child who wets the bed may get teased or bullied at school and their siblings may also ridicule them. Waking up in a cold wet bed is unpleasant and interrupts the child's sleep. As a result they may be unable to concentrate and this could affect their progress in school. Socially, they may be unable to sleep over with friends due to the embarrassment of being woken frequently during the night.

Amanda Page writing under a pseudonym shared her experience of bringing up a daughter with urinary incontinence and how the stigma of incontinence impacted on their relationship to the extent that at the age of 16 her daughter chose to go into the care of the local authority. Reflecting on her experiences Amanda felt the need to be better informed about urinary incontinence to have been able to support her daughter. She also recognised that she herself needed support and the opportunity to speak to other parents in similar situations (Page 1999).

For more information on effective interventions for managing childhood enuresis access the NHS Centre for Reviews and Dissemination University of York CRD Report No. 11, or access National Library for Health (www.prodigy.nhs.uk).

Physical and mental disabilities

Some males may suffer from a condition know as phimosis. Phimosis is a situation where the foreskin or prepuce of the penis is too tight to be retracted over the glans penis. Natural separation of the two layers of the skin occurs around the age of 2 years. If this is attempted before the two layers have naturally separated then scar tissue will form which can lead to urinary retention, pain and discharge. Circumcision may also contribute to phimosis if it is incorrectly performed.

There are some children who are born with neurological lesions such as spina bifida. The location of the lesion will depend on the extent to which the child's ability to pass water is affected. High lesions will result in detrusor and sphincter overactivity and the inability to recognise when they have a full bladder. Many of these children may be wheelchair dependent and may have difficulty accessing toilets as well as managing their clothes without help. For some of these children intermittent catheterisation is usually considered the best option (McMonnies 2002). Children with learning difficulties such as Down syndrome and cerebral palsy may suffer from incontinence; however they respond well to behavioural toilet training sessions (Rogers 2001).

Encopresis

Faecal incontinence or soiling in children is known as encopresis and is defined as the passage of a normal consistency

stool or an incomplete or loose stool in a socially inappropriate place. It is common in children with best estimates suggesting that 1.5% of children still lack bowel control by their 7th birthday (see Box 7.1) (Royal College of Physicians 1995). There are a number of factors and health problems why children may not achieve faecal continence, including failure or delay in normal development, neurological deficiency, and abnormality of the anal sphincter muscles, faecal retention, incorrect laxative treatment and psychological and emotional problems. Children may suffer from one or more of these health problems and both they and their parents will require input and support from a multidisciplinary team. The possibility of invasive procedures and investigations can be very distressing and add to the psychological and emotional turmoil for both the child and their parents (Royal College of Physicians 1995).

Adulthood

In adulthood we are expected to have full control of our bladder and bowels. Incontinence is the inability to maintain voluntary control resulting in excretion of urine and/or faeces in inappropriate places or at inappropriate times (Royal College of Physicians 1995). Often associated with old age, incontinence is a taboo subject and has a significant impact on an individual's personal dignity, social and occupational activity, psychological functioning, and physical and sexual relations.

Around 200 million adults worldwide are estimated to be incontinent (Abrams 2002). The prevalence of incontinence increases with age and is associated with medical problems, injury, cognitive impairment or loss of functional ability and mobility (Sampselle et al 2004). A postal survey within two health authorities in the UK revealed that a large number of adults (23%) had experienced urinary incontinence at some time during their adult years, also those that were incontinent also had a lower health status (Roe & Doll 2000). A Royal College of Physicians (1995) report on incontinence suggested that the prevalence of urinary incontinence is widespread. Whilst it is difficult to measure accurately the prevalence because of the subjective nature of the problem and associated embarrassment, it has been estimated that in the region of six million people within the UK have continence problems (Willis 1999) and further estimations have been provided by the Department of Health (DoH 2000) (see Box 7.2).

Box 7.2	Statistics for the incontinence

For people living at home
- Between 1 in 20 and 1 in 14 w
- Between 1 in 13 and 1 in 7 wor
- Between 1 in 10 and 1 in 5 wom
- Over 1 in 33 men aged 15–64
- Between 1 in 14 and 1 in 10 men a

For people living in institutions
- One in three in residential homes
- Nearly two in every three in nursing h
- Half to two-thirds in wards for elderly a mentally infirm.

Source: Good practice in continence services (Do

Common symptoms of urinary incontin frequency of micturition, needing to go t in the night, a sense of urgency or need to urgently, leakage of urine when trying not to sneezing or coughing, and being incontinen sleep. Pregnancy and childbirth are cited as t cause of incontinence in women (Logan 2005). causes of urinary incontinence in adults include sity, chronic constipation, chronic chest problems weak pelvic floor muscles. Physical exercise, coughin sneezing may exacerbate the problem. The menopaus women is thought to increase the risk of urinary sym toms as a result of hormonal changes and reduction oestrogen levels. In males, diseases of the prostate ma lead to obstruction of the flow of urine. In both males and females retention of urine due to an obstruction can lead to incontinence. Males may also suffer from post-micturition dribble, this is when leakage of urine occurs as the penis is placed back in underclothes. A summary of the age-related disorders associated with incontinence in males is provided in Box 7.3.

Faecal incontinence

Faecal incontinence affects both males and females of all ages. Whilst less prevalent than urinary incontinence it is reported to affect about 2% of the adult population and 7% of healthy independent adults over the age of 65 (Nelson et al 1995, Johanson & Laferty 1996). Sufferers are caused a great deal of embarrassment (Herbert 1999).

Around 30% of women suffer damage to one or both anal sphincter muscles during their first vaginal delivery (Kamm 1998). Forceps deliveries, large baby, a long second stage of labour and occipitoposterior presentation of the fetus are all common risk factors. Of the women who have a third-degree tear during delivery, despite repair, a significant number develop anal incontinence (gas) or urgency (Sultan et al 1993). Anal surgery,

---

Box 7.1	Prevalence rates of children incontinent of faeces

- One in 30 of children aged four to five
- One in 50 of children aged five to six
- One in 75 of children aged seven to ten
- One in 100 of children aged 11 to 12.

Source: Good practice in continence services (DoH 2000).

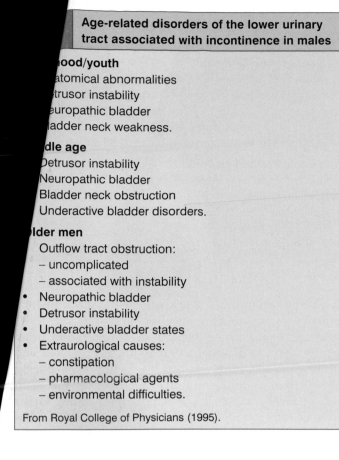

Age-related disorders of the lower urinary tract associated with incontinence in males

...ood/youth
- ...atomical abnormalities
- ...trusor instability
- ...europathic bladder
- ...ladder neck weakness.

...dle age
- Detrusor instability
- Neuropathic bladder
- Bladder neck obstruction
- Underactive bladder disorders.

...lder men
- Outflow tract obstruction:
  - uncomplicated
  - associated with instability
- Neuropathic bladder
- Detrusor instability
- Underactive bladder states
- Extraurological causes:
  - constipation
  - pharmacological agents
  - environmental difficulties.

From Royal College of Physicians (1995).

Box 7.4	Causes of faecal incontinence

Sphincter or pelvic floor damage
- Obstetric trauma
- Direct trauma or injury.

Diarrhoea/intestinal hurry
- Inflammatory bowel disease
- Irritable bowel disease.

Iatrogenic/post surgery
- Post haemorrhoidectomy
- Sphincterotomy for fissure
- Anal stretch.

Anorectal pathology
- Rectal prolapse
- Anal or rectal–vaginal fistula
- Congenital abnormalities.

Neurological disease
- Spinal cord injury
- Multiple sclerosis
- Spina bifida/sacral agenesis
- Parkinson's disease (often secondary to constipation)
- Secondary to degenerative disease, neurological disease, e.g. Alzheimer's, environmental.

Impaction with overflow
- Institutionalised or immobility
- Elderly
- Severe constipation in children.

Environmental
- Poor toilet facilities
- Inadequate care.

Idiopathic
- Unknown causes
- Psychological factors.

From Norton (1996).

structural damage to the internal sphincter, neurological disease and congenital anorectal malformations may also lead to faecal incontinence (Lunniss et al 2004). Faecal incontinence occurs in 50% of people who have multiple sclerosis and is the cause of significant distress (Hinds et al 1990). Norton (1996) provides a useful summary (Box 7.4) of the causes of faecal incontinence. For further information see Brooker & Nicol (2003) or Alexander et al (2006).

Older people

Whilst people at all ages may be affected by inability to remain in control of bladder and bowel functions it is more prevalent in the older person and in particular the frail older person due to the loss of muscular control, changes to the central nervous system, atrophic vaginitis, cerebrovascular disease, constipation, immobility and drug usage (see Box 7.5). Older people also tend to pass more during the night due to changes in homeostatic mechanisms controlling the production of urine. The prevalence of incontinence is higher in older people living in institutions than in those living in their own homes (Wald 2005). A recent pilot audit undertaken by the Royal College of Physicians (2004) showed that in care homes 46% of people were incontinent of urine and 43% incontinent of faeces.

Exercise
1. Reflect on your own personal views of elimination and the older person. It is important for you to appreciate your own views on this, as it will have a direct effect on the nature of your assessment of patients' needs and care planning.

The care of the older person is one of the key priorities for the NHS in England and in order to reduce inequalities the Government has published a National Service Framework for Older People (DoH 2001c). The framework sets out the standards for services for the older person and aims to ensure these are delivered to the same standard irrespective of geographical location (Box 7.6).

Box 7.5 | **Causes of faecal incontinence in later life**

1. Constipation/faecal impaction with overflow incontinence.
2. Neurogenic incontinence – due to loss of cortical inhibition in dementia.
3. Colorectal disease
   - colorectal cancer
   - diverticular disease
   - inflammatory bowel disease.
4. Causes of diarrhoea
   - drug-induced (e.g. laxatives, magnesium-containing antacids, iron preparations)
   - gastric and small bowel disorders
   - irritable bowel disease.
5. Anal sphincter defects, rectal prolapse.
6. Factors relating to access to toilets and handling clothing, in association with impaired mobility.

From Royal College of Physicians (1995).

Box 7.6 | **Integrated continence services**

Integrated continence services should:

- be in line with published guidance on good practice
- link identification, assessment and treatment across primary, acute and specialist care

and should include:

- primary and community staff giving general advice to older people and their carers about healthy living (in particular diet, and drinking appropriate fluids)
- staff in nursing and residential care homes to identify, assess, treat and review the needs of residents within agreed protocols
- hospital nurses to identify people with incontinence, and to ensure that treatment is provided and that continence needs are assessed and a plan agreed before discharge from hospital
- specialist continence services to provide expert advice and be available to people whose condition does not respond to initial treatment and care
- links to designated medical specialties such as urology and geriatrics
- links to regional and national units for specialist surgery to form part of the care pathway for continence services
- availability and provision of continence aids/equipment
- access to bathing and laundry services
- patients and carers in developing local services.

Source: Integrated Continence Services (DoH 2001c).

Exercise

1. Find out what services are available within your local area for older people who suffer from incontinence.
2. How does the service available reflect the guidance set out in the National Service Framework?
3. If you have access to continence services, arrange to spend some time with the team members during a clinical placement. Find out how patients are assessed and referred for treatment.

The influence of faecal and urinary incontinence on an individual's personal dignity, health, quality of life and self-respect is enormous. The health and social care issues and impact on the individual are summarised in Box 7.7. The National Institute for Health and Clinical Excellence has produced clinical guidelines on the treatment of urinary incontinence (NICE 2006) and on the management of faecal incontinence in adults (www.nice.org.uk). The Continence Foundation provides information for both patients and professionals (www.continence-foundation. org.uk) and the Department of Work and Pensions provides information on benefits available (www.dwp.gov.uk).

Box 7.7 | **Impact on the individual**

As a health issue incontinence can:

- cause skin breakdown which may lead to pressure sores
- be indicative of other problems in children, such as emotional problems rather than physical discorders.

As a social issue, faecal and urinary incontinence can:

- lead to bullying of children at school, adults in the workplace and older people in residential care and nursing homes
- in children, cause emotional and behavioural problems
- restrict employment, educational and leisure opportunities
- result in people moving to residential and nursing homes – incontinence is only second to dementia as an initiating factor for such moves
- cause conflict between the individual and their carer
- cause soiling and ruin clothes and bedding leading to extra laundry costs and increased expense for those items.

From DoH (2000).

DEPENDENCE/INDEPENDENCE IN THE AL OF ELIMINATING

Dependence/independence in the ALs is closely related to a person's lifespan (Roper et al 1996, 2000). Viewed as a continuum it is central to the concept of the model (see Chapter 1).

Babies and young children rely on adults to keep them clean and dry. From the age of five most children are able to undertake this activity independently during the daytime. However, in some cases it may take longer at night. Children who are physically disabled or suffer from learning difficulties may be dependent on others to assist them in elimination.

Likewise most adults remain independent in this activity for the most part of their life unless illness, injury or disability occurs.

Exercise

Mary is an 85-year-old lady who lives alone. She has recently been discharged from hospital following surgery for a fractured neck of femur. She walks with a walking frame and is finding it difficult to get upstairs to her toilet.

1. Find out what help is available for Mary. What might be put in place to help Mary be independent in the activity of elimination?

If physically or mentally disabled, individuals are likely to require help in the form of aids and adaptations to their accommodation to help them to be independent in the activity of elimination. In Mary's case you may have considered asking an occupational therapist, physiotherapist or social worker to visit her in her own home to assess how she might be helped to maintain her independence in the activity of elimination. Vickerman & Whitehead (2001) outline the benefits to patient care of adopting a multidisciplinary approach. Mary may benefit from adaptations to her home to enable her to maintain her independence, for example a stair lift may help Mary to get upstairs to the toilet. She may also require grab rails to assist her getting on and off the toilet. A social worker would be able to assess if she would be eligible for financial assistance to enable her to fund extra help or to access other resources.

Other patients may be unable to pass urine without the aid of a catheter or evacuate their bowels without the assistance of a nurse or carer. Within most cultures elimination is a very private activity and having to depend on others to assist in this private and personal Activity of Living can be very humiliating. Nurses must ensure privacy and dignity and take account of the patient's cultural needs and self-esteem when assisting with elimination.

Diseases of the intestinal tract and urinary tract may require surgical intervention or a temporary or permanent diversion on to the abdomen to enable passage of waste products from the body. In these cases patients are dependent on stoma appliances and the assistance from specialist nurses, e.g. stoma nurses, to teach them how to become independent in managing their stoma care, emptying their stoma bags and coping with the change in body image and functions. For further information see Alexander et al (2006) and Fillingham & Douglas (2004).

Exercise

1. Find out what services exist in your area for patients who have had a urostomy, ileostomy or colostomy.
2. What advice is given to patients on how to manage their stoma?
3. When is this advice given?
4. If you have access to a specialist team, make arrangements to spend some time with the team. Find out how patients are referred, managed and what support is available in the community.

You may have found out about a specialist nursing service within your local area. These nurses work as part of a multidisciplinary team including medical staff, physiotherapists, occupational therapists, clinical psychologists, surgical appliance officers and community nurses to provide a comprehensive service. Advice and counselling is provided prior to surgery and the patient is encouraged to be involved in their own care as soon as they are able following surgery.

FACTORS INFLUENCING THE AL OF ELIMINATING

This section will help you to understand the factors influencing the activity of elimination. Each of these will now be explored.

Biological factors

Any living organism must eliminate waste products. In human beings this is achieved through the renal system and urinary tract as urine and the intestinal tract as faeces. Elimination is also under neurological control.

Renal system

Normally each individual has two kidneys that lie on the dorsal wall of the abdomen. Each kidney consists of a million nephrons and collecting tubules and receives a supply of blood from the renal artery and a capillary network of arterioles (see Fig. 7.1). A good blood supply to the kidneys is crucial in maintaining their functioning (McLaren 2005) (see Fig. 7.2). The kidneys also play an important part in maintaining homeostasis by regulating the water and electrolyte content and acid–base balance of the body (see Box 7.8).

The removal of the waste products of metabolism is achieved through a process of ultrafiltration and

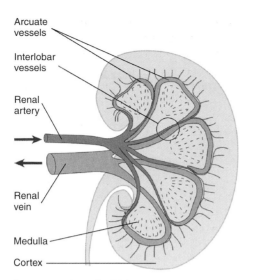

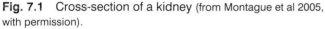

Fig. 7.1 Cross-section of a kidney (from Montague et al 2005, with permission).

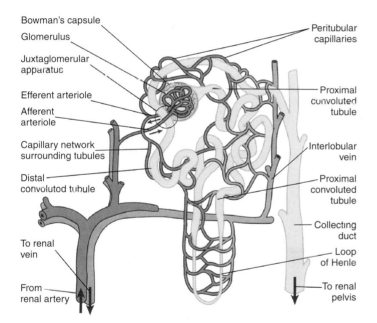

Fig. 7.2 Anatomy of a nephron with associated blood supply (from Montague et al 2005, with permission).

reabsorption in the nephrons and passed via the ureter into the bladder, before being excreted as urine. Urine consists of urea, creatinine, uric acid, sulphates and nitrates (Box 7.9) (see Appendix 2).

Each day an average healthy adult will excrete in the region of 1–1.5 litres of urine. The exact amount will depend on a number of factors such as how much fluid has been taken in, diet and the amount of water lost in sweat and expired air.

Exercise

1. Monitor your fluid intake and your urine output for 24 hours.
2. Is there any difference in volume in your intake and your output?
3. How many times did you pass urine?

You will have found that intake roughly matches output. However, this can depend on your activities during the day and the type of fluid that you drank. For example, if you are exercising your may lose more water in sweat and expired air. Some substances such as alcohol and caffeine act as diuretics and increase the urine flow. Recording a patient's intake and output of urine is an important responsibility for the nurse and will aid diagnosis and treatment. For instance, patients with heart failure may be unable to excrete fluid and because of this may develop dyspnoea and peripheral oedema. Recognising this early will enable timely medical intervention (Herbert & Sheppard 2005).

Urine

Observing and reporting the colour and odour of urine can inform diagnosis. For example, cloudy urine may indicate infection, whereas dark urine may indicate that a patient is dehydrated or the presence of bilirubin. Undertaking

Box 7.8	Principle function of the kidney

The kidney has four main functions:

1. The removal of the nitrogenous waste products of metabolism
2. Regulation of acid–base and other electrolyte balances
3. Maintenance of water balance
4. Production of erythrogenin (renal erythropoietic factor) and biologically active form of vitamin D.

Source: McLaren (2005).

Box 7.9	The composition of urine in an adult
pH	5.0–6.0
Osmolality	500–800 mosmol
Specific gravity	1.003–1.030
Urea	200–500 mmol/l
Creatinine	9–17 mmol/l
Sodium ions	50–130 mmol/l
Potassium ions	20–70 mmol/l
Organic acids	10–25 mmol/l
Protein	0–50 mg/24 h
Urochrome	Traces
Glucose	0–11 mmol/l
Cellular components (epithelial cells, leucocytes)	< 20 000/l

From Valtin (1979). Source: McLaren (2005).

urinalysis on the ward or in a clinic allows the nurse to measure the pH and test for the presence of protein, glucose, ketones, blood and bilirubin. Urine that smells offensive can often suggest the presence of an infection. Accurate recording of the results in the nursing care plan or patient record is essential. Often the nurse will be expected to obtain a specimen for laboratory testing. In this case, it is best obtained first thing in the morning before being diluted by fluid intake later in the day.

Exercise

1. If you are a student nurse undertaking a clinical placement, test a patient's urine, observe and report your findings to your mentor and discuss the significance of your results. Find out what should be recorded in the patient's nursing care plan or medical notes.
2. Find out what the presence of glucose in the urine (glycosuria) would indicate.

Examination and testing of urine can reveal a great deal of information about a patient's urinary and kidney function. The presence of protein in urine may be an indication of infection. Blood in the urine may indicate a urinary infection but also renal stones or cancer. The presence of glucose in the urine (glycosuria) may suggest that the patient has diabetes mellitus. A patient with diabetes may also pass large volumes of urine (polyuria); in severe cases the patient may become dehydrated. Glucose in the urine may also indicate an acute response to stress. Often further specimens of urine are required for laboratory investigations.

Exercise

1. Find out how to obtain the following for laboratory investigation:
   - early morning specimen of urine
   - midstream specimen of urine
   - catheter sample of urine
   - 24-hour urine collection.
2. Find out why these specimens are required and what the results of these tests may reveal.

You will have found out about the types of organisms and key metabolites that may aid diagnosis, as well as the need to reduce the possibility of contamination when obtaining specimens for culture and sensitivity, and maintaining asepsis when accessing a catheter drainage system.

Micturition

Urine is propelled down the ureters by peristaltic action into the bladder, which is a hollow highly muscular organ lined by epithelial cells (see Fig. 7.3). The bladder holds about 0.5

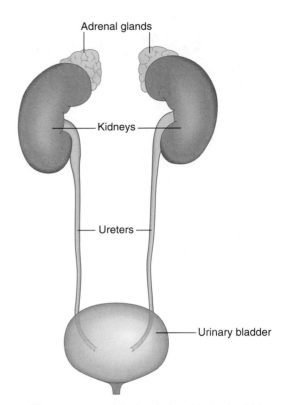

Fig. 7.3 The ureters and their relationship to the kidneys and bladder (from Waugh & Grant 2006, with permission).

litres. The detrusor muscle is a layer of smooth muscle, which lies beneath the lining of the bladder (Fig. 7.4). As the bladder fills the lining stretches and the detrusor muscle contracts, the internal sphincter also contracts. As the urethra widens, the muscles of the pelvic floor relax (Fig. 7.5). This allows the urine to flow into the urethra. For micturition to take place

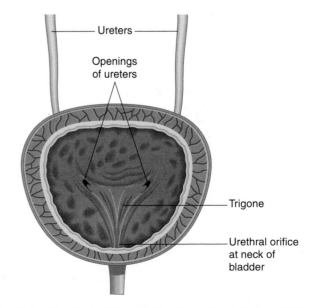

Fig. 7.4 Structure of the bladder (from Waugh & Grant 2006, with permission).

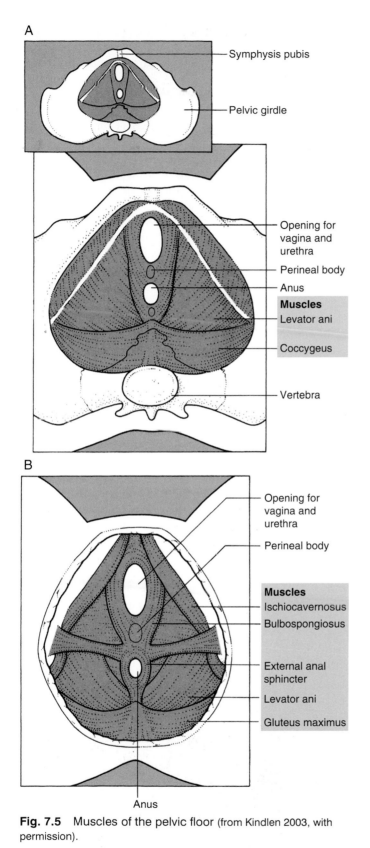

A

- Symphysis pubis
- Pelvic girdle
- Opening for vagina and urethra
- Perineal body
- Anus

Muscles
Levator ani

Coccygeus

- Vertebra

B

- Opening for vagina and urethra
- Perineal body

Muscles
Ischiocavernosus

Bulbospongiosus

External anal sphincter

Levator ani

Gluteus maximus

Anus

Fig. 7.5 Muscles of the pelvic floor (from Kindlen 2003, with permission).

normally the bladder must be healthy and its neural supply intact. Evacuation of urine from the bladder is controlled by both voluntary and involuntary systems (see Fig. 7.6). As the pressure in the bladder increases the bladder wall distends and stimulates the stretch receptors in the wall of the bladder. The external sphincter opens and urine passes into the urethra. As it is not always convenient to pass urine, the voluntary control mechanism via the pudendal nerve will prevent contraction of the external sphincter. There are a number of possible neurogenic causes of incontinence (see Fig. 7.7). For further information see Iggulden (2006).

When it is convenient to pass urine, contraction of the bladder is aided by contraction of the abdominal muscles. This effect of the contraction of the abdominal muscles can be seen when coughing or sneezing. This may result in a leakage, known as stress incontinence; it is usually found in females. The bladder may develop spontaneous contractions,

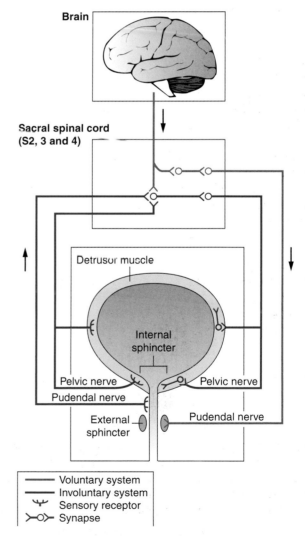

Brain

Sacral spinal cord (S2, 3 and 4)

Detrusor muscle

Internal sphincter

Pelvic nerve

Pelvic nerve

Pudendal nerve

External sphincter

Pudendal nerve

— Voluntary system
— Involuntary system
⋎ Sensory receptor
>○> Synapse

Fig. 7.6 Involuntary and voluntary systems (from Rutishauser 1994, with permission).

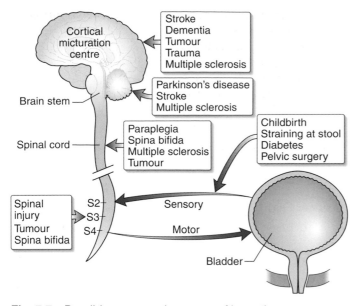

Fig. 7.7 Possible neurogenic causes of incontinence. (Reproduced with kind permission from Coloplast. From Alexander et al 2006, Fig. 24.3, p. 866.)

which result in the intravesical pressure exceeding the intra-urethral pressure, leading to involuntary leakage of urine. This is known as detrusor instability, or in cases where there is known neurological disease, detrusor hyperreflexia.

Urinary retention

In some cases a patient may be unable to empty their bladder or they might be passing frequent small amounts of urine or dribbling. On examination the abdomen might be distended and the bladder palpable, the patient might also be complaining of pain and be distressed. Retention of urine is usually due to an obstruction, e.g. prostatic disease or neurological disease and interruption of the nerve supply. Other reasons include patients who have undergone surgery, lack of privacy, pain and discomfort.

One of the commonest causes of urinary retention is seen in males over the age of 50 who suffer from benign prostatic disease (Selfe 2006). The prostate gland is enlarged and obstructs the normal flow of urine from the bladder (Fig. 7.8). Unable to empty their bladder completely they frequently experience dribbling and frequency. On examination of the abdomen the bladder may be distended. A comprehensive and sensitive nursing assessment is required when dealing with these patients.

Intermittent self-catheterisation may be an option for patients who have atonic bladders or dysynergia, and where the bladder contraction does not synchronise with opening of the urethral sphincter. These patients may be constantly wet or suffer pain from retention of urine that requires urgent medical treatment. Intermittent self-catheterisation involves passing a clean catheter into the bladder, draining the urine away and then removing the catheter. A patient is taught to pass the catheter several times a day; this puts the patient in control and improves their quality of life (Hunt et al 1996). Nevertheless, not all patients are able to self-catheterise and a thorough assessment of their manual dexterity, motivation and mental capacity is required before introducing intermittent self-catheterisation. Intermittent catheterisation in older people has been shown to be a valuable alternative to an indwelling catheter (Pilloni et al 2005). However, should a patient be unable to self-catheterise then with the patient's agreement a relative or carer may be trained to undertake the procedure.

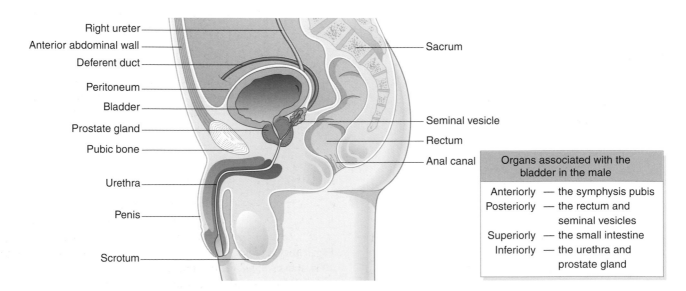

Organs associated with the bladder in the male	
Anteriorly	— the symphysis pubis
Posteriorly	— the rectum and seminal vesicles
Superiorly	— the small intestine
Inferiorly	— the urethra and prostate gland

Fig. 7.8 The male urinary system (from Waugh & Grant 2006, with permission).

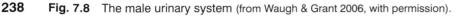

Urinary catheterisation

In some situations, following a full assessment and informed consent of the patient the bladder may be emptied by insertion of a urethral catheter on a continuous or intermittent basis. However, catheterisation should not be performed without routine and careful consideration as it poses a significant risk of infection for patients (Pratt et al 2001). Insertion of a catheter must be undertaken under strict aseptic technique and with care to lessen the risk of trauma. Depending on the reason for catheterisation, the catheter may be left in place or removed and inserted intermittently if necessary. If the catheter is left in place, the urine can be collected in a urine bag which is attached to the catheter and to the patient's leg or alternatively on a stand under the bed. It is important that urine bags are kept below the height of the bladder to encourage drainage and that catheters are observed for kinking so that the risk of retention is reduced. It is also important not to disconnect the catheter from the drainage bag unnecessarily so that the risk of infection is reduced. This is known as maintaining a closed system. Urinary catheterisation should not be undertaken without considering the risks involved. Catheterisation increases the risk of acquiring a urinary tract infection, increasing a patient's length of stay in hospital, increased use of antibiotics and increased morbidity (Tew et al 2005). The use of bladder ultrasound to assess urine volume has been shown to reduce unnecessary catheterisation in patients with neurological problems (Lee et al 2007).

Long-term catheterisation in the management of incontinence should only be undertaken after all other options have been explored. The nurse must consider the patient's wishes, lifestyle and likelihood of compliance.

Exercise

1. If you are a student nurse undertaking a clinical placement find out about the infection control guidelines and local policies for catheter care and how you would care for a patient with a catheter, and what you need to record in the patient's notes.
2. Discuss with your mentor and personal tutor the knowledge and skills you need to care for a patient with a catheter and undertake catheterisation safely and competently.
3. Find out what types of urine collection devices are available.

You may have discussed the following:

- importance of informed consent (DoH 2001a)
- principles of asepsis
- indication for catheterisation including advantages and disadvantages
- anatomy and physiology of both the female and male urethra and bladder
- counselling skills
- knowledge of the different types of catheters available, indications for use and product liability
- procedure for catheterisation
- recording observations
- problems that might arise, e.g. blocked catheter, leaking urine and how to deal with these
- patient self-management
- other options and alternatives to catheterization.

For further information see Selfe (2006) and Colpman & Welford (2004).

Urinary tract infections

Infection of the urinary tract is common in women. The close proximity of the vagina to the urethra allows the passage of organisms normally found in the bowel and perineum into the urinary tract more easily than in males (Selfe 2006) (Fig. 7.9).

Normally the route of the infection is through the bladder but in some cases the infection may enter through the bloodstream. Pyelonephritis is an infection of the renal pelvis. Patients may present with a sudden onset of pain in the loin radiating to the iliac fossa. They may also have pyrexia, rigors, nausea and vomiting. A midstream specimen of urine should be collected and sent for bacteriological examination. Once the bacterial organism is identified then the doctor will prescribe the appropriate antibiotic. However, it is important that further diagnostic investigations are undertaken to understand the underlying cause of the infection.

Exercise

1. Find out which organisms are likely to cause a urinary tract infection.
2. What are the predisposing factors for urinary tract infection?
3. What other investigations would be undertaken to assist diagnosis?
4. What advice would you give to a patient to prevent recurrence of a urinary tract infection?

Organisms likely to be involved are *Escherichia coli*, *Klebsiella*, proteus, pseudomonas, *Streptococcus faecalis* and *Staphylococcus albus*. Some of the factors which predispose to urinary infection are listed in Box 7.10.

Urinary investigations for urinary tract infections

Investigations may include:

- routine ward testing using a dipstick
- collection of a midstream specimen of urine (MSU), which is sent to the laboratory for culture and sensitivity. The MSU should be collected under clean conditions to reduce the risk of contaminants
- a full blood count, urea and electrolytes
- an ultrasound scan to identify any obstruction.

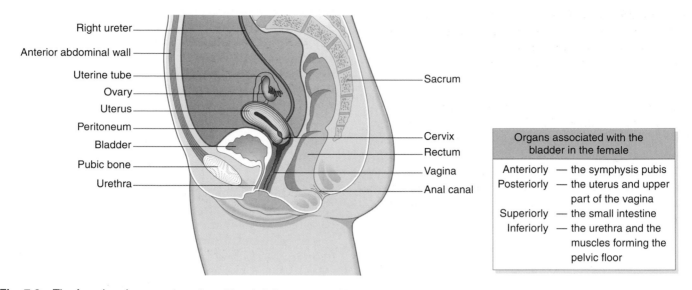

Fig. 7.9 The female urinary system (from Waugh & Grant 2006, with permission).

The nurse has an important role in health promotion and the prevention of recurrence of urinary tract infections by providing advice to patients on handwashing and personal hygiene, in particular after defecation.

Box 7.10	Urinary infection: predisposing factors

Vesico-ureteric reflux
This may be congenital or acquired.

Obstruction such as stricture, tumours of the bladder, prostate or kidneys
The inability to empty the bladder (urinary retention) due to stricture or abnormality of neighbouring organs may result in a build-up of pressure and backflow on the kidneys. This predisposes the individual to urinary tract infection, formation of stones and possible renal impairment.

Fistula
An abnormal opening between the bowel and the bladder will allow organisms to pass into the urinary tract.

Sexual trauma
The female ureter may suffer trauma during sexual intercourse and allow the passage of organisms.

Personal hygiene
Lack of attention to personal hygiene, contamination from the rectal area or inadequate hygiene facilities may also predispose to urinary tract infection.

Surgical and diagnostic procedures
Unless strict asepsis is maintained medical and nursing interventions such as catheterisation can introduce organisms or indeed exacerbate an existing infection.

Adapted from Selfe (2006).

Pelvic floor muscles
The pelvic floor muscles support the bowel, the bladder and in women the uterus (see Fig. 7.5). The muscles are attached to the inner surface of the pelvic girdle. The urethra, anus and the vagina in women pass through openings in these muscles. Weak pelvic floor muscles due to repeated heavy lifting, surgery, obesity, constipation, chronic cough and lack of general fitness both in men and women can lead to incontinence. In women, childbirth and the menopause are also major factors. Pelvic floor exercises can help to increase the power of the pelvic floor muscles to aid urinary continence.

Exercise
1. If you are female, find your pelvic floor muscles by placing the tip of your finger in or against your vagina. Try to contract the muscle against your finger.
2. If you are male, find your pelvic floor muscles by placing your finger just behind your scrotum. When you try to contract your muscles you will feel them tighten away from your fingers. This should give you some idea of the strength of your pelvic floor muscles.
3. Now find out how to do pelvic floor exercises and how often they need to be done.

You will have discovered that pelvic floor exercises need to work against gravity and so they should be done either standing or sitting upright. Sitting on a chair you should concentrate on lifting your perineum off the chair by tightening the muscle inwards and lifting up at the same time. Make sure you are not moving your leg or thigh muscles and buttocks or pulling in your abdominal muscles. Pelvic floor exercises should be done regularly. The pelvic floor muscles consist of different muscle fibres, which need to be

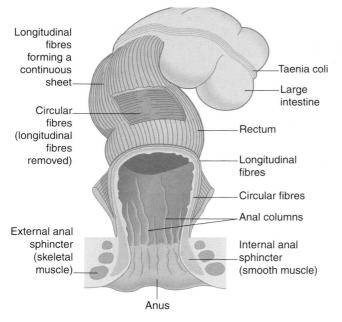

Fig. 7.11 Arrangements of muscle fibres in the colon, rectum and anus (from Waugh & Grant 2006, with permission).

Exercise

1. Find out why people who have had a stroke are likely to suffer from faecal incontinence.

You will have found out those patients who have damage to their pudendal nerve or spinal cord because of a stroke, due to loss of voluntary sphincter control, may not be able to inhibit defecation until a time when it is convenient. This may result in faecal incontinence whilst in some cases patients may need to evacuate their rectum manually in order to eliminate faeces. In addition to neurogenic causes, patients who have had a stroke may experience functional factors including immobility, medication, communication etc.

Kamm (1998) suggests that faecal incontinence affects 2% of all adults and 7% of all adults over the age of 65 years and is more prevalent in females and patients with multiple sclerosis, spinal injuries and congenital disorders. A summary of the causes of faecal incontinence can be found in Box 7.12.

Stool assessment

The colour and consistency of faeces and any alteration in a person's pattern of defecation may indicate a potential health problem. Hence, the importance of assessing the patient's normal bowel habits and reporting any abnormal findings to the doctor. Careful assessment and recording of the frequency and appearance of stools in the patient's nursing care plan or health record is an important part of nursing care. The Bristol Stool Chart devised by Dr KW Heaton

Box 7.12	**Causes of faecal incontinence in adults**
Causes of faecal incontinence in adults	Common examples
Sphincter or pelvic floor damage	Obstetric trauma Direct trauma or injury
Diarrhoea	Inflammatory bowel disease Irritable bowel syndrome
Iatrogenic/post surgical	Post haemorrhoidectomy, sphincterotomy for fissure or anal stretch
Anorectal pathology	Spinal cord injury Multiple sclerosis Spina bifida Parkinson's disease (usually secondary to constipation) Secondary to degenerative neurological disease, e.g. Alzheimer's disease, dementia (environmental, see below)
Impaction with overflow 'spurious diarrhoea'	Institutionalised or immobile elderly
Environmental	Poor toilet facilities Inadequate care
Idiopathic	Unknown cause Possible psychological factors

From Norton (1996).

is a tool used in some areas to aid accurate and descriptive recording in the patient's notes; this ensures consistency between members of the clinical team (Heaton 1999).

Exercise

The following are abnormal types of stools that you may come across. Find out what each indicates:

- black and tarry (malaena)
- maroon
- bright red (blood)
- putty coloured
- black stool
- diarrhoea.

You may have found out that the first three types of stools indicate some form of bleeding in the gastrointestinal tract. A malaena stool is an indication of bleeding from the upper gastrointestinal tract caused by oesophageal varices, bleeding duodenal ulcer or peptic ulcer. Malaena has a characteristic smell of altered blood due to the action of digestive enzymes. The maroon stool indicates bleeding from the lower gastrointestinal tract, possible causes include inflammatory bowel disease and malignancy. The presence of fresh blood is usually due to haemorrhoids but could also indicate malignancy or inflammatory bowel disease.

A bulky, pale foul-smelling coloured stool is indicative of an obstruction to the flow of bile into the duodenum.

Diarrhoea

Diarrhoea, a loose watery stool, or a stool that assumes the shape of its container, may be the result of an infection, medication, e.g. antibiotics, laxative abuse, inflammatory conditions such as ulcerative colitis or irritable bowel syndrome, malabsorption syndrome, stress, tumours or thyrotoxicosis. Diarrhoea is a distressing and embarrassing condition for patients, who will require reassurance and support from nursing staff to help relieve the problems. Strict attention of the nurse and the patient to handwashing and personal hygiene is essential to reduce the risk of cross-infection. Diarrhoea can also be present in patients who are constipated as a result of faecal overloading and irritation of the lining of the intestine. For further information see Brooker & Nicol (2003) or Montague et al (2005).

Constipation

The food residue can remain in the colon for 2–3 days as water and salts are gradually reabsorbed. The longer the residue remains the more water is absorbed and the faeces will become compact and hard, possibly leading to constipation.

Everyone has an individual pattern of defecation. Constipation is when that pattern is less frequent than normal and stools are hard and difficult to pass. A frequency of less than three times a week has been used as an objective measure to define constipation (Wald 2005). Symptoms associated with constipation include flatulence, bloating, abdominal pain and a feeling of incomplete evacuation, nausea, headaches and fatigue. Factors which may increase the likelihood of constipation include: diet, fluid intake, lack of exercise, poor dental health, pain on defecation, drug regimes and psychological factors such as impaired cognitive function and anxiety, and socioeconomic status (Miller et al 2006). Constipation in women can also cause incontinence of urine due to pressure of the loaded rectum on the urethra (see Fig. 7.12). Again an accurate nursing assessment should be made including questions about frequency and consistency of stools, access to a toilet or commode, mobility and dexterity and any urinary incontinence or leakage. The nurse should be aware that the patient may feel embarrassed to talk about their bowel and therefore should ensure privacy when undertaking a nursing assessment.

Treatment for constipation may include a change in dietary habits and increase in the fibre content in the diet such as wholemeal bread, bran and fruit and intake of fluids.

Any medication should be reviewed regularly, especially analgesics such as opiates as a common side-effect is constipation (British National Formulary 2006). Laxatives remain the most common choice of treatment; they work by (a) increasing the bulk of the stool, (b) stimulating the intestinal motility, or (c) softening the stool by increasing water absorption by osmosis.

In some instances it may be necessary for a nurse to undertake a rectal examination to examine for faecal loading. Whilst every attempt should be made to avoid manual evacuation, Powell & Rigby (2000) point out that it may be the only viable method of evacuating the bowel in some cases. This should only be undertaken by a nurse who is professionally competent to do so, following individual assessment and with the informed consent of the patient (Nursing and Midwifery Council (NMC) 2004, Royal College of Nursing (RCN) 2003, DoH 2001a, 2001b). The nurse should also take account of the cultural and religious beliefs of the patient.

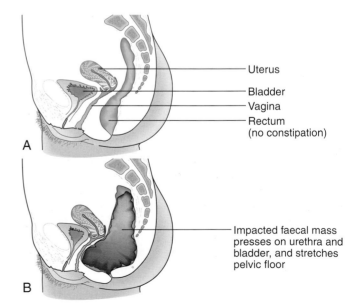

Fig. 7.12 How constipation can cause incontinence. Female, side view, (A) normal, (B) impacted. (Reproduced with kind permission from Coloplast.)

Useful resources to guide you in this exercise are the *Royal Marsden Manual of Nursing Procedures* (Dougherty & Lister 2004) and *Digital Rectal Examination and Manual Removal of Faeces* (RCN 2003).

Psychological factors

Psychology is concerned with explaining the way people think, behave and experience the world. Roper et al (1996, p. 25) state that 'psychological factors cannot be considered in isolation; they are related to biological and also sociocultural, environmental and politicoeconomic factors'. Psychological factors and perspectives influence individuality and the way a person undertakes each AL across the lifespan.

Kenworthy et al (2002) outline four main psychological theories or perspectives, which seek to explain human psychological development:

- the psychodynamic perspective
- the behaviourist perspective
- the cognitive perspective
- the humanist perspective.

Nurses will need to draw on these psychological theories and perspectives when assessing planning, implementing and evaluating care. Psychological problems which nurses may consider include: stress of coping with elimination problems, altered body image, self-esteem and sexuality.

Eliminating is a personal Activity of Living and patients may be too embarrassed to talk about their urinary and bowel functions. Incontinence has an impact on the quality of life and psychological wellbeing of individuals (Shaw 2001). The extent to which people with incontinence seek help depends on their knowledge of the problem and treatment options, how severe they believe the symptoms to be and the resources they have available to deal with the problem (Shaw 2001). As a result they may delay seeking help until they feel more able to do so or they feel unable to cope by which time the problem will have been present for a few days if not longer.

Health beliefs

Each of us may hold a different view or belief of what is health and what is illness. A patient's health beliefs will guide how they access health services and take responsibility for their own health. For example, an older person who believes that problems with eliminating are part of the natural process of ageing may not seek the help of professionals believing that nothing can be done or the problem is outside their control. Equally people may associate old age with incontinence and accept it as the norm.

Health locus of control

The extent to which individuals will take responsibility for their own health is dependent on what they regard as controllable by themselves or others (Ogden 2004). The extent to which a person will take responsibility for their own health will depend upon their locus of control (Wilkinson 2002). Consequently a person who has a problem with incontinence may decide to seek out the help of a health professional to assist in making a decision about how they can take responsibility for managing or taking ownership of the problem (internal locus of control). Alternatively, if they believe that their situation is outside their control, they may hand over the responsibility for making decisions for their health to the health professional (external locus of control). A literature review by Shaw (2001) found evidence to suggest that different personality types might also influence the outcome of treatment for incontinence, with introverted patients responding better to bladder training than extroverts. Consider the following exercise.

Firstly, by adopting an internal locus of control she would want to begin to understand her problem and question how she might work with the physiotherapist to manage the problem. She would seek out other sources of information and would possibly join self-help groups.

In the second scenario, she would adopt a more passive role and expect the physiotherapist and GP to provide information and take ownership of her problem. She may also fail to comply with the instructions and exercises provided by the physiotherapist. Understanding a patient's health belief will assist the nurse when planning care and providing health education.

The concept of classical conditioning developed by Pavlov in the late 19th century and operant conditioning by BF Skinner in the mid 1900s underpins the behaviourist perspective (Wilkinson 2002). Nurses may choose to use these theories by positively reinforcing activities that contribute to achieving continence, for example giving rewards and praise for remaining dry or prompts to confused patients to visit the toilet at regular intervals. Research undertaken by McDowell et al (1999) showed that behaviour therapies could reduce incontinence in older people who were cognitively intact. Using a randomised crossover trial the intervention group received behaviour therapies, e.g. pelvic floor exercises, bladder retraining and urge and stress strategies. Nurses also visited them at regular intervals and spent much more time with them than those patients in the control group. The control group of patients received the information on the exercises without the behaviour therapy interventions. Patients who received behaviour therapies and increased input from nursing staff had fewer incidences of incontinence than those who were in the control group.

Stress

Problems associated with the activity of elimination can be a source of shame and stigma and a source of stress. People experience stress in many different ways (Ogden 2004). Requiring help with the activity of elimination can result in loss of a person's sense of dignity and a feeling of 'being like a child', which may lead to anxiety and/or depression. Caring for an incontinent person can be a major source of stress for carers who are required to help with toileting, faced with constant laundry and lack of personal time.

There is a relationship between stress and disease (Wilkinson 2002). As well as certain types of food, stress is thought to be an important factor in irritable bowel disease (Heitkemper et al 1998, Smith & Fawcett 2003). Stress management and counselling and dietary advice are helpful. In some cases where the patient is anxious or depressed, psychotherapy may be helpful, although in all cases investigations should be undertaken to exclude more sinister bowel disease.

Exercise

1. Think about a stressful situation you may have experienced.
2. What impact did the stressful situation have on your urinary and intestinal systems?

You may have thought about an exam situation, an interview for a new post or a presentation to a group of people. Prior to the event or situation you may have visited the toilet frequently or experienced loose stools.

Sociocultural factors

Elimination is undertaken in private and in some cultures separate facilities are provided for males and females. The facilities provided can, however, differ depending on the country. Facilities also differ according to economic, religious and cultural needs, for example in many places in Europe and in Asia the toilet facility is a hole in the ground.

Exercise

Think about a country that you may have visited.

1. What toilet facilities were there?
2. Did they differ from what you were normally used to and if so how?
3. How did you feel about this?

You may have visited a country where men and women share the same toilet facilities and felt embarrassed. In some countries you may have experienced urinating or defecating into a hole in the ground. If you are used to sitting on a toilet you may have found the experience uncomfortable or difficult. Likewise a person who is used to this way of life will find sitting on a toilet uncomfortable.

Attitudes to continence are influenced by several factors, including the ability to access appropriate medical help, expectations and education. Country of origin is also thought to influence the attitude of women to their incontinence. A study of migrant women in Australia revealed that Vietnamese and Chinese women were reluctant to discuss their incontinence problems with their families (Burton 1996). It is important to remember that in any community discussing continence is a very sensitive topic and consideration must be given to those people whose first language is not English. Many Muslim women will not disclose their continence problems in the presence of their husbands or a male interpreter (Haggar 1997). They may also refuse to be examined by a male doctor. Incontinence poses specific religious problems for practising Muslim women as passing of urine or faeces during prayer would render them 'unclean' (Wilkinson 2001).

People who suffer from incontinence problems or who require assistance from another to enable them to pass urine or faeces can experience social and cultural isolation, embarrassment and lack of self-esteem, and may isolate themselves from their family and friends. It can also impact on their quality of life, including sleep disturbance, mobility problems and discomfort.

Environmental factors

What is acceptable in one culture and/or religion may not be acceptable in another. Some cultures place emphasis on respecting a person's modesty and segregation. Within England in the late 20th century many wards were designated mixed-sex wards in an attempt to maximise the use of beds. However, for many patients, irrespective of their religious beliefs, being nursed in mixed-sex accommodation caused anxiety and distress. More recently, attempts have been made to eradicate mixed-sex accommodation and improve single-sex accommodation, including separate washing facilities and lavatories in hospitals.

> **Exercise**
> 1. Take some time to walk around the clinical environment.
> 2. Assess how the layout, accommodation and availability of toilet facilities meet the needs of the patients.

Patients whose cultures require strict modesty will find the collection of bodily fluids and substances (e.g. faeces and urine) and investigations involving the rectum or urethra very distressing (Henley & Schott 1999). Facilities that do not afford patients privacy or dignity (e.g. using a bedpan in hospital or in the presence of another person) may lead to constipation and stress. Access to washing facilities is required for South Asians and Muslims who using their left hand wash their perineal area with running water after going to the lavatory. The right hand is reserved for handling food and clean things. These patients need access to a bidet, basin or a jug to be able to pour running water over them.

> **Exercise**
> 1. Undertake an assessment of the toilet and washing facilities in your practice setting. What arrangements are in place for patients who are confined to bed, or use commodes, to wash their hands before eating and after using the toilet?
> 2. Does the environment afford your patients privacy and dignity?
> 3. What facilities are there for patients who are Muslim or have other religious beliefs about elimination activity?

Individuals need access to suitable toilet facilities. In the event of disability, toilet facilities will need to be adapted. For example, a person suffering a stroke will need assistance to go to the toilet until such time as he or she is able to function independently. Adaptations may include raised toilet seats, grab rails and easy access to a suitably placed call bell. Toilets will need to be of sufficient width to allow the carer and person enough space to manoeuvre, including if needing wheelchair access. They should be warm and private. Adequate washing facilities are also required either within the person's own home or within an institution in order to reduce any risk of infection.

Patients who have continence problems should be positioned within easy access of a toilet and assessed regarding their dexterity and ability to mobilise with or without assistance. Assessment and input from physiotherapy and occupational therapy may be helpful here. Adaptations to the environment may be needed to enable the patient to function independently within their own home.

Politicoeconomic factors

Incontinence affects large numbers of people in the UK yet it remains a hidden problem by comparison with other conditions. Despite incontinence being underreported because of embarrassment, stigma and lack of understanding and awareness of treatment available the Continence Foundation (2000) estimated 5 million people over the age of 30 have experienced urinary incontinence and 0.6 million have experienced faecal incontinence. The risk of hospitalisation is greater in people who are aged 65 and over and who suffer from incontinence (RCP 1995). The cost to the NHS in 1997 was reported to be in the region of £47 million (Petticrew 1998).

A number of problems have been previously identified with continence services including variation in type and access to NHS services, the number of staff trained to provide specialist care, lack of involvement of users in determining how services should be provided and variation in the range of treatments provided, and the time patients spent waiting for treatment (DoH 2000). In some areas, because of lack of access to the continence advisor, incontinence pads were offered without assessment and attempting curative treatment. Continence aids are available on the NHS but only after comprehensive assessment and implementation of an evidence-based care plan by a specialist nurse.

> **Exercise**
> 1. Visit your local pharmacy and make a note of the products on sale for people who are incontinent.
> 2. Consider what might be the cost to a person suffering from an incontinence problem.
> 3. What information is available?
> 4. Find out what services are available for people with incontinence problems within your local area.
> 5. What can a patient expect from the service?
> 6. Whilst on a clinical placement find out if there are any standards or benchmarking activities being undertaken for continence.

The Department of Health's *Good Practice in Continence Services* (DoH 2000) sets out a Charter for Continence outlining what a person suffering from incontinence can expect. Delivering the rights outlined in the Charter requires different professionals working at different levels of practice to work in unison. In undertaking the previous exercises you may have found out about a specialist team involving continence nurses and continence physiotherapists working to common policies, procedures and guidelines. They also have a role in supporting and working alongside other practitioners providing expert advice and raising awareness. There may also be a continence service supplying continence aids and providing education and training to both patients and professionals. They may also be working with different community groups to raise awareness of the service and incontinence.

You may also have discovered that some clinical areas are undertaking clinical benchmarking activities based on *Essence of Care* (DoH 2003) to ensure that patients'/clients' bladder and bowel needs are met. More information on this initiative can be found at www.dh.gov.uk.

Exercise

1. Using the *Essence of Care* benchmarks for continence discuss with your mentor how these are being used within the clinical area.
2. Are there any action plans, initiatives or projects underway to ensure that these benchmarks are being met?

Within the first part of this chapter the factors influencing the Activities of Living within the model of living and lifespan have been used to illustrate the activity of eliminating in health and everyday life. By engaging in the exercises and reflective activities it is hoped that the reader has begun to appreciate the complexity of the model and its interrelatedness of the AL of eliminating to the other 11 ALs.

SUMMARY POINTS

1. The ability to eliminate relies on mature physiological systems.
2. Illness or disability can have an impact on elimination.
3. The activity of eliminating is influenced by societal and cultural norms.
4. The prevalence of urinary and faecal incontinence is high.

THE MODEL FOR NURSING

INTRODUCTION

Within this part of the chapter, you will be encouraged to transfer your understanding of eliminating and consider its relationship to other ALs. Using the model for nursing and a main case scenario you will consider what information you will need to develop an assessment framework, identify patient problems and develop a plan of care. If you wish you may choose to record the information on the Patient Assessment Sheets provided in Appendix 3.

Assessing individual needs and problems

If patients' expectations are to be understood and their problems (whether actual or potential) with this AL are to be addressed then an assessment must be undertaken. Assessment involves the following three phases:

- collecting information from the patient and nursing history
- interpreting the information collected
- identifying the patient's actual and potential health problems.

However, to undertake a comprehensive and holistic nursing history it is essential to take account of all the Activities of Living as seen in Chapter 1. This is not only undertaken at the beginning of the patient's episode of care or admission to hospital but is an ongoing and dynamic process. However, before assessing the AL of elimination in ill health the nurse must first of all understand and have knowledge of the AL of elimination in health.

Roper et al (1996) provide us with an *aide mémoire* of areas which may be considered in relation to each of the components of the model of living; these will serve as a reminder of the many dimensions and components of the model which underpin a nursing assessment.

Assessing the individual

Assessment is the cornerstone on which the patient's care is planned, implemented and evaluated. In most cases the nurse undertakes an initial nursing assessment within the first few hours of admission to hospital by gathering information that informs the nursing assessment without overburdening the patient and duplicating assessments. However, it must be remembered that nursing assessment is continuous and patients must be reassessed as their condition changes or in response to the outcome of evaluation.

Using the model of living as a framework to collect information on the patient's normal habits and routines and any factors that might cause the activity to be altered is the first step in applying the Roper et al (1996) model for nursing in practice. Box 7.13 provides a summary of the key factors which may be considered when assessing the activity of elimination.

In most cases the nurse undertakes an initial nursing assessment within the first few hours of admission to hospital. Assessment is the cornerstone on which the patient's care is planned, implemented and evaluated. As stated in Chapter 2 nurses work in partnership with other professionals to deliver an integrated and collaborative approach to care delivery. The introduction of nurse-led pre-assessment clinics within the UK and NHS Direct provide a unique opportunity for early holistic assessment of a patient being admitted to hospital for elective surgery.

Working in collaboration with other health care professionals, nurses are able to gather information that informs the nursing assessment without overburdening the patient and duplicating assessments. This is particularly important where different agencies are involved in providing packages of care for older people. A single assessment process has been introduced in England to ensure that older people are treated as individuals and aims to cut down the number of times a person is required to give information to different agencies regardless of health and social care

Box 7.13	Assessment framework for the activity of elimination

Lifespan
- consider the effect of age on the activity of elimination.

Dependence/independence
- dependence is linked to lifespan and age, e.g. childhood/old age
- dependence is linked to specific needs, e.g. disability
- ill health affects the dependence–independence balance, e.g. trauma, paralysis.

Factors affecting elimination
Biological
- muscle tone
- neurological impairment
- muscular damage, e.g. childbirth
- medication.

Psychological
- attitudes to elimination
- emotional state
- cognitive state.

Sociocultural
- sociocultural similarities/differences
- religion.

Environmental
- access to toilets
- privacy
- home circumstances.

Politicoeconomic
- diet
- access to aids
- finance
- access to health services.

Exercise
1. Arrange to spend some time with a nurse working in a pre-assessment clinic.
2. Find out the purpose of pre-assessment.
3. What information does the nurse collect at pre-assessment?
4. What information is given to the patient prior to admission?
5. How might this information prepare the patient for admission?
6. How might this information be used by the ward nurses?
7. How might this information be used to prepare the patient for discharge?

boundaries (DoH 2001c). The single assessment process is important in ensuring a timely and appropriate discharge process. An ill-planned discharge has the potential to cause great difficulty and stress for patients, their relatives and carers.

Exercise
1. Find out how the single assessment process is undertaken within your clinical area.
2. What do you need to know to contribute to the single assessment process?
3. How does the information collected inform the nursing care plan and discharge?
4. Discuss these with your mentor and tutor.

When assessing the patient the nurse will need to use interviewing, observational and listening skills. In addition she will also need to understand the anatomy and physiology associated with eliminating. Poor or incomplete assessment subsequently leads to poor care planning and implementation of the care plan (Sutcliffe 1990).

Exercise
Consider the following activities and identify which skills you have already and the ones you need to develop when undertaking an assessment of eliminating. In your personal development plan identify how you plan to further develop these skills.

1. **Interviewing**
   - asking open and closed questions relevant to the health status of the patient
   - use of appropriate language
   - determining the priority of the questions to be asked
   - giving information relating and checking understanding
   - involving relatives and carers.
2. **Observation**
   - verbal and nonverbal responses
   - body language
   - appearance
   - vital signs and urinalysis
   - skin condition
   - pain
   - anxiety and stress.
3. **Listening**
   - verbal and nonverbal cues
   - checking out, understanding and giving explanation.

Box 7.14	Using the assessment framework in practice

Lifespan
- How old is the patient?
- Do they have a life history of health problems?
- Is there anything in their life history that may affect the way in which they view their present health problems?

Independence/dependence
- Has the individual experienced any difficulties in relation to independent living?
- Are they able to go out and meet other people or are they dependent on others to transport them?
- Will they experience difficulties in the future as a result of their current health problems?

Factors affecting health
Biological
- From what specific health problem are they suffering?
- What do they understand about their present health status?
- Are there any disabilities?
- Do they take any medication?

Psychological
- Are there any cognitive problems?
- What effect is their health problem having on their emotional wellbeing?
- Is the patient suffering from stress?

Socioeconomic
- Are there any specific spiritual or religious needs that the patient may have?
- How does the health problem impact on working and playing?
- Is the health problem impacting on financial security?

Environmental
- Does the individual have any environmental needs that will affect future care?
- Are there any environmental hazards or risks of infection?
- Is there a need for adaptations or resources?

Politicoeconomic
- What resources could be required to help the individual manage their health problems both in hospital and at home?
- Is the patient aware of the resources that are available?
- Are there any financial constraints compromising recovery or maintenance?
- What effect is this having on their other Activities of Living?

PATIENT ASSESSMENT

A relevant and realistic individualised nursing care plan is founded on a thorough patient assessment. The nursing care plan should aim to:

- solve actual problems
- prevent potential problems becoming actual problems
- prevent solved problems from recurring
- alleviate problems which cannot be solved
- help the person cope with temporary or permanent altered states.

Within this chapter, in addition to the main case scenario, you will be encouraged to transfer your understanding of eliminating to other individual patients and consider its relationship to other ALs. Using the assessment guide consider what information you would obtain from Case study 7.1. You can record the information on the Patient Assessment Sheets provided in Appendix 3.

> **Exercise**
> 1. Consider the questions in Box 7.14 and reflect on how you might use this framework and your knowledge of pre-assessment as a basis for your assessment of this patient in your care.
> 2. Make a list of the questions you might ask and check your answers against those listed below.

Case study 7.1

Cyril

Cyril, a 63-year-old man with a history of recurrent urinary tract infections and an enlarged prostate is admitted to your ward for a transurethral resection of the prostate (TURP).

Using the Activities of Living as a framework for assessment you may consider the questions in Box 7.14.

You may have decided to ask the following questions to identify what the patient's needs are in relation to the ALs, taking account of the lifespan, dependency and factors which contribute to health.

Lifespan
- Benign prostatic hyperplasia is a condition associated with ageing in males.
- Urinary tract infections in men are associated with tumours of the prostate, bladder and kidney (Selfe 2006).
- There is an increase in prostatic cancer in the older male in the West.

Dependency
- Does he require help to get to the toilet?
- How does he manage at home?
- Does he have any help in the home?

Physical
- How long has the problem existed?
- When did the problem start?
- Does he have any pain?
- Does he have any problems starting to micturate?
- Does he have any difficulty stopping micturition?
- Does he have any frequency or urgency?
- Does he have dribbling or incontinence?
- Does he have any nocturia?
- Does he have any haematuria?
- What do his urinalysis and vital signs tell you?
- What medication is he taking?

Psychological
- What does he think the problem is?
- Is the problem worrying him?
- Does he understand the nature and outcome of his proposed treatment?
- Has he had any information?
- How does he feel about being in hospital?
- Is he anxious?
- Is he embarrassed?
- How is he coping with the situation?

Socioeconomic
- How has his problem impacted on his everyday activities?
- Does it affect his ability to interact with other people?
- Has the problem impacted on his family and social life?
- How has he managed at home?
- What support is available from family and carers?
- Does he have any specific cultural or religious practices or needs?

Environmental
- What toilet facilities are there at home, where are these located and are they suitable?
- Are there any risks of further infections?
- Are there any environmental hazards?

Politicoeconomic
- Does the health problem impact on his ability to work?
- Does he need access to resources in the community to enable independent living?
- Are there any financial constraints?

> **Exercise**
> 1. Are there any other questions that you consider relevant to this scenario?

You may have considered his understanding of his condition and his understanding of the treatment for which he has been admitted.

Roper et al (2000) point out that each Activity of Living is interrelated and it is the interaction of each of these that contributes to the individualisation of nursing. Hence it is necessary to assess the patient's other Activities of Living to obtain a holistic view.

> **Exercise**
> 1. Now consider the remaining ALs and identify how you might assess each of these to provide a holistic assessment of the patient.
> 2. Make a list and check these against the suggestions below.

You may have considered and observed the following.

1. **Breathing**
   - Does he have any problems breathing?
   - Does he smoke and if so how many and how often?

2. **Eating and drinking**
   - How much fluid is he drinking?
   - What does his intake and output chart tell us?
   - Does he need any help to eat and drink?
   - How is his appetite?
   - Does he have any dislikes or allergies to food?
   - What is his weight?
   - Has he suffered any weight loss?
   - Does he have any problems with oral hygiene, e.g. dentures, crowns, gum disease?

3. **Eliminating**
   - Is he continent?
   - Does he need to use a urinal, if so how often?
   - What does his urinalysis tell you?
   - What are his urinary symptoms?
   - Is he able to recognise when he needs to void urine?
   - How often does he open his bowels?
   - Does he have any diarrhoea/constipation?
   - Does he have any pain?

4. **Mobilising**
   - Has he any disability that restricts his mobility?
   - If so how does this impact on his ability to eliminate?
   - Is he able to get to the toilet with or without assistance?

5. **Expressing sexuality**
   - What has been the nature of the problem on his relationship with his partner?

6. **Personal cleansing and dressing**
   - Is he able to shower or bathe?
   - How frequently does he bathe or shower?
   - Does he require any assistance to dress/undress and if so who helps?

7. **Working and playing**
   - Does the health problem impact on his work, home and social life?

- Does he need help in the home?
- What support is provided by family carers?

8. Maintaining a safe environment
- Does he have any pain?
- Does he have any visual or auditory impairment?
- Are there any risks, e.g. infection, pressure sore development, falls, and moving and handling?
- Does he take any medication and if so does he understand his medication regime?

9. Sleeping
- Does he get up to go to the toilet or have any episodes of incontinence at night?
- Does this disturb his sleep?
- Does this affect his performance at work or leisure?

10. Controlling body temperature
- Does he have a temperature because of the infection?
- What sources of heating does he have at home?

11. Dying
- What does he understand the prognosis to be?
- Does he have any religious and cultural beliefs about dying?

Using the information presented so far in this chapter, think about the following short case studies and plan your assessment of the activity of eliminating. There may be other questions that you consider relevant and you may use the template in Appendix 3.

Case study 7.2

A patient with inflammatory bowel disease

Mary is a 30-year-old secretary who has inflammatory bowel disease.

Irritable bowel disease or inflammatory bowel disease (IBD) is a term used to describe ulcerative colitis or Crohn's disease, which usually affects younger adults in the Western world (for more information on IBD see Alexander et al 2006).

1. Biological
- How long has she suffered from IBD?
- What are her symptoms?
- Does she suffer from any pain?
- What treatment does she take?
- Does she suffer from incontinence?
- If so how does she manage her incontinence?
- What is her weight?
- How is she sleeping?

2. Psychological
- Is she suffering from stress or anxiety?
- What is her mood?
- Is she depressed?
- How is she coping with the situation?

- What does she understand about her illness?
- Does the problem impact on her sexual relationships?

3 Sociological
- How does the problem impact on her social life?
- What support does she have?
- How does she cope with everyday living?
- How does her problem impact on her family and relationships?

4. Environmental
- What facilities are at home?
- How does she cope with the problem in the community and at work?

5. Politicoeconomic
- How does the problem impact on her working life?
- Are there any economic factors that may be causing stress and anxiety?

Case study 7.3

A patient with urinary incontinence

Ellen is an 82-year-old lady with congestive cardiac failure who has recently become incontinent of urine. She is slightly deaf and has poor eyesight.

One of the symptoms of heart failure is generalised oedema. One objective is to reduce fluid excess by prescribing diuretics (for further information on heart failure see Herbert & Sheppard 2005 and Webster & Thompson 2006).

1. Biological
- How long has she suffered from urinary incontinence?
- What are her symptoms?
- How does she manage her incontinence?
- Does she suffer from any pain?
- What treatment does she take?
- When does she take her treatment?
- Is she constipated?

2. Psychological
- Is she suffering from stress or anxiety?
- What is her mood?
- Is she depressed?
- How is she coping with the situation?

3. Sociological
- Does she live alone?
- What support does she have at home?
- How does she cope with everyday living?
- Does she manage to do her shopping?
- Does she go out?
- How does her problem impact on her family?

4. Environmental
- What facilities are at home?
- What type of accommodation?
- Does she have an upstairs toilet?

- Can she climb the stairs?
- Does she have a commode downstairs?
- Does she have any adaptations to her house?

5. **Politicoeconomic**
   - Does she have access to resources to help her cope with her incontinence?
   - Are there any economic factors that may be causing stress and anxiety?

> **Exercise**
> 1. Having reflected on the clinical application of heart failure and the above questions, are there any other questions that you might consider and why?
> 2. Discuss these with your mentor or tutor.

PLANNING NURSING ACTIVITIES AND CARE

Planning nursing activities and care involves the following:

- identifying the problems or needs
- identifying priorities
- establishing short- and long-term goals
- determining the nursing actions and interventions required
- documenting the care plan.

Having undertaken a thorough assessment the nurse is now able to identify any problems or patient needs and determine the nursing interventions required in order to meet those needs. It is important to stress that such problems and needs must be patient-focused, and relate to the nursing assessment and what is needed to aid recovery in the immediate, short and long term. They may be actual or potential problems or needs that should be prioritised to take account of life-threatening situations.

Whilst undertaking the initial nursing assessment the nurse may obtain a considerable amount of information; it must be remembered that assessment is an ongoing and interactive process. Roper et al (2000) seek to clarify the use of the word assessment in relation to their model for nursing as follows:

- collecting information from or about the person
- reviewing the collected information
- identifying a person's problems with Activities of Living
- identifying priorities amongst the problems.

Assessment is an iterative and ongoing process and involves the patient. Having undertaken a thorough assessment, you should be able to identify any problems or patient needs and determine the nursing interventions required in order to meet those needs. It is important to stress that such problems and needs must be patient-focused, relate to the nursing assessment and what is needed to aid recovery in the immediate, short and long term. They may be actual or potential problems or needs and should be prioritised to take account of life-threatening situations.

Once the patient's problems or needs have been identified the nurse can review these and plan the nursing interventions required to:

- solve actual problems
- prevent potential problems occurring
- prevent solved problems from reoccurring
- develop positive coping strategies for any problem that cannot be solved.

> **Exercise**
> 1. Consider what skills and knowledge you will need to plan care for a patient.
> 2. Check your knowledge and skills against your list and those listed in Box 7.15. Identify any learning needs and/or skills development; discuss these with your mentor and personal tutor.

Box 7.15	**Knowledge and skills for care planning**

- Analytical skills
- Problem-solving skills
- Knowledge of the illness
- Knowledge of anatomy and physiology
- Decision-making skills
- Negotiating skills
- Priority setting.

Identifying problems and needs

Having undertaken a nursing assessment let us consider what actual and potential problems have been identified and how these might be prioritised. Within the context of this chapter we will focus on those problems, actual and potential in relation to the activity of elimination during a patient's admission to hospital.

Return to Case study 7.1 (details continue overleaf). Using the 12 Activities of Living as a framework for assessment the nurse might discover that:

1. **Breathing**
   - Cyril smokes 10 cigarettes a day

2. **Communicating**
   - Cyril is slightly deaf and wears a hearing aid.
   - He wears spectacles for reading.

3. **Eating and drinking**
   - Cyril has restricted his fluid intake recently for fear of not making it to the toilet on time and becoming incontinent.
   - He normally has a good appetite and eats three meals a day. He has no food allergies or special dietary needs.
   - He weighs 90 kg but feels he might have lost a little weight recently.

4. **Eliminating**
   - He has frequency of micturition.
   - He has some incontinence of urine and dribbling.
   - Ward urinalysis shows the presence of blood and protein.

Case study 7.1 (continued)

Cyril

Having undertaken a nursing assessment and taking account of the lifespan, dependency and factors that contribute to health we have now learned that Cyril is married to Janet and has three grown-up children. He works for an insurance firm and is looking forward to his retirement in 2 years. He is a keen gardener and supports his local football team. He lives in a two-storey house, with an upstairs bathroom and toilet. Eighteen months ago he noticed that he was having difficulty in starting and stopping the passage of urine. He had also noticed that he was going to the toilet more frequently and he had noticed slight dribbling of urine. This became a problem when he was at work and attending football matches. He believed that the problem was a result of his age and had tried to cope with it. Initially, he was embarrassed and had been reluctant to discuss his problem with anyone. More recently, he had noticed blood in his urine and had been treated by his GP for urine infections with antibiotics. When taking the antibiotics he had also suffered from diarrhoea. On further investigation he had been diagnosed with benign prostatic hyperplasia. He has read some information on the disease and is worried that he may have cancer.

- He usually opens his bowels once a day but has experienced diarrhoea when on antibiotics.

5. **Mobilising**
   - He is fully mobile and can manage to climb the stairs to the upstairs bathroom without difficulty.
   - He drives a car.

6. **Expressing sexuality**
   - He is concerned about how his problem would impact on his sexual relations with his wife.
   - He is also concerned about being incontinent during the night whilst sharing a bed with his wife and has moved into a single bed in the spare room.

7. **Personal cleansing and dressing**
   - He is able to shower and bathe independently and usually does so each day.
   - He dresses smartly and is careful about his appearance.

8. **Working and playing**
   - His health problem has impacted on his work, home and social life. He used to like going to the pub to have a drink with his friends.
   - Over the past few months he has purchased some incontinence pads from the local chemist to wear under his underpants.

9. **Maintaining a safe environment**
   - He is pain-free at the moment.
   - He is short-sighted and wears glasses.

- He is not at risk from pressure ulcer development, his Waterlow score is 10.
- He has been orientated into the ward environment.
- A risk assessment reveals he is not at risk from falls but will require a moving and handling risk assessment if he becomes dependent.
- He understands his medication regime but is concerned that any further antibiotic treatment will result in him suffering from diarrhoea.

10. **Sleeping**
    - He gets up to the toilet two or three times a night. Lately he has experienced some dribbling incontinence at night.
    - He has been tired during the day and in the evening he has been sleeping in his chair in front of the television and is reluctant to go out.

11. **Controlling body temperature**
    - His temperature is normal on admission.

12. **Dying**
    - He has read some information on prostate problems and benign prostatic hyperplasia. He has also read in the newspaper about cancer of the prostate and is worried that he might have cancer.
    - Whilst he does not go to church regularly he regards himself as a Christian and believes in God.

Identifying actual and potential problems

Having undertaken a nursing assessment and reviewed the information it is now possible to consider what actual and potential problems have been identified and how these might be prioritised.

Whilst undertaking the nursing assessment the nurse should be able to detect potential problems which the patient may not be aware of. This is where the nurse's knowledge of the factors relating to ill health, socioeconomic, biological, psychological and environmental is important.

It must be remembered that assessment is an ongoing and interactive process. Having undertaken a thorough assessment you should be able to identify any problems or patient needs and determine the nursing interventions required in order to meet those needs. It is important to stress that such problems and needs must be patient-focused, relate to the nursing assessment and what is needed to aid recovery in the immediate, short and long term. They may be actual or potential problems or needs and should be prioritised to take account of life-threatening situations.

Prioritising problems

Prioritising problems is an important component of care planning. By using the independence/dependence continuum of the model of living we are able to identify and prioritise those problems that patients require nursing care and assistance to regain or maintain their independence, or where the patient is totally dependent on the nurse (Roper et al 1996). You may choose to do this by listing the problems in priority order in the nursing care plan, by dependency or by level of risk. As there may be local systems of prioritising problems it is advisable to check these out with your mentor.

Having now undertaken a thorough nursing assessment you will have already begun to identify a number of potential and actual problems. Taking account of lifespan, and factors which influence the Activities of Living, i.e. psychological, sociocultural, environmental and politicoeconomic, make a list of what you think these might be in relation to the activity of elimination and check your list against those below. This list might not be exhaustive but will give some indication of those you might consider.

Before planning the nursing care, Roper et al (1996, 2000) suggest that the nurse in collaboration with the patient, or with the patient's consent the patient's family, determines and agrees the priority of each of the problems. Of course problems that are life-threatening take precedence over those of less importance. The nurse may choose to number these according to the level of priority or simply by listing the problems in order of priority in the nursing care plan. There are a number of ways in which you might do this, for example numbering in order of priority or simply by listing the problems in the nursing care plan in order of importance. However, it is important to take account of the patient's view, as their priority may not be the same as yours (Roper et al 1996).

> **Exercise**
> 1. Review Cyril's nursing assessment, begin to identify any actual and/or potential problems and place them in order of priority.

When determining the priority you must consider the patient's priorities. As a nurse you may have decided that the risk of chest infection, deep vein thrombosis and haemorrhage are potentially life-threatening and therefore given priority. However Cyril's priorities might be very different. He is worried that he has cancer and requires reassurance and information. He may also be concerned and embarrassed about the possibility of being incontinent whilst in hospital and how to gain access to the toilet in time. Box 7.16 provides some possible actual and potential problems which emerged during the assessment of Cyril.

Goal setting

Returning to Case study 7.1 and taking into consideration the nursing assessment and actual and potential problems

Box 7.16	Actual and potential problems	
Activity of Living	**Actual problem**	**Potential problem**
Breathing	Cyril smokes and is at risk of developing a chest infection following anaesthetic	Chest infection
Communicating	Cyril has difficulty hearing and needs to have his hearing aid in situ	Misunderstanding of information, advice and instructions aimed at increasing his recovery from surgery
Eating and drinking	Cyril is reluctant to drink fluids due to his dribbling incontinence Difficulty eating in bed due to IVI	Electrolyte imbalance Constipation Nausea due to anaesthetic drugs
Elimination	Cyril is embarrassed about his dribbling incontinence He will have a catheter in situ after surgery Pain from excision site in bladder or catheter	Increased stress levels will delay recovery Blocked catheter due to blood clots Urine bypassing catheter Urinary tract infection Constipation due to period of immobility following surgery
Mobilising	Reluctant to mobilise due to pain	At moderate risk of developing deep vein thrombosis and pulmonary embolism Constipation
Expressing sexuality	Cyril is worried about the outcome of his surgery on his sexual relations with his wife	
Personal cleansing and dressing	Cyril will be unable to attend to his personal hygiene in the immediate postoperative period	*(continued)*

Box 7.16	Actual and potential problems (continued)	
Activity of Living	Actual problem	Potential problem
Working and playing		Anxiety about the impact of his ill health on his ability to earn a living and his future pension
Maintaining a safe environment	Cyril will need to be prepared for theatre and anaesthetic	Risk of infection
	Risk of bleeding from the transurethral site	Risk of haemorrhage Risk of pressure ulcer development due to immobility and surgery
Sleeping	Cyril has difficulty sleeping and gets up two or three times a night	Lack of sleep due to postoperative vital signs, monitoring and pain
Controlling body temperature		Potential drop in body temperature during surgery
Dying	Cyril is anxious about his prognosis	Increased stress which might delay recovery

identified, it is necessary to agree long- and short-term goals or outcomes for Cyril's nursing care.

Goals should be realistic, achievable and measurable. It is advisable to include dates and times to indicate when the goal is to be achieved. This enables the nurse to evaluate progress and achievement and demonstrate how nursing has benefited the patient (Roper et al 1996). In some cases it may be necessary to agree long-term goals, i.e. those goals that might take longer to achieve than those that can be achieved within a shorter timescale. Roper et al (1996, 2000) liken goals to signposts on a journey indicating when you have arrived at your destination.

Box 7.17 provides examples of how goals might be set.

Exercise
1. Revisit Cyril's actual and potential problems.
2. What goals might you identify in relation to the activity of elimination?

Statement of intentions/aims

In some clinical areas you might find that nursing staff prefer to identify statements of intentions or aims rather than goals in which case these would be written in a slightly different way. For example, consider problem 2 in Box 7.17; an aim might be identified as shown in Box 7.18.

Box 7.17	Examples of how goals might be set		
Actual problem	Potential problem	Goals	
1. Cyril feels embarrassed about his dribbling incontinence	Increased stress levels	Cyril states he feels less embarrassed about his dribbling incontinence	
2. Cyril is at risk from developing a urinary tract infection due to catheter in situ after surgery	Urinary tract infection	Cyril will not develop a urinary tract infection during his hospital stay	
3. Risk of bleeding from the excision site	Blocked catheter due to blood clots Urine bypassing catheter	Cyril's catheter remains patent whilst in situ Urine drains via the catheter and not via the urethra	
4. Cyril will be immobile due to surgery	Constipation due to period of immobility following surgery	Cyril will have his bowels opened and report no pain or discomfort within 2 days following surgery	
5. Cyril has undergone surgical excision of his prostate gland	Pain from excision site in bladder or catheter	Cyril will confirm that his pain is controlled postoperatively	
6. Cyril feels reluctant to drink fluids due to his dribbling incontinence	Dehydration	Cyril understands why he is required to drink 2–3 litres of fluid a day Cyril's intake and output are recorded on his daily chart and demonstrate an intake of 2 litres within 24 hours Cyril will contribute to recording his intake and output	

Box 7.18	Example of how an aim might be identified	
Actual problem	**Potential problem**	**Aim/s**
2. Cyril has a catheter in situ	1. Risk of infection	To reduce the risk of infection
	2. Catheter may become blocked due to bleeding from the excision site and blood clot formation in the catheter	To observe for any blockage of the catheter
	3. Pain at catheter site	To ensure Cyril remains pain free

Whether you decide to use goals or aims you should be able to evaluate the outcomes of the nursing care plan and nursing interventions.

> **Exercise**
> 1. Now consider Cyril's remaining problems in relation to the other Activities of Living and identify goals or aims that you might set.
> 2. Discuss these with your mentor or personal tutor.
> 3. Reflect on how the activity of elimination impacts on the other Activities of Living and vice versa.

PLANNING CARE

Having undertaken a nursing assessment and identified actual and potential problems the nurse has information which will inform a plan of care and nursing interventions. It is important to remember to involve the patient fully in planning their care.

Roper et al (2000) state that the objective of the plan is:

- to prevent identified problems with any of the ALs from becoming actual ones
- to solve identified actual problems
- where possible, to alleviate those that cannot be solved
- to help the person cope positively with those problems that cannot be alleviated or solved
- to prevent recurrence of a treated problem
- to help the person to be as comfortable and pain-free as possible when death is inevitable.

Availability of resources

When planning the care and determining nursing actions and interventions the nurse must take account of the resources available, including staffing levels, knowledge and skills available, the environment and equipment and any evidence-based guidelines, protocols or policies. They will also need to take account of any interventions and care prescribed by other members of the health care team and incorporate these in to the nursing care plan where necessary. A registered nurse remains at all times accountable for the appropriate delegation to unregistered staff and making sure that the person is competent to undertake the task or duty (NMC 2004).

Care pathways

The introduction of clinical governance into the NHS in the UK (DoH 1998) has placed greater emphasis on ensuring quality care to patients and effective outcomes. A care pathway is a tool that sets out the evidence-based care a patient should receive for an episode of care (Ellis & Johnson 1999). Care pathways are normally developed for high-volume cases. Ellis & Johnson (1999) developed a care pathway for transurethral resection of the prostate (TURP) in Ashford and St Peter's Hospitals NHS Trust. The benefits they identified were that: all staff were able to understand how patients undergoing this procedure should be cared for, care was consistent, risks to patients were reduced and auditing by variance reporting informed education and enabled patients to be discharged earlier. You will be able to locate examples of care pathways on the National Library for Health (www.library.nhs.uk/pathways).

When planning the nursing care of a patient it is necessary to consider where care pathways have been developed and take account of these when determining the nursing interventions and individualising nursing care.

> **Exercise**
> 1. Are there any integrated care pathways being used in your clinical area?
> 2. In what way do these take account of the Activities of Living?
> 3. Discuss your findings with your mentor or personal tutor.

Collaboration

Nurses do not work in isolation, they work in teams and in collaboration with others. In hospital, nurses are with the patients for 24 hours a day and in many cases they may take the lead role in coordinating the care of the patient, referring if necessary to specialist nurses and health care professionals.

You may have considered the following:

- medical staff including consultant urologist
- junior medical staff
- physiotherapist
- chaplain
- anaesthetist
- health care assistant.

Other professionals who may input indirectly or at a later date include:

- pharmacist
- phlebotomist
- dietitian
- social worker
- discharge liaison coordinator.

When preparing a nursing care plan you will need to take account of the input and assessments undertaken by these professionals.

Nursing interventions

The nursing care plan details the nursing interventions required to achieve the stated goals or aims. The plan should enable other staff including other health care professionals to provide continuity of care for the patient (Roper et al 2000). The nursing care plan may be paper-based or computerised.

When determining the nursing interventions you will need to consider where the patient is on the independency–dependency continuum as identified in the model of living (Roper et al 2000). The nurse provides nursing interventions for a dependent patient whereas nursing interventions

in an independent patient aim to encourage and maintain independence. As discussed in the first part of this chapter, dependency may be influenced by the factors associated with living across the lifespan.

Breathing

Cyril smokes 10 cigarettes a day and is therefore at risk of developing a chest infection following a general anaesthetic. During surgery the patient is unable to cough or sigh and thus expectorate or move any sputum from the lungs. This will pool and become a focus for bacterial infection. Patients who smoke should be advised to stop smoking at least 10 days prior to undergoing a general anaesthetic (Gibson 2006). It is important that all patients are referred, prior to undergoing surgery, to a physiotherapist and taught deep breathing exercises and how to clear stagnating fluids from their lungs.

In many cases, patients being admitted to hospital for elective surgery attend a nurse-led pre-assessment clinic where routine investigations are performed and the patient receives information on the procedure and health education advice. If Cyril had attended a pre-assessment clinic he would have been given advice on giving up smoking and the anaesthetic risks involved (see Chapter 3 for pre- and postoperative care).

Nursing interventions   These might include:

- reinforcing information on the risks of smoking prior to surgery
- arranging access to nicotine replacement patches if prescribed
- referring to the physiotherapist for deep breathing exercises
- encouraging deep breathing exercises pre- and postoperatively
- monitoring his temperature, pulse and respirations.

Communicating

Cyril wears a hearing aid. He can hear with difficulty without it and may misunderstand or misinterpret what is being said to him. This may result in increasing stress levels and lack of compliance and cooperation in relation to preoperative fasting and advice on postoperative recovery (see Chapter 4).

Nursing interventions   These might include:
- ensuring that Cyril understands information and does not misinterpret instructions or health advice
- ensuring that Cyril has his hearing aid in place and that it is working when communicating with him
- checking that he has understood any instructions or information
- ensuring that other health professionals are aware that Cyril wears a hearing aid.

Eating and drinking

Whilst Cyril's appetite is fairly good he is reluctant to drink fluids. Cyril will need to have at least 2 litres of fluid a day. An adequate fluid intake is essential to achieve fluid and electrolyte balance prior to surgery. Following surgery Cyril will have an intravenous infusion of fluid and bladder irrigation in situ. TUR syndrome is an uncommon but serious complication following surgery and occurs when the irrigation fluid enters the circulation and leads to circulatory overload (see Forristal & Maxfield 2004). The nurse should monitor the patient's intake and output carefully to ensure that the patient's output is greater than intake. When Cyril has recovered from the anaesthetic he will need to drink at least 2–3 litres of fluid a day to ensure that the catheter does not become blocked by blood clots and prevent infection, unless medical advice is to the contrary.

Nursing interventions   These might include:
- encouraging Cyril to drink at least 2 litres of fluid each day when recovered from anaesthetic
- monitoring and recording Cyril's fluid intake and output
- maintaining hydration and ensuring the safe administration of intravenous fluids
- monitoring the amount and colour of urine drainage from the catheter
- where necessary providing assistance to enable Cyril to eat his meals
- observing any nausea or vomiting
- encouraging a high-fibre diet if constipated.

Eliminating

Initially on admission Cyril will need to be able to find his way round the ward and know the location of the toilets. He will need reassurance regarding his dribbling incontinence and access to any incontinence aids or adaptations. He will also need information on how the activity of elimination will be affected initially post surgery.

Following surgery he will have a catheter inserted and undergo continuous irrigation until his urine is clear. Preventing infection and maintaining the dignity of the patient are the two key principles in caring for a patient with a urethral catheter (see Dougherty & Lister 2004, p. 330, for further information on the principles of catheter management). It is essential to maintain a closed system to reduce the likelihood of infection. Following removal of the catheter some patients may suffer from dribbling incontinence and be advised to perform pelvic floor exercises. Cyril's mobility following surgery will be restricted initially and this may result in Cyril becoming constipated. He may also complain of pain due to bladder spasm or the catheter in situ.

Nursing interventions   These might include:
- ensuring that Cyril is orientated into the ward and knows where the toilets are
- ensuring that Cyril has access to any incontinence aids for his dribbling incontinence prior to surgery
- maintaining Cyril's privacy and dignity when attending to catheter and continuous bladder irrigation
- monitoring, observing and recording his urine output
- maintaining and observing his bladder irrigation as prescribed
- maintaining asepsis when changing urine drainage bags
- attending to catheter toilet
- administering pain relief as prescribed
- ensuring that Cyril understands the need for good personal hygiene
- monitoring Cyril's bowel movements and taking action if Cyril complains of constipation
- recording temperature, blood pressure and pulse, and reporting any changes
- advising on pelvic floor exercises if necessary

Mobilising

Normally Cyril is able to mobilise independently. However, following surgery he will undergo a period of bed rest and his mobility will be restricted by the intravenous infusion and continuous irrigation of fluid. He will also need assistance when mobilising for the first time following surgery. Cyril's privacy and dignity may be compromised due to being catheterised and having to carry around a urine bag.

Surgery and a period of immobility may increase the risk of deep venous thrombosis and pulmonary embolism. Whilst Cyril's risk may be moderate he would benefit from application of compression stockings and advice on leg exercises whilst in bed and early mobilisation (see Gibson 2006). In some cases prophylactic anticoagulants prior to surgery may be prescribed.

Nursing interventions   These might include:
- recording Cyril's temperature and pulse and reporting any rise in temperature
- applying compression hosiery prior to surgery
- explaining to Cyril the need for early mobilisation following surgery
- encouraging passive movements whilst in bed
- encouraging gentle exercise following surgery
- referral to the physiotherapist for advice and support pre- and postoperatively
- explaining the hazards associated with mobilising whilst catheter and infusion are in situ.

Expressing sexuality

Cyril is concerned about how his operation will impact on his sexual relations with his wife. Following a TURP most men will suffer from retrograde ejaculation; however, this does not mean that the man will be impotent. A small percentage of men may suffer from long-term incontinence. It is important that men undergoing this procedure are given adequate information and reassurance about the procedure and if necessary counselled prior to surgery. Failure to provide this information and support may lead to anxiety and stress and lack of informed consent. It is important to remember to consider what information his wife will require.

Nursing interventions These might include:
- providing written and verbal information on the side effects of prostatectomy
- listening to Cyril's concerns
- checking that he has understood the information
- arranging access to a clinical nurse specialist if available
- liaising with medical staff regarding informed consent.

Personal cleansing and dressing

Normally fully independent in washing and dressing, Cyril will need help to undertake this Activity of Living in the immediate postoperative period. He may also find it difficult to dress himself as a result of the intravenous infusion and catheter drainage (see Chapter 8).

Nursing interventions These might include:
- assisting Cyril to maintain his personal and oral hygiene
- providing advice on how to manage his catheter care.

Working and playing

Cyril has arranged for sick leave from work. But because of his sickness and absence record any further absences will have financial implications for his family (see Chapter 11).

Nursing interventions These might include:
- referral to social worker for advice on financial support and benefits available during periods of illness.

Maintaining a safe environment

Cyril is scheduled for surgery. He will require preoperative preparation and safe transfer to theatre. Haemorrhage or bleeding from the excision site is a major risk following TURP. Therefore one of the nurse's major roles is to record the patient's blood pressure, pulse and observe the urine for clots and signs of bleeding (see Chapter 3).

Whilst an assessment for the risk of pressure ulcer development showed that Cyril was not at risk, his transfer to theatre, surgery and subsequent recovery period will increase his risk status and it will be necessary to review his score following surgery.

Nursing interventions These might include:
- preparing Cyril for theatre and complete preoperative assessment
- providing anti-embolic stockings

- observing for bleeding on return from theatre
- monitoring Cyril's temperature, pulse, respiration and blood pressure
- monitoring and observe for bleeding via the catheter
- reassessing risk of pressure ulcer development, providing pressure reduction mattress if required, encouraging and supporting Cyril to turn or move his position at least 2 hourly
- monitoring and observing pressure points, paying particular attention to heel pressure points and ensuring that his skin is clean and dry
- maintaining strict aseptic technique when dealing with the catheter, irrigation system and intravenous site.

Sleeping

Cyril may find it difficult to sleep in hospital at first due to the unfamiliarity of his surroundings, noise and anxiety about his surgery (see Chapter 13). Following surgery, postoperative checks carried out by nurses to monitor his vital signs and observe for complications will result in Cyril's sleep being disturbed.

Nursing interventions These might include:
- orientating Cyril into his surroundings and environment
- reducing the amount of noise within the ward wherever possible.

Controlling body temperature

Normally Cyril is able to control his body temperature by thermoregulation. However, during surgery consideration should be given to ensuring a warm environment to prevent unnecessary heat loss and aid recovery. Following surgery his temperature should be monitored. A rise in his temperature may indicate an infection and should be reported to medical staff (see Chapter 9).

Nursing interventions These might include:
- monitoring his temperature
- ensuring a warm environment.

Dying

Cyril has indicated that he is very worried about the outcome of his surgery and prognosis. He does not openly talk about dying but when asked he would like to speak to a chaplain or counsellor (see Chapter 14).

Nursing interventions These might include:
- referral to the chaplain or counsellor
- reassurance and information on the possible outcomes of his surgery.

IMPLEMENTING NURSING CARE

Successful implementation relies on a thorough initial nursing assessment (Sutcliffe 1990), a comprehensive nursing care plan, well-organised care delivery systems and competent staff.

The nursing care plan provides a written guide and instructions on implementing the care for the patient. It also provides an accurate record of the care given to the patient.

Record keeping is an integral part of nursing care. It is a tool for professional practice and one which should help the care process. There is no single model or template for a nursing record but it must follow a logical sequence with clear milestones and goals (NMC 2007).

Nursing records are an integral part of the patient's health care record and can be called in evidence before a Court of Law, Health Service Commissioner or in order to investigate a complaint about care at a local level. The NMC Professional Conduct Committee may also use patient records when considering complaints about professional misconduct.

Whilst it is preferable that nursing records are completed contemporaneously, workload pressures, stress and being too busy are reasons given why nurses find it difficult to do so (Mason 1999). Mason also found that the verbal report, direct observation and bedside charts guided practice rather than the nursing care plan. In response to the concerns expressed, the Department of Health (2003) has published a Clinical Practice Benchmark for Record Keeping. (This may be accessed at www.doh.gov.uk.)

Exercise

Return to Cyril's nursing care plan.

1. What factors might influence implementation?
2. What knowledge and skills would you need to implement these nursing interventions?

You may have considered that the following factors might influence implementation:

- the philosophy of care on the ward or department (beliefs and values, advocacy)
- the nursing model used
- the care delivery system (primary nursing, team nursing, case management or task allocation)
- resources available (skill mix of staff available, equipment, support staff and other health care professionals).

You may have considered that the following knowledge is required when implementing nursing activities:

- anatomy and physiology of urinary and intestinal systems
- psychological effects associated with elimination
- sociocultural issues relating to elimination
- environmental issues and concerns
- political and economic concerns.

You may have considered that the following skills are required when implementing nursing activities:

- caring skills (listening, comforting, reassuring, helping)
- clinical psychomotor skills (catheterisation, intravenous infusions, rectal examination, urine testing, specimen collection, etc.)
- management skills (organisational, supervision, delegation skills)
- counselling skills (listening, problem solving, advising)
- teaching skills
- research skills (literature searching, critical appraisal)
- problem solving skills (problem identification, goal setting, priority setting)
- leadership skills (advocacy, teamwork, transformational leadership skills, networking).

Exercise

1. Reflect on these and assess your current knowledge and skills.
2. Record your reflections in your diary.
3. Identify those areas in which you need further development.
4. Take these to your next tutorial or clinical supervision session. Discuss with your mentor or preceptor how you plan to develop these further.

EVALUATION OF NURSING ACTIVITIES

Evaluation of nursing care is an important part of professional practice and provides feedback on the patient's progress and effectiveness of nursing care. It is an ongoing process, which should be undertaken by the nurse in conjunction with the patient and his or her relatives or carers and other health care professionals (for further information refer to Chapter 1).

Evaluating care consists of checking the patient's progress against the identified goals and timescales to determine whether these have been fully or partially met or indeed not met at all.

When evaluating the care plan you will need to establish if the goals have been completely met, partially met or not met at all. If the goal has not been met or has partially been met then the nurse must consider if the agreed timescale was realistic. If not then you may decide to extend the timescale. Alternatively you may need to reassess the problem and modify the plan. In some cases the problem may have changed or the goal may have been inappropriate. Not all goals will be achievable during a hospital stay. In which case you might need more information on the problem. Is it worse or has it changed?

You should also reconsider the appropriateness of the prescribed nursing actions and interventions – do these need to be changed or modified? By involving patients in their nursing care planning and evaluation it is possible to identify and agree realistic goals and meaningful evaluation of outcomes.

Not all goals or aims will be achievable during an episode of care. In such cases these may form the basis of discussion with colleagues in primary or secondary care settings and family or carers. Nursing care plans can be a useful tool to provide information on discharge or transfer of care between secondary, tertiary and primary care.

DISCHARGE PLANNING

A comprehensive nursing assessment using the Roper et al (1996, 2000) model of living and model for nursing will also provide the basis of a well-developed discharge plan and facilitate safe and effective discharge (DoH 2004).

> **Exercise**
> 1. Revisit Cyril's care plan. What information and or support will he need to ensure a safe discharge home?
> 2. Discuss is with your mentor and tutor.

In your discussions you may have considered: advice on avoiding heavy lifting, drinking plenty of fluids and ensuring a high-fibre diet to prevent constipation, avoiding sexual activity for a period of time, and what to do and who he should call if there are signs of infection. Depending on his physical condition he may need a little extra help around the house until he has fully recovered. As his toilet is upstairs consideration should be given to checking if he is able to climb the stairs unaided.

PERSONAL AND PROFESSIONAL DEVELOPMENT

Having worked through this chapter and the exercises, you need to reflect on what you have learnt and how you might use this to inform your personal and professional development.

You may like to consider your needs under the following headings:

- What do I need to see now?
- What do I need to do now?
- What do I need to know now?
- Who can help me?

SUMMARY POINTS

> 1. This chapter introduced the fifth Activity of Living – elimination, as described by Roper, Logan and Tierney in their model for nursing (Roper et al 1996, 2000). It systematically explored the framework of the model and its application in clinical practice, the use of a case scenario, exercises, and reflection and further reading. It has been impossible within this chapter to cover every aspect in relation to the activity of elimination and health issues associated with elimination. Therefore, it is important that you keep up to date with new information and evidence-based practice in order to be able to meet the changing needs of patients and health care delivery.
> 2. Nurses have a very important role in ensuring the quality of the patient experience, and that patient needs are met in relation to the activity of elimination. Throughout the chapter we have shown how, by applying the Roper, Logan and Tierney model for nursing in practice, the nurse is able to recognise and take account of the patient's individual needs in relation to elimination when assessing, planning, implementing and evaluating holistic patient care.

References

Abrams P, Cardozo L, Khoudy S, Wein S 2002 Incontinence. In: Abrams P, Cardozo L, Khoudy S, Wein S (eds) 2nd International consultation on incontinence, 2nd edn. Health Publications, Plymouth

Alexander MF, Fawcett J (Tonks) N, Runciman PJ (eds) 2006 Nursing practice hospital and home (the adult), 3rd edn. Churchill Livingstone, Edinburgh

Beaton S 2001 How foot and mouth disease affected a rural continence service. Nursing Times 97(40):59, 70

British National Formulary 2006 No. 52 (www.bnf.org, last accessed 25 January 2007)

Brooker C, Nichol M, 2003 Nursing adults. The practice of caring. Mosby, London

Burton G 1996 An assessment of attitudes to incontinence in different migrant groups. Australian Continence Journal March:4–6

Colpman D, Welford K 2004 Urinary drainage systems. In: Fillingham S, Douglas J (eds) Urological nursing, 3rd edn. Baillière Tindall, Edinburgh

Continence Foundation 2000 Making the case for investment in an integrated continence service. A source book for continence services. The Continence Foundation, London (www. continence-foundation.org.uk)

Department of Health 1998 A first class service: quality in the new NHS. The Stationery Office, London

Department of Health 2000 Good practice in continence services. HMSO, London

Department of Health 2001a Good practice in consent: implementation guide. HMSO, London

Department of Health 2001b Reference guide to consent for examination or treatment. The Stationery Office, London

Department of Health 2001c Modern standards and service models of older people: national service framework for older people. The Stationery Office, London

Department of Health 2003 The essence of care: patient-focused benchmarking for health care professionals. The Stationery Office, London

Department of Health 2004 Achieving timely simple discharge from hospital. A toolkit for the multidisciplinary team. (www.dh.gov.uk last accessed January 2007)

Department of Health 2006 The Health Act 2006. Code of practice for the prevention and control of healthcare associated infactions. (www.dh.gov.uk/publications)

Dougherty L, Lister S 2004 The Royal Marsden Hospital manual of clinical nursing procedures, 6th edn. Blackwell Publishing, Oxford

Ellis BW, Johnson S 1999 The care pathway: a tool to enhance clinical governance. British Journal of Clinical Governance 4(2):61–71

Fanning H 2003 Nursing patients with urinary disorders. In: Brooker C, Nichol M (eds) Nursing adults. The practice of caring. Mosby, London

Fillingham S, Douglas J 2004 Urological nursing, 3rd edn. Baillière Tindall, Edinburgh

Forristal H, Maxfield J 2004 Prostatic problems. In: Fillingham S, Douglas J (eds) Urological nursing, 3rd edn. Baillière Tindall, Edinburgh

Gibson CE 2006 The patient facing surgery. In: Alexander MF, Fawcett J (Tonks) N, Runciman PJ (eds) Nursing practice hospital and home (the adult), 3rd edn. Churchill Livingstone, Edinburgh

Glazener CN, Evans JH, Peto RE 2003 Effects of interventions for the treatment of nocturnal enuresis in children. Quality and Safety in Health Care 12(5):390–394

Glazener CN, Evans JH, Peto RE 2004 Treating nocturnal enuresis in children: a review of the evidence. Journal of Wound, Ostomy and Continence Nursing 31(4):223–234

Haggar V 1997 Continence. Foreign policy ... minority ethnic communities ... continence problems. Nursing Times 93(15):78

Heaton K 1999 The Bristol stool form scale. In: Understanding your bowels. Family Doctor Series. BMA, London

Heitkemper MM, Jarret M, Caudell KA et al 1998 Women with gastrointestinal symptoms. Implications for nursing research and practice. Gastroenterology Nursing 21(2):52–58

Henley A, Schott J 1999 Culture, religion and patient care in a multi-ethnic society. A handbook for professionals. Age Concern Books, Glasgow

Herbert J 1999 Faecal incontinence: the last taboo? British Journal of Therapy and Rehabilitation 6(9):453–458

Herbert RA, Sheppard M 2005 Cardiovascular function. In: Montague SE, Watson R, Herbert RA (eds) Physiology for nursing practice, 3rd edn. Elsevier, Edinburgh

Hinds JP, Eidelman BH, Wald A 1990 Prevalence of bowel dysfunction in multiple sclerosis. Gastroenterology 98:1538–1542

Hjalmas K, Arnold T, Bower W et al 2004 Nocturnal enuresis: an international evidence based management strategy. Journal of Urology 171(6 Pt 2):2545–2561

Hunt GM, Oakeshott P, Whitaker RH 1996 Fortnightly review: Intermittent catheterisation: Simple, safe, and effective, but underused. British Medical Journal 312:103–107

Iggulden H 2006 Care of the neurological patient. Blackwell Publishing, Oxford

Johanson JJ, Laferty J 1996 Epidemiology of faecal incontinence: the silent affliction. American Journal of Gastroenterology 91(1):33–36

Kamm MA 1998 Faecal incontinence. British Medical Journal 316:528–532

Kenworthy N, Snowley G, Gelling C 2002 Common foundation studies in nursing, 3rd edn. Churchill Livingstone, Edinburgh

Kindlen S 2003 Physiology for health care and nursing. Churchill Livingstone, Edinburgh

Lee YY, Tsay WW, Lou MF et al 2007 The effectiveness of implementing a bladder ultrasound programme in neurosurgical units. Journal of Advanced Nursing 57(2):192–200

Logan K 2005 Incontinence and the effects of childbirth on the pelvic floor. British Journal of Midwifery 13(6):374–377

Lunniss PJ, Gladman MA, Hetzer FH et al 2004 Risk factors in acquired faecal incontinence. Journal of the Royal Society of Medicine 97(Mar):111–116

McDowell BJ, Engberg S, Serika S et al 1999 Effectiveness of behavioural therapy to treat incontinence in home bound older people. Journal of the American Geriatrics Society 47:309–318

McLaren SM 2005 Renal function. In: Montague SE, Watson R, Herbert RA (eds) Physiology for nursing practice, 3rd edn. Elsevier, Edinburgh

McMonnies G 2002 Paediatric continence in children with neuropathic bladders. British Journal of Nursing 11(11):765–772

Mason C 1999 Guide to practice or 'load of rubbish'? The influence of care plans on nursing practice in five clinical areas in Northern Ireland. Journal of Advanced Nursing 29(2):380–387

Miller M, Crawshaw A, Logan L, et al 2006 Disorders of the gastrointestinal system, liver and biliary tract. In: Alexander MF, Fawcett J (Tonks) N, Runciman PJ (eds) Nursing practice: hospital and home (the adult), 3rd edn. Churchill Livingstone, Edinburgh

Montague SE, Watson R, Herbert RA (eds) 2005 Physiology for nursing practice, 3rd edn. Elsevier, Edinburgh

Nelson R, Norton N, Cautley E et al 1995 Community based prevalence of anal incontinence. JAMA 274(7):559–561

NICE 2006 Urinary incontinence. The management of urinary incontinence in women, Clinical Guideline 40 (www.nice.org.uk, downloaded January 2007)

NICE 2007 Faecal incontinence: the management of faecal incontinence in adults. Clinical Guideline 49 (www.nice.org.uk, downloaded September 2007)

Norton C 1996 Faecal incontinence in adults 1: Prevalence and causes. British Journal of Nursing 5(22):1366–1374

Nursing and Midwifery Council 2004 Code of professional conduct: standards for performance and ethics. NMC, London (www.nmc-uk.org)

Nursing and Midwifery Council 2007 NMC record keeping guidance. (www.nmc-uk.org, downloaded October 2007)

Ogden J 2004 Health psychology: a textbook, 3rd edn. Open University Press, Maidenhead

Page A 1999 Twelve years of hell. Nursing Times 95(18):65–66

Petticrew M, Watt I, Sheldon T 1998 Systematic review of the effectiveness of laxatives in the elderly. Executive summary, vol 13. NHS Research and Development Health Technology Assessment Programme. HMSO, London

PHLS Advisory Committee on Gastrointestinal Infections 2000 (www.phls.co.uk)

Pilloni S, Krhut J, Mair D et al 2005 Intermittent catheterisation in older people: a valuable alternative to an indwelling catheter. Age and Ageing 34(1):57–60

Powell M, Rigby D 2000 Management of bowel dysfunction: evacuation difficulties. Nursing Standard 14(47):47–51

Pratt RJ, Pellowe C, Loveday HP et al 2001 The Epic Project: developing national evidence-based guidelines for preventing healthcare-associated infections. Journal of Hospital Infection 47(Suppl):S3–S82

Roe B, Doll H 2000 Prevalence of urinary incontinence and its relationship with health status. Journal of Clinical Nursing 9:178–188

Rogers J 2001 Fast-track toilet. Training Nursing Times 97(40):53–54

Rogers J 2002 Managing day-time and night-time enuresis in children. Nursing Standard 16(32):45–52

Roper N, Logan WW, Tierney AJ 1996 The elements of nursing: A model for nursing based on a model for living, 4th edn. Churchill Livingstone, London

Roper N, Logan WW, Tierney AJ 2000 The Roper–Logan–Tierney model of nursing based on activities of living. Churchill Livingstone, Edinburgh

Royal College of Nursing 2003 Digital rectal examination and manual removal of faeces. Guidance for nurses. Royal College of Nursing, London

Royal College of Physicians 1995 Incontinence: causes, management and provision of services. Royal College of Physicians, London

Royal College of Physicians 2004 Pilot of the National Audit of Continence for Older People (England and Wales) Executive Report. Available from www.rcplondon.ac.uk (last downloaded March 2007)

Rutishauser S 1994 Physiology and anatomy: A basis for nursing and health care. Churchill Livingstone, Edinburgh

Saker LR Wagner K Pearson A 2006 Changing burden of Clostridium difficile associated disease in England 2004–2005. In: Interscience Conference on Antimicrobial Agents and Chemotherapy, 26–30 September San Francisco USA Health Protection Agency (www.hpa.org.uk, last downloaded 22 January 2007)

Sampselle C, Palmer MH, Boyington AR et al 2004 Prevention of urinary incontinence in adults. Population based strategies. Nursing Research 53(6S):61–67

Selfe L 2006 The urinary system. In: Alexander MF, Fawcett J (Tonks) N, Runciman PJ (eds) Nursing practice: hospital and home (the adult), 3rd edn. Churchill Livingstone, Edinburgh, pp 357–393

Shaw C 2001 A review of the psychosocial predictors of help seeking impact on quality of life in people with urinary incontinence. Journal of Clinical Nursing 10:15–24

Smith GD 2003 The digestive system. In: Kindlen S (ed) Physiology for health care and nursing. Churchill Livingstone, Edinburgh

Smith GD, Fawcett J (Tonks) 2003 Stress. In: Alexander MF, Fawcett J (Tonks), Runciman PJ (eds) Nursing practice hospital and home (the adult), pp 633–713. Churchill Livingstone, Edinburgh

Sultan AH, Kamm MA, Hudson CN et al 1993 Anal sphincter disruption during vaginal delivery. New England Journal of Medicine 329:1905–1911

Sutcliffe E 1990 Reviewing the process progress: a critical review of the literature on the nursing process. Senior Nurse 10(a):9–13

Tew L, Pomfret I, King D 2005 Infection risks associated with urinary catheters. Nursing Standard 20(7):55–62

Valtin H 1979 Renal dysfunction: mechanisms involved in fluid and solute imbalance. Little Brown, Boston

Vickerman J, Whitehead J 2001 Continence management: an occupational therapist and physiotherapist perspective. Nurse May:34–36

Wald A 2005 Faecal incontinence in the elderly: epidemiology and management. Drugs and Aging 22(2):131–139

Waugh A, Grant A 2006 Ross and Wilson anatomy and physiology in health and illness, 10th edn. Churchill Livingstone, Edinburgh

Webster RA, Thompson DR 2006 Disorders of the cardiovascular system. In: Alexander MF, Fawcett J (Tonks) N, Runciman PJ (eds) Nursing practice: hospital and home (the adult), 3rd edn. Churchill Livingstone, Edinburgh

Wilkinson K 2001 Patkistani women's perceptions and experiences of incontinence. Nursing Standard 16(5):33–39

Wilkinson J 2002 The psychological basis of nursing. In: Kenworthy N, Snowley G, Gelling C (eds) Common foundation studies in nursing, 3rd edn. Churchill Livingstone, Edinburgh, pp 197–224

Willis J 1999 The future beckons. Nursing Times 95(18):61–63

Further reading

Brocklehurst J (ed) 1999 Health outcome indicators: urinary incontinence: report of a working group to the Department of Health. National Centre for Health Outcomes Development, Oxford

Brocklehurst J (ed) 1999 Report to the Department of Health working group on outcome indicators for urinary incontinence. National Centre for Health Outcomes Development, Oxford

Royal College of Physicians 1998 Clinical incontinence: A clinical audit scheme for the management of urinary and faecal incontinence compiled by the Research Unit of The Royal College of Physicians. Royal College of Physicians, London

Useful websites

www.continence-foundation.org.uk (Continence Foundation)

www.dh.gov.uk (Department of Health Essence of Care)

www.disabilitybenefits.co.uk (Disability Benefits)

www.enuresis.org.uk (Enuresis Resource and Information Centre)

www.hpa.org (Health Protection Agency)

www.library.nhs.uk/pathways (National Library for Health)

www.nafc.org (National Association for Continence)

www.nelh.nhs.uk/cochrane (Cochrane Library)

www.nhsdirect.nhs.uk (NHS Direct)

www.nhshealthquality.org (NHS Quality Improvement Scotland)

www.nhshealthquality.org (NHS Quality Improvement Scotland)

www.nice.org.uk (National Institute for Health and Clinical Excellence)

www.nmc-uk.org (Nursing and Midwifery Council)

www.npsa.nhs.uk (National Patients Safety Agency)

www.rcn.org.uk (Commissioning Continence Advisory Services: An RCN Guide)

www.rcplondon.ac.uk (Royal College of Physicians)

Personal cleansing and dressing

Karen Holland

INTRODUCTION

The way in which people dress and maintain personal cleanliness is inextricably linked to the society and culture in which they live. Clothing is influenced by many factors such as the weather, customs and social expectations of men and women. In Western societies it is also linked to what people can afford. Being 'clean' is also a relative concept, in that it depends on whose standards and beliefs it is being measured against. It is important to take account of this when we are assessing individual needs in both personal cleansing and dressing, in particular as to how it affects the health of the individual.

This chapter will therefore focus on the following:

1. **The model of living**
   - Personal cleansing and dressing in health and illness across the lifespan.
   - Dependence/independence in the AL of personal cleansing and dressing.
   - Factors influencing the AL of personal cleansing and dressing.

2. **The model for nursing**
   - Nursing care of individuals with health problems affecting the AL of personal cleansing and dressing, i.e. application of the Roper et al (1996, 2000) model in practice.

THE MODEL OF LIVING

What is meant by personal cleansing and dressing? Roper et al (1996) associate personal cleansing (personal hygiene) with several different activities, i.e. washing and bathing, hand-washing, perineal toilet, care of the hair, care of the nails and care of teeth and mouth. Dressing is used to refer to 'putting on of clothes' which are seen as a medium of nonverbal communication 'and are also essential for living in different environments and social and cultural contexts' (Roper et al 1996, p. 234).

PERSONAL CLEANSING AND DRESSING IN HEALTH AND ILLNESS – ACROSS THE LIFESPAN

Childhood

When babies are first born they are unable to care for themselves, requiring an adult to both clothe them and take care of their personal hygiene. Clothing is required for both warmth and protection, whilst washing is required to remove urine and faeces from contact with their bodies. This will prevent their skin from becoming sore. As children grow they will come to learn to control their own bladder and bowel activity, learning also to use appropriate toilet facilities depending on the culture in which they live. Children in some cultures will use the more natural environments whilst others will learn to use bathrooms and indoor toilet facilities. The effect of not washing children's skin from urine and faeces can be seen in extreme cases of physical abuse – with severe burns and skin damage through neglect and nonwashing.

Other personal cleansing behaviours learnt by young children include combing or brushing their hair, cleaning their teeth and bathing or showering. Lawler (1991) indicates that our cultural beliefs about the body, its functions and products will be reflected in our practice in managing childhood personal cleansing behaviour.

Adolescence

As children grow up their bodies also undergo changes that necessitate additional personal cleansing behaviours. Underarm perspiration and growth of body hair are two changes that occur at puberty, as are the potential problems of dandruff of the scalp and facial acne. In many societies whole industries have developed, aimed at managing these changes and problems. Products such as shampoo, deodorant and soap have become an essential part of living in the modern world and for many, having to go without these becomes stressful. Roper et al (1996, p. 235) point out that:

> *Adolescence can be the period for experimenting with way out fashions and new hairstyles and provided that they do not cause any harm, tolerance and good humour reap better rewards all round than continual derisory remarks. It can be seen as part of a young person's bid for independence and a means of communication, both with peers and other groups.*

Examples of these fashions are nose and lip rings, tattoos and shaved heads. Fashion magazines have a significant influence on how and what we do at all ages but none more so than in young adults. For example, one of the major influences is linked to how we express our sexuality (see Chapter 12), in particular the impact on what we do with and to our bodies, both in terms of dressing and personal hygiene.

Exercise

1. Consider your own adolescent years. What kind of clothes did you wear?
2. Discuss with colleagues how your culture expects you to behave in the period before reaching adulthood.
3. Consider the above quote by Roper et al (1996) and consider your views on their opinion of adolescence.
4. Obtain a wide variety of magazines aimed at the 15–19-year-old age bracket. What do they tell you about how we see the body in Western society?

Adulthood

Reaching adulthood will probably require a different lifestyle, as many adults undertake employment, which will give them financial rewards, and the wherewithal to spend money on both clothes and personal cleansing products. The kind of clothes that people wear can tell us much about both their culture and their lifestyle. Henley & Schott (1999, p. 112) state that 'standards of modest behaviour and decency vary enormously' and that 'what is perfectly acceptable to some, shocks others deeply' (see Box 8.1).

Exercise

Consider the issues identified by Henley and Schott.

1. How would the issue of modesty be affected in mixed-sex wards or mixed-sex washing and toilet facilities?
2. How would you ensure that cultural practices were taken into account in your health care practice?

Box 8.1	Modesty and health care

Some cultures place a particularly high value on personal modesty. Care must be taken to ensure that people always feel decently covered during examinations, treatments and everyday practical care. It is also important to ensure that the patient's environment takes their requirements for modesty into account.

- Many people, especially women of conservative communities, never undress fully except when they are alone. They may be used to uncovering only the relevant part for a medical examination or for treatment.
- Some people never undress completely even to wash. They shower in their clothes, changing into clean dry clothes afterwards.
- For some people it is important that all intimate treatments, examinations and practical care are carried out by someone of the same sex. When there is no health professional of the same sex, some patients may prefer to be washed or helped with washing and using the lavatory by a family member of the same sex if possible.
- For some people the idea of being seen in bed or in nightclothes by strangers, and particularly by people of the opposite sex, is very shocking. This is especially likely for people who normally have little contact with people outside their own family. Women and some men of many communities may feel immodest and exposed in their nightclothes and in a public area. Some may want to keep their curtains closed all the time so that they are not exposed to public gaze.

From Henley & Schott (1999), p. 114.

It is interesting to note that the UK Government decreed that mixed-sex wards are no longer appropriate in a modern hospital, and funds were made available to abolish 95% of them by 2002. The Department of Health has made every attempt to comply with this and agreed three objectives to do this:

1. to ensure that appropriate organisational arrangements are in place to secure good standards of privacy and dignity for hospital patients
2. to achieve the Patient's Charter standard for segregated washing and toilet facilities across the NHS
3. to provide safe facilities for patients in hospital who are mentally ill which safeguard their privacy and dignity (DoH 2007).

A significant number of trusts have complied with this request (DoH 2007).

The National Service Framework for Older People (DoH 2001a, p. 57a) also stated that 'mixed sex wards can be embarrassing and for some people culturally insensitive'. This is also outlined in the DoH (2000a) guidance on mixed-sex accommodation for mental health services which will 'ensure that the safety, privacy and dignity of in-patients are protected'.

Old age

As people get older some tasks may become more difficult to undertake. In many cases these difficulties are linked to underlying health problems such as arthritis. Roper et al (1996, p. 235) also state that:

> 66 *Failing eyesight and shaking hands may make it increasingly difficult for older people to retain their independence with conventional clothing. Back fastenings of garments are difficult to reach and front fastenings are therefore preferable; zips and Velcro tapes are much easier to manipulate than small buttons or hooks and eyes. Many older people more readily feel the cold and may need to wear extra clothing to keep warm. Two layers of thin material (because of the entrapped air which is a bad conductor of heat) are warmer than one thick layer. Adequate warm clothing is a simple but important means of preventing hypothermia, which is a particular threat to old people in severe winter weather.* 99

Clothes, however, provide more than physical comfort and protection. They also help provide a positive self-image and clothes that make us 'feel good' about ourselves can boost our sense of wellbeing. This is as important to the older person as it is to other age groups.

Exercise

1. Talk to someone in your family, or a friend, who is over 70 years old and ask them to describe what it is like to be that age in relation to how they dress and how they manage their personal cleansing and dressing activities.
2. Find out what has influenced any changes in their patterns of behaviour or their own personal preferences.
3. Compare their responses with your own experience and discuss with colleagues from different cultural groups to see if there any differences or similarities between age groups.

DEPENDENCE/INDEPENDENCE IN THE AL OF PERSONAL CLEANSING AND DRESSING

Dependence or independence in this Activity of Living will depend on both age and health and illness status. In infancy there is a total dependence on others, which would also be apparent in later life if the individual was no longer able to physically or mentally cope with their own personal cleansing and dressing needs. Being physically disabled from a traumatic illness, e.g. tetraplegia, is one such example, as are the effects of a chronic illness such as multiple sclerosis. Some children may also be affected by such illnesses, thus prolonging their childhood and infancy dependency.

FACTORS INFLUENCING THE AL OF PERSONAL CLEANSING AND DRESSING

Biological

Roper et al (1996, p. 236) identify the skin 'as the largest physical body structure which relates directly to the Activity of Living of personal cleansing and dressing'. However, as with all Activities of Living, the influence of other physiological systems must be considered. For example, we can see that the physiological changes brought about at puberty have a significant affect on adolescent fashion and their body perceptions (see Chapter 12), and that being physically incapacitated by rheumatoid arthritis will prevent the person from being able to dress themselves without help.

The skin

The skin is the largest organ in the body, and has an important role in the defence of the body (Montague et al 2005). It covers a 'surface area of about 1.5 to 2 square metres in adults and contains glands, hair and nails' (Waugh & Grant 2006, p. 358). Its main structures can be seen in Figure 8.1. Its two main layers are:

- the epidermis
- the dermis.

In addition there is a layer of subcutaneous tissue between the skin and the underlying structures, known as the hyperdermis (Montague et al 2005). The skin has many functions:

- protection
- regulation of body temperature
- formation of vitamin D
- sensation
- absorption
- excretion.

An understanding of the structure and function of the skin is important when considering the personal cleansing and dressing needs of individuals both in health and illness. It is also important when considering the needs of patients who experience breakdown in normal skin functions and structure, for example serious burns or the skin disorder psoriasis.

Structure of the skin

As can be seen from Figure 8.1, the skin has many structures in the dermal layers. The epidermis or outer layer:

> 66 *is the most superficial layer of the skin and is composed of stratified keratinised squamous epithelium (see Fig. 8.2) which varies with thickness in different parts of the body. It is thickest on the palms of the hands and soles of the feet. There are no blood vessels or nerve endings in the epidermis but its deepest layers are bathed in interstitial fluid from the dermis, which provides oxygen and nutrients, and is drained away as lymph.*

> *There are several layers (strata) of cells in the epidermis that extend from the deepest germinative layer to the*

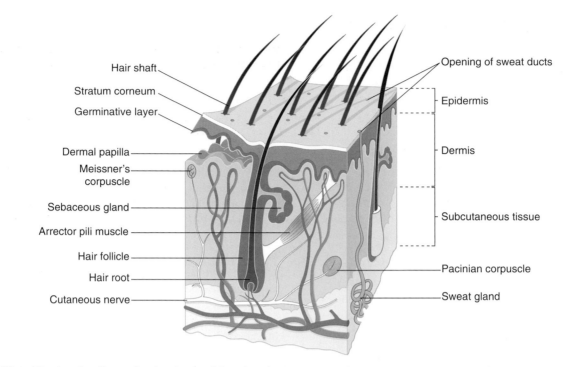

Fig. 8.1 The skin showing the main structures of the dermis (from Waugh & Grant 2006, with permission).

surface stratum corneum (a thick horny layer). The cells on the surface are flat, thin, non-nucleated, dead cells, in which the cytoplasm has been replaced by the fibrous protein keratin. These cells are being rubbed off and replaced by cells that originated in the germinative layer and have undergone gradual change as they progressed towards the surface. Complete replacement of the epidermis takes about 40 days. 〞 (Waugh & Grant 2006, p. 358)

One health problem where this process is altered is psoriasis. Psoriasis is a skin condition 'characterised by rapid and excessive production of keratinised cells which form silvery flakes on the skin surface and which result in excessive desquamation' (shedding of skin cells) (Montague et al 2005, p. 653).

Skin colour will vary according to how much melanin (a dark pigment) is in the skin and this varies 'between members of the same race and between races'. Melanin also protects the skin from the harmful effects of the sunlight (Waugh & Grant 2006, p. 358). The observation of skin colour is an important part of a nurse's observation skills and in particular there is a need to understand how certain signs and symptoms of illness need to be particularly observed in both normal and abnormal skin colour. Examples of skin assessment observations can be seen in Box 8.2.

The dermis or inner layer is tough and elastic in structure.

〞 *It is formed from connective tissue and the matrix contains collagen fibres interlaced with elastic fibres. Rupture of elastic fibres occurs when the skin is overstretched, resulting in permanent striate, or stretch marks that may be found in pregnancy and obesity. Collagen fibres bind water and give the skin its tensile strength, but as this ability declines with age, wrinkles develop.* 〞 (Waugh & Grant 2006, p. 358)

The main structures found in the dermal layer are:

- blood vessels
- lymph vessels
- sensory nerve endings
- sweat glands and their ducts
- hairs, erector pili muscles and sebaceous glands.

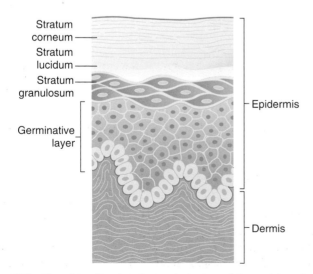

Fig. 8.2 The skin showing the main layers of the epidermis (from Waugh & Grant 2006, with permission).

| Box 8.2 | Physiological assessment (observing skin problems in dark skin) |

1. Pallor

There is an absence of underlying red tones; the skin of a brown-skinned person appears yellow–brown and that of a black-skinned person appears ashen, and the lips and nail beds are similar.

2. Erythema

Inflammation must be detected by palpation; the skin is warmer in the area, tight, and oedematous, and the deeper tissues are hard. Fingertips must be used for this assessment, as with rashes, since they are sensitive to the feelings of different textures of skin.

3. Cyanosis

Cyanosis is difficult to observe in dark-coloured skin, but it can be seen by close inspection of the lips, tongue,

conjunctiva, palms of the hands and the soles of the feet. Slow blood return is an indication of cyanosis. Another sign is ashen grey lips and tongue.

4. Ecchymosis

History of trauma to a given area can be detected from a swelling of the skin surface.

5. Jaundice

The sclera are usually observed for yellow discolouration to reveal jaundice. This is not always a valid indication, however, since carotene deposits can also cause the sclera to appear yellow. The buccal mucosa and the palms of the hands and soles of the feet may appear yellow.

From Spector (1996), p. 206.

Each of these will be considered in relation to the functions of the skin. It is recommended that you read specialist anatomy and physiology books for more detail in relation to the skin and its structure and function (see Further Reading).

Functions of the skin

Protection As well as protecting the deeper and more delicate structures of the body, the skin is an important defence mechanism against: 'invasion by microbes, chemicals, physical agents, e.g. mild trauma, ultraviolet light, dehydration' (Waugh & Grant 2006, p. 360).

Regulation of body temperature The normal temperature of the body 'remains fairly constant at about 36.8°C (98.4°F), although it is slightly raised in the evening, during exercise and in women just after ovulation' (Waugh & Grant 2006, p. 361). In order to ensure this normal measurement the body has to balance heat produced with heat lost from the body. Heat is produced in a number of ways, mainly through muscle activity, liver function and digestion. Heat is lost from the body through the skin, although 'small amounts are lost in expired air, urine and faeces' (Waugh & Grant 2006, p. 360.). The mechanisms of heat loss can be seen in Box 8.3 and the control of body temperature can be seen in Chapter 9.

Formation of vitamin D A substance called 7-dehydrocholesterol found in the skin is converted to Vitamin D by the action of ultraviolet light from the sun. This is then transported in the blood and used in the formation and maintenance of bone (see Chapter 10).

Sensation The dermal layer of the skin consists of nerve endings (sensory receptors) that are 'sensitive to touch, pressure, temperature or pain', and some parts of the body have more of these receptors than others, making them more sensitive, for example the lips and fingertips.

| Box 8.3 | Mechanisms of heat loss |

Evaporation

The body is cooled when heat is used to convert the water in sweat to water vapour.

Radiation

Exposed parts of the body radiate heat away from the body.

Conduction

Clothes and other objects in contact with the skin take up heat.

Convection

Air passing over the exposed parts of the body is heated and rises, cool air replaces it and convection currents are set up. Heat is also lost from the clothes by convection.

From Waugh & Grant (2006), p. 361.

Absorption Waugh & Grant (2006, p. 362) state that:

    ❝ *This property is limited but substances that can be absorbed include:*

- *some drugs, in transdermal patches, e.g. hormone replacement therapy during the menopause, nicotine as an aid to stopping smoking*
- *some toxic chemicals, e.g. mercury.* ❞

Excretion The skin is only a minor excretory organ. Substances that it excretes include sodium chloride in sweat, urea and aromatic substances, e.g. garlic.

Other structures associated with the skin are hair, the sebaceous glands and nails. A brief overview is given of these in order to enable them to be considered when assessing patients' needs with regard to personal cleansing and dressing.

Hindu beliefs

Women must cover their legs, breasts and upper arms. They usually wear a sari and the midriff is very often left bare. Some Hindu women may wear a shalwar kameez both during the day and night. Women wear jewellery in the form of bracelets and a brooch known as a mangal sutra, which is strung on a necklace. These must not be removed unnecessarily. Men usually wear a kameez and pajamas (trousers with drawstring) or a dhoti. This is a cloth about 5–6 metres in length that is wrapped around the waist and drawn between the legs. Older men may also wear a long coat (Achkan) or a shirt with a high collar and buttons down the front known as a kurta. Some men may wear a bead necklace or other jewellery of religious significance.

Sikh beliefs

As an act of faith Sikhs wear what is known as the 5 Ks.

- Kesh – long hair. Men wear this in a bun (jura) under a turban. Women may wear plaits and cover their hair with a scarf (dupatta or chuni); Sikh boys will usually wear their hair in a bun on top of their head covered with a small white cloth (rumal) or a large square cloth (patka)
- Kanga – small comb worn at all times
- Kara – steel bracelet worn on right wrist
- Kacha – special type of underwear, white shorts
- Kirpa – symbolic dagger/sword.

Women wear the salwar (trousers) and kameez (shirt) with a long scarf (chuni); the salwar and kameez are worn day and night. They will also wear glass or gold wedding bangles that are never removed unless they are widowed. (Their removal symbolises the loss of a husband.) Men wear a kameez and pajama or kurta (a long shirt with a high collar and buttons down the front).

From Holland & Hogg (2001), pp. 198, 205.

The climate will also influence personal cleansing and dressing behaviour. Living in a hot climate, for example, may require one to wear light cotton clothing which absorbs perspiration more readily, or if in a very cold climate 'garments made from man-made fibres and wool are useful for providing warmth' (Roper et al 1996, p. 239). Continual exposure to sun, however, can lead to an increased risk of skin cancer (Peters et al 2003), whilst in some skin diseases, e.g. psoriasis, exposure to ultraviolet light is one form of treatment. Skin cancers are preventable. Collier (2002, p. 956) recommends the following 'health-seeking behaviours' in their prevention:

- the avoidance of unnecessary sun exposure, especially between 10.00 and 14.00 hours when the ultraviolet rays are strongest
- the application of sunscreens and/or sunblocks with levels of para-aminobenzoic acid (PABA) whenever exposure to the sun is unavoidable; PABA-free lotions are available for people who are allergic to it
- the wearing of protective clothing, e.g. long-sleeved shirts and broad-brimmed hats, but to recognize that sunscreens and blocks are still necessary
- the treatment of moles if they are particularly prone to repeated friction and irritation
- an awareness of indicators of potential malignancy, i.e. an increase in size, ulceration, bleeding or serous exudates from a mole or other skin lesion.

Uniforms and protective clothing are also encouraged in those work areas where people need to be protected from the physical effects of some activities, e.g. men who work with asbestos or coal dust.

Exercise

Examine your own home and work environments.

1. Consider how they affect your personal cleansing and dressing needs.
2. Compare your own living expectations with those of your colleagues and discuss how cultural needs are also influenced by the environment.
3. Compare evidence of skin cancers in different countries and determine how environmental factors have influenced this (see **www.who.int**).

Politicoeconomic

The political factors associated with personal cleansing and dressing needs are those associated with both housing and access to employment and therefore financial remuneration. In some countries even providing adequate shelter is all that is possible, for example following a severe flood or other disaster. We have often seen pleas for clothes and blankets as well as money from aid agencies in order to ensure basic protection from the elements. Economic factors are interlinked with the political, for without adequate funds no government can hope to ensure that their policies with regard to meeting basic needs can be implemented. We can also see the economic cost of failing to prevent some avoidable skin problems when we see the cost to the National Health Service of pressure ulcer development. Collier (2002, p. 927) states that the Department of Health in 1992 and 1993 reported that the cost to the NHS of pressure ulcers was between £60 million and £321 million. The importance of pressure ulcer prevention to the NHS can be seen in the way that it is one of the nine fundamental aspects of care identified in the *Essence of Care* report (DoH 2003). This offers a set of benchmarking standards, underpinned by an evidence base, to help improve the quality of care in relation to pressure ulcer prevention.

SUMMARY POINTS

1. Both personal cleanliness and dressing are affected by our culture, gender, age and environment.
2. Personal cleanliness includes caring for our skin, nails, hair, teeth, mouth and hands.
3. Maintaining privacy and dignity for individuals to carry out personal hygiene and dressing activities is an essential part of health care.

THE MODEL FOR NURSING

In order to enhance your understanding of how health and illness affect this Activity of Living this section will focus on specific case studies, and will utilise the Roper et al (1996, 2000) model of nursing as a framework to assess, plan, implement and evaluate care. (See Chapter 1 for a full explanation of the nursing process.)

ASSESSING THE INDIVIDUAL IN THE ALs OF PERSONAL CLEANSING AND DRESSING

It is important to remember that every individual must be considered 'holistically' and that personal cleansing and dressing will be affected by health problems specific to other Activities of Living. The summary of life span, dependence/independence and factors affecting personal cleansing and dressing can be seen in Box 8.7.

Assessing the individual

Assessment involves three phases:

- collection of data when taking a nursing history
- interpretation of the data collected
- identification of the individual's actual and potential health problems.

Collection of data when taking a nursing history

The nursing history will involve all Activities of Living and, as seen in Chapter 1, all must be taken into account in the holistic assessment of individuals. If patients' expectations are to be understood and their problems (whether actual or potential) with this AL are to be addressed then assessment must be undertaken. A résumé of topics addressed in relation to each of the components of the model is provided in Box 8.7 and will serve as a reminder of the many dimensions of the AL of personal cleansing and dressing which underpin nursing assessment.

Assessment of the ALs of personal cleansing and dressing

When assessing the ALs of personal cleansing and dressing the following questions can be considered, which also take account of the whole life of the individual.

Box 8.7	Assessing the individual in the AL of personal cleansing and dressing

Lifespan: effect on personal cleansing and dressing
Infancy
- skin care (incontinent state)
- suitable clothing for mobility/safety
- growth of teeth.

Childhood
- developing independence and individuality
- developing concept of modesty
- importance of care of teeth.

Adolescence
- increased underarm perspiration
- problems of acne, greasy hair, dandruff
- expression of feelings/individuality/sexuality through clothes, make-up, hairstyle
- puberty (menstruation/ejaculation).

Adulthood
- routines related to working and playing
- reflection of personality in appearance and clothes.

Old age
- skin dryness
- difficulties with bathing, care of nails and feet
- difficulties with dressing
- physical disability.

Dependence/independence in personal cleansing and dressing
- dependency in infancy/old age/illness
  - on people
  - on aids and equipment.

Factors influencing personal cleansing and dressing
Biological
- stage of physical development
- physical changes with ageing
- individual physical differences
- skin state – colours, bruising/scars/blemishes/dry/moist/turgid/wrinkled areas of discontinuity, cleanliness
- state of hands and nails cleanliness
- handwashing habits   *(continued)*

| Box 8.7 | Assessing the individual in the AL of personal cleansing and dressing *(continued)* |

- state of mouth and teeth
  - moist/dry mouth
  - odour of breath
  - teeth (number/condition/dentures)
  - teeth cleaning routine
- condition/style of hair, type (dry/greasy), dandruff/lice/hairwashing routine
- dress style/appropriateness
- standard of cleanliness/odour/quality
- speciality clothing for work and play
- physical hazards
- physical sex differences
- female – perineal toilet, breast care, menstruation, body hair
- male – cleansing foreskin, shaving.

Psychological
- sex differences/sexuality
- standards related to personality/emotional states

- knowledge (e.g. handwashing, dental care)
- intelligence.

Sociocultural
- values concerning cleanliness/appearance
- social norms for cleansing/dressing routines
- cultural influences/rules on dress
- religious influences/rules on cleansing, dressing.

Environmental
- bath/shower in the home
- piped hot/cold water in home
- exposure at work to substances damaging to the skin
- availability of bathing/handwashing facilities at work
- climate.

Politicoeconomic
- adequacy of necessary facilities for low-income groups
- personal income for articles for personal cleanliness
- personal income for essential clothing and footwear.

From Roper et al (1996).

Lifespan
- How old is the person?
- Do they have a life history of health problems?
- Is there anything in their life history that may affect the way in which they view their present health problems?

Dependence/independence
- Has the individual experienced any difficulties in relation to independent living?
- Are they able to go out and meet other people or are they dependent on others to transport them?
- Will they experience difficulties in the future as a result of their current health problems?

Factors affecting the AL of personal cleansing and dressing
- What specific health problem are they suffering from?
- What do they understand about their present health status?
- What effect is this having on their other Activities of Living?
- What effect is their health problem having on their emotional wellbeing?
- Are there any cultural needs to be taken into account prior to assessment?
- Are there any specific spiritual or religious needs that the patient may have?
- Does the individual have any environmental needs which will affect future care?
- What resources could be required to help the individual manage their health problems both in hospital and at home?

Exercise
1. Reflect on how you have assessed patients' personal cleansing and dressing needs in your practice.
2. Did you use a similar set of questions and a model for nursing?
3. Discuss with your mentor or preceptor how you intend to assess an individual patient's personal cleansing and dressing needs by using the Roper et al model for nursing framework and the above questions.

Consider the following case study and using the same approach consider which questions would be appropriate in the assessment of the patient's needs. Given the sensitive nature of her health problem these questions will have to be asked, as with all questioning and all patients, sensitively and with understanding.

Case study 8.1

Assessment focusing on the ALs of personal cleansing and dressing

A girl, aged 16, attends the Dermatology Clinic in the Outpatient Department for her second appointment. Her GP had diagnosed psoriasis and had referred her to the Consultant at the hospital for further tests and treatment. She is to be seen by both the Consultant and the Specialist Dermatology Nurse. As the Clinic Nurse on the day of her appointment you are required to undertake the initial assessment and history. She is accompanied by her mother.

The following questions might have been asked in relation to the ALs.

Questions as part of the assessment

- When did she first notice the patches of psoriasis?
- Where are the largest ones?
- Do they cause her any irritation?
- Has she been scratching them?
- Has she noticed any scalp irritation or flaky dandruff?
- Has she noticed any flaking of her skin in the bed or on her clothes?
- How does she feel about this?
- Do any of her clothes make the irritation worse?
- Does swimming make her skin more or less irritable?
- Has she any painful lesions anywhere?
- Has any member of her family the same or similar problem?

Other questions that the nurse or doctor may ask include:

- Has she had a throat infection recently?
- Has she found that being in the sun makes the problem better or worse?
- Has she found that the problem gets worse during menstruation?

The responses to the above questions may also give an indication of how she has been dealing psychologically with the appearance of this skin condition, as well as whether she has been trying to hide lesions which have appeared on her arms and legs (by wearing long-sleeved shirts and not going bathing). Assessment may also reveal other problems reported by patients with skin disorders (see Box 8.8).

The following information may be helpful for your assessment of this young girl's needs and also to understand the relevance and importance of some of the questions.

Psoriasis

Psoriasis is a skin disease that causes much psychological distress, mainly because of its appearance and the side-effects of some of the treatments. It is a 'chronic, noninfectious inflammatory skin disorder, characterised by well demarcated erythematous plaques with adherent silver scales' (Page 2006, p. 530). In psoriasis there is an increased production of epidermal cells that do not have time to keratinise completely. This causes 'the build-up of a white waxy silver scale as immature skin cells remain adherent to the skin' (Page 2006, p. 530). There is a genetic predisposition to the disease and it occurs in 2% of the UK population. The precipitating factors can be seen in Box 8.9.

The link can now begin to be seen between the questions asked at assessment, the underlying physiological changes and precipitating factors. The consultant will then make a diagnosis as to which type of psoriasis she has and the subsequent treatment, which could contribute to further psychological stress. Treatments could include coal tar products, which are messy, smelly and can stain clothes, dithranol (suppresses cell proliferation) which if applied to the skin

Box 8.8	Problems reported by patients with skin disorders

Emotional problems
- low self-esteem
- feel body is 'unclean'
- relationships can be problematic
- feel people stare – real and imagined
- regarded as infectious or contagious.

Clothing restrictions
- avoid short sleeves
- avoid dark clothes due to skin shedding
- avoid summer clothes where skin is exposed
- clothes get stained or ruined due to messy creams.

Social restrictions
- skin gets itchy in hot pubs/clubs
- avoid swimming or sports as people stare
- avoid communal changing rooms when shopping.

Financial implications
- routine prescriptions are expensive but essential
- no allowances to replace clothing or bedding
- no allowances available for fuel bills due to extra laundering and bathing, etc.

From Page (2006), p. 533.

Box 8.9	Precipitating factors in psoriasis

- Infection – streptococcal throat infection
- Medication – can exacerbate or trigger psoriasis
- Sunlight – in some patients, psoriasis improves during the summer and relapses during the winter; however others report that sunlight aggravates the condition
- Hormonal – psoriasis can get better or worse during pregnancy or menopause
- Psychological stress – can exacerbate psoriasis but the condition itself is recognised as a stressful condition
- Trauma – creates the 'Koebner effect' where psoriasis is triggered in damaged skin, e.g. the site of an injury or surgical scar.

From Page (2006), p. 530.

also stains the skin and clothing, and emollients to lubricate and moisturise the skin. Other treatments will depend on the precipitating cause and the type of psoriasis (see Box 8.10). Examples of topical therapies used in the management of psoriasis can been seen in Box 8.11.

It can be seen from the questions asked at the initial assessment how important it is for the nurse to know not only the nature and cause of the skin condition but also the normal and abnormal physiological responses of the body.

Box 8.10	Classification of psoriasis

Guttae psoriasis

Presents as drop-like symmetrical lesions on the trunk and the limbs. It is most common in adolescents and young adults and is often triggered by a streptococcal throat infection. It responds well to therapy.

Plaque psoriasis

Presents as well demarcated erythematous plaques covered in dry, white-waxy scale often localised to the knees and elbows. Removal of this build up of keratin leaves small bleeding points. Plaques vary considerably in size and can extend to cover the trunk and scalp. Plaque psoriasis tends to be chronic with exacerbations and periods of remission.

Flexural psoriasis

Affects the axillae, submammary and anogenital areas and looks different from typical psoriasis. Plaques are sharply defined but the skin has a thin glistening redness, often with painful fissures in the skin folds.

Pustular psoriasis (palmoplantar pustulosis)

Localised form of psoriasis affecting the hands and feet. It is characterised by yellow/brown pustules which dry into brown scaly macules. It is a painful condition and difficult to treat.

Generalised pustular psoriasis

Rare yet serious form of the disease. Sheets of sterile pustules develop, merging on an erythematous background. These areas of skin shear and the patient will be unwell. It is often triggered when attempts are made to withdraw oral or topical steroids or may just reflect the instability of the condition.

Scalp psoriasis

Can often be the sole manifestation of the disorder. Thick scale adheres to the scalp and can extend to the edges of the scalp margin and behind the ears.

Nail changes

In psoriasis can involve pitting of nails and onycholysis when the distal edge of the nail separates from the nail bed. There is no effective topical treatment for psoriatic nail changes.

Erythrodermic psoriasis

Rare but severe form. The skin becomes uniformly red with a high blood volume flushing it. The patient feels unwell and maintaining body temperature is difficult. It can be triggered by the irritant effects of therapies (e.g. dithranol, tars), by withdrawal of systemic/oral steroids or by a medication reaction. Erythrodermic psoriasis is an unstable state that is potentially life threatening and warrants urgent hospital admission. The condition can progress to general pustular psoriasis.

Psoriatic arthropathy

Psoriasis can be complicated by psoriatic arthropathy, a 'rheumatoid-like arthritis' affecting about 5% of psoriasis patients. Joint changes occur in hands, feet, spine and sacroiliac joints. This rheumatoid-like arthritis mimics rheumatoid disease but notably the rheumatoid test factor is negative. Psoriatic arthropathy is a difficult combination to treat, meriting the combined expertise of a rheumatologist and dermatologist.

From Page (2006), p. 531.

Box 8.11	Examples of topical therapies used in psoriasis management

- Emollients – emulsifying ointment, 50/50 (white soft paraffin/liquid paraffin)
- Bath additives – Aveeno, Dermol 600, Hydromol, Oilatum
- Soap substitute – aqueous cream, emulsifying ointment, Epaderm
- Coal tar ointments – Alphasol HC, coal tar solution, crude coal tar solution, Carob-Dome
- Dithranol – Micanol, Dithrocream, Dithranol in Lassar's paste
- Vitamin D analogues – calcipatrol, tacalcitol, calcitrol
- Scalp therapy – olive oli, Cocois scalp application, Capasal shampoo, Polytar liquid, Alphosyl shampoo
- Phototherapy – ultraviolet light B (UVB)
- Photochemotherapy – oral: psoralen tablets + ultraviolet light A (UVA); bath: trimethylpsoralen + UVA.

From Page (2006), p. 533.

Understanding these will enable the nurse to offer support during the subsequent treatment of the patient, in particular when it comes to personal cleansing and dressing activities such as which clothes she might find more comfortable to wear and how she will cope with the possible staining of them by skin preparations. The condition as can be seen is one that has exacerbations and remissions and is unlikely to go away entirely. She will have to live with its presence for the rest of her life and learn how to cope with its visual and systemic appearance.

Undertaking a health history is therefore an essential part of any nursing assessment, and an understanding of the elements of the nursing model that comprise the living aspects will enable you to ensure that the questions directly affecting this young girl will be relevant. However, what is not possible within this example is to identify how her other Activities of Living are affected by what is happening due to the fact that we have no further information about her life and health. If it does indicate that she has psoriasis then we can only surmise how her life could be affected.

For example, her symptoms may prevent her from going out socially with her friends as she may worry about her skin appearance and wearing the clothes that she would have normally gone out in, e.g. short-sleeved shirts (working and playing). Understanding the physiological factors affecting psoriasis will enable you to explain to her why she has the skin problems; understanding about the psychological factors will enable you to give her support to cope with having a skin disease. To be able to explain and offer effective support however will require the nurse to have, and be able to use, good communication skills (see Chapter 4).

Exercise

1. Given the information about the girl's health problem and taking into account the abnormal physiology and types of psoriasis, how would you advise her and her mother about how to manage the condition in the short term and long term?
2. Find current research on the care of patients with psoriasis and other skin conditions you have come across in order to ensure that your practice is evidence based.

SUMMARY POINTS

1. Personal cleansing and dressing is affected by lifespan, dependence/independence and biological, psychological, sociocultural, environmental and politicoeconomic factors.
2. Assessment of a patient/client in the daily activity of personal cleansing and dressing needs to be holistic.
3. Sensitive questioning and a knowledge of normal physiology is essential in caring for patients with health problems such as skin disorders which affect personal cleansing and dressing activities.

APPLICATION OF THE ROPER, LOGAN AND TIERNEY MODEL IN PRACTICE

Using all the information in the previous sections of this chapter we will now explore how the model can be used in the care of two patients who have a health problem that affects their personal cleansing and dressing needs (see Case studies 8.2 and 8.3).

Case study 8.2

Focus on health problem in the ALs of personal cleansing and dressing

An evidence-based total care approach
Mrs Joan Wells, an 84-year-old lady, is admitted to hospital with pneumonia.

Health history
She has a daughter living in Canada and a son living in America, and lives on her own. Her husband Bob had died 5 years previously. She is normally a very physically and socially active healthy person but since she had a fall the previous month she has been unable to look after herself as normal. She had not required hospitalisation but it had made her lose confidence and reduced her mobility. She has been feeling very depressed and has neglected herself. Her present illness has increased this feeling. Her neighbour called the doctor's surgery when she had not seen her for a week and she would not answer the door. Her son and daughter had also contacted her when their mother had not made contact with them as she normally did once a week. When the district nurse and General Practitioner (GP) arrived they were also unable to get a response and the police had to be called to break down the door. They found Mrs Wells in her bed, looking very ill and she was obviously dehydrated. (Her eyes appear sunken and her skin has lost its natural elasticity and is 'wrinkled' in appearance.) Her mouth is encrusted with sores and she has been incontinent of both urine and faeces – due to not having the strength to get out of bed to go to the toilet. She is also slightly confused and it is apparent that she has not been eating either. Her neighbour was also upset to see her in such a mess as she was normally a very fastidious lady and kept herself and her house very clean. The GP decides that she needs admitting to hospital for care and treatment of both the bronchopneumonia and related health problems.

On admission
Mrs Wells is admitted to the ward directly from home following the GP referral and has clearly been unable to maintain her own personal cleansing and dressing needs. Her neighbour has arrived with her and has agreed to contact Mrs Wells' son and daughter regarding their mother, once it has been decided on the course of treatment and care plan. Mrs Wells appears to be confused and cannot remember what has happened to her. She is visibly distressed when she is admitted to the ward.

You may have considered the following.

LIFESPAN

Mrs Wells is an older person and, like all patients, requires her personal dignity and modesty to be considered. However, as the Nursing and Midwifery Advisory Committee Report *Caring for Older People* (DoH 2001b) shows, negative attitudes to older people in the acute care sector generally have influenced the way in which nurses ensure this essential care is undertaken. Mrs Wells is very ill with pneumonia and as an older person is more vulnerable to its effects. As a result she has been unable to maintain her normal standards of personal cleansing and dressing. Acknowledgement of her age and her normal capabilities will be vital in restoring her dignity.

DEPENDENCE/INDEPENDENCE

As seen in the brief profile of Mrs Wells, her neighbour has informed us that she is normally a very active lady who lives on her own. It will be important to determine during the assessment her normal pattern of independent living and, in preparation for her discharge home from hospital, how she is going to manage during her recuperation from her current illness. She appears to have the support of her neighbour but her immediate family is not available. The way in which she recovers from her present illness will also affect her situation in the future, as it is apparent that her recent depression has contributed to the deterioration in her general health.

FACTORS AFFECTING PERSONAL CLEANSING AND DRESSING

As we get older there are many physiological changes that occur in our bodies all of which will have an effect on our response to illness. It can be seen that, due to her fall, Mrs Wells has been unable to be as mobile as she is normally. She was fortunate that she had not sustained a fracture, given that osteoporosis is a common occurrence in older women (see Chapter 10).

It can also be seen from the brief health history that the depression that affected Mrs Wells following her fall had contributed to her current state of ill health. Her normal independence was compromised by this. This feeling of isolation can in turn lead to loss of confidence and 'self-worth'.

Mrs Wells' son and daughter live abroad and therefore are unable to offer their immediate support. It is apparent that they are, however, in regular contact with their mother and have been concerned that she has not been in communication with them. This lack of immediate support from her son and daughter will be crucial when nurses are planning for her discharge home from hospital, as it will mean that Mrs Wells will need to probably rely on the health and social services for her future support. If she owns her own home and has savings it may also mean that she will have to contribute to her own care. Her home environment will also be a contributing factor in her aftercare – in particular how easy it is for her to use toilet and bathroom facilities, especially as it appears that she has been unable to do so during her prehospital admission. All these factors will influence the assessment of her needs in all areas of her normal living activities.

ASSESSMENT OF NEEDS

Using this knowledge of her background and potential influencing factors assess Mrs Wells' individual needs on admission to hospital. Use the questions on p. 276 as a guide.

Collection of data on admission

As well as gathering information from Mrs Wells herself, her neighbour and her GP will also have a contribution to make. It is also pertinent to note that all data obtained concerning Mrs Wells and her care will need to be documented in her medical notes and her nursing care plans. You may work in an environment that has integrated care pathways, in which case the multidisciplinary team will be responsible for documenting care and treatment planned and implemented (see Chapter 1 for further details on care plans).

Assessment of Mrs Wells' actual problems on admission to the ward: using the model for nursing as a framework

Ensuring a safe environment in which to carry out the initial assessment of Mrs Wells' needs will be an important aspect of the nurse's role. It is also important to remember that she is very ill and may be unable to answer questions in the immediate post-admission period. Some details will be essential in order to plan her immediate care but other data can be gathered over the following 48-hour period. Using the questions on p. 276 and her pre-admission history we can see that some details have already been obtained from her neighbour, the GP and the district nurse. These are:

- *Lifespan*: she is 84 years old; she is normally a very active healthy person.
- *Independence/dependence*: she has been independent until her minor fall when she appears to have lost her confidence, become depressed and neglected herself to the point that she is now dependent on the health care team.
- *Factors affecting the AL of personal cleansing and dressing*: she has pneumonia which has affected her ability to care for herself and she has become incontinent of both urine and faeces; it is her previous minor fall that affected her emotional wellbeing initially; we are not aware of her religious nor spiritual beliefs at this stage nor her own health beliefs; as she currently lives on her own, there will be resources, both physical and human that she will require during her stay in hospital and in preparation for her future discharge from hospital.

Based on this initial information an assessment of her needs at various stages of care will now be explored using an evidence-based approach (see Chapter 2). It will be seen that problems in one Activity of Living cannot be easily separated from others, in that each activity is directly linked to another (see Chapter 1 for further information).

Activities of Living: an evidence-based approach
Personal cleansing and dressing
Given that Mrs Wells is seriously ill and has neglected herself as a result of this and her depression, it can be seen that she is unable to care for her own personal cleansing and dressing needs. As she normally did so she will probably be very distressed that she is now dependent on others to manage this for her. An assessment of her tissue breakdown risk also needs to be undertaken as she has been doubly incontinent and her skin integrity is therefore at risk. She has mouth sores and will need mouth care and hygiene. Older people such as Mrs Wells are at a higher risk of developing pressure sores, especially if they are also undernourished and incontinent. The nurse may decide to use one of several risk assessment scoring systems available, ensuring that reassessment is undertaken at identified intervals following admission. Bale (2006) argues that 'it is only useful if it is used regularly'. Assessing risk on admission is essential also to ensuring that Mrs Wells has the correct mattress and other pressure-relieving devices as part of her care plan.

Actual problem   Mrs Wells is unable to manage her own personal cleansing and dressing activities. She is also at risk from developing pressure sores.

Communication
From the health history it can be seen that Mrs Wells is probably very depressed and may well have withdrawn from communicating with her friends and neighbour. She is normally in contact with her children but has failed to communicate with them recently due to her illness and its consequences. She is also confused on admission, possibly due to the dehydration. This makes it difficult for the nurse

admitting her to obtain informed consent to any treatment or care she may require at this stage. The doctor may talk to her next of kin if Mrs Wells continues to be confused and unable to make decisions about her own care. However, the Department of Health (2001c, p. 9) point out that:

> 66 *If a person is not capable of giving or refusing consent it is still possible for you lawfully to provide treatment and care, unless such care has been validly refused in advance. However this treatment or care must be in the person's 'best interests'.*
>
> *No one (not even a spouse or others close to the person) can give consent on behalf of adults who are not capable of giving consent for themselves. However those close to the incapacitated person should always be involved in decision-making, unless the older person has earlier made it clear that they don't want such involvement. Although legally the health professional responsible for the person's care is responsible for deciding whether or not particular treatment is in that person's best interests, ideally decisions will reflect an agreement between professional carers and those close to the older person.* 99

Thomson & Norman (2006) note that it is important for confusion to be correctly defined and that causes are many in older people. Treatment will depend on the cause, as in Mrs Wells' situation that has arisen because of her dehydration and her respiratory infection.

Actual problem   She is unable to communicate why she has been admitted to hospital. She is unable to articulate her understanding of what is happening to her and to give her informed consent.

Working and playing
According to her neighbour Mrs Wells is normally a very active and healthy lady. However, since her fall and her depression she has withdrawn from her normal social activity. This is quite a normal occurrence for someone of her age. The Department of Health Report *Caring for Older People* (2001b) stresses the importance of assessing the mental health needs of older people and points out that 'older people often (35%) present with co-morbidity of physical and mental problems, most commonly dementia and depression'. They identified a set of standard statements and indicators which could guide nurses in their attempts to ensure that mental health needs were assessed (see Box 8.12).

Actual problem   She is unable to undertake her normal social activities.

Expressing sexuality
It is known that Mrs Wells was normally a very fastidious lady, taking pride in herself and her home. She was also very socially and physically active. Her present illness has led to her neglecting her normal personal cleansing and dressing behaviour which would normally enhance her wellbeing and her self-image. She may also be worried about her future and how

Box 8.12	Standards in specific clinical aspects of care: mental health needs

Standard statement

The older person's mental health needs form an important part of nursing assessment and care planning, as part of the multidisciplinary approach to care during the acute phase of illness.

Criteria

1. Nursing assessments take account of the older person's mental health status and needs and these are translated into nursing care plans.
2. Nurses work in partnership with other members of the multidisciplinary team to meet the older person's mental health needs.

Indicators

Examples of indicators in each criterion are given below:

1. (i) Local guidance is available on assessment appropriate to the mental health needs of the older person. This recognises that the person has a biography and that psychological aspects of care are an integral part of assessment in general.

   (ii) Nursing staff are aware of local specialist mental health colleagues (e.g. liaison nurse, community psychiatric nurse, dementia care specialist) to whom they refer older people for further assessment and advice.

2. (i) A nurse on each ward or unit is designated to act as a contact point in respect of the mental health needs of the older person and to liaise with other members of the multidisciplinary team and specialists.

   (ii) Specialist advice on the mental health needs of the older person is available on the ward/unit.

From Department of Health (2001b).

---

she is going to cope with caring for herself as she gets older and less able to deal with illness. According to Rutter (2000, p. 204) this is quite often a normal response to coping with the effects of old age. In relation to sexual activity (people are sexual beings – see Chapter 12) it is not known if Mrs Wells is still sexually active and this is not immediately relevant to her care. However, it cannot be assumed that she has not been sexually active prior to her illness. Roper et al (1996, p. 345) point out that 'although sexual activity generally decreases with age, many older adults continue to be sexually active and human beings do not cease to be sexual beings in old age'. This knowledge would be of value in her post-illness rehabilitation and would possibly be discovered as part of the ongoing care of Mrs Wells. She may, however, decide not to disclose this kind of personal information and that is her right.

Actual problem Mrs Wells has lost interest in herself and her self-image.

Dying

Mrs Wells is seriously ill with pneumonia. She is also suffering from depression and confusion on admission to hospital. She may also have memories of her husband dying in a hospital environment and this may have increased her awareness of her own vulnerability. Roper et al (1996, p. 402) point out that 'for the elderly there is a constant realisation that they are approaching the end of the lifespan and they are made aware of this by an increasing number of deaths in their peer group'. Her religion may also be important to her but because of her confusion and distress this type of information can be obtained at a later time when her condition is improved. She may express her fears of dying to the nurse.

Actual problem Mrs Wells is seriously ill.

Elimination

Mrs Wells has been incontinent of both urine and faeces due to her illness and lack of mobility. This is not normal behaviour for her. On admission the nurse needs to determine the extent of her problem and once the patient is made comfortable offer an opportunity for Mrs Wells to use either a bedpan or commode as soon as possible. The nurse needs to assess her level of confusion at the same time to see whether she is capable of asking for help to go to the toilet. Her skin may already have started to break down. Nurses caring for older people in acute care areas may wish to refer to the Department of Health's (2001d) *Practice Guidance* on continence care to support their assessment and subsequent care of patients such as Mrs Wells. These standards are part of a resource tool developed as a result of the findings of the Nursing and Midwifery Advisory Committee report *Caring for Older People* (DoH 2001b, p. iii) which reported that there were 'major deficits in the standards of nursing care given to older patients in acute hospitals, with some of their most fundamental needs remaining unmet' (see Box 8.13 for standards recommended and Chapter 7).

Actual problem Mrs Wells is incontinent of urine and faeces on admission.

Eating and drinking

As Mrs Wells has been unable to care for herself due to her illness and poor mobility she has obviously not been eating and drinking as normal. She has become dehydrated. It will be important for the nurse to determine as soon as possible following admission what her food and drink preferences are, in order to ensure that when she has recovered from the pneumonia her dietary needs are met. What people eat is very often linked to their age and their culture (DoH 2001b). Mrs Wells will probably need an intravenous infusion of fluid in order to ensure that her immediate needs are met, which will also improve her confusion if it has been caused by an associated sodium imbalance (Gobbi et al 2006). An effective assessment of her eating and drinking needs will be key to her

---

Box 8.13 **Standards in specific clinical aspects of care: continence**

Standard statement

Continence forms an important part of nursing assessment and care planning in relation to the older person. The subject is handled with sensitivity by the nursing staff.

Criteria

1. Nursing assessments take account of the older person's previous, current and desired continence status and health needs and these are translated into nursing care plans.
2. Nurses work in partnership with other members of the multidisciplinary team to meet the older person's continence needs.

Indicators

Examples of indicators for each of the criteria are given below. See also *Good Practice in Continence Services* (DoH 2000b).

1. (i) A continence assessment is carried out as part of the initial nursing assessment. While the nurse may use a checklist to ensure that the relevant subjects are covered, this is used discreetly with recognition that many older people may find the subject in general a very embarrassing one. Time and as much privacy as possible are allowed for the assessment, to go at the older person's pace and put them at their ease.

   Examples of subjects to be covered include:

   a. current difficulties with continence and nature of difficulty
   b. any accompanying symptoms, e.g. burning, itching or pressure

   c. relevant past medical/surgical history
   d. possibly related areas such as use of medications
   e. activities of daily living: ability to reach and/or find a toilet, finger and wrist dexterity (affecting management of clothing)
   f. usual bowel movement pattern
   g. any recent changes in bowel movement patterns, e.g. constipation or diarrhoea.

   (ii) Where a problem is discovered, a management and treatment plan is started. The named nurse or their substitute acts in an advocacy role for the older person, ensuring that the older person has an explanation of this plan. The nurse introduces the subject sensitively and tactfully, taking time to explain it to the older person and to discuss any psychological issues.

2. (i) A nurse on each ward or unit is designated to act as a contact point in respect of continence care and to liaise with other members of the multidisciplinary team and specialists (e.g. a urologist) about the continence service they provide to older people. The service is reviewed regularly.

   (ii) All nurses are knowledgeable and skilled in the management and promotion of continence and promotion of continence and the continence service provided to older people.

   From Department of Health (2001d).

---

recovery. (See Box 8.14 for recommendations and standards of care for older people's nutrition and hydration needs.)

Actual problem Mrs Wells is dehydrated and malnourished.

Maintaining a safe environment

As it is known that Mrs Wells had a minor fall before her present illness and it was a contributing factor in her inability to look after herself, an assessment of how this will put her safety at risk in hospital will be essential. A nursing care plan will need to be devised which will ensure that her need for independence is taken into account but that this is gradually achieved over time as her illness and her self-esteem improve. She will clearly need to be dependent on the nurses and others until her strength is improved and this will mean ensuring her external and internal environments are safe (see Chapter 1).

Actual problem She is unable to maintain her own safe environment.

Breathing

Mrs Wells has bronchopneumonia (see Box 8.15). She will have difficulty breathing properly and may already have been given oxygen prior to her admission. (See Chapter 3 –

Breathing, for details of the normal physiology.) This is also the main cause of her inability to care for herself and her personal cleansing and dressing needs, which are significant considering that she is incontinent of urine and faeces and she will also be sweating due to the pyrexia associated with such an illness.

Actual problem Mrs Wells is having difficulty breathing due to the bronchopneumonia.

Mobilising

Due to the fall she has been unable to be as mobile as she normally is – she is therefore at risk of further falls and immobility. Assessment of her mobility capability will need to be undertaken in order to ensure her safety and also any rehabilitation needs she may have. Her illness will also prevent her from being as mobile and she will probably be dependent on the nurses for many activities, including maintaining her own personal cleansing and dressing needs, until she has recovered. An assessment by the physiotherapist will be essential in order to identify her capability for movement and determine a plan for her physical rehabilitation. At some point an assessment with the occupational therapist will be necessary, in order to determine how she will manage when she is discharged and if she may require aids to help her with her personal cleansing and dressing needs,

---

Box 8.14 | **Standards in specific clinical aspects of care: nutrition and hydration**

Standard statement

The older person's nutritional needs, including hydration, form an important part of nursing assessment and care planning, as part of the multidisciplinary approach to dietary care during the acute phase of illness.

Criteria

1. There is evidence that nursing assessments take account of the older person's physical, cultural and individual preferences when considering nutritional status.
2. Nurses work in partnership with others to meet the nutritional needs of the older person. This includes clinical and nonclinical support staff and involves input from carers, where indicated. It also includes working in direct partnership with the older person.

Indicators

Examples of indicators for each criterion are given below.

1. (i) All older people are screened on admission by nurses to determine their nutritional 'risk' status, using evidence-based protocol. Screening of individual people for past and/or potential difficulties in eating and drinking is also undertaken. This screening needs to include aspects such as:
   a. height and weight

   b. recent weight loss
   c. reduced appetite
   d. eating and digestive difficulties
   e. excessive weakness, apathy, fatigue
   f. other risk factors – infection, recent surgery, radiotherapy, pain
   g. cultural or religious eating habits and taboos.

   (ii) If risk is identified, a dietary care plan is devised with appropriate members of the multidisciplinary team to ensure that older people receive adequate nutrition and hydration. This includes physical assistance with eating and drinking. Nursing staff will ensure that this is provided.

2. (i) A nurse on each ward or unit is designated to act as a contact point in respect of dietary care and to liaise with clinical and nonclinical staff involved in dietary care to review the nutritional service to individual people and to the ward/unit as a whole.

   (ii) All nurses are knowledgeable and skilled in the management and promotion of good dietary care in the context of religious and cultural practices and the dietary care service provided to older people.

From Department of Health (2001d).

---

e.g. bathroom aids such as handles for getting in and out of the bath. As she lives on her own and has been unable to look after herself, it will be essential that an agreement is reached with her and her family prior to her being discharged home as to how her aftercare will be managed. Her immediate family live some distance away. At this stage the Social Services may have to be contacted in order to assess aspects of future care. The involvement of the multidisciplinary team is an essential aspect of her post-hospital recovery. It is essential that discharge becomes an integral part of initial assessment following admission to hospital to ensure that both intermediate care needs as well as long-term care needs are considered in partnership with families and the patient (Manthorpe 2006, p. 91).

Actual problem   Mrs Wells is unable to mobilise by herself.

Controlling body temperature

The pneumonia will mean she is pyrexial in the early stages of the illness. Observations of her temperature and pulse on admission should reveal the extent of this. As seen in Box 8.15, personal hygiene will be essential to her wellbeing, especially as she will be sweating as a result of the pyrexia (see Chapter 9).

Actual problem   Mrs Wells is pyrexial.

Sleeping

Given her health history it is not difficult to imagine that Mrs Wells has been having difficulty sleeping. Older people

need less sleep than younger ones (Le May 2006) and anxiety and depression together with physical illness will exacerbate this (see Chapter 13).

Actual problem   Mrs Wells may have difficulty in sleeping due to anxiety, depression and breathing difficulties.

Conclusion

Caring for Mrs Wells will require a plan that incorporates every Activity of Living. We can see clearly the difficulties in trying to tease apart the effects of her illness and other predisposing factors. Mrs Wells is a unique individual who has to be seen as a whole person, taking account of the fact that a model for nursing used in the assessment process is there to guide the nurse in ensuring that all her needs are taken into account in the planning, implementing and evaluating stages of her care.

Exercise

1. Based on the above assessment and an evidence base, plan Mrs Wells' care for the duration of her stay in hospital, with particular reference to her personal cleansing and dressing needs.
2. Plan her care for discharge home or alternative care arrangements. Refer to Chapter 1 for goal setting and evaluation of care.

| Box 8.15 | Bronchopneumonia |

Pathophysiology

Bronchopneumonia is characterised mainly by patchy areas of consolidated lung tissues. Causative organisms are bacterial and fungal and include staphylococci, pneumococci, streptococci, *Haemophilus influenzae* and Candida. It usually occurs in individuals weakened by other conditions and often in the very old, the very young, and the unconscious and as a result of a pre-existing disease, such as chronic bronchitis, atelectasis or carcinoma in adults or infectious diseases in infants.

Clinical features

These vary in severity depending on the overall condition of the patient but include varying degrees of pyrexia, cough with copious purulent sputum, exhalatory rales, dyspnoea and tachypnoea. Consolidation of the lower lobes is found on auscultation.

Medical management

The causative organism is isolated by sputum culture and sensitivity and appropriate antibiotic therapies are commenced. The patient's general condition is improved by attention to nutrition, hydration and physiotherapy.

Nursing priorities and management

The patient with bronchopneumonia will be very ill and she and her family will need a great deal of comfort and reassurance. Attention to personal hygiene and physical comfort is important. The patient should be turned or encouraged to move regularly. A sitting position, where possible, will make breathing easier and, if oxygen is prescribed, this therapy should be monitored carefully. Aids to prevent pressure sores developing should be selected judiciously.

Bronchopneumonia can be prevented in many hospitalised high-risk patients by thorough nursing assessment and meticulous nursing care.

From Edmond et al (2006) pp. 73–103.

SUMMARY POINTS

1. An understanding of the ageing process is essential for assessing the personal cleansing and dressing needs of the older person.
2. Health problems affecting the ALs of personal cleansing and dressing can be seen to be interdependent on other Activities of Living.
3. Effective discharge planning and outcome begin as soon as the patient is admitted to hospital.

Exercise

1. Before assessing his needs on admission to the ward following surgery, consider what knowledge of bilateral amputation and care of patients following such trauma you will need to help Mr Upton with his personal cleansing and dressing needs postoperatively and on discharge home from hospital.

| Case study 8.3 |

Health problem in the AL of personal cleansing and dressing

This case study focuses on a health problem not directly connected to ALs of personal cleansing and dressing, but one which has major implications for assessment of need in relation to the individual's specific personal cleansing and dressing functioning.

Mr John Upton, a 42-year-old married man, is admitted to an orthopaedic ward for amputation of both legs following a car accident in which he sustained a crush injury to both his legs.

Health history

Mr Upton is a self-employed director of his own clothing company. His 38-year-old wife works for him as a fashion buyer and they have two children – boys aged 10 and 15 years. They had just returned from their annual holiday to their villa in the south of France when the accident happened. He plays football for a local team and keeps fit at the sports centre. His work involves meeting different people and he always ensures that his company is promoted by the smart clothes he wears, in particular his sports range and business suits. He is a very social person and enjoys going out with his wife and family for meals and other social events. The family live in a large five-bedroomed house with a large garden. He was travelling home from a business appointment when the accident happened. An articulated lorry went out of control on the motorway and hit a number of vehicles. Mr Upton unfortunately became trapped in his vehicle during the 'pile-up'.

He has been made aware of the extent of the surgery undertaken to save his life. An above-knee amputation was necessary on both legs.

The following may have been considered:

- knowledge of the anatomy and physiology of the lower limbs, including the blood and nerve supply
- knowledge of what happens during surgery, i.e. the procedure for amputation
- current evidence-based practice for caring for patients who have had amputations
- current medication and treatment for bilateral amputations
- knowledge of care from admission to discharge home and follow-up rehabilitation programmes.

FACTORS AFFECTING PERSONAL CLEANSING AND DRESSING FOLLOWING BILATERAL AMPUTATION

For any patient, removal, or partial removal, of two of their limbs will be a traumatic experience. Mr Upton, however, has not had the opportunity to be prepared for this eventuality and will therefore require additional support following surgery (Lucas 2006). Consider the issues in relation to postoperative care of a patient who has been prepared for the eventuality following amputation of a lower limb (see Exercise box and Box 8.16).

In relation to question 1 the following have been considered:

- Mr Upton has not been prepared for the surgery.
- He has had two lower limbs amputated at the same time.
- He is severely shocked due to the trauma of the accident and the emergency surgery.
- Mobility will be difficult as he has had two lower limbs amputated.

In relation to question 2 the following have been considered:

- Mr Upton has been a physically active man who has taken an interest in his own dressing requirements, partly as a result of his own clothing business. He has probably enjoyed swimming as well as playing football and playing with his children. This has now come to an end for the time being, as he is no longer able to stand or undertake any of the physical activities he was capable of. As we can see in Box 8.16 he will need to adapt his clothing to take account of the fact that until he has his prostheses fitted he will be unable to walk and will be confined to a wheelchair. The clothes that he previously wore will still be able to be worn, but the trousers will need to be tucked up when he is sitting in a wheelchair. A great deal of his management will depend on how he responds to the postoperative shock of finding he no longer has his lower limbs and that he will be unable to move and exercise as he previously did. The response of his family at

---

Exercise

1. What will you need to consider in relation to Mr Upton that is different from the issues in Box 8.15?
2. Given Mr Upton's previous lifestyle what will be the major changes he will be required to make with regards to his personal cleansing and dressing needs?
3. Consider your own experiences of caring for people who may have had an amputation. How did they cope with this?

| Box 8.16 | Caring for a patient following amputation of a lower limb |

Mobilisation

The patient will normally sit out of bed within 12 hours of surgery and may use a wheelchair initially to assist with mobilisation. Practice in standing, and transferring from bed to chair and from wheelchair to toilet will be given. This increases the patient's independence and improves their morale. The physiotherapist will supervise walking. The patient may find that their sense of balance has been temporarily altered, but with advice and support this problem will be overcome.

Clothing

The patient's clothing may need to be adapted temporarily until the prosthesis is supplied. The tucking of an empty arm of a jacket or the leg of a pair of trousers into the body of the garment is an apparent detail but failure to do this can often be the last straw for a patient who until then, has been coping well.

Promoting independence

The patient should be taught how to care for the stump once the sutures are removed by maintaining skin hygiene, moisturising the skin surface if required, and twice daily inspecting the whole stump for any skin discolouration, which may indicate the potential development of a pressure sore. This care will be reinforced during visits to the prosthetic department where information about care of the prosthesis will be given. The patient or a relative should be taught how to apply the stump bandage so that necessary compression is maintained, to help mould and firm the tissue in preparation for fitting the definitive prosthesis at a later date. (For further information see Smith 2003.) Stump bandaging is an area of changing practice and the elastic bandage soft dressing traditionally used may be replaced by other types of dressing, for example semirigid dressings (Wong & Edelstein 2000).

From Jamieson et al (2000).

this time will also be crucial to how he manages to come to terms with his initial dependence on them and health carers. Caring for his stump, with the help of his wife will also depend on a number of other factors, including how he sees his own sexuality and body image. However, as we can see, making sure the stumps are kept clean and moist will be essential if the prostheses are to be fitted properly.

- Successful rehabilitation in all Activities of Living and caring for Mr Upton and his family will require the involvement of the multidisciplinary team.

SUMMARY POINTS

1. Personal cleansing and dressing needs can be affected by indirect health problems in other Activities of Living, e.g. severe trauma causing difficulties with mobility.
2. Meeting patients' personal cleansing and dressing needs is the responsibility of the multidisciplinary team and can also involve the patient's family.
3. Promoting self-care with personal cleansing and dressing needs is an important part of patient rehabilitation.

References

Bale S 2006 Wound healing. In: Alexander MF, Fawcett JN, Runciman PJ (eds) Nursing practice – hospital and home (the adult), 3rd edn. Churchill Livingstone, Edinburgh, pp. 833–860

Collier M 2002 Caring for the patient with a skin or wound care need. In: Walsh M (ed) Watson's clinical nursing and related sciences. Baillière Tindall, Edinburgh, pp. 925–959

Department of Health 2000a Guidance on mixed-sex accommodation for mental health services. DoH, London

Department of Health 2000b Good practice in continence services. DoH, London

Department of Health 2001a National service framework for older people. DoH, London

Department of Health 2001b Caring for older people: a nursing priority, Nursing and Midwifery Standing Committee. DoH, London

Department of Health 2001c Seeking consent: working with older people. DoH, London

Department of Health 2001d Practice guidance: principles, standards and indicators – a resource tool – Caring for older people: a nursing priority. DoH, London

Department of Health 2003 Essence of care – patient focused benchmarking for health care practitioners. DoH, London

Department of Health 2007 Privacy and dignity – a report by the chief nursing officer into mixed sex accommodation in hospitals. DoH, London

Edmond CB, McClean J, McGlone J et al 2006 The respiratory system. In: Alexander MF, Fawcett JN, Runciman PJ (eds) Nursing practice – hospital and home (the adult), 3rd edn. Churchill Livingstone, Edinburgh, pp. 73–103

Gobbi M, Cowen M, Ugboma D 2006 Fluid and electrolyte balance. In: Alexander MF, Fawcett JN, Runciman PJ (eds) Nursing practice – hospital and home (the adult), 3rd edn. Churchill Livingstone, Edinburgh, pp. 763–786

Henley A, Schott J 1999 Culture, religion and patient care in a multi-ethnic society, Age Concern, London

Holland K, Hogg C 2001 Cultural awareness in nursing and health care, Arnold, London

Jamieson L, McFarlane CM, Brown JM 2000 The musculoskeletal system. In: Alexander MF, Fawcett JN, Runciman PJ (eds) Nursing practice hospital and home (the adult). Churchill Livingstone, Edinburgh, pp. 393–427

Jamison JR 2001 Maintaining health in primary care guidelines for wellness in the 21st century. Churchill Livingstone, Edinburgh

Lawler J 1991 Behind the screens – nursing, somology and the problem of the body. Churchill Livingstone, Edinburgh

Le May 2006 Sleep. In: Alexander MF, Fawcett JN, Runciman PJ (eds) Nursing practice – hospital and home (the adult), 3rd edn. Churchill Livingstone, Edinburgh, pp. 883–898

Lucas B 2006 The musculoskeletal system. In: Alexander MF, Fawcett JN, Runciman PJ (eds) Nursing practice – hospital and home (the adult), 3rd edn. Churchill Livingstone, Edinburgh, pp. 443–478

Manthorpe J 2006 Policy developments in the organization of support for older people (eds). In: Nursing older people, 4th edn. Redfern SJ, Ross M. Churchill Livingstone, Edinburgh, pp. 86–102

Montague SE, Watson R, Herbert RA 2005 Physiology for nursing practice, 2nd edn. Baillière Tindall, London

Page BE 2006 Skin disorders. In: Alexander MF, Fawcett JN, Runciman PJ (eds) Nursing practice – hospital and home (the adult), 3rd edn. Churchill Livingstone, Edinburgh, pp. 525–552

Peters J, McKeon S, Pringle F et al 2003 Nursing patients with skin problems. In: Brooker C, Nicholl M (eds) Nursing adults – the practice of caring. Mosby, Edinburgh

Roper N, Logan W, Tierney A 1996 The elements of nursing, 4th edn. Churchill Livingstone, Edinburgh

Roper N, Logan W, Tierney AJ 2000 The Roper–Logan–Tierney model of nursing based on activities of living, Churchill Livingstone, Edinburgh

Rutter M 2000 Life experiences and transitions in adolescence and childhood. In: Wells D (ed) Caring for sexuality in health and illness. Churchill Livingstone, Edinburgh, pp. 135–149

Sharpe J, Bostock J 2002 Supporting people with debt and mental health problems: research with psychological therapists in Northumberland. Community Psychology 2002 (www.haznet.org.uk)

Smith M 2003 Nursing patients with musculoskeletal disorders. In: Brooker C, Nichol M (eds) Nursing adults – the practice of caring. Mosby, Edinburgh, pp. 793–839

Spector R 1996 Cultural diversity in health and illness, 4th edn. Appleton Lange, Stamford

Thomson H, Norman IJ 2006 Delirium (acute confusional states) in later life. Redfern SJ, Ross M (eds). In: Nursing older people, 4th edn,. Churchill Livingstone, Edinburgh, pp. 475–490

Waugh A, Grant A 2006 Ross and Wilson anatomy and physiology in health and illness. Churchill Livingstone, Edinburgh

Wong CK, Edelstein JE 2000 Unna and elastic post-operative dressings: comparison of the effects on function of adults with amputation and vascular disorders. Archives of Physical Medicine and Rehabilitation 81(9):1191–1198

Further reading

Jamieson EM, McCall JM, Whyte LA 2002 Clinical nursing practice, 5th edn. Churchill Livingstone, Edinburgh

Walsh M (ed) 2002 Watson's clinical nursing and related sciences. Baillière Tindall, Edinburgh

Useful websites

www.alzheimers.org.uk (Alzheimer's Association)

www.dohgov.uk/essenceofcare (Essence of Care – Benchmarking Toolkit)

www.icn.ch/matters_ageing (International Council of Nurses)

www.nhsdirect.nhs.uk (NHS Direct)

www.psoriasis.org.sg (Psoriasis association of Singapore)

www.psoriasis-asociation.org.uk (Psoriasis association in UK)

www.psoriasiskenya.org (Psoriasis association of Kenya)

Controlling body temperature

Susan Walker

INTRODUCTION

The body should be considered as being made up of inter-dependent parts, each part interacting physiologically with others. When one part is impaired in its function, all other body systems are affected. As living individuals, we have homeostatic mechanisms, which assist us to maintain a constant internal environment in the body, so enabling optimum function (see Chapter 3).

Core body temperature is usually maintained within a narrow range of 36.1–37.8°C (Marieb 2006). This is regardless of external environmental temperature or the amount of heat being produced by the body. It is when deviation from this core body temperature occurs that body dysfunction becomes inevitable. With extreme deviations comes the increased likelihood of death.

It is relevant for any interventions to bring the temperature back within normal limits to be based on solid underpinning knowledge. This supports a holistic approach to assessment, planning, implementation and evaluation of care.

This chapter will therefore focus on the following:

1. **The model of living**
   - controlling body temperature in health and illness across the lifespan
   - dependence/independence in the AL controlling body temperature
   - factors influencing the AL controlling body temperature.

2. **The model for nursing**
   - nursing care of individuals with health problems affecting the AL controlling body temperature (i.e. application of the Roper et al (1996, 2000) model for nursing in practice).

THE MODEL OF LIVING

CONTROL OF BODY TEMPERATURE

Body temperature reflects the balance between heat production and heat loss. Body temperature of 36.1°C–37.8°C is maintained to enable optimum function by homeostatic mechanisms (Marieb 2006). Extremes of body temperature have an effect on biochemical reaction rates, particularly enzyme activity, which is impaired when temperature changes occur.

An increase in temperature leads to faster chemical reactions. As temperatures rise higher and higher beyond homeostatic range, neurones become depressed and proteins degrade. With a temperature of 41°C convulsions are usually experienced. A temperature of 43°C is likely to precede death (Lloyd 1994).

A decrease in temperature reduces metabolic rate and symptoms associated with the condition of hypothermia may occur. Hypothermia is a condition associated with a body temperature of 35°C or below (Lloyd 1994).

The vascular system contributes to control of body temperature, with the blood serving as an exchange agent between the core and the shell. When referring to the core body temperature we refer to the organs of the skull, thoracic cavity and abdomen, the skin providing a shell. Whenever the skin is warmer than the external environment, heat is lost from the body through vasodilation. The hypothalamus is the part of the brain most responsible for thermoregulation. Vasodilation is triggered via the parasympathetic (heat loss) centre in the anterior hypothalamus when the temperature of circulating blood rises.

In vasodilation the peripheral blood vessels are dilated to allow more blood to flow to the periphery. This is accompanied by structures called the precapillary sphincters relaxing, allowing blood to flow into peripheral capillaries bringing it close to the surface of the body (Hinchliff et al 2005). Blood flow through the skin increases, depending upon the need for temperature control.

The skin plays an important role in body temperature control (see Chapter 8). It protects against invading microorganisms and through the processes of radiation, conduction, convection and evaporation it helps regulate body temperature. These processes are described below.

- *Radiation* – This is loss of heat in the form of infrared waves. The flow of energy is always from hot to cold. The body can also gain heat by radiation, for example warming of the skin during exposure to strong sunshine.

- *Conduction* – As in radiation, conduction involves the transfer of heat from the body, but to objects that the body may have contact with, such as a floor or chair. Loss of heat by conduction can be minimised by wearing clothes that are poor conductors of heat. Trapped air provides thermal insulation, so layers of light clothes are better than one heavy garment.
- *Convection* – As heat is generated and transfers from the body surface to the surrounding air it rises and cool air falls. The warm air surrounding the body is constantly replaced by cooler air molecules. Strong winds and electric fans, which move air quickly across the body surface, aid the processes of conduction and convection.
- *Evaporation* – This is the process of converting the water in sweat, to water vapour, by heat production.

Most of the heat lost from the body is through the skin though some heat is lost through excretion in urine and faeces and some through expiration from the lungs. It is the sweat glands in the skin that are the mechanism for heat reduction when the environmental temperature is higher than that of the body; this will be discussed further within this chapter.

Vasoconstriction will occur when there is a need to conserve body temperature. This results in peripheral shutdown and is associated with shivering. Shivering is an involuntary spasmodic contraction and relaxation of the skeletal muscles. It contributes to the generation of heat and is associated with the pilomotor reflex, which makes the hairs on the skin surface stand up to trap air, producing 'goosebumps'.

Vasoconstriction is triggered via the sympathetic (heat-promoting) centre in the posterior hypothalamus when the temperature of circulating blood falls (see Fig. 9.1 for heat loss/gain balance).

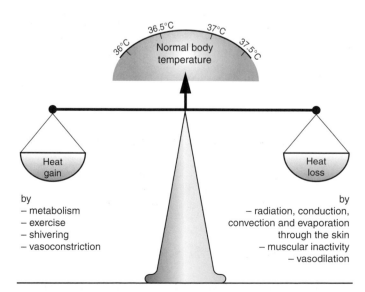

Fig. 9.1 Heat gain/heat loss balance (from Roper et al 1996, with permission).

Biological factors related to physiology and temperature control will be discussed throughout the chapter.

Exercise

1. Revise the structure and function of the skin and vascular system.
2. Consider your own experiences of radiation, conduction, convection and evaporation processes.
3. Consider how this would differ if you lived in a country where temperatures were either very cold or very hot.

CONTROLLING BODY TEMPERATURE IN HEALTH AND ILLNESS – ACROSS THE LIFESPAN

Childhood

Body temperature reflects the balance between heat production and heat loss. All body tissues produce heat, those producing the greatest amount being those that are most metabolically active. Infants and young children have higher metabolic rates than adults and smaller body masses. This is relevant as they are generating more body heat, but have a smaller body surface from which to lose it, enhancing the likelihood of temperature deviations. In the newborn infant, heat loss is rapid after birth (Blackburn & Loper 1992, cited in Sganga et al 2000).

Temperature can fall 2–3°C after birth and interventions such as providing warm towels and blankets, skin-to-skin contact, or an incubator are vital (Sganga et al 2000). A young child is dependent on warm clothes, adequate diet and a warm environment to prevent a hypopyrexia.

Fisher & Warren (1999) refer to the fact that infants' and children's regulatory reflexes are likely to be underdeveloped, hence an irregular or recurrent rise in temperature may be of little significance. A transient hyperpyrexia may occur following a tantrum, prolonged crying or a physical display of excitement. The resulting discomfort is a hot, sticky and sweaty child, who is dependent on an adult to offer a cold drink, remove an item of clothing and encourage rest, until the child has reached an age where they are able to manipulate their own environment.

Prolonged temperature rise in a child is usually associated with fever as a result of infection from bacteria or viruses.

Exercise

Think of a child you have nursed/cared for who had a fever.

1. Without the aid of a thermometer how did you establish if the child was pyrexial?
2. What over-the-counter medications are available to ease the symptoms of fever?

Fever is recognised as having a positive effect on the immune system. Fullick (1998) refers to the fact that most pathogens reproduce best at 37°C or lower. Therefore a raised temperature will affect reproduction of the pathogen causing less damage. Also, the immune system works better at higher temperatures, and so will be more successful at combating the infection by the raised temperature. By developing knowledge of the immune response and the physiological events that occur during fever we are able to provide appropriate and effective care, recognising when a fever may place a child at risk. Consider the following brief case study.

Case study 9.1

Emma – an 18-month-old baby girl

Emma is an 18-month-old baby girl – normally fit and well. Over the last few days Emma has been unusually sleepy and uninterested in her toys and surroundings. When Emma's mum attempts to encourage food, drink and play, Emma becomes distressed and uncooperative. Sarah, Emma's mum, is 17 and a single parent living in local council accommodation. She is supported by her parents who see her and her baby twice weekly. Recently Sarah and Emma joined a weekly mother and baby group.

Sarah is a sensible and loving parent to Emma. She has checked Emma for a rash and a temperature; neither is noted.

Emma – 18-month-old baby

18 December 2006 2.00 p.m.

Emma Smith 18-month-old baby girl brought to Accident and Emergency by her mother. No previous medical/surgical history. Normally fit and well. Normal delivery at birth, lives with mother, no other siblings. Has social contact with other children.

History of sleeping more than usual over last 3 days, when awake often crying and uninterested in her toys and surroundings. Refusing diet, but taking small amounts of oral fluid. Seen by GP yesterday – no active treatment.

Today anxious mum, very concerned. This a.m. child vomited × 2, mum noticed shivering. Also number of wet nappies reduced. On examination – she is awake but quiet, skin hot and dry, refusing oral fluids. Her pulse is 108 and tympanic temperature 38.8°C.

Exercise

1. To whom can Sarah take her concerns? Some services are available for Sarah to access quickly and easily for advice regarding baby Emma (consider health visitor, NHS Direct, Accident and Emergency or other facilities you may be aware of in your local community).
2. Do you consider the baby's presenting symptoms to be significant?

Emma may be reacting to an invading pathogen.

Pathogens and the active immune response

Pathogens are invading organisms that do not belong to the normal body flora. Pathogens transmitted from one person to another result in infectious disease. They may be mild or result in severe illness and death. Human viral disease includes amongst others, polio, influenza and acquired immune deficiency syndrome (AIDS).

Viruses are only able to replicate if inside a host cell. Once inside a cell, the virus will take over the cellular biochemistry and use it to produce new viruses, until the host cell is completely destroyed, leaving the virus free in the circulation to affect other cells (Fullick 1998). Human bacterial diseases include tuberculosis, salmonellosis and cholera. Bacteria can latch on to host cells and live and reproduce independently. Not all bacteria are harmful, and some can help us develop natural resistance (Fullick 1998).

Defence responses to invading pathogens are provided by the immune system. Leucocytes (white blood cells) are manufactured in the bone marrows of the long bones of the body. As they mature they become known as phagocytes. Phagocytes are able to move in and out of capillaries and engulf dead cells and foreign material. Other types of leucocytes are T cells and B cells; these are produced in the lymph glands.

Once a pathogen is inside the body it is recognised by its antigens. These are specific proteins on its outer surface identifying it as foreign material. T cells attach to the antigen and destroy it. Phagocytes will engulf the foreign material. The role of the B cell is to multiply in large numbers and secrete antibodies. Antibodies are proteins specific to a particular antigen, which bind to it and destroy it, the remaining material of destruction being then engulfed by the phagocytes. These immune responses are referred to as the cell-mediated response and the humeral response (see Fig. 9.2). As part of the humeral response, B memory cells remain in the body providing a long-term immunology memory. Should the same disease-causing antigen be encountered again, protective antibodies will be released. Fullick (1998) refers to this fact explaining why diseases such as chicken pox or measles are usually only encountered once (see also Waugh & Grant 2006, Ch. 5).

Exercise

1. Consider why individuals may regularly contract a cold or flu.
2. What signs and symptoms did you experience?
3. Discuss with friends and family members their experiences and compare them to yours.

You may have considered the following issues.

Flu Influenza is a virus that is highly contagious. It affects the nose, throat and lungs. In the United Kingdom, 3000–4000 deaths are attributed to 'the flu' each year

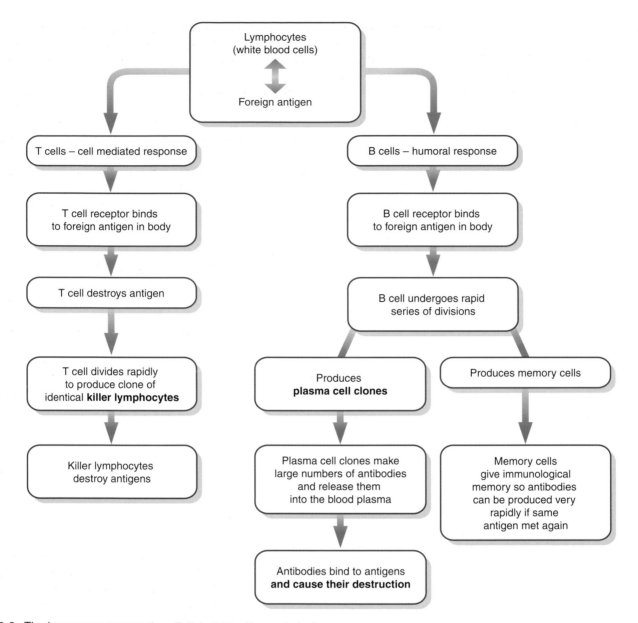

Fig. 9.2 The immune response (from Fullick 1998, with permission).

(Gupta 1999). Gupta goes on to say that this figure is increased tenfold during epidemics. There are two strains of the virus, Influenza A and Influenza B. Type A strain is responsible for more severe illness, often resulting in pneumonia, hospitalisation and death (Miller 2001). The flu viruses are antigenically unstable and mutate constantly (Miller 2001). This is why people contract the flu often, as the immune system will not necessarily recognise the new virus strain.

The Public Health Laboratory Service (1998) states that the bigger the change in the viral strain, then the greater the likelihood of a larger outbreak. Management of the flu is largely based on relief of symptoms that have a sudden onset. Symptoms include: headache, coughs, fever, appetite loss, tiredness, aches and pains and chills.

The upper respiratory tract may be affected and you may have experienced the following:

- constant runny nose
- sore throat
- sneezing
- irritated, watery eyes.

Gastrointestinal symptoms may include:

- nausea
- vomiting
- often diarrhoea.

When gastrointestinal symptoms occur, it is often referred to as 'stomach flu'.

Miller (2001) states that the period of infectiousness from the onset of symptoms is usually 3–5 days in adults and up to 7 days in young children. The World Health Organization monitors the worldwide influenza situation (WHO 1999). In the United Kingdom, vaccination is available to prevent much of the illness and death attributed to influenza. The vaccine components are dependent on the strains expected to develop in the coming season (Miller 2001).

Symptom management includes rest, increased fluid intake and antipyretic medications to relieve the symptoms of fever. To distinguish flu from other respiratory diseases, laboratory tests are necessary. In the United Kingdom, increased surveillance is underway which links laboratory and community data, so that response to any emerging flu epidemic is quick and coordinated. It is the very young and the elderly and those who may be immunosuppressed due to chronic illness that are most at risk.

Avian influenza According to the Department of Health (2006), since 2003 avian influenza or 'bird flu' has affected poultry and other birds in several countries. By November 2006, 285 people were known to have caught the infection through direct contact with infected birds, and over half of these people have subsequently died. There is great concern that the bird flu virus called H5N1 may mix with human flu viruses and create a new virus which may lead to a human flu pandemic, due to its ability to jump the species barrier (WHO 2005).

An epidemic is an outbreak of disease which is widespread, occurring in a single community, region or population (DoH 2006). In the UK, epidemics of ordinary flu are often experienced, and planned for through seasonal flu vaccination programmes. A pandemic occurs on a much greater scale, spreading from country to country, across the world, affecting hundreds of thousands of people, resulting in many deaths and causing social and economic disruption in the countries affected (Box 9.1). According to the Department of Health (2006) the WHO has developed a global alert system, to indicate in advance the seriousness of the risk of an influenza pandemic. This global alert system has six phases; the world is currently at phase three, indicating that although disease is not efficiently sustained, there is a new virus subtype that is causing disease

and deaths in humans. The UK has had a national influenza pandemic plan since 1997, based on a framework for national pandemic plans, recommended by the WHO. This plan is continually updated.

According to the Department of Health (2006) there is evidence that recent H5N1 viruses have been susceptible to a certain class of antiviral drugs; based on this evidence, as part of their pandemic plan, the UK Government has purchased an antiviral drug called Tamiflu, and has a strategy for stockpiling, distribution and use of this drug in the event of a pandemic. Further manufacture of drugs would be required once the pandemic virus strain was identified.

Immunisation For the newborn infant, immunity is provided when antibodies and antitoxins circulating in the mother's blood are passed via the placenta to the fetus. This natural passive immunity usually only lasts a few months following birth. Until the active immunity through immunisation is taken up, the child is vulnerable to infectious disease.

Controversy exists about the safety of the triple MMR (measles, mumps, rubella) vaccine and its link to the incidence of autism and bowel disease occurring post-vaccination (Patja et al 2000, Taylor et al 1999).

Exercise

1. Talk to parents of young children about decisions they made regarding immunisation of a child.
2. What influenced their decisions regarding immunisation?

MMR protects against measles, mumps and rubella (German measles). Measles is usually a mild disease; however, it can cause fever, rash and chest infection. The danger is that if fever is not controlled it may lead to convulsions which if not treated immediately may lead to brain damage. It is a very infectious virus.

In 1987, the year prior to MMR being introduced to England, 86 000 children caught measles and this resulted in 16 deaths. There are now fewer than 100 cases of measles per year reported (NHS 2001).

Mumps is a virus that causes headache, fever and painful swollen neck glands. It can also cause inflammation of the brain and permanent deafness. Due to vaccination, mumps, which is the most common cause of viral meningitis of children under 15 years, has now resulted in hospital admissions for children with mumps meningitis becoming almost eradicated.

Rubella (German measles) is recognised by a rash and can be a mild infectious disease in children; however, if contracted by a woman during early pregnancy it can cause serious damage to the unborn baby. Any damage resulting is known as congenital rubella syndrome (CRS) (NHS 2001) (Table 9.1).

Box 9.1	**Pandemics during the last century**

- 1918–1919: Spanish flu, affected healthy young adults, estimated 20–40 million deaths globally
- 1957–1958: Asian flu, affected very young and very old, estimated 1 million deaths globally
- 1968–1969: Hong Kong flu, affected the very old and those with underlying medical conditions, estimated 1–4 million deaths globally.

From Department of Health (2005).

Table 9.1 Childhood vaccination

When to immunise	What is given	How is it given
2–4 months old	Polio	By mouth
	Diphtheria, tetanus, pertussis and Hib (DTP-hib)	One injection
	MenC	One injection
Around 13 months old	Measles, mumps and rubella (MMR)	One injection
3–5 years old (pre-school)	Polio	By mouth
	Diphtheria, tetanus and acellular pertussis (DtaP)	One injection
	Measles, mumps and rubella (MMR)	One injection
10–14 years old (and sometimes shortly after birth)	BCG (against tuberculosis)	Skin test, then, if needed, one injection
13–18 years old	Diphtheria and tetanus (Td)	One injection
	Polio	By mouth

From NHS (2001).

Prevention is always better than cure, and immunisation of a child against infective diseases that can be prevented is considered vital (see Box 9.2).

Tuberculosis Tuberculosis (TB) is an example of a human bacterial disease that can affect anyone at any age. *Mycobacterium tuberculosis* is transmitted from human to human; it causes chronic granulomatous lesions, mainly in the lungs, but often also in bones and the brain.

Box 9.2	Diseases preventable by vaccination

- Anthrax
- Poliomyelitis
- Cholera
- Rubella
- Diphtheria
- Smallpox
- Hepatitis B
- Tetanus
- Measles
- Tuberculosis
- Meningitis C
- Typhoid
- Mumps
- Whooping cough.

From Waugh & Grant (2006), p. 382.

There has been an increase worldwide, and this is reflected in the UK, particularly in respiratory TB, which increased by 13% between 1996 and 1997 (Public Health Laboratory Service 1998 cited in Mallett & Dougherty 2004). The Department of Health (2006) reports that in the UK the incidence of TB has increased from 5745 cases a year to over 7000.

The World Health Organization predicts that by 2020 nearly one billion people will be infected with TB; of them, 70 million will die. TB blackspots include Eastern Europe, South-East Asia and sub-Saharan Africa (BBC News 1999).

Immigrant subgroups have been highlighted as an attributable cause for the increase in the UK (Public Health Laboratory Service 1998 cited in Mallett & Dougherty 2004). This particular group of people proves to be a difficult target for TB prevention programmes due to cultural and language difficulties and ability to access health care professionals. Those who are immunosuppressed due to disease or drugs, along with those suffering with alcoholism or living in poverty are most susceptible to TB, as these conditions tend to predispose its development.

Primarily, tuberculosis is spread by inhalation of the bacteria. When an infected person coughs, droplets are produced which can be inhaled by another person. Once infected the host's immune response is activated; it can usually destroy the TB bacilli – preventing development of the disease but producing a calcified granuloma. However, some TB bacteria may survive the host's immune response after primary infection, and lie dormant in any body site, especially the lungs, for many years. They can be reactivated by debilitative disease or by later exposure to TB itself (Medico 2001).

The Department of Health (1998) suggests that TB should be suspected in all people who have a cough lasting for 3 weeks or more, accompanied by weight loss, anorexia, haemoptysis, fever and night sweats. A provisional diagnosis is based on 'smear-positive' findings of acid-fast bacilli in sputum or other bodily fluids. Patients who have a smear-positive result are considered as infectious while those with a smear-negative result are noninfective.

Further investigation is required to identify the specific strain of disease by bacterial growth in culture (Medico 2001).

Prevention and control of spread of TB is necessary. All forms of TB are statutorily notifiable to the consultant in communicable disease control (Medico 2001) or the medical officer for environmental health in the UK. A person with a smear-positive result is a primary source for spread of the disease and contact tracing is an important means of identifying secondary cases (Medico 2001). TB is found in 19% of all contacts; about 10% of notified cases each year are found through contact tracing (Ejidokum et al 1998 cited in Mallett and Dougherty 2004). Besides laboratory testing to diagnose TB, X-rays can be taken. A chest X-ray may show damage in the lungs. A Heaf or Mantoux test to which an individual will react if they are infected or have active disease will be used. This is a common test in children, but is not considered effective in adolescents and adults.

Prevention is through vaccination with Bacillus Calmette–Guérin (BCG). In the UK the vaccine is given to schoolchildren and has been shown to give 70–80% protection lasting at least 15 years. The vaccine is given to new UK entrants from high-risk countries and to infants born to families from these countries (Public Health Laboratory 2001).

Treatment for those found to have infectious (active) TB includes antibacterial drugs. Those who are infectious will also be isolated at the start of the drug therapy. The drugs used to treat TB are: isoniazid, rifampin, pyrazinamide, ethambutol, streptomycin (www.lung.ca.drugs2001).

A combination of these drugs is usually necessary during treatment, as the TB bacteria can be resistant to one or more of the drugs. Drug therapy can last for 6–8 months. It is essential that the prescribed amount be taken at the prescribed time, for the full length of time prescribed. This is because TB is a slowly developing disease and therefore the desired results may take some time to achieve.

Where severe damage has been caused to an organ of the body, i.e. the lung, surgical intervention may be necessary. This may have a greater long-term effect on an individual and their lifestyle and Activities of Living. For example:

- time spent in hospital
- loss of independence during recovery period
- ability to return to work will all depend on the degree of surgery undertaken and the individual's recovery to the illness and the surgical intervention.

Exercise

1. Find out the incidence of TB in your community.
2. What simple practice can minimise the risk of spread of infection within a community?
3. Discuss with colleagues how you would care for someone with TB.

Adolescence and adulthood

In adolescence and adulthood we experience changes in body temperature as part of the lifecycle or in relation to lifestyle choices we have made.

Around 12 years of age female menstruation occurs; it ceases at menopause, which usually occurs when a woman has reached her forties. Gould (1994) refers to the fact that a slight temperature rise may occur at the time of ovulation, but can be as little as 0.3°C. This slight rise in temperature is considered as a method of indicating the time of ovulation and is used by some to aid fertility. There is also a slight temperature rise during the first trimester of pregnancy. These slight variations in temperature are due to the influences of the female sex hormones.

During health diurnal variations can be noted in body temperature. Recordings are lowest in the early hours of the morning, rising steadily throughout the day, reaching a peak in the late evening. This is influenced by the day and night patterns of activity and rest. Roper et al (1996) state that the converse is true for people who regularly work at night and sleep in the day.

It is relevant to note that during adolescence and early adulthood social grouping and social activity are important, as these affect the social activities a young person may choose. Peer pressure should be noted as playing a part in our socialisation.

Some social drugs are known to increase metabolic rate, such as nicotine and caffeine, and an increased metabolic rate will lead to a rise in body temperature. Caffeine is legal and socially accepted, but it can be addictive, especially if taken in large amounts. Withdrawal symptoms when coffee drinking stops include lethargy and headache and an inability to concentrate. Nicotine is a mild stimulant, although it is known to cause vasoconstriction of the peripheral blood vessels. This raises the heart rate slightly and leads to an increase in blood pressure. Nicotine is addictive, and when nicotine levels are reduced, there is a physical craving for the drug. Fullick (1998) states withdrawal symptoms include irritability, lack of concentration, restlessness, hunger and sadness or depression, the later 'feeling low' contributing to a reduction in body temperature. (For effects of smoking on the activity of breathing see Chapter 5.)

Alcohol taken in excessive amounts is associated with a lowering of body temperature as cooling is increased due to vasodilatation of blood vessels in the skin (Roper et al 1996).

Freedom of maturity and managing one's own lifestyle may also permit foreign travel. There may be a greater risk of contracting a tropical infectious disease. Chiodini (2001) refers to the fact that the increase in the number of visitors to exotic locations has pushed travel medicine to the forefront of primary care. Access to travel and immunisation advice has become essential. Detailed information can be obtained from the World Health Organization website at www.who.int.

We have so far considered the need for immunisation and the body's immune defence system; now we consider general health advice when in a hot climate, at home or abroad.

Consider the scenario described in Case study 9.2.

You may have considered the following information regarding skin cancer to support your advice on prevention of sunburn.

Skin cancer

If you have revised the function and structure of the skin you will have identified that melanin can provide some protection from the harmful effects of sunlight. Waugh & Grant (2006) state that the amount of melanin in the skin is genetically determined and varies between parts of the body, between members of the same race and between races.

Sarah – 18-year-old

Sarah is 18 years old, a fashion fanatic and a keen sunbather, believing a suntan to be the ultimate fashion accessory. She is planning her first holiday abroad, with friends and is excited about the opportunities for partying and obtaining that ultimate tan.

What advice could you offer Sarah in relation to prevention of sunburn and heatstroke?

Sarah has spent her morning joining in an exercise class around the pool, at her holiday hotel. She has done this under duress, as she would rather have stayed in bed following a late night of partying and drinking excessive alcohol. It is the third day of the holiday and temperatures have soared in the last week.

During a walk to a restaurant for lunch Sarah complains of headache and nausea. She looks flushed, her skin is dry and her breathing is rapid. On reaching the restaurant Sarah goes straight to the toilet (rest room). Twenty minutes later Sarah has not returned. A friend finds Sarah lying on the rest room floor. She is not responding. Sarah is known to be normally fit and well.

Having made a safe approach and assessment of Sarah's airway, breathing and circulation, all of which are present, consider the information below on heatstroke.

Exposure to sunlight promotes synthesis of increased amounts of melanin and this affects the differences in colour. However, it does not give ultimate protection, and exposure to ultraviolet (UV) radiation can damage the skin. UVA ages the skin and UVB burns the skin. Both types of ultraviolet radiation can lead to cancer (jas 2001).

There are three types of skin cancer; basal cell and squamous cell carcinomas are easily treated and rarely fatal, but malignant melanomas grow uncontrollably and these are the most dangerous, and can cause death. About 1500 people die from melanomas in Britain every year (jas 2001). Fortunately melanoma is curable when detected and treated early.

Melanoma cancers contain melanin, which causes them to be mixed shades of brown; they can appear suddenly or may begin in or near a mole or dark skin spot. Melanomas occur on sun-damaged skin and those particularly at risk are those having sudden short bursts of sunlight, on holiday, in places where the sun is very strong (jas 2001).

People most at risk include those with:

- a high number of moles
- red or fair hair
- fair skin or freckles
- blue eyes
- who tan with difficulty and burn in the sun.

It is important for people to recognise that a tan is not healthy, rather that it is indicative of damage to the skin by UV radiation. The melanin moves to the surface of the exposed skin, to provide protection. Remember that even dark skin can burn. To reduce risk of melanoma and sunburn requires adaptation of behaviour. This involves:

- avoiding exposure during midday temperatures
- enjoy the sun before 10 a.m. and after 3 p.m. local time
- wear a wide-brimmed hat to protect eyes, ears, head and neck.
- sit in the shade (remember sand, water and snow all reflect UV radiation) but shade may not give complete protection
- use sunglasses that block UV rays to protect the eyes (UV rays can cause cataracts)
- cover the body with light clothing
- use sun-protective creams/lotions/sprays that guard against both UVA and UVB rays
- protect children – keep them out of direct sunlight as much as possible.

It may be assumed that a person who has little knowledge regarding sunburn, and so places him or herself at risk, is also likely to fail to recognise symptoms of heat-related illness.

Heatstroke

During high environmental temperatures and humidity we are all at risk of heat-related illness and heatstroke without appropriate education and management.

Batscha (1997) refers to three major types of heat-related illness:

- Heat cramps, caused by sodium depletion in the body.
- Heat exhaustion, which generally occurs as a result of dehydration and accompanies untreated heat cramps. It is characterised by profuse sweating, fatigue, thirst and headache, which may lead to nausea and vomiting. An elevation in body temperature will be present. It is insidious in onset.
- Heatstroke, which occurs in two forms. It develops when the body is unable to dispel heat through normal physiological mechanisms. Exertional heatstroke occurs as a result of strenuous physical exercise, leading to excessive internal heat production, particularly during periods of extremely hot weather. Highest incidence is in the first few days of a heatwave when people have had little chance to acclimatise. Classic heatstroke is often seen in elderly people and the infirm and results from a combination of a hot environment and ineffective heat-loss mechanisms Heatstroke is considered a medical emergency. It requires an immediate response should it occur; this will be discussed later in this chapter.

Prevention of heat-related illness, again, involves behavioural adaptation such as:

- avoid exercise
- drink plenty of water

- stay cool, by seeking shade and wearing light single-layered clothes
- try to access a heat-conditioned building
- take a tepid shower or bath.

Keeping cool may be more difficult for an overweight person. Reasons for this include the decreased vascularity of adipose tissue which inhibits heat loss by increasing the difficulty of blood moving to the skin surface. Adipose tissue also acts as an insulator (Sidebottom 1992, cited in Batscha 1997). Additional weight also increases the work of the heart when activity is undertaken, which tends to raise body temperature further (Batscha 1997).

Metabolic rate, body temperature and weight control

Fullick (1998) refers to the fact that some lifestyle factors that can cause, or increase the likelihood of suffering, a particular disease or illness are under our control, others are not. Fullick (1998) states that babies and young children have little choice about what they eat, yet foundations of diet-related illnesses may well be laid in early childhood.

However, adolescents and adults can make lifestyle choices about diet. Food is required to provide the body with sufficient energy to maintain basic body functioning, and to carry out the Activities of Living. The amount of energy the body requires on a daily basis will depend on the basal metabolic rate (BMR) and the level of activity. The BMR can affect body temperature. The BMR is greater in babies and young children, as they use a great deal of energy in growth. In newborn babies brown fat is a form of fat in adipose tissue that is a rich source of energy and can be converted rapidly to heat. It is a useful source of heat production contributing to maintenance of body temperature in babies, where a smaller body surface area can contribute to difficulties with the normal processes of conduction, convection, radiation and evaporation in relation to heat production and heat loss.

This adipose tissue is found around the viscera, the back and the neck. It is controlled by the sympathetic nervous system (Imrie & Hall 1990). The BMR is also related to the total body mass and the lean body mass. People with a higher proportion of muscle tissue require more energy for maintenance than fat. Fullick (1998) states that one reason why men have a higher BMR than women is because they tend to have a higher proportion of muscle to fat.

Marieb (2006) defines the metabolic rate as the sum of heat produced by all the chemical reactions and mechanical work of the body. It can be measured directly or indirectly.

Using the direct method it is necessary for a person to enter an enclosed chamber where heat produced by the body is absorbed by water circulating around the chamber. The rise in the temperature of the circulating water is directly related to the heat produced by the body (Marieb 2006).

The indirect method involves use of a respirator measure of oxygen consumption, which is directly proportional to heat produced. For each line of oxygen used, the body produces about 4.8 kcal of heat (Marieb 2006).

By multiplying the BMR with a factor reflecting an individual physical activity level (PAL) the estimated average requirements (EAR) for energy can be obtained. In the UK a PAL of 1.4 is used for adults (Fullick 1998). If energy intake is not matched to the requirements of the body then weight gain or loss will occur as a result of eating too much or too little.

With a greater body surface area, heat loss to the environment increases and the metabolic rate must be higher to replace the lost heat. With ageing and as the body shrinks in relation to the amount of skeletal muscle, the BMR declines. Decreasing calorie intake can help prevent obesity in later life.

Physical activity and exercise which increase skeletal muscle activity result in the most significant rise in the BMR and body heat production. The combination of increased physical activity and exercise with a reduced calorie intake remains the most acceptable way to reduce weight. This often means a change in lifestyle and/or lifelong habits.

Surface area, age, gender, stress and hormones are all factors influencing BMR. Although body weight and size are related, it is body surface area that is the vital factor. A greater body surface area to body volume means a higher BMR, as heat loss to the environment is greater. Body temperature will rise and fall with BMR.

Exercise

Consider the following based on the information presented.

1. Two people weigh the same. One is tall and thin and one is short and fat. Who has the greater BMR? Read up on the hormone thyroxine and its effect on BMR in relation to body temperature, weight gain and weight loss.

2. Assess the amount of physical exercise undertaken by
   - a school-age child
   - an adult (over 18 years)
   - an older person (over 60 years)

   as part of their normal living activities; consider exercise involved in work, hobbies, school activities, etc.

Old age

A study conducted on exercise and older people at the University of Indiana's Institute for Aging Research (Environmental News Network 1999) reported that older individuals felt less able to engage in exercise, with females being less confident than males. A total of 729 senior citizens spoke with researchers about environmental obstacles that prevented exercise. All respondents were low-income, urban residents.

The elderly people referred to barriers such as bad weather, crime, poor walking paths and facilities, when considering outdoor exercise, whilst those considering indoor exercise were concerned they would experience chest pain or respiratory problems and had fear of injury.

Self-confidence, desire and motivation were also identified as significant factors, even when the person knew that exercise would improve their health and wellbeing.

Researchers at the University's Bechman Institute studied 124 previously sedentary men and women between the ages of 60 and 75 years (Environmental News Network 1999). The group was randomly divided into two; one group gradually worked up to walking an hour a day, three times a week (aerobic exercise), the other group did anaerobic exercises such as stretching and toning. Over the course of 6 months the groups were given a variety of simple tests which measured their ability to plan, establish schedules, make and remember choices and rapidly reconsider them if the circumstances change. The walkers showed an improved ability to complete the tests compared with the nonwalkers.

The researchers were focusing on the areas of the brain responsible for 'executive control processes', these being the frontal and prefrontal lobes of the brain, which are known to be the areas of the brain which decline earliest with ageing.

The better the executive control processes, the better someone can complete day-to-day tasks such as driving, cooking, etc., as these tasks require a person to keep track of more than one thing at once. Hence, the more independent they can be.

The Environment News Network (1999) notes that exercise could help delay the time at which older people become more dependent on others.

In relation to body temperature control, ill health and dependency are clearly significant especially when considering an elderly person's ability to respond to variations in temperature. With this in mind, it is important in older age to remain alert and as independent as possible. The thermoregulation system becomes less efficient making it more difficult to detect temperature variations from the norm.

This can be due to a number of factors:

- physiological changes such as a reduction in the ability to constrict peripheral blood vessels, and a possible reduction in the shivering threshold (Collins et al 1977, Macmillan et al 1967, cited in Roper et al 1996)
- increased risk to be medication-dependent
- obesity, increased risk in advanced age due to reduced mobility and exercise
- possible mental impairment affecting judgement and decisions regarding appropriate actions during temperature variations
- possible social isolation, poorer housing.

Old age accompanied by acute or chronic illness/disease will increase the risk of an older person experiencing heat- and cold-related illness.

Exercise

1. Talk to an elderly family member or neighbour about how they adapt to high and low environmental temperatures.

In order to explore the issues of older people and the AL of controlling body temperature consider the following case study.

Case study 9.3

Marjory – a 78-year-old widow

Marjory is a 78-year-old, who has been widowed for 12 months. During the last 12 months she has become increasingly isolated and reliant upon her only daughter for social contact and support. Her daughter makes great effort to visit Marjory every other day.

Although physically able Marjory has considerably reduced her mobility and spends much time sitting in her armchair, some days not even bothering to get dressed. She has a hot meal on the days her daughter visits and although a meal is left for the next day Marjory chooses to eat something cold. Marjory has seen the doctor at her daughter's request, but has refused any help from social services in the form of a home help or meals on wheels. She insists she is grieving – as confirmed by the doctor, and will come round in her own time. Her only physical complaint is myxoedema for which she takes regular medication (thyroxine).

Christmas is approaching and Marjory has refused to stay with her daughter and family over the Christmas period saying she prefers the peace and quiet of her own home.

When her daughter next visits she finds Marjory lying on the floor in the hall. Marjory is semi-conscious; she has been incontinent of urine. Her daughter is unable to make sense of Marjory's verbal responses. Marjory has a blue tinge to her lips and hands. She feels very cold to the touch but is not shivering. Marjory's daughter dials for the emergency services to attend. Marjory is transferred to the Accident and Emergency department.

Exercise

Consider the following based on the information presented:

1. What physical and psychological factors may increase Marjory's risk of hypothermia?
2. Why are older people considered to be more susceptible to hypothermia?
3. What measures could Marjory and her daughter have employed to prevent hypothermia?

Marjory's psychological state clearly affected her behaviour. It is necessary to recognise the effect of an individual's psychological state on body temperature.

Psychological factors

When there is an increase or a decrease in the environmental temperature information is sent to the cerebral hemispheres where behavioural and psychological responses are triggered. In response to feeling hot a person may have a cold drink, open a window or remove an item of clothing, alternatively if feeling cold, they may take exercise, walk, or rub hands together in an attempt to create heat and increase blood supply to muscles. They may also add an item of clothing or turn up the heating; however, this behavioural response is linked closely to their psychological state. Bringing the environmental temperature back to a comfortable level has the immediate effect of making one feel better.

If an individual's psychological state is impaired through illness such as depression, or affected through medication/drugs such as sedatives, they may neglect to respond appropriately and therefore any increase or decrease in temperature will become exaggerated. The sluggishness, lack of mobility and lethargy associated with 'feeling low' will contribute to a decreased metabolic rate and reduction in temperature, while the increased heart rate and activity associated with the excitement and euphoria of 'feeling good' may contribute to an increased metabolic rate and rise in body temperature.

Other psychological states which may lead to a rise in temperature are anxiety, nervousness, displays of anger and fear. The apocrine sweat glands are those triggered by emotional stimuli. They secrete sweat in the hair follicles of the armpits and groins (Kerry 1999 cited by USA Today

---

Exercise

1. Recall your own psychological state prior to sitting an exam, an important interview and a visit to the dentist, or on your wedding day.
2. What physiological events occurred?
3. Talk to a successful slimmer about the 'feel good' factor related to a weight loss.

1999).

Psychological state linked with 'feeling low' leads to consideration of seasonal affective disorder (SAD). This is a type of depression that tends to occur and reoccur during autumn and winter months when there is deprivation of sunshine, daylight hours are reduced, and there is exposure to colder temperatures. Medical recognition of this condition is relatively recent.

Symptoms may include:

- weight gain due to overeating
- feeling low, desperate, anxious
- lethargy

- recurrent infections due to lowered resistance
- behaviour difficulties in children.

The first four of these symptoms might affect body temperature.

It is estimated that 2% of people in Northern Europe suffer considerable symptoms, with more than 10% coping with milder symptoms. Across the world incidence increases with distance from the equator (Medicinenet 1999). It is thought that bright light makes a difference to brain chemistry. Treatment involves light therapy known as phototherapy and sufferers would obviously benefit from living in brighter, sunnier climates (although this for many is not an alternative).

Environmental factors

Seasonal variations and extremes in environmental temperature can also cause variations in an individual's body temperature, which can cause them to feel hot or cold. These variations may be mild or extreme. The most common conditions related to extremes in environmental temperature are hyperpyrexia (heatstroke) or hypothermia.

Heatstroke is a medical emergency requiring an immediate response. Body temperature may be 40°C or greater (Hinchliff et al 2005). Hypothermia is defined as a body temperature of 35°C or below (Lloyd 1996).

So why can high and low environmental temperatures have such a profound effect on body temperature?

Worfolk (2000) refers to the fact that the body's dominant means of losing heat in a hot environment are radiation and evaporation. But for heat to radiate from the body, the body temperature must be greater than that of the environment. However, when the environmental temperature is higher that that of the body, evaporation of water from the sweat glands forms the only mechanism available for the reduction of body temperature (Green 1989).

Heat is needed to convert water to water vapour. The vaporisation of 1 ml of water needs 0.58 calories. The heat is termed the latent heat of vaporisation. This is the amount of heat lost by the evaporation on the skin of 1 ml of sweat. If sweat falls off the skin without evaporating there is no cooling effect (Green 1989). It is the eccrine sweat glands that are triggered by heat and aid cooling (Kerry 1999).

Evaporation is aided by convection. Light winds on an unusually hot day can speed the evaporation of heated moist air next to the body, however on days of extreme humidity, with still air, sweat evaporation becomes impossible. This is because the body's thermoregulatory mechanisms have become overwhelmed. In high heat and humidity it is voluntary acts based on knowledge that will prevent the body temperature rising too high, i.e.

- moving to an air-conditioned building
- turning on a fan
- removing clothing.

Remember that these actions are dependent upon a person's ability to respond to the discomfort they are feeling.

In a cold environment, heat production by the body is necessary to maintain core body temperature within normal limits. Heat loss in a cold outdoor environment may be exacerbated by wind chill. This is a term used to describe the rate of heat loss from the body from the combined effect of low temperature and wind. As wind speed increases it carries heat away more quickly. High winds even on cool days can significantly affect body temperature (Noa 2002). Should an individual be exposed to a combination of moderately low temperature, wind and wet, loss of heat from the body is enhanced and the risk of hypothermia is increased. Heat production will depend on internal metabolism, hot food and drink, exercise, and the body's ability to maintain heat through vasoconstriction. Again it is the very young and the very old at risk from extremes in environmental temperature, as this is linked with their perception of temperature change and their independent ability to respond accordingly.

Exercise

Consider the environment in which you work (hospital-based, community staff, those within schools of nursing).

1. If exposed to the outdoors, how do you adapt to environmental temperature variations?
2. If an indoor worker, find out about legislation governing temperatures and ventilation in your work place.

Roper et al (1996) refer to the fact that environmental factors cannot be considered in isolation, they are related to biological, psychological, sociocultural and politicoeconomic factors. They also state that environmental factors influence living throughout the lifespan and have a bearing on the person's independence and dependency status, and influence the individuality in a person's way of living.

Politicoeconomic factors

There is a need to recognise that politicoeconomic factors link clearly to the environment, as living conditions and income clearly play a part. For example, low-quality housing and low income will mean inadequate levels of heating as people worry about being able to 'meet the bills', whilst failure to pay may lead to disconnection, increasing the risk of hypothermia. Low income also dictates diet, and poor nutrition can also affect our ability to keep warm.

According to Help the Aged (www.helptheaged.org.uk) it is difficult to give an exact figure for the number of people affected by hypothermia and cold-related deaths, as other illnesses are more likely to be recorded as the main cause of death should they be present, i.e. heart disease or pneumonia. What is clear is that the risk of hypothermia rises sharply during winter months (see Tables 9.2 and 9.3). A direct correlation between cold weather and higher death rates is evident from these figures.

Keeping warm costs money. Fuel, food, insulation and upkeep of homes all come at a price, as does social activity such as holidays during winter months to warmer climates,

Table 9.2 Deaths related to hypothermia in England and Wales

Year	65+	80+	All ages
1996	365	244	414
1997	215	138	277
1998	212	135	273
1999	225	166	325

Office for National Statistics 1999/2000.

Table 9.3 Excess winter deaths

	1996/7	1997/8	1998/9	1999/2000
65+	38 000	21 000	44 000	45 000
All ages	45 000	23 000	48 000	49 000

Office for National Statistics 1999/2000.

or visiting a luncheon club on regular occasions to ensure a hot meal, good company and a warm environment. Help the Aged (www.helptheaged.org.uk) state that 48% of the households in the poorest tenth of the population are single, retired households.

A recommended room temperature for an older person in the United Kingdom is 21°C compared to that of 18°C for others. The government offers a winter fuel allowance to all those over the age of 60 years to support older people with fuel bills. A person living alone will qualify for a payment of £200, married couples both eligible for a winter fuel payment should receive £100 each, whilst a payment of £300 is available to those aged over 80 years (Department for Work and Pensions 2006).

Age Concern (2006) reports that older people are more likely than any other age group to be affected by fuel poverty with more than one in five (22%) of those over 70 years eligible for pension credit living in fuel poverty, compared with only three in 50 people (6%) of the population as a whole. In the UK since 2003 domestic gas prices have risen by 87% and domestic electricity by 56%. This is a rise not reflected in the winter fuel payment from the government.

In 2004/05, 31 250 people over 65 years of age died from cold-related illnesses in England and Wales (Age Concern 2006).

In the winter of 2005/06 (December to March) there were an estimated 25 700 more deaths in England and Wales, compared to the non-winter period (Office for National Statistics 2006). Most of these deaths were amongst those aged 75 and over. (The non-winter period is defined as the months April to July of the current year and August to November of the previous year (see Fig. 9.3).)

Outside the United Kingdom for many people politicoeconomic factors can be considered as the extremes of

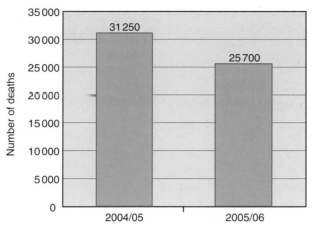

Fig. 9.3 Winter mortality (www.statistics.gov.uk).

poverty, isolation and war. We have seen many images of refugees whose homes have been destroyed, and who exist in refugee camps, living under canvas with little food, water and nonexistent sanitary facilities. (See the World Health Organization website for further information on refugee camps and conditions (www.who.int) and the BBC News website for images (news.bbc.co.uk).)

Warmth is provided by communal living and sleeping, and by the meagre food, clothing and blanket rations provided. Refugees run the risk of death by hypothermia, as temperatures drop dramatically at night. There is little in the way of sustenance and comfort to prevent it. Poor sanitation, in large overcrowded populations such as those in refugee camps lead to a greater chance of developing an infectious disease and the accompanying symptom of fever.

Politicoeconomic factors clearly have an indirect effect on body temperature control.

Exercise

1. Think about your own home circumstances and living conditions. Consider:
   - the type of accommodation you have
   - how much of your (or family) expenditure is spent on food, clothes and keeping warm
   - how you keep warm during low environmental temperatures
   - how you keep cool during heatwaves.

Sociocultural factors

It is easy to make an assumption about sociocultural factors which may influence the AL of controlling body temperature, particularly in relation to customs concerning clothing,

e.g. some religious customs require full covering of a woman's body despite extreme heat. However, a person may be conditioned regarding behaviour that enables them to cope with extreme heat. For example, people may stay indoors in cool stone-built houses in midday temperatures, drink plenty and avoid activity which will increase body temperature further during the greatest heat in the day.

An object's colour and texture as well as its temperature will aid heat loss by radiation (Green 1989). Dark rough surfaces radiate maximally while light smooth surfaces at the same temperature do not lose heat as quickly. The same is said in relation to heat gain by radiation. However, the human skin irrespective of colour is able to radiate heat away from the body. This does not apply to clothes worn. White clothes are more suitable than black in the tropics where it is very hot (Green 1989).

Everyone is socialised into acceptance of norms regarding the extent to which clothes can be shed in hot weather. Roper et al (2000) state that this is socioculturally determined rather than by need for comfort and body temperature control.

In the United States where summers are renowned for being hot and humid, great effort is made to prevent heat-related illness. Education regarding application of measures to avoid heatstroke and exhaustion plays a vital part in its prevention. These have been discussed earlier within this chapter. In 1995 Chicago experienced a summer heatwave, which sent 3300 people to the emergency department and killed more than 600 (Dematte et al 1998 cited in Worfolk 2000).

Acclimatisation can produce beneficial physiological changes. Adaptation occurs over 10–14 days of heat exposure. Lloyd (1994) states that acclimatisation to heat results in increased work output, endurance, plasma volume and sweat production, with a decrease in heart rate, oxygen consumption, electrolyte concentration and core and skin temperature. This timescale indicates why some of us suffer heat exhaustion whilst on foreign holidays to hot exotic destinations.

But what about countries which have colder winters than the UK? In countries such as Sweden and Canada, there is a much smaller difference between the number of deaths in the summer and in the winter. One reason for this is that houses in these countries are better insulated and heated than homes within the UK.

Sociocultural factors do have an effect on the AL of controlling body temperature, but they are limited. When a person is in good health the homeostatic and physiological mechanisms will assist in the maintenance of a core body temperature which will enable optimum function, but it is important to note that they are connected.

DEPENDENCE/INDEPENDENCE IN THE AL OF CONTROLLING BODY TEMPERATURE

In wellness the body is able to regulate its own body temperature. However, in infancy and early childhood, the immaturity of the thermoregulatory system and the child's dependency on others to provide suitable clothing and adequate diet, increase opportunities for deviations from normal temperature to occur. In adulthood, in health, changes in body temperature are related to diurnal variations and hormonal influences. Thermoregulation in older age is less efficient and older people are more susceptible to extremes of heat and cold. Nonphysiological contributing factors may be lack of mobility, poor diet and inadequate heating and often underlying pathological disease.

SUMMARY POINTS

1. Lifespan
The age of the patient will have great bearing on this Activity of Living. The very young have an immature thermoregulatory system and the elderly possibly an impaired thermoregulatory system. Both groups will have some dependency on others to maintain body temperature. During puberty and menstruation it is important to note there may be some slight rise in body temperature. Also, during female menopause, due to hormonal changes, the person may experience hot flushes and hot sweats that disrupt normal living activities.

2. Dependency
At any time during the lifespan an individual may develop dependency due to ill health.

3. Independence
Linked to health and control of body temperature. It is important to remember that choices are made in health about lifestyle, which may affect body temperature, i.e.
- immunisation
- foreign travel
- diet and weight control
- addictive substances – alcohol, nicotine, caffeine
- amount of exercise taken.

4. Factors affecting control of body temperature
Biological
- age
- underlying pathological illness/disease, i.e. carcinoma, myxoedema, thyrotoxicosis
- trauma

- damage to the hypothalamus or vascular system or skin
- weight and food intake
- physical activity
- medication
- diurnal variations
- puberty, pregnancy, menstrual cycle and menopause
- social drugs.

Psychological
- emotional state – anxiety, depression, fear, euphoria
- seasonal affective disorder.

Sociocultural
- exposure of the skin, traditional clothing linked to religion
- bathing habits (see Chapter 8).

Environmental
- outside temperatures/exposure to heat and cold
- windchill
- exposure to sunlight and UVA/UVB rays
- inside temperatures, air conditioning, draughts, damp.

Politicoeconomic
- standards for living
- housing
- income
- lifestyle choices
- education for health
- political agendas, i.e. war.

Yet at any age injury or illness can occur, and body temperatures deviating from the norm may be experienced. During this time there is dependence upon others to provide an environment and interventions which will encourage the body temperature to return within the normal range.

Roper et al (1996) refer to this concept as the dependence/independence continuum component of the model of living.

It is important that the caregiver has an understanding of factors influencing the AL of controlling body temperature to enable them to make an individualised assessment.

THE MODEL FOR NURSING

Using the model for nursing to individualise nursing in the AL of controlling body temperature, this part of the chapter will demonstrate how the components of the model of living are applied in nursing situations in ill health. The case scenarios introduced earlier in this chapter will be developed further. The nursing process (see Chapter 1) will be used to demonstrate application of the Roper et al model for nursing (1996, 2000) in practice.

It has already been demonstrated that in health body temperature is something that is very much taken for granted. Control of body temperature is maintained through a complex feedback system, and behavioural and physiological mechanisms.

So what can cause things to go wrong?

Exercise
1. Review the issues discussed earlier in this chapter in the model of living.
2. List possible causes of disruption to thermoregulation.

ASSESSMENT

Assessment of the individual is a dynamic ongoing process. Assessment is the first phase of the nursing process (see Chapter 1) and without this phase it is impossible to proceed with nursing care. Assessment facilitates the collection of information about the individual's past and current health status and life situation. Collier et al (1996) refer to the fact that the extent or depth of assessment may range from being focused to developing a comprehensive database. This will depend upon the situation in which nursing assessment takes place. For example, in an emergency or life-threatening situation, rapid focused assessment of airway, breathing and circulation may be called for, and identified problems addressed before further comprehensive assessment is possible.

In less acute situations, the nurse will collect data, which will be both subjective and objective in nature. Subjective data are experiences or phenomena experienced by the client and recounted by the nurse. It is an account of how the patient is feeling or a description of symptoms the patient may have experienced.

Collier et al (1996) state that subjective data are not generally observable or measurable by the nurse. The amount of subjective data collated is dependent on the nurse's communication skills (see Chapter 4) and ability to build a therapeutic nurse–patient relationship (Peplau 1952).

The phenomena that can be observed and measured by the nurse are referred to as objective data. The collection of objective data involves the nurse's use of the skills of observation, examination and measurement.

Complete and thorough assessment involves all of these components.

The first part of this chapter (p. 291) introduced Emma, an 18-month-old child. In this section it is disclosed that Emma's health status has deteriorated.

Exercise
1. Can you differentiate between the subjective and objective data presented?
2. Can you identify any phases of fever?
3. What nursing interventions may promote patient comfort?
4. At what point would a prescribed antipyretic agent be useful?

The following may be considered.

Fever management in children

Those involved in caring for a child as a parent or a professional will be aware of how quickly a child can become unwell. In children illness is commonly accompanied by a rise in body temperature. When the rise in body temperature is prolonged physical signs and symptoms of fever will be present.

In children under 5 years pyrexia is the most common cause of convulsions. Convulsions are life-threatening, yet early management of symptoms of fever can prevent a convulsion occurring. A temperature above 38°C may place a child at risk. So what is fever?

Porth (1994) cited in Casey (2000) refers to four phases of fever.

The prodromal phase consists of a feeling of being unwell, however body temperature will be normal. A young baby or child may be quiet, wanting to sleep more than usual and refusing food or generally 'cranky' and unsettled. In this stage pyrogens (chemicals) are released by inflamed and damaged cells. They travel via the bloodstream to the hypothalamus, which releases prostaglandins which raise the hypothalamic thermostat to a higher temperature.

In the second phase, the chill phase, although the body temperature is now rising the child will complain of cold and shivering will occur. The body is responding to the rise in the hypothalamic thermostat by activating heat-promoting mechanisms, until the higher temperature is reached.

During the flush phase, although the body temperature is elevated, the child may feel better. The skin will feel hot and dry. The child's temperature has reached that of the raised hypothalamic thermostat. To bring the body temperature back within the normal range removal of the causative agent or pharmaceutical intervention is required (Casey 2000). The body will assist by activating heat-loss mechanisms when the hypothalamus detects an increase in temperature.

The final phase is referred to as diaphoresis. The child will begin to sweat profusely. Sweat needs to evaporate for cooling to occur (Green 1989). Use of fanning and sponging will aid the cooling process. (Further explanation for these interventions is given in the section relating nursing knowledge to best practice for fever management (p. 307).) The skin will be pink and flushed due to vasodilatation. With the profuse sweating, and evaporation of water from the skin surface, comes the risk of dehydration and electrolyte imbalance. Careful monitoring of the infant/child is paramount.

> ### Exercise
> 1. Besides shivering, which other heat-promoting mechanism will be activated?
> 2. List the physical signs of dehydration.
> 3. Consider the effects of a fever on an adult and elderly person as well as Emma.

By applying the information given regarding baby Emma to the model of living it is possible to build a holistic, individualised picture, which supports the nursing approach (see p. 305 for potential nursing care plan for Emma).

Lifespan
Emma at 18 months old is still dependent on an adult to provide a suitable safe environment in relation to body temperature control. Also she is dependent on the provision of suitable clothing for environmental temperature and fluids to promote comfort on hot days and replace fluid lost through sweating.

Dependence
Having developed a fever, Emma is dependent on recognition of her symptoms of illness by an appropriate adult who will provide suitable interventions or seek medical advice.

Independence
For Emma independence in relation to body temperature control is only in relation to biological and physiological feedback systems during health.

Biological
As part of the immune response Emma has developed a fever. Remember that fever can play a positive part in the immune response, affecting the ability of the invading pathogen to reproduce and enabling better function of the immune response (Fullick 1998). Emma has recently joined a mother and baby group. She has been exposed to other children through social contact; this may be relevant. Her age will play a part in her ability to respond and should her fever not be well controlled then risk of convulsion is increased. Application of nursing interventions must be appropriate to the stages of fever and the biological and physiological responses of the body.

Psychological
As Emma's temperature increased, her thermoregulatory system raised the thermostat to a higher level – this produced a shiver response. As Emma then felt cold, seeing the shiver her mother provided extra clothing, increasing Emma's temperature further. This would result in a hot, sticky and distressed baby. It is imperative that parents are provided with information about fever management to ensure they respond appropriately. Although Emma's mum noted shivering, touch would have told her that Emma was pyrexic.

Sociocultural
Consider the culture that has been created in relation to the use of GPs and emergency services. People must feel comfortable about accessing help and advice. Emma's mum took the correct action in utilising A&E when her child's condition deteriorated.

Environmental
It has already been identified that environmental temperatures can affect control of body temperature. A health visitor can be involved to provide further information regarding Emma's home environment. A suitable safe environment is provided in which to nurse Emma. Control of her body temperature to prevent convulsion is paramount. The internal environment of the body in relation to homeostatic mechanisms must be maintained.

Politicoeconomic
This scenario has considered only Emma and her mum. It is relevant to consider the amount of support offered to single parents. Housing, income and lifestyle all need to be considered in the assessment. It is neccessary to ascertain that when Emma is discharged her mum has all the relevant support to continue to care for her daughter to the best of her ability.

Assessment skills
Nurses carry with them unique tools that will aid patient assessment and on-going evaluation in relation to body temperature control. These tools are the interpersonal and communication skills with which the nurse can obtain information. These same skills enable the development of a therapeutic nurse–patient relationship (Peplau 1952).

Nurses may also develop an acute use of their special senses to aid assessment. These special senses involve the use of touch to ascertain if the patient's skin feels hot, cold, dry or clammy.

Nursing care plan for Emma Smith –18 months

Assessment	Goal/aim	Planning	Implementation	Evaluation
Maintaining a safe environment Emma is dependent on others to keep her safe	Keep safe from harm	Ensure side room is at a constant comfortable temperature and free from draughts Ensure observation is continuous Nurse with cot sides raised Keep mum with child as much as possible Observe intravenous cannula site for signs of infection Maintain IV as prescribed	Mum present with Emma at all times Named nurse identified for continuous observation Document interventions affecting IV site Report and document any evidence of infection	Mum and Emma settled on ward
Breathing Maintaining own airway	To recognise any early disruption with breathing	Record 4 hourly Observe rate, depth Note any audible cough or wheeze	4 hourly observation of temperature, pulse and respiration recorded	Maintaining own airway Breathing rate within normal limits
Communication Emma is quiet and not willing to respond to smiles etc. – possibly due to lethargy Appears content when nursed by mum	To promote positive communication for Emma's stage of development	Observe Emma's communication as temperature returns to normal limits Keep mum in contact with Emma Use gentle tone of voice and smile when talking to Emma Utilise touch to provide comfort Provide information for mum regarding Emma's condition, nursing interventions and treatment	Mum with Emma at all times Side room next to nursing office Tolerating nursing intervention	Good relationship between mum and nursing staff Emma now responding positively with simple words/smile, e.g. naming familiar objects and toys
Eating and drinking Continues to refuse diet, but now taking small amounts of oral clear fluids Not vomiting at time of assessment	For Emma to tolerate fluids and diet	Record input and output Monitor physical signs of dehydration Encourage clear fluids orally Maintain intravenous fluids as prescribed	Tolerating oral clear fluids well Continuing to record input and output Urea and electrolyte balance recorded Intravenous therapy continuing	Now graduated to mixed fluids and light diet Urea and electrolyte balance within normal limits Intravenous therapy discontinued
Mobilising Able to walk normally unassisted Today prefers to lie still and quiet	To be mobilising as normal	Allow Emma to mobilise as she feels able	Provide a safe environment for mobilisation – keep with adult at all times	Now mobilising
Sleep and rest Awake for short periods of time only Normally sleeps 7 p.m.–7 a.m. with afternoon nap	Return to normal sleep patterns	Allow to sleep as required Ensure observation Ensure quiet periods Record temperature during rest periods	Nurse in side room	Takes an interest in her surroundings Responding positively to others Still experiencing disrupted nights sleep
Work and play Uninterested in favourite toys	To be stimulated by play activities	Provide stimulus in the environment, e.g. pictures to look at, mobiles Provide toys which are relevant for Emma's development Keep favourite toy close	Nursed in paediatric side room Environment and toys provided to encourage play when required Favourite toy present	Playing for short periods Still sleeping a little more than normal

(continued)

Nursing care plan for Emma Smith –18 Months *(continued)*

Assessment	Goal/aim	Planning	Implementation	Evaluation
Personal cleansing and dressing Dependent on others to provide care for cleansing and dressing	To promote physical comfort	Cleanse Emma as necessary, recognising associated lethargy and possible need for tepid sponging Dress Emma appropriate to climate and body temperature	Promote comfort Encourage mum with this activity Wearing T-shirt, vest and nappy Covered with a light sheet when sleeping Cleanse by bed bath	Emma appears settled and comfortable Mum involved in all aspects of care Skin is cleansed and intact
Eliminating One wet nappy today 2.30 p.m. Urine in this nappy observed to be dark in colour and strong in odour	To improve urine output to normal limits	Record output, number of wet nappies Obtain specimen of urine for culture and sensitivity Check bowels moved	Input and output measured Urine specimen obtained for culture and sensitivity	Input and output improved Urine infection isolated Oral antibiotic treatment commenced as prescribed
Expressing sexuality		Allow mum to provide appropriate comfort with love and hugs, etc.	Mum and staff providing comfort with appropriate use of touch	Emma is responding to comfort shown
Maintaining body temperature Raised tympanic Temperature of 38.8°C	To bring temperature back within normal limits (36.5–37.5°C)	Nurse in a suitable environment, free from drafts Give prescribed antipyretic Monitor temperature Promote patient comfort by using tepid sponging at an appropriate time in the fever phase	Paracetemol given as prescribed at 2.10 p.m. Hourly temperature recording implemented skin exposed	Temperature now within normal limits Fever management information provided for mum
Dying Emma due to her stage of development will not be familiar with the concept of death	To promote recovery	Provide information for mum regarding Emma's condition and her treatment Reassure	Mum informed of all nursing action and involved in care delivery	Responding positively to nursing and medical interventions

Touch may also enable detection of dehydration should the skin have lost elasticity (usually tested by a skin stretch on the back of the hand). Touch (or movement) of the patient may be associated with pain indicating inflammation.

By using sight to observe the patient, the nurse will notice if the colour of the skin is pink, red, flushed, pale, mottled or cyanosed. The nurse may also notice the presence of a rash, indicating infection, or breaks in the surface of the skin. The nurse will observe and note the level of activity or lethargy with which the patient presents, and the presence or absence of shivering. The nurse's sense of smell may be used to recognise the presence of infection and excessive sweating. Fetid (stale) breath on the patient may be a symptom of dehydration. The patient may be able to tell the nurse if they feel uncomfortably hot or cold. The nurse must hear the patient and respond accordingly. The nurse may hear moans/cries of discomfort, or the chattering of teeth if shivering is present.

If the patient is conscious, nurses will use their communication and interpersonal skills to ask open and closed questions as appropriate, depending on the patient's ability to respond (see Chapter 4).

The following are examples of useful questions to ask should a patient present with symptoms of fever. They can be adapted for an adult or child.

- Are you normally fit and well?
- For how long have you felt unwell?
- How long have you been aware of fever?
- Do symptoms worsen at night and can you describe the symptoms?
- Have you any other symptoms, e.g. cough, cold, headache, sore throat, pain passing urine, stomach pain, vomiting, diarrhoea, joint point, urethral or vaginal discharge?
- Have you recently received a vaccination or travelled abroad?

- Is anyone else you closely associate with unwell?
- How have you managed the fever, e.g. has an antipyretic been taken?
- Is the fever worse at night?
- What is your current fluid intake?
- When did you last pass urine?
- Have you been involved in any new social activity recently?
- Is there any previous history (or family history) of convulsion?

It has been identified that fever can occur whenever the immune system is attacked. It carries greater risk in children as their febrile state may lead to convulsions, but its management in an adult patient is equally important.

Consider the following case study.

Case study 9.4

Lynn – a 28-year-old primary school teacher

Lynn is 28 years old, living in an inner city with a high immigrant population. She works as a primary school teacher. For some weeks Lynn has found work increasingly difficult, as she has been unable to shake off a bad cold, in which she experienced flu-like symptoms and a persistent cough. Her partner is concerned, as he has noticed that Lynn has lost weight and appears constantly tired. Lynn is having difficulty sleeping at night due to night sweats. She has treated her flu-like symptoms with over-the-counter medications but has experienced little relief. Following a severe bout of night coughing and fever her partner calls the emergency GP, who arranges admission for Lynn to the local hospital.

Exercise

1. List physical symptoms which may lead you to suspect tuberculosis.
2. Identify environmental and politicoeconomic factors which are significant.
3. If Lynn's laboratory test proves 'smear-positive' can you identify those who may require contact surveillance?
4. Using the example of baby Emma, apply the information you have regarding Lynn to the model of living.
5. Devise a nursing care plan for Lynn which addresses her needs on admission to hospital.

Relating nursing knowledge to best practice for fever management

Pyrexia, as previously explained, is usually the result of an invading pathogen. Watson (1998) states that pyrexia should be considered to be present when body temperature is 38°C or above. If the cause of the pyrexia is bacterial, it can be treated with antibiotics. Should an inflammatory response be present, anti-inflammatory drugs (steroids) will prove useful. Should the invading pathogen be a virus it will need

to run its own course. However, the symptoms of pyrexia can be treated regardless of cause, to promote patient comfort. This will require skilled nursing intervention and use of antipyretic medications, with thorough knowledge of the physiological phases of fever (Porth 1994). A mild temperature of less than 38°C in an otherwise healthy person will have a positive effect on the immune system (Fullick 1998) (see Fig. 9.2, p. 292).

A temperature of greater than 38°C carries with it risk of rigors, convulsions in children, electrolyte imbalance and the destruction of body proteins.

In the chill phase of fever, Porth (1994) explained that the body's temperature is increasing to the higher thermostat set point. The patient feels cold and the thermoregulatory system initiates vasoconstriction and shivering (heat-generating mechanisms) until the circulating blood reaches the new temperature set point.

Casey (2000) suggests that cooling measures such as tepid sponging are not appropriate at this stage, as cooling the shell of the body will encourage further generation of heat. At this stage pharmacological intervention is recommended to bring the raised thermostat set point back within normal limits. Previous reference has been made to the fact that pyrogens travel via the bloodstream to the hypothalamus, which produces prostaglandins that act on the hypothalamus, raising the set point. Casey (2000) states that prostaglandin synthesis can be inhibited by paracetemol and non-steroidal anti-inflammatory drugs (NSAIDs).

Paracetamol causes temporary disruption of the enzymes which manufacture the prostaglandins associated with fever and pain responses in the body, and so reduces temperature and helps aid patient comfort. NSAIDs such as aspirin are helpful in reducing fever, but they can cause side-effects such as gastric irritation and indigestion. As they act to permanently inhibit the prostaglandins, side-effects can be widespread throughout the body (Casey 2000).

As body temperature returns to within normal limits during the flush and diaphoresis phases (Porth 1994), nursing interventions may be initiated to quicken the return of normal body temperature. These may be by the use of an electric fan or tepid sponging.

The rationale supporting the use of electric fans is that they encourage convection of heat from the body surface (Watson 1998) so lowering body temperature. This is the same effect as wind chill, which enhances drops in body temperature during low environmental temperatures. Watson (1998) advises that fans are not directed at the patient as they can cause discomfort, which may lead to shivering and to reflex vasoconstriction that will enhance heat generation. It is only necessary to ensure adequate ventilation, ensuring patients are not in draughts.

Tepid sponging is less aggressive than sponging with cold water, so vasoconstriction is lessened. However, latent heat will still cause evaporation, and cooling will result (Watson 1998). For evaporation to occur the body must be hotter than the temperature of the surrounding environment.

The optimal time to measure temperature is 8 p.m. but this can be affected when patients are hospitalised, and pain, trauma and sleep disturbance all affect normal sleeping patterns. Temperatures recorded at other times during the day are equally valuable, but diurnal/circadian rhythms must be considered (Edwards 1997).

Best practice in relation to method, rate and regularity for body temperature measurement will be a direct result of an accurate and individualised patient assessment. Remember that assessment is an ongoing process to be performed regularly throughout an episode of patient care.

SUMMARY POINTS

1. Caring for a person who has a deviation from normal body temperature involves thorough knowledge of the body's physiological responses. By understanding these physiological responses it is possible to provide safe and effective nursing interventions that promote patient comfort.

2. This knowledge also assists in providing advice for others regarding prevention of temperature deviations which can cause great harm. Accurate assessment, followed by the setting of achievable goals, facilitates a plan of care that addresses individualised patient needs. Nursing interventions must be based on best practice, and knowledge of equipment which may be used to measure body temperature is essential. The choice of equipment will be based upon individual patient assessment.

3. Evaluation of nursing interventions must be ongoing, so practice can be altered should the patient's condition change. By using the model for nursing alongside the model of living a holistic view of a person's lifestyle can be developed. Ultimately this should result in an episode of skilled caregiving which is beneficial and therapeutic in both the prevention and treatment of illnesses related to deviations in body temperature control.

References

Age Concern 2006 (www.ageconcern.org.uk)

Batscha C 1997 Heat stroke. Keeping your client cool in the summer. Journal of Psychosocial Nursing 35(7): 12–17

BBC News 1999 (news.bbc.co.uk/hi/english/health/medical)

Blackburn E 1994 Prevention of hypothermia during anaesthesia. British Journal of Theatre Nursing 4(8): 9–14

Blackburn S, Loper D 1992 Maternal, fetal and neonatal physiology. A clinical perspective. WB Saunders, Philadelphia

Blumenthal D 2000 Fever and the practice nurse: measurement and treatment. Community Practitioner 73(3): 519–521

British National Formulary 2006 (www.BNF.org)

Casey G 2000 Fever management in children. Paediatric Nursing 12(3): 38–43

Chiodini J 2001 Where do we get our travel health information from? Nursing in Practice 2: 139–140

Closs J 1987 Oral temperature measurement. Nursing Times 83: 136–139

Collier I, McCash E, Bartram J 1996 Writing nursing diagnosis: A clinical thinking approach. Mosby, London

Collins K, Dore C, Exton-Smith AN 1977 Accidental hypothermia and impaired temperature homeostasis in the elderly. British Medical Journal 1: 353–356

COSHH 2002 Health & Safety Executive regulations (www.hse.gov.uk/hthdir/noframes/coshh)

Dematte J, O'Mara K, Buescher J et al 1998 Near fatal heatstroke during the 1995 heat wave in Chicago. Annals of Internal Medicine 129: 173–181

Department of Health 1998 The prevention and control of tuberculosis in the United Kingdom. HSC 1998/196. Stationery Office, London

Department of Health 2006 Heatwave plan for England (www.dh.gov/publications)

Department of Work and Pensions 2001, 2006 (www.dwp.gov.uk/winterfuel)

Edwards S 1997 Measuring temperature. Professional Nurse 13(2): 253–258

Edwards S 2003 Temperature regulation. In: Brooker C, Nicol M (eds) Nursing adults the practice of caring, Chapter 5. Mosby, London

Ejidokun O, Ramaiah S, Sandhu S 1998 A cluster of tuberculosis cases in a family. Communicable Disease in Public Health 1(4): 245–300

Environmental News Network 1999 (www.enn.com/ennnewsarchive/1999)

Erickson RS, Woo TM 1994 Accuracy of infrared ear thermometry and traditional temperature methods in young children. Heart and Lung 23: 181–193

Fisher B, Warren C 1999 Walk-in-clinic fever. Practice Nursing 10(15): 31–34

Fraden J, Lackey RP 2000 Estimation of body site temperatures from tympanic measurements. Clinical Paediatrics Supplement 30: 65–70

Fullick A 1998 Human health and disease. Heinemann Advanced Science, Oxford

Gould D 1994 Controlling patients' body temperature. Nursing Standard 8(35): 29–31

Green JH 1989 An introduction to human physiology, 4th edn. Oxford Medical Publications, Oxford

Gupta A 1999 Influenza: Improving uptake of vaccination in older people. Geriatric Medicine 11: 13

Handley AJ, Swain A (eds) 1996 Advanced life support manual, 2nd edn. Resuscitation Council UK, London

Heidenreich T, Giuffre M, Doorley J 1992 Temperature and temperature measurement after induced hypothermia. Nursing Research 419(5): 296–300

Hinchliff S 2005 Innate defences. In: Hinchliff S, Montague S, Watson R (eds) Physiology for nursing practice. Baillière Tindall, London,

Hinchliff S, Montague S, Watson R (eds) 2005 Physiology for nursing practice, 3rd edn. Baillière Tindall, London

Imrie M, Hall G 1990 Body temperature and anaesthesia. British Journal of Anaesthetics 64: 346–354

Jamieson EM, McCall JM, Whyte LA 2002 Clinical nursing practice, 4th edn. Churchill Livingstone, Edinburgh

jas 2001 (www.jas.tj/skincancer/facts)

Keane C 2000 Physiological responses and management of hypothermia. Emergency Nurse 8(8): 26–31

Kelly M, Ewens B, Jevan P 2001 Hypothermia management. Nursing Times 97(9): 36–37

Kerry 1999 USA today (www.usatoday.com/weather)

Krikler S 1990 What to do about temperatures. Nursing Standard 4(25): 37–38

Kunihiro A, Foster J 1998 Heat exhaustion and heat stroke (www.emedicine.com/EMERG/tropic236.htm)

Lloyd E 1994 Temperature and performance II: Heat. British Medical Journal 3096954: 587

Lloyd E 1996 Hypothermia and cold stress. Croom Helm, London

Luckman J 1997 Saunders manual of nursing care. Saunders, Philadelphia, PA

Macmillan A, Corbett JL, Johnson RH et al 1967 Temperature regulation in survivors of accidental hypothermia of the elderly. Lancet 22: 165–169

Mallett J, Dougherty L 2004 The Royal Marsden Hospital manual of clinical nursing procedures, 6th edn. Blackwell Science, Oxford

Manian F, Griesenauer S 1998 Lack of agreement between tympanic and oral temperature measurements in adult hospitalised patients. American Journal of Infection Control 26. 428–430

Marieb E 2006 Human anatomy and physiology, 7th edn. Addison Wesley, California

Medicinenet 1999 (www.medicinenet.com)

Medico 2001 (Medico.uwcm.ac.uk)

Miller D 2001 The flu: current treatments and future strategies. Nursing in Practice 2: 87–90

Murphy P 1998 Handbook of critical care. Science Press, London

Newman J 1985 Evaluation of sponging to reduce body temperature in febrile infants. Canadian Medical Association Journal 132: 641–642

NHS 2001 A new guide to childhood immunisation. Health Promotion England, London

Nichols G, Kucha D 1972 Oral measurements. American Journal of Nursing 72(b): 1091–1093

Noa 2002 (www.erh.noa.gov/den/windchill)

Office for National Statistics 1999/2000 (www.statistics.gov.uk)

Office for National Statistics 2006 (www.statistics.gov.uk)

Patja A, Davidkin I, Kurki T 2000 Serious adverse events after measles, mumps, rubella vaccination during a 14 year prospective follow up. Pediatric Infectious Disease Journal 19: 1127–1134

Peplau HE 1952 Interpersonal relations in nursing. GP Putnam, New York

Porth M 1994 Pathophysiology – concepts of altered health states, 4th edn. Lippincott, Philadelphia

Pransky SM 1991 The impact of technique and condition of the tympanic membrane upon infrared tympanic thermometry. Clinical Paediatrics Supplement 30: 50–52

Public Health Laboratory Service 1998 Communicable Disease Surveillance Centre Supplement. Infectious disease in England and Wales: April 1966–June 1992. Communicable Diseases Report 8(2): 53

Public Health Laboratory Service 2001 (www.phls.co.uk/facts/influenza/flu.html)

Pugh-Davis S, Kassab JY, Thrush AJ et al 1986 A comparison of mercury and digital clinical thermometers. Journal of Advanced Nursing 11(5): 535–543

Pursell E 2000a The use of antipyretic medications in the prevention of febrile convulsion in children. Journal of Clinical Nursing 9: 473–480

Pursell E 2000b Physical treatment of fever. Archives of Diseases in Childhood 82: 238–239

Roper N, Logan W, Tierney A 1996 The elements of nursing – a model for nursing based on a model of living, 4th edn. Churchill Livingstone, Edinburgh

Roper N, Logan W, Tierney A 2000 The Roper–Logan–Tierney model of nursing based on activities of living. Churchill Livingstone, Edinburgh

Sganga A, Wallace R, Kiehl E et al 2000 A comparison of four methods of normal newborn temperature measurement. The American Journal of Maternal/Child Nursing 25(2): 76–79

Sharber J 1997 The efficacy of tepid sponge bathing to reduce fever in young children. American Journal of Emergency Medicine 15: 188–192

Sidebottom J 1992 When it's hot enough to kill. RN 55(8): 31–34

Taylor B, Miller E, Farrington C et al 1999 Autism and measles, mumps, rubella vaccine: no epidemiological evidence for a causal association. Lancet 353: 2026–2029

Tinker J, Zapol W 1992 Care of the critically ill patient, 2nd edn. Springer-Verlag, New York

Torrence C, Semple MC 1998 Recording temperature. Nursing Times 94(3): Practical Procedures for Nursing Supplement

Watson R 1998 Controlling body temperature in adults. Emergency Nurse 6(1): 31–39

Waugh A, Grant A 2006 Ross and Wilson anatomy and physiology in health and illness, 10th edn. Churchill Livingstone, Edinburgh

Wells, King J, Hedstrom C et al 1995 Does tympanic temperature measure up? American Journal of Maternal Child Nursing 14: 88–93

While A 2000 Putting fever in perspective. British Journal of Community Nursing 5(10): 517

Wilshaw R, Beckstrand R, Ward D et al 1999 A comparison of the use of tympanic, axillary and rectal thermometers in infants. Journal of Paediatric Nursing 4(2): 88–93

World Health Organization 1999 (www.who.int/inf-fs/en/fact.html)

World Health Organization 2005 International travel and health – vaccination requirements and health advice. WHO, Geneva

Woollens S 1996 Temperature measurement devices. Professional Nurse 11: 541–547

Worfolk J 2000 Heat waves: Their impact on the health of elders. Geriatric Nursing 21(2): 70–77

Yetman R, Coody DK, West MS et al 1993 Comparison of temperature measurement by an aural infrared thermometer with measurements by traditional rectal and auxiliary techniques. Journal of Paediatrics 122: 769–773

Further reading

Childs C 2006 Temperature control. In: Alexander M, Fawcett J, Runcimann P (eds) Nursing practice – hospital and home – the adult. 3rd edn. Chapter 22. Churchill Livingstone, Edinburgh,

Desborough J 1997 Body temperature control and anaesthesia. British Journal of Hospital Medicine 57(9): 440–442

Edwards S 2003 Temperature regulation. In: Brooker C, Nicol M (eds) Nursing adults: the practice of caring. 1st edn, Chapter 5. Mosby, London,

Hinchliff SM, Montague SE, Watson R 2005 Physiology for nursing practice, 3rd edn. Baillière Tindall, London

Jamieson EM, McCall JM, Whyte LA 2002 Clinical nursing practice, 4th edn. Churchill Livingstone, Edinburgh

Jones JG, Needham M, Roberts E et al 1999 A history of Abergele Hospital – confronting the white plague, Gee & Son (Denbigh), Denbigh

Mallett J, Bailey C 2000 Manual of clinical nursing procedures, 4th edn. Blackwell Science, Oxford

Useful websites

www.age.concern.org.uk (Age Concern)
www.helptheaged.org.uk (Help the Aged)
www.resus.org.uk (Resuscitation Council)
www.statistics.gov.uk (Office for National Statistics)

Mobilising

Julia Ryan

INTRODUCTION

A characteristic of living things is the ability to move independently of external forces. Movement is important for many reasons – to find and prepare food, to get away from danger, and to make the environment safe, comfortable and enjoyable. Mobilising is not only about obvious behaviours such as walking, running or swimming – it's also about being able to use a computer keyboard, gardening or painting. Movement provides the means for personal contact with other people and the surroundings.

Many illnesses and injuries can cause mobility problems, diminishing the capacity to move freely around the environment, be that a room, a chair or even a bed. Loss of mobility, even for a short time, can have devastating effects on physical wellbeing. Being in control of movement can be a source of autonomy, pride and dignity, so mobility problems can have significant psychological and emotional effects.

This chapter explores the Activity of Living 'mobilising' described by Roper, Logan and Tierney in their model for nursing (Roper et al 1996, 2000). The model of living will be used to look at mobilising in everyday life. Concepts of lifespan, independence/dependence and important factors influencing mobility will be explored. The model for nursing will examine how the Activities of Living can be used in practice.

Using the components of the model, the chapter will focus on the following:

- mobilising in health and illness across the lifespan
- dependence and independence in mobilising
- factors influencing mobilising
- nursing care of individuals with health needs associated with the Activity of Living, mobilising.

This chapter does not intend to be a definitive account of all the knowledge and skills you will need to effectively meet the mobility needs of the patients you will come across in practice – rather the intention is to help you to make sense of your previous experiences, challenge your current ideas, and help you to identify further learning.

THE MODEL OF LIVING

MOBILISING IN HEALTH AND ILLNESS ACROSS THE LIFESPAN

Infancy and childhood

Learning how to move independently begins even before birth. Mothers are often all too aware of the movement of their baby in the uterus, and whilst this might mean sleep-disturbed nights, it also indicates that the baby is developing as expected. Fetal movement can be seen on an ultrasound scan in very early pregnancy, and the mother can often feel movement from around 16 weeks gestation onwards.

The newborn human baby is not able to mobilise independently. The development of basic mobility skills is very complex and takes a considerable time, a much longer time, relatively speaking, for humans than other animals. This is principally due to the human infant's immature nervous system which does not allow for purposeful coordinated movement. Throughout infancy and childhood great importance is attached to the development of independent movement. Rolling, crawling, standing, walking and running are greeted with joy by the child's family, and are important milestones noted during the monitoring of a child's development. As children attain greater neuromuscular dexterity they can use their mastery of mobilising to develop skills in the other Activities of Living such as playing, eating, drinking and personal cleansing and dressing.

> **Exercise**
> 1. List the child development milestones related to mobility.
> 2. What factors might influence a child's ability to achieve these milestones?

Adolescence and adulthood

Good mobility habits, as with so much else, are established in the early years. Exercise/sport is often a compulsory element of education, with the intention of developing healthy living skills from early in the life course. Increasing independence in mobility reflects increasing personal independence. A sign of maturity is the ability to go out into the world; a symbol of this is the young person being given the keys to the car (rather than the keys to the door!). Young adulthood is often seen as a 'risk-taking' time of life. This applies to mobilising as well as other activities and is illustrated by the high levels of road traffic and other accidents and sporting injuries amongst young people.

In adulthood the increasing pressures of work, maybe parenthood or other family commitments can make regular exercise difficult. This might be especially problematic if one has a sedentary occupation. Mobility as such is taken for granted, and it is only when something happens to reduce one's ability (an accident or illness for example) that the individual might be made aware of how mobility affects many aspects of life.

Late adulthood

Much of the world is experiencing demographic change as both the numbers and proportions of older people increase. Globally the proportion of people over 60 years is growing faster than any other age group. It is estimated that in 2025 there will be 1.2 billion people worldwide, rising to 2 billion in 2025, 80% of whom will be living in developing countries (World Health Organization (WHO) 2002a). In the UK around a fifth of the population is over 60 years of age (Department of Health (DoH) 2001). Whilst there is predicted to be a continued increase in the number and proportion of people reaching late adulthood, the most significant rise will amongst the oldest old (Soule et al 2005).

Whilst the majority of older people live fulfilling, independent lives, there are a number of age-related changes that impact on mobility in late life, and increase the likelihood of problems in mobilising. It is for this reason that much of the material in this chapter will relate to the older adult. As an example, falls are a common occurrence in later life and are associated with significant levels of morbidity (disease and disordered function) and mortality (death) (Stuck & Beck 2001).

Purposeful mobilising depends on a functioning sensory ability, central nervous system coordination and musculoskeletal system. Physiological changes in late life which affect mobilising include: a reduced sense of balance, reduced righting reflex, reduced reaction time and speed of response. Despite these changes, impaired mobility is not inevitable in late life.

There are a number of factors, other than the biological, which impact on an older person's mobility levels. Ayis et al (2006) propose that psychosocial factors are as strongly associated with significant decline in mobility in later life as physical factors. Perceptions and beliefs about levels and types of activity appropriate for older people can be important. Old age can be seen as a time to take it easy and retire to a sedentary life, indeed there is evidence that detraining starts fairly early in the life course. Whilst Brown-Wilson

(2002) claims that ageist attitudes amongst nursing staff can promote immobility and dependency.

Whilst some physiological changes might be inevitable, the extent to which they impact on mobility and broader function are modifiable. Even a fairly moderate reduction in mobility can have serious implications, for frail older people in particular. Problems with mobilising can mean that the individual can't get out to do the shopping, stand up to cook, or get to the toilet in time. The good news is that appropriate interventions can increase mobility and functional independence, and reduce admissions to long-term care.

Exercise

Take some time to observe how people move: for example how individuals stand, get up from a sitting position, walk or run.

1. Can you see any similarities and differences in the patterns you observe?
2. How are these similarities and differences related to lifespan?
3. You might want to think about why people move in the way they do.
4. Think about how the way someone stands or sits (posture), or the way they walk (gait) can project an image of who they are (or maybe who they would like to be).

You may have noted:

- How a baby learns to stand, balance and walk unsupported. Whilst initially movement is clumsy and the child has to concentrate, with practice movement becomes smooth and automatic.
- Children running, skipping and jumping as they use movement to expend reserves of energy and explore the world around them.
- Young people, as they become more self-conscious are often aware of their bodies and this can affect posture and gait.
- Perhaps you thought about how pregnancy can affect mobility. Try and recall how a pregnant woman stands and walks, especially in the latter stages of pregnancy.
- You might have noticed some differences in gait amongst older people. Older women often develop a narrow base when standing or walking, which leads to a 'waddling' gait. Older men often develop a wider walking base.
- Very old people tend to walk more slowly and deliberately. This might be due to physical changes, but also might be related to a lack of confidence or fear of falling. It's also interesting to think about societal views of mobilising in later life – for example, in the UK the road sign for 'older people crossing' shows a bent-over figure with a stick.
- Some people have a characteristic posture or gait which means you can recognise them even at a distance.

People move in a variety of ways. Some of these differences may be due to age, but others are not. They may be due to temporary changes, for example physical factors such as a waddling gait in pregnancy, or psychosocial factors such as the way in which people who are attracted to each other mirror the other's posture. Some of these points will be revisited later in the chapter when looking in detail at assessment.

DEPENDENCE AND INDEPENDENCE IN MOBILISING

At a simple level the dependence–independence continuum might be equated with lifespan: dependency existing at both extremes of age, and independence the norm in-between. A wider consideration of mobilising might challenge some notions inherent in this opinion. There is a view that equates physical mobility with independence in its broadest sense – leading to perceptions of people who have impaired mobility as being wholly dependent. Consider a young woman who uses a wheelchair and a modified car to enable her to get to work, go to a club, or to do her shopping. On one hand she might be considered dependent because she relies on her wheelchair, yet the wheelchair enables her independence in living. Yet again, the young woman might also be an elite athlete with an extremely high level of physical fitness.

It is evident that independence in many of the other Activities of Living is closely related to independence in mobilising.

> ### Exercise
> Have you ever had an illness or accident that has affected your mobility? If not, imagine that you are not able to move without help.
>
> 1. Make a note of the effects reduced mobility had on your other Activities of Living.
> 2. What sort of help did you need?
> 3. How did you feel?

You might have thought about:

- the frustration of not being able to do what you want, when you want
- the embarrassment of needing help to go to the toilet, or having to urinate or defecate in bed (have you ever sat on a bed pan? If not then try it!)
- feelings of loneliness and isolation with everyone else getting on with their lives whilst you are in bed or in hospital, not able to join in.

Now it might be that you have had or have imagined very different feelings. That is understandable, we are all individuals. It is just worth remembering that even a limited alteration in mobility can have a big impact on one's experience and quality of life (see Case study 8.2, p. 279).

Dependence in mobility can occur as a result of disease or trauma, for example injury following a road traffic accident. For most people this will be temporary and so, with time, mobility will be regained; however, for some there will be long-lasting problems. Other people have impaired mobility from birth because of altered body structure and/or function, for example lack of muscle tone is a common feature in Down syndrome.

There are a number of mobility aids that can be used to support independence in mobilising. Walking aids, such as sticks and crutches can be used to:

- improve balance and stability by widening the person's base
- relieve pain from fractures or arthritis, for example by transferring weight through the upper limbs to the ground
- give confidence.

As with any piece of equipment used in patient care, the nurse should understand the principles of use. Walking aids should be of the correct length, so when one is standing and holding the aid the elbows should be slightly flexed (30° angle). The exception to this is a gutter aid, which keeps the elbow at a right angle. Walking aids should be checked regularly to make sure that ferrules (caps) on the end of the aid are tightly fitting and not worn down. Metal aids should be checked for bends in the frame, and wooden ones for splits and cracks.

People might need to use a wheelchair to maintain or restore independence. Each person will have specific requirements, which must be taken into account. Wheelchair use might be temporary, intermittent or regular. There are many types of wheelchair including: self-propelled and electrically controlled, those for indoor use or outdoor use, lightweight or heavyweight, one-arm or two-arm drive, high seat or low seat. From this short list of potential differences it is clearly important to match the person's individual requirements with an appropriate wheelchair.

> ### Exercise
> 1. What do you think the consequences of inadequate wheelchair provision might be?
> 2. Have you ever used a wheelchair to transport people? Do you know what to check to make sure that the wheelchair is appropriate and fit for the task?
> 3. How are mobility aids provided in your locality? Think about walking sticks, crutches, wheelchairs, calipers and prosthetic limbs.

The impact of inadequate provision can be significant, as Table 10.1 indicates. In some situations, for example in some nursing homes or rehabilitation wards, there is a pool of wheelchairs that are used for everyone. Not only might these not be suitable for a particular individual, but they might also be poorly maintained and hazardous to both the patient and the nurse.

Table 10.1 Potential consequences of poor wheelchair provision

For the wheelchair user	Impairment or loss of mobility Reduced choice of lifestyle Reduced quality of life Increased dependence Discomfort and pain Pressure sores Poor posture Permanent deformity (especially in children)
For carers	Fatigue Back pain Impact on personal relationship
For service providers	Increased dependency of service user Increased need for care Health problems for wheelchair user and carer

Exercise
1. Find a model skeleton in either your educational establishment or clinical area.
2. Take your time to look at and handle the bones.
3. Note the shapes of the bones and how they fit together, find out where the main muscles would be attached, and see how and where the joints articulate.

FACTORS RELATING TO MOBILISING

Biological factors

The first question to ask might be 'how do we move?' To fully answer this question requires a deep understanding of the central and peripheral nervous systems, as well as the musculoskeletal system. It is also important to think about the way that genetics and the external environment can impact upon the anatomy and physiology needed for normal movement. It should also be remembered that we are always moving: your eyes are moving as you read this book, your gut is slowly moving digestive products along its length, the diaphragm and your intercostal muscles are moving your ribcage causing air to move in and out of your lungs.

The Activity of Living 'mobilising' is principally concerned with purposeful voluntary movement. This chapter will provide a basic overview of how bones, muscles and joints work together to produce movement. You might find it helpful to use Chapter 4 'Communication' to review your knowledge of the nervous system.

The skeleton

The skeleton (see Fig. 10.1) has a number of functions which include:

- providing the body with a supporting framework
- protecting soft vital organs such as the brain, spinal cord, heart and lungs from injury
- storing a reserve of minerals such as calcium, phosphorus and magnesium; around 99% of the calcium content (1kg) of the body is contained in the skeleton
- developing blood cells in bone marrow
- allowing movement by providing a base for the attachment of muscles and tendons, and the formation of joints.

Bone

It is sometimes easy to forget that bone is living tissue. Bone is made up of 20–30% water; so living bones are soft and slightly flexible. Bone has its own blood and nerve supply, which is why fractures are painful and can cause significant blood loss. Bones are not solid, but are made up of small tubes arranged in concentric circles. This means that bone is strong but lightweight, and weight for weight healthy bone is stronger than concrete or steel. If you can, arrange to attend an orthopaedic operation and see for yourself what living bone looks like.

Types and classification of bone There are two types of bone. Compact bone appears to be solid, but is made up of the tubes referred to earlier, which are closely packed together. These tubular arrangements are called Haversian systems.

Figure 10.2 illustrates the features of a typical Haversian system, which consists of:

- a central canal containing blood vessels, lymph vessels and nerves
- concentric plates of bone (called lamellae)
- spaces between the lamellae called lacunae; these are filled with lymphatic fluid and contain osteocytes (bone cells)
- small channels called canaliculi which link lacunae with the lymphatic system.

The second type of bone is called cancellous or trabecular bone. The Haversian systems are much larger and there are fewer lamellae than in compact bone. This gives a honeycomb or spongy appearance. Cancellous bone contains red bone marrow.

Bones can be classified, according to shape, as long, short, flat or irregular. Figure 10.3 shows a longitudinal section of a mature long bone. The shaft (diaphysis) is made up of compact bone, and contains yellow bone marrow. The shape of the bone is such that it allows for maximum strength whilst reducing weight. The two ends (epiphyses) have an outer covering of compact bone over cancellous bone. Bone is almost always covered with a fine but tough membrane called the periosteum which gives it some protection. The periosteum also provides for the attachment of ligaments and tendons, and contains cells to help maintain the shape of the bone. At the ends of the bones – where the

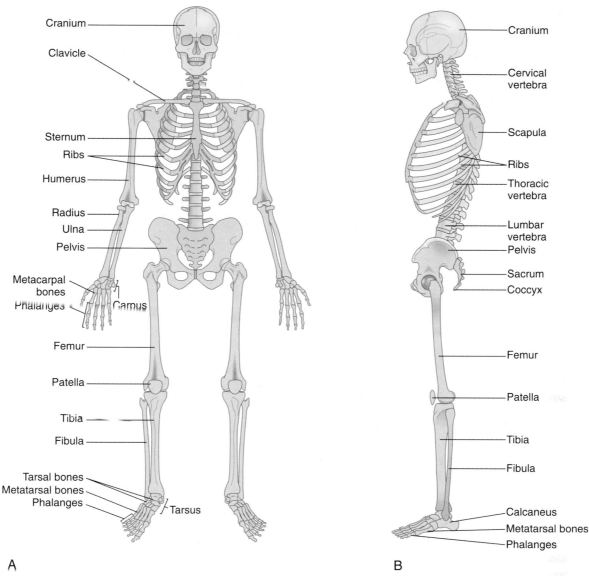

Fig. 10.1 The skeleton (from Waugh & Grant 2006, with permission).

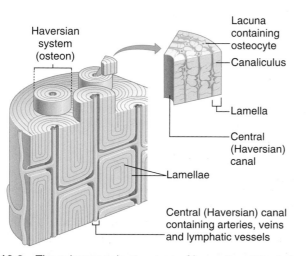

Fig. 10.2 The microscopic structure of bone (from Waugh & Grant 2006, with permission).

joint is formed – periosteum is replaced by a tough, smooth substance called hyaline cartilage.

Short, irregular and flat bones are made up of a thin layer of hard compact bone surrounding an inner mass of cancellous bone. The latter contains red bone marrow.

Bone formation (osteogenesis) and maintenance The development of bone begins before birth and is usually completed by the mid twenties. In the skeleton of a baby many of the bones are made up of cartilage. During childhood the cartilage is replaced by true bone, during which process many bones fuse together, leaving an adult skeleton of around 206 bones. Whilst the number and gross structure of bones normally remain fairly constant in adulthood, bone tissue is constantly being replaced. The rate at which this replacement takes place varies, but can be quite rapid. For example it is estimated that, over a

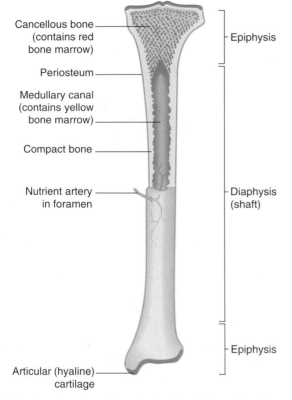

Cancellous bone (contains red bone marrow) — Epiphysis

Periosteum

Medullary canal (contains yellow bone marrow)

Compact bone

Nutrient artery in foramen — Diaphysis (shaft)

Epiphysis

Articular (hyaline) cartilage

Fig. 10.3 A mature long bone in longitudinal section (from Waugh & Grant 2006, with permission).

6-month period, the distal (hip) end of the femur is gradually replaced.

The cells responsible for bone formation are osteocytes (bone cells) and chondrocytes (cartilage cells). There are two types of osteocyte, osteoblasts which build bone up, and osteoclasts which remove bone tissue by reabsorption. There has to be a fine balance between the activities of these two types of cells so that the structure of the bone is maintained. Imagine the consequences if osteoblasts became more active than osteoclasts (or vice versa).

Balance in the growth, development and maintenance of bone tissue is governed by hormones. Growth hormone and thyroid hormones are important during infancy and childhood. Excessive or deficient secretion of these hormones can cause skeletal deformities, such as dwarfism, gigantism and acromegaly. During puberty both testosterone and oestrogen play a part in bone development. In adulthood, regulation is governed by the action of calcitonin, which is released by the thyroid gland increasing bone production, whilst parathyroid hormone, which is secreted by the parathyroid glands, causes calcium to be released from bone. It is deficiency in oestrogen in particular which contributes to the development of postmenopausal osteoporosis. Weight-bearing exercise also stimulates local bone growth, and loss of weight bearing results in a loss of calcium from the bone – an important fact to remember when considering the effects of immobility.

Bone healing   Following a fracture the broken ends of the bone are joined together by new bone (see Fig. 10.4). This occurs in a number of stages:

1. A haematoma (blood clot) is formed at the site of injury.
2. There is an acute inflammatory response. Large numbers of macrophages (cells which engulf and devour damaged tissue, bacteria and other foreign bodies) enter the injury site and phagocytose (engulf and digest) exudate from the haematoma and small fragments of bone.
3. Granulation tissue develops and new blood vessels infiltrate the site.
4. Large numbers of osteoblasts invade the areas and form new bone or callus.
5. Osteoclasts shape the callus, removing excess bone.

It might have been surprising to learn how much 'broken' bones vary, and how many different factors can influence the rate and effectiveness of bone healing. There are many serious complications associated with fractures, for example fat emboli. The nurse needs to know what to do to promote bone healing, and minimise the risks associated with fractures. Consider Case study 10.1.

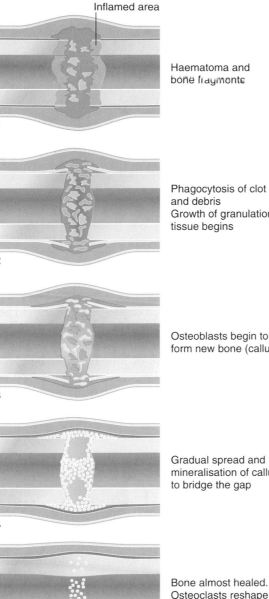

Inflamed area

Haematoma and bone fragments

1

Phagocytosis of clot and debris
Growth of granulation tissue begins

2

Osteoblasts begin to form new bone (callus)

3

Gradual spread and mineralisation of callus to bridge the gap

4

Bone almost healed. Osteoclasts reshape and canalise new bone

5

Fig. 10.4 Stages of bone healing (from Waugh & Grant 2006, with permission).

Case study 10.1

Young man with an injured arm

Pete Marshall, a 19-year-old young man, was on his way home from college when he fell and injured his right arm. Pete is brought to Accident and Emergency by ambulance. It is suspected that he has sustained a fracture. Pete has Down syndrome and lives at home with his parents. He is in pain and distressed.

Exercise

1. Review your skills and knowledge in relation to this scenario and the care that Pete may require. Identify any learning needs you might have.
2. How would you explain the fracture and the process of bone healing to Pete?
3. Pete has a simple fracture of the radius, which is to be treated with a plaster splint. What advice will you need to give him before discharge home?

Joints

A joint occurs where two bones meet. Joints can be classified as:

1. fixed or ossified joints, such as those between the bones of the adult skull
2. slightly movable, cartilaginous joints, such as the symphisis pubis of the pelvis
3. free moving or synovial joints, which are important in movement.

Figure 10.5 illustrates the structure of a typical synovial joint. The bones of the joint are held together by a tough band of fibre (ligament) which is able to give protection to the joint, but is loose enough to allow movement. The articulating surfaces of the bones, which match each other in shape, are covered in smooth durable hyaline cartilage. Synovial membrane lines the internal surface of the joint, and those parts of the bone which are not covered in hyaline cartilage. The synovial membrane secretes a thick viscous fluid (synovial fluid) which provides lubrication. Synovial joints can be further classified according to the range of movements they make (see Box 10.1).

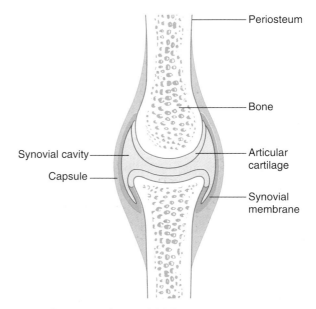

Periosteum

Bone

Articular cartilage

Synovial membrane

Synovial cavity

Capsule

Fig. 10.5 Structure of synovial joint (from Waugh & Grant 2006, with permission).

Muscle structure Skeletal muscle is made up of numerous fibres (muscle fibres). These fibres are of varying length and lie parallel to each other. Each muscle fibre is filled with a special cytoplasm (sarcoplasm) which contains many nuclei. The outer membrane of the muscle fibre is called the sarcolemma. Each muscle fibre contains many fine threads (myofibrils) which run along its length (see Fig. 10.8). When viewed through an electron microscope, the structure of the myofibril is revealed as consisting of sets of thick and thin filaments. The thick filaments are made up of a protein called myosin, and the thin filaments of a protein called actin. Muscle contraction is caused by the interaction of these proteins.

Actin and myosin have a natural attraction for one another. Where filaments of actin and myosin overlap, they bond to form crossbridges. The sliding filament theory of muscle movement proposes that when a bond forms the myosin crossbridge bends, pulling the myosin filament along the actin filament. The conversion of the chemical ATP to ADP releases the energy needed to straighten the myosin crossbridge to its former position. This means the myosin can reattach to the actin filament further along its length. This repeated action pulls the two ends of the muscle fibre together, causing it to contract (see Fig. 10.9).

Muscles have a very rich nerve supply. Motor neurones (nerve cells) travel from the central nervous system and carry an electrical impulse to muscle fibre. The impulse is transferred from the motor neurone to the muscle at the neuromuscular junction or motor end plate through the release of a chemical (acetylcholine) which stimulates the contraction of the muscle fibre.

Under normal circumstances, at any one time, some muscle fibres will be contracted, whilst others will be relaxed. This state is called muscle tone. Muscle tone is particularly important for maintaining posture. Disorders of muscle tone are often the result of muscular or neurological disorders. Loss of muscle tone means the muscles are floppy or

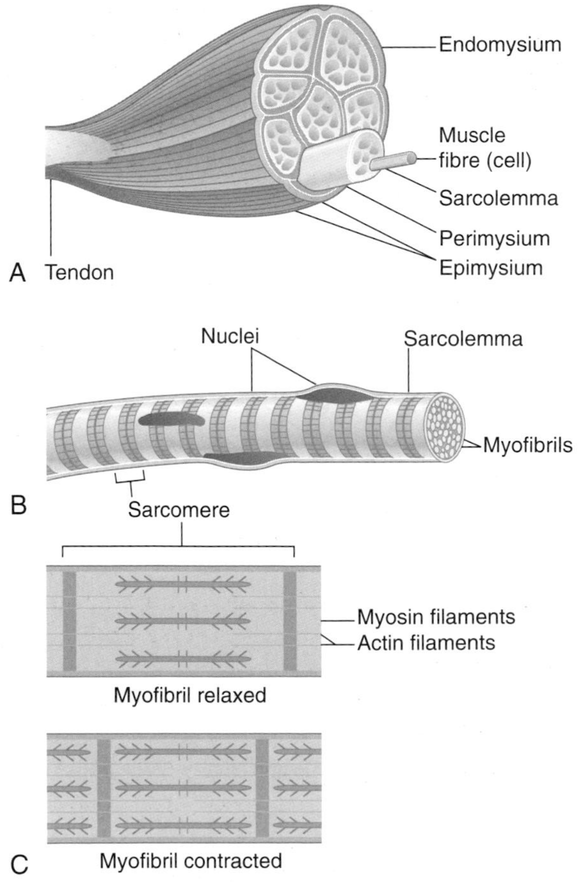

Fig. 10.8 Microscopic structure of a skeletal muscle fibre (from Waugh & Grant 2006, with permission).

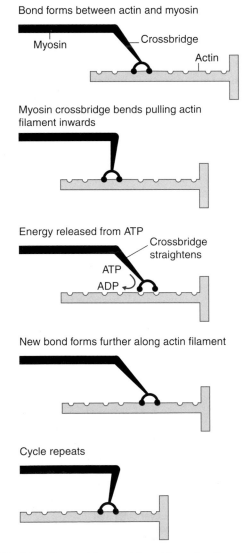

Fig. 10.9 How the making and breaking of actin and myosin bonds causes muscle contraction (ATP = adenosine triphosphate, ADP = adenosine diphosphate) (from Rutishauser 1994, with permission).

flaccid. Flaccid muscle tone can be the result of prolonged reduced mobility (such as bed rest for example). Excessive muscle tone results in spasticity which can cause the formation of contractures

---

Exercise

1. What are the effects of exercise and endurance training on muscle?
2. What effects do steroids have on muscle?
3. What are the short- and long-term effects of lack of muscle use?
4. What happens in rigor mortis?
5. Look up the following conditions and find out: (a) the cause of the pathology, (b) the effects it has on the individual (c) the implications for health and health care:
   - motor neurone disease
   - Parkinson's disease
   - myasthenia gravis
   - myopathy
   - myositis.

Mobilising therefore is a complex process which depends on the coordinated functioning of nerves, bones, joints and muscles. Further reading will be necessary to gain sufficient knowledge of biological factors influencing mobilising and a range of recommended texts are given at the end of the chapter.

Psychological factors

There are many psychological factors that can influence how an individual mobilises. Further, impaired mobility can have serious psychological and emotional effects.

The ability to mobilise allows infants and young children to discover who they are and where they fit into their environment. Lack of ability or opportunity to explore can affect psychological wellbeing. Even for adults movement can act as an outlet for emotional expression. Indeed the link between our emotional state and mobility is complex. Think of the behaviours you might see in someone who is anxious – an archetypal picture might be someone who is not able to keep still, who is pacing up and down, 'like a cat on hot bricks'. People who are depressed often feel a desperate lack of energy, overwhelming fatigue and lack of motivation, which prevents them from mobilising.

People may hold beliefs and attitudes which influence mobilising patterns. In the past, beliefs about people with physical disabilities underpinned exclusion from mainstream society. It was commented on earlier that there are beliefs regarding mobility in late life, which can impact on the lives and wellbeing of older people.

Knowledge for practice: physical activity and health

It might be that the relationship between beliefs and mobilising is best illustrated by considering attitudes and behaviour in relation to physical activity. Physical activity is associated with positive effects on both mental and physical wellbeing (summarised in Box 10.2). The effects of increasing physical activity can be wide-ranging, for example as a therapeutic intervention for people with dementia (Eggermont & Scherder 2006, Teri et al 2003), or in the maintenance of social networks and friendships.

The effects of an inadequate level of activity are equally significant. The World Health Organization (2002a, 2002b, 2004) describes lack of sufficient physical activity as an underlying cause of disability, disease and death. It is estimated that, in 2000, very low levels of physical activity caused 1.9 million deaths and 19 million disability-adjusted life years across the globe.

It would appear that many people fail to take sufficient physical exercise; over 60% of adults are not active enough to benefit health (WHO 2004). The 2003 Health Survey for England (Joint Health Surveys Unit 2003) identified that seven out of ten women, and six out of ten men were not taking sufficient exercise to maintain general health and wellbeing. There is evidence that children are becoming increasingly sedentary, especially in poor urban areas. These concerns are not confined to the developed world. In large cities in the developing world, issues such as overcrowding, poverty, crime, traffic, reduced air quality, lack of green areas and recreation space are having an effect.

Increasing physical activity is seen as a key element of the WHO global health promotion strategy (WHO 2004). The aim of this strategy is 'to promote higher levels of physical activity in the world population' and is applicable to all ages,

---

Box 10.2	The preventative effects of exercise

Regular physical activity can:
- decrease the risk of death from cardiovascular disease, coronary heart disease and stroke
- prevent, delay and help control high blood pressure
- help people control body weight
- help reduce risk of developing diabetes
- reduce the risk of colon cancer and maybe other forms of cancer
- enhance the immune system
- have positive effects on mental health, promoting psychological wellbeing
- reduce feelings of psychological stress and anxiety
- enhance mood, self efficacy and self esteem
- enhance cognition
- help in the prevention and treatment of low-back pain
- prevent osteoporosis.

Specific forms of physical activity can:
- reduce the risk of falls and other accidents by improving the health of bones, maintaining body strength, balance and coordination and cognitive function.

From DoH 2001b.

of older people in hospital. Indeed, a study by Callen (2004) in acute care in the US reported that only 27% of 118 patients walked, and then only for a mean time of 5.5 minutes. Nurses have a central role in developing a hospital environment and care plans which maintain and mobility.

Politicoeconomic factors

Maintaining and promoting physical mobility and activity are part of many policy initiatives to enhance wider social participation and inclusion as well as promote other aspects of health and wellbeing. This is especially so for groups who are traditionally seen as marginalised, for example older people, people with disabilities and people living in poverty.

Increasing urbanisation is leading to a reliance on the private car as a principal means of transport. This is exacerbated by the proliferation in many industrialised countries of 'out of town' shopping. The closure of small, local facilities such as banks, post offices, chemists and other shops disadvantages those people without private transport. This can contribute to the sense of social exclusion in many disadvantaged communities.

Knowledge for practice: moving and handling

Back pain and back injury have a significant personal and economic cost. A National Audit Office (2003) report in the UK reported that 24% of NHS staff regularly have back pain. One in four nurses reported experiencing a work-related back injury, with moving and handling given as the most common cause (NAO 2003). Nurses are an occupational group at significant risk of back injury. In some fields of practice the nurse undertakes numerous moving and handling activities, increasing the likelihood of developing back problems (Pheasant 1998).

Moving and handling activity can be defined as 'any transporting or supporting of a load (including the lifting, putting down, pushing, pulling, carrying or moving thereof) by hand or bodily force' (Health and Safety Executive (HSE) 1998). Throughout the European Community there are a range of legal requirements in relation to moving and handling. These international requirements are supported by national legislation and guidelines, and local policies.

Exercise

1. Find out what the legal requirements for safe moving and handling are in your country.
2. Find any national policies or guidelines which support the implementation of the above. These guidelines might be developed by government, trades unions, professional associations, for example.
3. Now look at local policy and procedure, to see how the legal framework and national initiatives can affect everyday practice.

When this exercise has been completed you might want to spend some time reflecting on your own moving and handling practice.

In the UK, moving and handling is regulated through The Manual Handling Operations Regulations 1992 (HSE 1998), under the terms of the Health and Safety at Work Act (1974). These comply with EU directives aiming to standardise the various and varying national safety directives/legislation. The directive makes clear what can be reasonably expected of employers and employees. Employers should, as far is reasonably practicable:

- avoid the need for employees to undertake manual handling which involves the risk of injury. The legislation recognises that there are 'special situations' involving manual handling which carry a higher risk, such as assisting people with mobility
- make sure that a 'suitable and sufficient' written assessment is undertaken by a designated person of all manual handling operations that involve the risk of injury, including patient handling. The assessment must take into account: the task, the load, the working environment and the capabilities of individuals involved
- take appropriate steps to reduce risk of injury to the lowest level possible
- provide suitable equipment and training in its use.

Employees have a responsibility to:

- obey 'reasonable and lawful instruction' and 'act with reasonable care and skill'
- use the process and implement policy as designed
- use equipment in accordance with their training
- report any hazards and changes in circumstances which may impact upon the assessment. This includes individual or personal changes (for example back injury or pregnancy).

There are a range of policies and guidelines available to support nursing practice in relation to patient handling. Many 'safer handling policies' share common features:

- eliminating manual and patient handling as much as possible
- encouraging the use of lifting equipment
- encouraging patient independence and self-care
- robust risk assessment and response processes.

For a moving and handling activity to be successful, it needs to address two objectives, minimal effort on the part of the handler and the experience of minimal discomfort for the patient (Dougherty & Lister 2004). This is dependent on a comprehensive and accurate assessment, clear recording and communication of the subsequent plan of action (Royal College of Nursing (RCN) 1996, 1999, 2003a, 2003b).

There are some key principles to remember whilst moving and handling. When you stand at rest, most of the force of gravity is applied through your head, trunk and spinal column. You need exert little effort to maintain stability, and there is little damaging pressure on the spine. When the trunk moves away from this midline, the spinal column experiences harmful shearing forces. So any twisting motion can exert harmful pressure on the spine and seriously damage the vertebral discs. So when moving and handling any load (not only people) you need to think about:

- moving with the natural curves of the spine maintained as much as possible
- holding the object as close to the body as possible to avoid stretching
- making use of large, strong hip and thigh muscles, rather than the muscles of your back and arms
- keeping a wide stable base to help maintain your balance and reduce the risk of twisting your spine – usually about a hip width apart
- avoiding tensing your muscles
- keeping your knees slightly bent

Exercise

1. What factors must you think of when planning to move/handle a patient?

The following might have been considered:

- assessing the patient's need
- assessing risk
- recognising your own level of skill and expertise
- working as a team
- using appropriate equipment
- communicating and gaining cooperation
- using touch and recognising any taboos on touch
- conveying respect, developing trust and promoting the patient's dignity.

Individuality in living

Individuality in mobilising is a result of the ways in which influencing factors come together. The capacity for mobilising depends on the possession of physical ability, the motivation to move and the provision of a nonrestrictive, enabling environment. Alterations in any of these elements can affect an individual's mobilising behaviour.

The model of living framework gives us an idea of how and why people mobilise in the way they do. It also highlights the complexity of the model and the extent to which the individual Activities of Living are interrelated. Consider the following case study and undertake the exercise.

Exercise

1. Read through the case scenario given below.
2. Use the components of the model to consider individuality in the Activity of Living mobilising.

Case study 10.3

Individuality in mobilising

Three generations of the Abram family live together. Cilla, aged 70, is the grandmother. She worked as a nurse before she had to retire at the age of 56. Cilla has osteoarthritis, which particularly affects her spine and hips making it difficult for her to walk. Whilst she manages to mobilise in the house and garden, she often uses an electrically powered wheelchair outside. Jeanie is her daughter, she works full time as a nursing sister on a rehabilitation ward. Craig who is 13 and Paula aged 10 make up the family.

You might have considered the following points:

Lifespan

The Abram family represent a range of ages across the lifespan. The expectation is that all members of the family would be independent in mobilising. Although joint stiffness and some discomfort might be perceived as 'normal' ageing, Cilla's degree of mobility impairment is greater than the majority of people her age expect. Jeanie has a busy job which although active, does not guarantee sufficient physical exercise. Her work and family commitments might make it difficult for her to maintain healthy levels of physical activity. The young people will be expected to take part in physical activity at school.

Dependence/independence

Cilla is dependent upon members of her family for help with mobilising, and some other Activities of Living. However, Jeanie depends on her mum to provide childcare and emotional support. The interdependence of the family unit is an important factor to consider. Cilla sometimes uses a wheelchair to aid her independence.

Factors influencing the Activity of Living

Biological The changes associated with 'normal' development including ageing. Osteoarthritis is a painful, long-term, degenerative condition that restricts mobility. Cilla's mobility is likely to become more impaired in the future.

Psychological Higher risk of depression in older people with long-term health problems. Attitudes of family members to physical activity.

Sociocultural Maintenance of social roles in the family. Beliefs about disability and handicap.

Environmental The impact of domestic and community space on Cilla's mobility, and the ability of the family to undertake joint activities. Accessibility of safe transport for all members of the family.

Politicoeconomic Financial concerns for the future. Ability to access appropriate services and facilities. Jeanie at risk of back injury.

SUMMARY POINTS

The information and the exercises in this chapter so far should have demonstrated a number of important aspects to this Activity of Living. These are summarised below. It is important that you understand the model of living, as this is the basis for individuality of care using the model for nursing.

1. Mobilising is a complex activity.
2. Individuality in mobilising can be illustrated through the components of the model of living.
3. Mobilising is affected by all the other Activities of Living.
4. Mobilising affects all the other Activities of Living.
5. Problems in mobilising can have a detrimental effect of health, wellbeing and quality of life.

THE MODEL FOR NURSING

INTRODUCTION

The aim of the model of living is to identify individuality in Activities of Living leading to individuality in nursing care. In the model for nursing, the role of the nurse is to provide person-centred nursing care which can prevent, alleviate, solve or help people come to terms with problems (actual or potential) related to Activities of Living. Chapter 1 of this book gives more detail on the overall model. This chapter will now focus on how you can use the model for nursing to care for people with actual or potential mobility problems.

This section also uses the nursing process as a vehicle to discuss the organisation and delivery of nursing care. It is intended to use the nursing process as a way of illustrating how you might 'think' about assessing, planning, implementing and evaluating the nursing care for an individual, rather than completing specific documents or care plans. Chapter 1 provides a more detailed description of the nursing process.

In this part of the chapter Miss Roberts and her experiences will be used as a case study to explore how to use the Activities of Living model in practice (see p. 336). Miss Roberts is based on the story of an older woman who was a participant in a research study on the nurse's role in rehabilitation (Long et al 2001). Permission has been given to share her story in this context. Miss Roberts' path, from admission to hospital after fall, through treatment and care for a fractured hip to her discharge home will be explored. The case study will look at the process as it relates to mobilising; it is not intended to give a comprehensive account of Miss Roberts' care. The interrelatedness of both the Activities of Living and the stages of the nursing process will be illustrated – demonstrating the complexity and skill of nursing practice.

Before starting to think about using the model in more detail, it might be useful to think broadly about some of the health problems related to mobilising.

Exercise
Using the components of the Activities of Living model, your life experiences and clinical experience to date, note down a list of health problems people might have in relation to the activity of mobilising.

1. Reflect on these and identify your learning needs.
2. You may wish to discuss these with your teachers or mentor to identify a learning plan to meet these needs.

Table 10.2 gives a list of some of the health problems you might have identified. You can probably add to this list from your own. What this exercise illustrates is the wide range of health problems that can cause (or be caused by) reduced or impaired mobility. It also gives an indication of the depth and breadth of knowledge and skill needed by the nurse in order to deliver effective nursing care to people with a range of mobility problems.

ASSESSING THE INDIVIDUAL

Whilst this chapter is looking specifically at mobilising, it must be borne in mind the extent to which mobility problems affect other Activities of Living and vice versa. A comprehensive

Table 10.2 Components of the Activities of Living model and health problems related to mobility

Lifespan	Congenital problems, e.g. congenital dislocation of the hip, congenital dystrophy Hormonal effects on development Trauma Sports injury Osteoporosis
Dependence/ independence	Use of mobility aids Effects of the environment
Biological factors	Arthritis Infections Trauma Tumours Neurological disease (e.g. stroke, Parkinson disease)
Psychological factors	Fear of falling Learning disabilities Cognitive impairment Depression
Sociocultural	Lifestyle choices Lack of exercise Social isolation
Environmental	Road traffic accidents Falls Limited local amenities for exercise
Politicoeconomic	Work-related injury Finance Limited access to resources and services

nursing assessment must also address all the other Activities of Living. It is through understanding a person's individuality in living that the nurse is able to provide individualisation in nursing (person-centred care).

Box 10.4 provides a summary of factors related to individuality in mobilising and their relationship to assessment.

The core processes in assessment are:

- collecting data
- reviewing and interpreting the data
- identifying problems related to Activities of Living
- identifying priorities amongst identified problems.

The primary source of information in any assessment is the patient. Secondary sources include the patient's family and friends, other professionals and the patient's records and notes. There are two types of information collected as part of the assessment process, biographical data and data related to the Activities of Living. The main methods of data collection are interview, observation and measurement.

It is important to remember that assessment is a continuous process and an initial assessment often needs to be built upon. For example, if somebody is suffering an acute exacerbation (worsening) of rheumatoid arthritis, they are likely to be in pain and extremely tired, and it may be neither possible nor desirable to undertake a comprehensive assessment in one sitting. Patients must also be reassessed in relation to change in condition or as a result of the evaluation of care.

The nurse also works in collaborative ways with other members of the multidisciplinary team to deliver comprehensive care based on comprehensive assessment. There is a danger that the patient can become overburdened with duplicate assessments (DoH 2001). In Miss Roberts' case, for example, she was assessed a number of times by people who asked some identical questions. Failure to share information gained through assessment can also lead to the patient failing to receive the most effective and appropriate package of care.

Collecting and interpreting data

The aim of the assessment process is to answer the following questions in relation to the Activity of Living:

- What was the person's previous routine?
- What can the person do independently?
- What can't the person do independently?
- What were the person's previous coping behaviours?
- What actual and potential problems does the person have?

Exercise

1. Using the components of the model, identify the sort of data you need to conduct a comprehensive assessment of an individual with an actual or potential mobility problem.
2. What sorts of skills and knowledge do you need?
3. Reflect on your current knowledge and skills base and identify your learning needs. Write these in your learning plan.

Box 10.4	Assessing the individual in the AL of mobilising

Lifespan: relationship to the AL of mobilising
- infancy and childhood – increasing skills
- adolescence and young adulthood – peak performance
- later years – decreasing agility and stamina.

Dependence/independence in mobilising
- increasing independence in childhood, to adulthood
- dependence on another person
- body-worn aids/external aids (for aided independence)
- transport mode – to school, work, shops, for leisure.

Factors influencing mobilising
Biological
- adequacy of musculoskeletal and nervous systems
- body posture/gait
- muscle strength/mass/tone
- congenital/hereditary interference with function
- effects of trauma, disease.

Psychological
- intelligence, temperament, values, beliefs, motivation
- knowledge about benefits of exercise and prevention of injury
- general attitudes
- attitudes to dependence and disability.

Sociocultural
- social class, tradition, religion
- work activities/transport
- effects of mechanical advances on lifestyle
- dependence affecting role in relation to family, work, leisure.

Environmental
- housing conditions and environs
- local climate and terrain: influence on work/hobbies
- effect of man-made energy on transport of people and goods.

Politicoeconomic
- community amenities
- safety of streets/crossings and prevention of injury
- legal requirements for access to and mobility in buildings
- availability of exercise facilities for leisure.

From Roper et al (1996), p. 293.

You should have generated a range of ideas on the sorts of data you might need to collect. Obviously, assessment in practice has to be relevant and appropriate to the individual person and the context of care, but think very broadly about the most complete and comprehensive data collection you might ever make in relation to mobilising! To begin with, identify the questions you might want to answer.

Lifespan
- How old is the person?
- How might age influence their mobility?
- Does the person have a history of mobility problems?
- How have they managed mobility problems in the past?
- Is there anything in their life history that might influence their current experience?

Dependence/independence continuum
- How dependent/interdependent/independent is the person in mobilising?
- What form does any dependency take?
- What effect does this have on the other Activities of Living?

Biological factors
- Are there deficits or deficiencies in the bones, muscles or joints?
- Are there any deficits or deficiencies in any other body system that might affect the person's mobility, or experience, or possible treatment?
- When/how does the individual undertake physical activity?

Psychological factors
- What is the person's level of knowledge and understanding about their current problem?
- How is the mobility problem affecting their psychological wellbeing?
- How is the mobility problem affecting their personal relationships?
- What is the person's level of knowledge and understanding of the relationship between health and mobility?

Sociocultural factors
- How is the mobility problem affecting the person's usual roles and behaviours?
- How might the person's cultural background influence their experience of a mobility problem or any possible treatment or intervention?

Environmental factors
- What effect is the mobility problem having on the person's ability to mobilise in their own social environment, at home and in their community?
- What access does the individual have to forms of transport?

Politicoeconomic factors
- Does the mobility problem affect the person's ability to work or play?

You might want to reflect on how and when you might ask these questions and the skills you need (see Chapter 4).

Some elements of data collection will now be considered in a little more detail. A large amount of data can be collected about an individual's mobility through observation. Other sorts of physical data also need to be identified, for example from examination and measurement. However, in order to undertake an effective and comprehensive assessment, the nurse not only needs to know what to look for, but also what a particular piece of data might mean.

Exercise

Look at Table 10.3.

1. Fill in the third column. You need to find out what the observational data might mean.
2. You might want to add other observational data of your own.

It is evident that there is a wide range of data available when assessing an individual's mobility. For some observational data (these may be referred to as cues), there might be a number of possible explanations. A core skill of nursing practice is the ability to integrate and interpret a number of cues and so come to an understanding of exactly what the patient's problem is and what has caused it.

Standard assessment scales which assess aspects of mobility and/or function may also be used. Commonly used tools include the Barthel Index (Mahoney & Barthel 1965) and the Functional Independence Measure (Oczkowski & Barreca 1993) which both use scoring systems to assess functioning in a range of activities. Other tools can be used to measure specific aspects of mobility, for example Table 10.4 which can be used to grade the degree of spasticity in an affected part, and Table 10.5 which can be used to assess the degree of contracture.

A more detailed view of assessment can now be examined using a case study.

Case study 10.4

Assessment following a fall

Elizabeth Roberts is 84 years old. She is single and until recently lived with her brother. He died about 6 months ago and now she lives alone. Miss Roberts has been admitted to a medical ward from Accident and Emergency following a fall which left her lying on the floor for several hours. You have been told there is no bony injury, but that Miss Roberts is bruised and distressed, and remains very unstable when she tries to walk.

You should have identified a wide range of data needed for a comprehensive assessment of Miss Roberts. In addition, you will have recognised the knowledge and skills base needed to support your assessment. Part of that knowledge base is an understanding of falls, particularly as experienced by older people (see also Chapter 3).

Table 10.3 Observations made during the assessment of the AL of mobilising

When you observe	You might see	Which might mean
Posture	A lateral S curve (scoliosis) A rounding of the thoracic spine (kyphosis) An increase in the curve at the lumbar spine causing the shoulders to be thrown back (lordosis)	
Gait	Poor balance Unsteadiness Irregular movements Weakness and fatigue	
Joints	A restricted range of movement Instability or stiffness Swelling Tenderness Nodules Crepitus	
Muscles	Differences in muscle strength Changes in muscle tone	
Limbs	Differences in size and shape of hands, feet, arms, legs, digits Alteration in reflexes	
Skin	Pallor Cyanosis	
Pulses	Faint or absent pulse	

Exercise

You have been asked to assess Miss Roberts.

1. What sort of data will you want to collect? Why do you want that data? How will you collect it?
2. What sort of knowledge base will you need to undertake the assessment?
3. What sorts of skills will you need to use?
4. Identify any learning needs in relation to the case study and develop a learning plan to meet these needs.

Table 10.4 The modified Ashworth scale for spasticity

0	no increase in muscle tone
1	slight increase in tone (catch and release)
2	slight increase in tone (catch and resistance through less than half of the range of movement)
3	marked increase in tone through most of range of movement
4	considerable increase in tone (passive range of movement difficult)
5	rigidity (flexion or extension) of affected part

From Davies & O'Connor (1999).

Knowledge for practice: falls in later life

Active people fall at any age. Slips, trips and falls are part of normal life. However, for some people the consequences of a fall can be severe. An increasing number of injurious falls are a worldwide major public health issue (Tinetti 2003). Some (but not all) of this rise can be accounted for by the ageing population. The risk of falling increases with age: one in three people over 65 fall at least once per year, increasing to half of those over 80 years (National Collaborating Centre for Nursing and Supportive Care 2004).

Falls are the most serious and frequent home accident. They are a common reason for admission to hospital and residential care (Tinetti 2003, American Geriatric Society (AGS) 2001), and are associated with high levels of morbidity and mortality, being a major cause of death for people over 65 years (Scuffham & Chaplin 2002). Todd & Skelton (2004), in a review of the literature, report 30% people over 65 years fall each year. Between 20% and 30% of those falls result in injury leading to long-term loss of mobility and dependence.

There is evidence that many falls can be prevented by multifactorial intervention (Gillespie et al 2003). The development of multifactorial prevention strategies is a common feature of many health and social care systems. Examples include the Australian 'Stay on Your Feet' campaign (Kempton et al 2000), and The National Service Framework for Older People (DoH 2001) identifies the prevention and effective management of falls as a key strategic target.

Table 10.5 Contracture assessment scale

Area	Severe (3)	Moderate (2)	Mild (1)	None (0)
Pain	Pain most of the time, with or without movement Overt facial signs of pain Guarding while performing passive ROM exercises Analgesia may not relieve	Pain with passive ROM exercises Sometimes pain at rest, relieved by analgesic	Pain at end of range of passive ROM exercises, resolved by rest Activity may be slowed Analgesia not usually required	Occasional or no pain
Function	No function possibly due to lack of innervation or fixed nature of the contracture No active of purposeful movement	Limited function Poor coordination due to limited movement Random joint movements may be present Limited grasp and release but no strength	Independent function possible Gross movements are easy, finer movements may be difficult Some incoordination may be present Movements may be uncoordinated Adaptive devices my be used	Independent function without assistive devices Fine movement unimpaired
Ease of movement	Fixed joints or limbs Passive range of movement absent or very limited (less than 25%)	Some passive joint movement (up to 50%) May or may not be able to initiate movement Joint returns to contracted position	Nearly full range of passive movement Some resistance at the end of the range	Full range of active movement
Nursing	Very difficult to clean skin and to prevent breakdown Nail cutting impossible Skin may be macerated	Difficult to complete skin care and reposition after care Odour may be present	Skin care is easy Limited ability to reposition	Easy to clean skin and to reposition after care

From Davies & O'Connor (1999).

Primary prevention of falls can include a number of population-based initiatives. These may comprise: raising awareness of safety amongst the general public, encouraging lifelong healthy eating habits, and healthier levels of physical activity and exercise. Increased physical activity has a positive effect on balance, strength, coordination and flexibility. Of particular benefit to older people can be those low-level preventative services (such as help with some household tasks) which are characterised as 'that bit of help' (Joseph Rowntree Foundation 2005).

There is a growing range of evidence from which to identify effective interventions specific to the prevention of falls (e.g. Gillespie et al 2003, Honkanen 2004, Todd & Skelton 2004, Chang 2004). There are also a number of evidence-based practice guidelines (e.g. NICE 2004, AGS 2001). Common elements in the above include:

The identification of people most at risk of falling Central to the prevention of falls and related injury is the identification of those individuals who are at high risk of falling and subsequent injury. This includes both routine screening by health care professionals and more complex multifactorial risk assessment for those more at risk or who have fallen. Alongside this there should be the identification of people who have, or who are at risk of developing, osteoporosis.

Multifactorial, multidisciplinary interventions Whilst specific risk factors and individual deficits should be screened for and addressed, it is important to consider the interaction of factors (Chang 2004). Interventions may include:

- strength, balance and gait training
- home hazard assessment and modification
- vision assessment
- medication review.

There are multiple risk factors for falls and osteoporotic fracture which are illustrated in Table 10.6. Look at the risk factors in relation to the previous exercise. Is there anything you want to add to your data collection?

It is known that some older people are more at risk of falling. They are the very old, those who are admitted to acute hospital care, or those who are in nursing or residential care (Rubenstein 2006). It is estimated that around 50% of people in residential care fall once per year, with 40% falling more than once (Salkeld et al 2000). Falls in hospital are a worldwide problem, and a falls risk assessment is increasingly

Table 10.6 Falls and osteoporotic fracture: risk factors

Risk factors associated with falls	Risk factors associated with osteoporotic fracture
• Impaired gait, balance or mobility • Polypharmacy (particularly drugs acting on the central nervous system or those causing hypotension) • Visual impairment • Impaired cognition • Depression • Stroke, Parkinson's, lower limb disease, arthritis • Postural hypotension • Environmental hazards • Living alone • Use of pharmacological or physical restraints • Sedentary lifestyle • Foot problems • Fear of falling	• Evidence of bone thinning (osteopenia) • Loss of height associated with vertebral deformity • Previous fragility fracture • Gender • Age • Prolonged corticosteroid treatment • History of early menopause • History of maternal hip fracture • Smoking • Low body mass index/malnutrition • Sedentary lifestyle

part of routine practice (Hayes 2004). Systematic reviews of studies of hospital falls (Oliver et al 2001, Evans et al 2001) identified the at-risk patient to be one with a history of previous falls, gait instability, lower limb weakness, urinary incontinence, frequent toileting needs, cognitive impairment and polypharmacy. Whilst older people are more likely to fall than younger people, this is a function of factors such as poor mobility or confusion rather than simply age itself.

The consequences of a fall are numerous, with physical injury common, which can include pressure injury, other consequence of reduced mobility. Between 20% and 30% of people who fall suffer physical injury, 10% of which result in serious injury (Freeman et al 2002). Such injuries reduce mobility and independence and increase the risk of premature death. Psychologically, the older person's confidence can be undermined and the fear of falling and fear of the consequences of a fall may severely curtail mobility. This can lead to functional deterioration and even institutionalisation. It should also be recognised that a fall is often a sign of an unidentified health problem, and should always be taken seriously and followed up (Chang 2004).

Exercise

Find out what resources are available in your locality for the prevention and treatment of falls.

1. On your next practice placement ask about the process used for falls risk assessment.
2. If there is a specialist falls service find out how it works. Identify what the referral mechanisms are to and from the falls service.
3. Identify the nurse's role in the prevention and treatment of falls in the primary, secondary and tertiary care settings.

Now, return to the assessment of Miss Roberts. Review and add to the notes from the last exercise and include the process of falls risk assessment.

As part of the data collection process the following questions might have been asked:

- Have you fallen before? If so, when? How often? What happened?
- Tell me about this latest fall.
- Do you normally have any trouble walking or getting around?
- Do you ever feel like you are losing your balance?
- Do you use anything to help you walk? Inside the house? Outside the house?
- Are you afraid of falling?
- Are there any activities you would like to do but don't because you can't get around?
- Do you ever have pain or discomfort in your joints and/or muscles?
- Are you seeing the doctor for anything at the moment?
- What medications are you taking?
- How much exercise do you get? (In particular, weight-bearing exercise such as walking.)
- How much do you smoke and drink?

In order to identify the risk of osteoporosis the following might have been considered:

- Do you have any blood relatives who have, or have had, osteoporosis, or who have had broken bones (fractures) late in life?
- Have you had any broken bones (fractures) in adult life?
- Do you take any vitamin D or calcium supplements?
- Have you ever had your bone density measured?
- Do you take any medication for osteoporosis?

These observations might have been undertaken:

- height measurement and comparison to peak height
- lying and standing blood pressure
- walking, posture and gait pattern
- moving from lying to sitting, and from sitting to standing

- creating a therapeutic environment which facilitates rehabilitation
- integrating therapy into the Activities of Living.

Discharge home

Systematic discharge planning is common in many health care systems. It is linked with decreased hospital stay and unplanned readmissions, and improved coordination of services after discharge (Shepperd et al 2005). Effective, timely and appropriate discharge relies on good assessment and team working, and the nurse's role can be vital. Nurses often act as discharge coordinators, a key role when complex packages of care are required.

In the NHS in the UK it is a requirement that all hospitals must have a clear discharge policy. Shepperd et al (2005) discuss the difficulty in identifying the impact of discharge planning when it is often part of a complex package of care, but comment that even a small reduction in hospital stay/readmission can have significant impact on the individual and the organisation.

Key principles of planned discharge for a person recovering from a fractured hip include:

- The patient, their needs and aspirations should be central to planning. Sometimes older people feel rushed into making decisions about their life after discharge from hospital (CSCI 2004).
- Effective liaison between organisations and agencies. CSCI (2004, 2005) report that older people value continuity of service provision between hospital and community, particularly if there is one point of contact to give support and advice after discharge.
- A date of discharge should be identified as soon as possible and communicated to all relevant parties including the patient, carer and community services.
- Information available to the patient and carers in appropriate and accessible format. This may include information on mobility, expected progress, medications, pain management and sources of help and advice.
- Relevant and timely information to community services.
- Prevention of another injurious fall; this may involve home adaptation and mobility equipment, as well as continuing rehabilitation.
- No discharge until community services are in place and the patient is fit to be discharged.

The above are particularly important in cases of supported or early discharge. Commonly this is mediated through a specialist team which assesses and identifies those who may be suitable for early supported discharge, facilitating rehabilitation, discharge and follow-up (SIGN 2002).

Despite there being a range of legislation and guidance on discharge, Parker (2002b) comments on the extent to which older people and carers have negative experiences. The complaints of older people and carers are similar to those factors identified as causes of delayed discharge:

- inadequate assessment, e.g. knowledge of patient's social circumstances
- poor organisation, e.g. arranging transport
- poor communication between hospital and community providers (DoH 2003)
- inadequate rehabilitation (Healthcare Commission 2006).

It might be the case that some patients are left with a long-term or permanent impairment in the activity of mobilising. The nurse has an important role to play in enabling the individual to adapt to this change in their lives.

It is important to recognise the varied potential reactions of the person, including a sense of loss or low self-esteem. Box 10.7 gives some potential effects of long-term impairment. It is important that you, as the nurse, can develop a trusting relationship with the patient; your attitude towards and acceptance of her/him is very important. You should always support participation and choice, enabling people to make decisions about their own care and their own lives.

Box 10.7	Potential effects of impairment and disability in mobilising

Physical
Loss of power, energy, impaired function.

Psychological
Mood swings (patient and family), boredom, depression, aggression, frustration.

Sociocultural
Impact on family and personal relationships, changed ability to fulfil roles, cultural interpretation of suffering as good, bad or punishing.

Environmental
Creation of dependence and handicap.

Politicoeconomic
Change in/loss of employment, reduced income.

EVALUATING

Systematic, rigorous evaluation enhances the overall quality of care. It enables us to understand what works and what does not work by constantly reviewing the patient's progress and the effectiveness of planned interventions. Evaluation emphasises the responsibility and accountability of nursing practice.

Exercise
Review the case study of Miss Roberts.

1. When and how would you evaluate Miss Roberts' care?
2. What sorts of skills, knowledge and resource might you need?
3. Identify any learning needs and develop a learning plan to meet your needs.

When evaluating, you should review the extent to which the nursing interventions you have planned and implemented have met the goals set. The skills needed to evaluate include:

- observing
- questioning
- examining
- testing
- measuring.

Miss Roberts achieved her overall goals – she went home to carry on her life much as before. She used a walking frame for about 6 weeks, then used a stick only when she went outside. Within 3 months she was fulfilling the same social roles she had previously. Her family replaced old and worn out carpets throughout her house. Her blood pressure medication was changed and she no longer felt dizzy and 6 months after discharge had suffered no further falls or trips.

CONCLUSION

Mobilising is a complex Activity of Living, the understanding of which requires a depth and breadth of knowledge. This complexity is reflected in the knowledge and skills needed to assess, plan, implement and evaluate effective, individualised nursing care. It is hoped that in working through part or all of this chapter, you have been able to recognise and value the knowledge and skills you already have and in addition that you have learned something new, and identified where you need to learn more.

References

American Geriatric Society, British Geriatric Society, American Academy of Orthopaedic Surgeons Panel on Falls Prevention 2001 Guidelines for the prevention of falls in older persons. Journal of the American Geriatric Society 49:664–672

Atkins WS 2001 Older people: their transport needs and requirements. Department of Environment, Transport and the Regions, London

Audit Commission 1995 United they stand: co-ordinating care for elderly patients with hip fracture. Audit Commission, London

Audit Commission 2000 United they stand: co-ordinating care for elderly patients with hip fracture. Commission Update. Audit Commission, London Audit

Audit Commission/District Audit 2002 Rehabilitation services for older people. A bulletin for trusts and social care organizations. Audit Commission, London

Ayis S, Gooberman-Hill R, Bowling A et al 2006 Predicting catastrophic decline in mobility among older people. Age and Ageing 35:382–387

Benner P 1984 From novice to expert. Addison-Wesley, Menlo Park, CA

Boore JRP, Champion R, Ferguson MC 1987 Nursing the physically ill adult. Churchill Livingstone, Edinburgh

Booth J, Hillier V, Waters K et al 2005 Effects of a stroke rehabilitation education programme for nurses. Journal of Advanced Nursing 49(5):465–473

Brown-Wilson C 2002 Safer handling practice: influence of staff training on older people. British Journal of Nursing 11(20):1332–1339

Burton C 2003 Therapeutic nursing in stroke rehabilitation: a systematic review. Clinical Effectiveness in Nursing 7:124–133

Callen BL, Mahoney JE, Grieves CB et al 2004 Frequency of hallway ambulation by hospitalised older adults on medical units of an academic hospital. Geriatric Nursing 25(4): 212–217

Chang JT, Morton SC, Rubenstein LZ et al 2004 Interventions for the prevention of falls in older adults: systematic review and meta-analysis of RCTs. British Medical Journal 328:680–687

Chilman AM, Thomas M 1987 Understanding nursing care, 3rd edn. Churchill Livingstone, Edinburgh

Commission for Social Care Inspection 2004 Leaving hospital – the price of delays. CSCI, London

Commission for Social Care Inspection 2005 Leaving hospital – revisited. CSCI, London

Cornuz J, Feskanich D, Willett WC et al 1999 Smoking, smoking cessation and risk of hip fracture in women. American Journal of Medicine 106:311–314

Davies S (ed) 2006 Rehabilitation. The use of theories and models on practice. Churchill Livingstone, Edinburgh

Davies S, O'Connor S 1999 Rehabilitation nursing foundations for practice. Baillière Tindall, Edinburgh

Department of Health 1995 More people, more active, more often. Physical activity in England: a consultation paper. HMSO, London

Department of Health 2001 National service framework for older people. HMSO, London

Department of Health 2003 The national service framework for older people. A report on progress and future challenges. DoH, London

Department of Health 2004 At last five a week: evidence on the impact of physical activity and its relationship to health. A report from the Chief Medical Officer. DoH, London

Department of Health 2005 Choosing activity. A physical activity action plan. DoH, London

Dougherty L, Lister S 2004 The Royal Marsden manual of clinical nursing procedures, 5th edn. Baillière Tindall, London

Eggermont LHP, Scherder EJA 2006 Physical activity and behaviour in dementia: A review of the literature and implications for psychosocial intervention in primary care. Dementia 5:411–428

Ethan K, Powell C 1996 Rehabilitation of the patient with hip fracture. Reviews in Clinical Gerontology 6:371–388

Evans D, Hodgkinson B, Lambert L et al 2001 Falls, risk factors in the hospital setting: a systematic review. International Journal of Nursing Practice 7:38–45

Freeman C, Todd C, Camilleri-Ferrante C et al 2002 Quality improvement for older people with hip fracture: experience from a multi-site audit. Quality and Safety in Health Care 11:239–245

Gillespie LD, Gillespie WJ, Robertson MC et al 2003 Interventions for preventing falls in elderly people (Cochrane Review). The Cochrane Library. Wiley, Chichester

Gillespie WJ, Walenkamp G 2001 Antibiotic prophylaxis for surgery for proximal femoral and other closed long bone fractures (Cochrane Review). The Cochrane Library. Wiley, Chichester

Gillis A, MacDonald B 2005 Deconditioning on the hospitalized elderly. Canadian Nurse 101(6):16–20

Hayes N 2004 Prevention of falls among older patients in the hospital environment. British Journal of Nursing 13(15):896–901

Health and Safety at Work Act 1974 Stationery Office, London

Health and Safety Executive 1992/1998 Manual handling operation regulations: guidelines on the regulations, 2nd edn. HSE Books, Sudbury

Healthcare Commission 2006 Living well in later life. A review of progress against the national service framework for older people. Commission for Healthcare Audit and Inspection, London

Hillsdon M, Foster C, Naidoo B, et al 2004 The effectiveness of public health interventions to increase physical activity among adult: a review of reviews. Health Development Agency

Honkanen L 2004 An overview of hip fracture prevention. Topics in Geriatric Rehabilitation 20(4):285–296

Joint Health Surveys Unit 2003 Health Survey for England, 2003. The Stationary Office, London

Joseph Rowntree Foundation 2005 The older people's inquiry: 'That bit of help'. Joseph Rowntree Foundation, York

Kannus P, Parkkan J 2006 Prevention of hip fracture with hip protectors. Age and Ageing 35–52:ii51–ii54.

Kempton A, van Beurden E, Sladden T, et al 2000 Older people can stay on their feet? Final results of a community based falls prevention programme. Health Promotion International 15:27–33

Kneafsey R 2007 Nursing contributions to mobility rehabilitation: a systematic review examining the quality and content of the evidence. Journal of Clinical Nursing (in press)

Long A, Kneafsey R, Ryan J et al 2001 Teamworking in rehabilitation: exploring the role of the nurse. Researching professional education, research reports series, number 19. English National Board for Nursing Midwifery and Health Visiting, London

Long AF, Kneafsey R, Ryan J et al 2002 The role of the nurse within the multi-professional rehabilitation team. Journal of Advanced Nursing 37(1):70–78

Mahoney FI, Barthel DW 1965 Functional evaluation: the Barthel Index. Maryland State Medical Journal 14:61–65

McKenna J, Naylor PJ, MacDowell N 1998 Barriers to physical activity promotion by general practitioners and practice nurses. British Journal of Sports Medicine 32:242–247

National Audit Office 2003 A safer place to work. Improving the management of health and safety risks to staff in NHS Trusts. National Audit Office, London

National Collaborating Centre for Nursing and Supportive Care 2004 Clinical practice guideline for the assessment and prevention of falls in older people. Royal College of Nursing, London

NICE 2004 Falls: the assessment and prevention of falls in older people. NICE, London

NICE 2006 Four commonly used methods to increase physical activity: brief interventions in primary care, exercise referral schemes, pedometers, and community based exercise programmes for walking and cycling. NICE, London

Nursing and Midwifery Council 2007 NMC Record keeping guidance. Nursing and Midwifery Council, London

Oczkowski W, Barreca S 1993 The Functional Independence Measure: its use to identify rehabilitation needs in stroke survivors. Archives of Physical Medicine and Rehabilitation 74: 1291–1294

Office of the Deputy Prime Minister 2006 A sure start to later life. Ending inequalities for older people. ODPM, London

Oliver D, Daly F, Martin C, et al 2004 Risk factors and risk assessment for patients in hospital: a systematic review. Age and Ageing 33:122–130

Parker MJ, Handoll HHG, Banghara A 2002a Conservative versus operative treatment for hip fracture. Cochrane Review, The Cochrane Library. Wiley, Chichester

Parker SG, Peet SM, McPherson A 2002b A systematic review of discharge arrangements for older people. Health Technology Assessment 6:4

Parker MJ, Gillespie LD, Gillespie WJ 2005 Hip protectors for preventing hip fracture in older people Cochrane Review. The Cochrane Library. Wiley, Chichester

Pheasant S 1998 Back injury in nurses – ergonomics and epidemiology. In: Lloyd P (ed) Guide to the handling of patients. National Back Pain Association/RCN, London

Robinson J, Batstone G 1996 Rehabilitation: a developmental challenge. Kings Fund working paper. Kings Fund, London

Roper N, Logan W, Tierney A 1996 The elements of nursing: a model for nursing based on a model for living. 4th edn. Churchill Livingstone, Edinburgh

Roper N, Logan W, Tierney A 2000 The Roper–Logan–Tierney model of nursing based on activities of living. Churchill Livingstone, Edinburgh

Royal College of Nursing 1996 Code of practice for patient handling. RCN, London

Royal College of Nursing 1999 Introducing a safer patient handling policy. RCN, London

Royal College of Nursing 2003a Manual handling assessments in hospitals and community. RCN, London

Royal College of Nursing 2003b Safer staff, better care. RCN manual handling training guidance. RCN, London

Rubenstein LZ 2006 Falls in older people: epidemiology, risk factors and strategies for prevention. Age and Ageing 35–52:ii37–ii41

Rutishauser S 1994 Physiology and anatomy: a basis for nursing and health care. Churchill Livingstone, Edinburgh

Salkeld G, Cameron ID, Cumming RG et al 2000 Quality of life related to fear of falling and hip fracture in older women: a time trade off study. British Medical Journal 320:341–346

Scuffham P, Chaplin S 2002 The incidence and costs of accidental falls inn older people in the UK. Journal of Epidemiology and Community Health 57:9740–9744

SIGN 2002 Prevention and management of hip fracture in older people. Clinical guideline 56. Scottish Intercollegiate Guidelines Network, Edinburgh

SIGN 2003 Management of osteoporosis A national clinical guideline 71. Scottish Intercollegiate Guidelines Network, Edinburgh

Shepperd S, Parkes J, McClaran J et al 2005 Discharge planning from hospital to home (Cochrane Review). The Cochrane Library. Wiley, Chichester

Soule A, Babb P, Evandrou M et al 2005 Focus on older people. Office of National Statistics/Department of Work and Pensions, London

Stuck A, Beck JC 2001 Preventing disability and death in old age. International Journal of Epidemiology 30(4):900–901

Teri L, Gibbons LE, McCurry SM, et al 2003 Exercise plus behavioral management in patients with Alzheimer disease. Journal of the American Medical Association 290:2015–2022

Tinetti ME 2003 Clinical practice. Preventing falls in elderly persons. New England Journal of Medicine 348:42–49

Todd C, Skelton D 2004 What are the main risk factors for falls amongst older people and what are the most effective interventions to prevent these falls. World Health Organization Regional Office for Europe, Copenhagen (Health Evidence Network report) (www.europe.who.int/document/E82552.pdf accessed 1 February 2007)

Wade DT, de Jong BA 2000 Recent advances in rehabilitation. British Medical Journal 320:1385–1388

Waugh A, Grant A 1996 Ross and Wilson anatomy and physiology in health and illness, 8th edn. Churchill Livingstone, Edinburgh

Wicker P, O'Neill J 2006 Caring for the peri-operative patient. Blackwell Publishing, Oxford

Woodhead K, Wicker P (eds) 2005 A textbook of peri-operative care. Churchill Livingstone, Edinburgh

World Health Organization 1980 International classification of impairments, disabilities and handicaps: a manual of classification relating to the consequences of disease ICIDH. WHO, Geneva

World Health Organization 1999 International classification of functioning and disability ICIDH-2. WHO, Geneva

World Health Organization 2002a Active aging. A policy framework. WHO, Geneva

World Health Organization 2002b Towards a common language for functioning, Disability and Health ICF. WHO, Geneva

World Health Organization 2002c Health promotion and healthy lifestyles. WHA 57.16. WHO, Geneva

World Health Organization 2003 Prevention and management of osteoporosis. WHO, Geneva

World Health Organization 2004 Global strategy on diet, physical activity and health. WHO, Geneva

World Health Organization 2006 Disability and rehabilitation action plan 2006–2011. World Health Organization, Geneva

Young J, Brown A Forster A et al 1999 An overview of rehabilitation for older people. Reviews in Clinical Gerontology 9.181–196

Further reading

Commission for Social Care Inspection 2004 Leaving hospital – the price of delays. CSCI, London

Commission for Social Care Inspection 2005 Leaving hospital – revisited. CSCI, London

Davies S (ed) 2006 Rehabilitation. The use of theories and models on practice. Churchill Livingstone, Edinburgh

Davies S, O'Connor S 1999 Rehabilitation nursing foundations for practice. Baillière Tindall, Edinburgh

Hillsdon M, Foster C, Naidoo B et al 2004 The effectiveness of public health interventions to increase physical activity among adult: a review of reviews. Health Development Agency

Hoeman SP (ed) 2002 Rehabilitation nursing: process, application, and outcomes, 3rd edn. Mosby, St Louis

Montague SE, Watson R, Herbert RA (eds) 2005 Physiology for nursing practice, 3rd edn. Elsevier, Edinburgh

Royal College of Nursing 2003a Manual handling assessments in hospitals and community. RCN, London

Royal College of Nursing 2003b Safer staff, better care. RCN manual handling training guidance. RCN, London

Useful websites

www.cochrane.org (The Cochrane Library)

www.doh.gov.uk/essenceofcare (Essence of Care Benchmarking Standard)

www.epid.unimaas.nl/cochrane/field.htm (Cochrane Rehabilitation and Related Therapies Field)

www.hda.nhs.uk/evidence (Health Development Agency)

www.hta.nhsweb.nhs.uk (Reports for the Health Technology Assessment Programme)

www.nelh.nhs.uk (National Electronic Library for Health)

www.nice.org.uk (National Institute for Health and Clinical Excellence)

www.rehabnurse.org (The Association of Rehabilitation Nurses)

www.rcn.org.uk (RCN website for policy on patient handling)

www.who.int/classification/icf (ICF home page)

Working and playing

Susan Whittam

INTRODUCTION

The activities of work and play are central to human development and motivation, influenced by individual opportunity, ability, necessity and desire, and as such there are enormous variations in the degree to which the activities are carried out. Throughout the lifespan people experience significant changes in their lives that are marked by events such as starting school, leaving home, starting work, changing jobs and reaching retirement. Although there are many differences throughout the world, play tends to be more commonly associated with childhood, and as we progress through life there is a sense that in adult life work takes priority over play. As societies have developed and paid work has become an important feature of life, in the interests of health and wellbeing, there is a growing recognition of the need to ensure that work and play are suitably balanced. In Britain this is referred to as the work–life balance, and following a national campaign launched by the Prime Minister in 2000, there have been a number amendments and additions to employment legislation such as the right to ask for flexible working (Department of Trade and Industry 2003, Work and Families Act 2006).

The importance of considering this activity is central to the notion that, on average, most people spend about two-thirds of their day engaging in activities that are associated with working or playing. The activity is complex and has many dimensions that are influenced by many factors such as age, gender, physical and intellectual ability, social organisation, culture, opportunities and experience. By using the Roper, Logan and Tierney model (Roper et al 1996, 2000), it becomes possible to broadly but systematically explore the activities that are associated with working and playing in order to develop an understanding of normal everyday living, the changes that occur during ill health and the impact this has on other Activities of Living (ALs). This chapter will therefore focus on the following.

1. The model of living

- working and playing in health and illness across the lifespan
- dependence and independence in the activity
- factors influencing the activity of working and playing.

2. The model for nursing

- nursing care of individuals with health problems that are affecting their ability to undertake the activity of working and playing.

THE MODEL OF LIVING

Working

It is important to appreciate that the word 'work' does not necessarily relate to a paid job. For example housework, schoolwork and voluntary work, whilst making a valuable contribution to the lives of individuals and society, do not result in financial gain. Given this understanding, work is best described as a meaningful, regular activity for which a person has responsibility, indicating their status, purpose and/or a sense of achievement. Whether the work is paid or unpaid, the activity provides a degree of daily structure, personal organisation and, in most cases, contact with other people. Paid work is generally associated with economic sufficiency and a means of providing for essential living needs. The type of work that is chosen is based upon individual abilities, circumstances and the availability and supply of jobs; hence there are many different attitudes towards the value of work. For many people work is a necessity rather than a desire and can sometimes be viewed and experienced negatively. For some people, however, financial gain is not the only key driver for work and some people are able to combine paid work with their particular skills, interests and ambitions, for example musicians or artists. As a paid activity, generally speaking, work features throughout the lifespan, beginning in adolescence through to adult life and gradually reducing in old age. Terms such as unemployment and retirement are used to describe cessation of paid employment and may be indicative of some loss of financial independence.

Throughout the world, there are many factors which influence the activity of working, based upon individual motivation, personal needs and circumstances, economic and social influences, and these will be discussed throughout this chapter.

Playing

Within the context of the model the activity of 'playing' is considered to be important at every stage of the lifespan, focusing upon activities that are pursued in the spare time that is not taken up by work. The importance of play in childhood development remains undisputed, but the model goes further to explore the importance that play has in adult life. Changing patterns of employment and wealth have increased the pursuit of leisure activities that have led to a significant growth in the leisure industry, providing facilities for sport, relaxation, hobbies, holidays and other personal interests.

The discussion so far has demonstrated that the degree to which individuals choose to, or are expected to, engage in work and play activities is influenced by many factors. The differences that occur will now be explored through the framework of the model, in order to help you develop your understanding of the following:

- why the AL is important to health and wellbeing
- what factors influence individual behaviour and choices within the AL
- how individuals might be affected by a temporary or permanent inability to carry out the activity
- why this knowledge and understanding is important to the quality of nursing care.

The topic is very broad and has close links to the AL of maintaining a safe environment. It will be necessary for you to refer back to Chapter 3 from time to time and further extend your knowledge by consulting the recommended reading list at the end of this chapter.

WORKING AND PLAYING IN HEALTH AND ILLNESS ACROSS THE LIFESPAN

Childhood/adolescence

The capacity for and importance of play in childhood is closely associated with learning and development. Through play a child learns to develop physically, intellectually, interpersonally and socially (Lindon 2005). Opportunities for play are provided through contact with other people and the provision of appropriate play equipment, toys, games, imaginative play and other stimulating environments both within and outside the home (Slater & Lewis 2002). The activity of play remains predominant into adolescence and early adulthood, but the notion of work takes on gradual emphasis as a child progresses through their school life, whereupon activities are referred to as 'schoolwork'. By the time a child completes their school career they will have been encouraged to achieve a basic level of knowledge and skill to prepare them for working life. Throughout childhood there will have been opportunities to engage in a vast number of play, sport and leisure activities, influenced by either school or the family. By the time an individual reaches adolescence, they are likely to have developed a preference for the type of play they enjoy, which they may then continue to pursue into adulthood. The presence of illness and disability will place some restrictions upon the ability to fully engage in some work and play activities. However, because of increasing recognition of the rights of disabled people, in Britain, public and private service providers and businesses such as schools, hospitals, employers and leisure facilities are governed by legislation to ensure that individuals have equal opportunity and access to work and play activities (Disability Discrimination Act 2005).

Adulthood/old age

In adult life there is generally a clear distinction between working life and leisure time, with the exception of those people who have the opportunity to combine their leisure activities or interests with paid work, such as sportsmen and women, actors, musicians, authors and artists. The ability to secure and sustain employment is a central feature of adult life, the nature of which will influence how much spare time, income and motivation there is to pursue leisure activities. It is estimated that most adults will spend more than half of their lives in work, the experience of which will vary enormously, dependent upon individual capability and availability of work. Some people will spend their entire working life pursuing one career path, whilst others may frequently change directions acquiring new knowledge and skills accordingly. By contrast, unemployment and redundancy are common events that can either have devastating effects or can produce opportunities to learn and use new skills and take up more meaningful work. Whilst unemployment and retirement essentially can create more personal free time to pursue leisure activities, a lack of income or physical health likewise can restrict activities. Generally in the UK, retirement occurs at the age of 65 years; however, in recognition of the experience and value that older people contribute to society, legislation influenced by the European Framework Directive has created the right for individuals to work beyond a compulsory age of retirement and it is illegal to discriminate against employing people on the grounds of their age (Employment Equality (Age) Regulations 2006). The Office for National Statistics (2005a) reported that over the previous 20 years the average life expectancy rates in the UK had been steadily increasing, to 82 years for men and 85 years for women. As a result older people make up an increasing proportion of the population, generally leading active, healthy lives and working longer. However, there is a view that whilst people are living longer they may not necessarily spend this time in good health and the quality of life is the subject of research and debate (Gabriel & Bowling 2003).

Preparation for life in retirement means that individuals will need to understand and cope with changes in health, work, social and leisure pursuits and financial security (Hartnell & Lyon 2003). A stereotypical view of retirement is that people are no longer required or able to undertake paid work, which contributes to the negative views of ageism. The World Health Organization (2002a) has shown that, worldwide, people over the age of 60 years play a critical role in contributing to society, through participation in the paid workforce by making significant contributions towards caring roles within the family and the community.

DEPENDENCY AND INDEPENDENCY IN RELATION TO THE ACTIVITY OF WORKING AND PLAYING

Children and adolescents spend most of their lives being dependent upon the family or society to help them develop the skills that enable them to engage in work and play activities for the remainder of their lives. For individuals with learning difficulties, physical or mental health disabilities, a degree of dependency upon the family or public services will to a certain extent remain, although the focus should always be to optimise independent living.

In adult life, there is an interdependency between employers and employees. Employers provide work opportunities and reasonable working conditions, and in return employees offer their knowledge, skills and experience. In old age particularly, where there are risks to health or safety, there can be a gradual return of dependence upon the family, friends and/or public services. It must be pointed out, however, that many older people do live quite independently through their older life. Although there are a number of reasons why independence at any given time across the lifespan might be affected, health and financial self-sufficiency are commonly identified.

Individual attitudes towards independence may also vary, for example some may view retirement as a loss of independence in terms of income, whilst others may see it as a welcome opportunity to pursue hobbies and leisure activities.

Exercise

How does society value people who are retired?

1. Consider your own personal views about retirement – what has influenced your views?
2. Think of someone you know who has been retired for some time. Ask them for their views about retirement as follows:
   - How well were they prepared for their retirement?
   - What different activities have they pursued since retirement?
   - How easy has it been to cope with retirement?

FACTORS INFLUENCING THE AL OF WORKING AND PLAYING

Given that the nature of the AL of working and playing has been identified through the common events that might occur across the lifespan, this section will help you to understand the differences that exist between individuals. This should help you to acknowledge the range of different circumstances that patients may face within the AL when they become ill and enable you to provide effective care that supports maximum individuality and independence.

Biological factors

All work and play activities will have some degree of biological link in relation to the following:

- physical ability to carry out work and play activities
- the extent to which activities are interrupted due to ill health.

It is important to understand that work and play activities will probably be associated with a number of body systems and that no one specific biological system can be aligned to this AL. However, work and play activities will essentially rely upon normal growth and development of all body systems, particularly the senses, movement, balance and coordination. Different activities will require varied degrees of physical health and fitness. Some activities are extremely physically demanding and the individual must have the required strength, energy and fitness to be able to sustain the activity over time. For a variety of reasons the ability to undertake the activity can be limited by disability, disease, injury or the ageing process. People who develop limitations within the AL may need help and support to engage in alternative activities that are compatible with their needs and abilities. Employers and leisure facility providers can make a range of adjustments to improve access to work and play activities by improving access to buildings, providing a range of specialised equipment and ensuring that staff have access to disability awareness training. Staff training plays an important part in changing attitudes towards disability and ensuring that individual needs and appropriate resources are provided. For some work and play activities, regular health checks may be required, in order to ensure that the individual can safely carry out the activity; for example, pilots, train drivers and individuals who join health and sports clubs. In sport, athletes undergo rigorous health checks, to detect if they have been taking drugs that enhance their sporting performance.

Exercise

Consider the following cases:

- a hay fever sufferer
- a person who requires regular renal dialysis
- a person with a hearing difficulty
- a person with irritable bowel problems.

1. How might their symptoms affect the AL?
2. What could be done in the work and play environment to accommodate their needs?
3. What advice could you give to each individual?

You will see that even the most minor health problems can influence the AL and that in all cases some adjustments within either the work or play environments would be required. It is important to recognise that disabilities are not only associated with mobility issues, and by increasing your awareness and understanding about the effects that ill health can have upon the AL of working and playing, you will begin to appreciate the importance of a holistic approach to nursing care.

Psychological factors

There are many different factors that influence an individual's choice of work and play activities, which are essentially related to levels of intelligence and personality. From birth, emotional and intellectual development is continued through play, to gradually help the development of communication and interpersonal skills that are essential to the AL (Lindon 2005).

In the world of work some jobs will require a certain level of knowledge and specific qualifications, whilst for others there may be a greater emphasis upon practical skills and experience. Many organisations are recognising the importance of recruiting the right staff and use a variety of psychological selection techniques ranging from simple interviews to sophisticated assessment exercises (Hall et al 2004). Some employers go to great lengths to appoint employees with the right knowledge, skills and experience to undertake the work, but also with the attributes to ensure organisational success. In response to a growing skills gap in Britain, the government published a white paper entitled *Skills: Getting on in business, getting on in work,* in order to ensure that people have the skills to make them employable and personally fulfilled (Department for Education and Skills (DfES)

2005). To this extent many organisations, including the NHS, are addressing essential workforce development issues in order to improve and sustain organisational reform and viability in a rapidly changing global economy (Department of Health 2000, 2001a, 2005a). In the UK, support for making career choices is available from school careers advisers (*connexions* service) and job centres, as well as some employer-based career advisers to help identify careers and further development opportunities that may best suit individual knowledge, skills, experience and personal attributes (see the Department for Work and Pensions website).

The ability to take part and be safe in play and leisure activities will similarly rely upon individual skills, abilities, interests and personality. Essentially there is a greater freedom of choice over play and leisure activities, although physical strength and in some instances financial cost may restrict participation. It is important that, in the pursuit of leisure, individuals remain safe and do not take risks that may endanger themselves or others; although, for some individuals it will be the risks that are the motivating factor for pursuing the activity, for example motor car racing, mountaineering and extreme sports.

Stress related to work and play

The subject of stress and its effects upon the body were introduced in Chapter 3. In relation to work, every individual has their own range of coping mechanisms, which helps us to understand why one person's stress can be another person's energiser. The subject of stress has been studied from many perspectives, and whilst it remains complex, the causes, effects and costs of work-related stress nationally, organisationally and individually are very well documented (Cox et al 2000). Stress in the workplace occurs when an individual feels overwhelmed and overburdened, resulting in a variety of physical and psychological illnesses. Certain types of jobs can cause workplace stress, related to workload, working conditions, working relationships, career opportunities, organisational culture, gender differences and the ability to sustain a work–life balance (WHO 2003). The effects of stress in the workplace can result in decreased job satisfaction, low morale, boredom, low performance and productivity, increased absenteeism and high staff turnover rates (Mullins 2004). However, it is important to recognise that stress is not exclusive to adults in the workplace. People who work at home, often in isolation, such as housewives, are also known to suffer from stress, resulting in many associated physical and mental health problems (Lombardi & Ulbrich 1997, Khan & Cuthbertson 1998). Alternatively unemployment caused by the inability to secure work, redundancy or retirement can be equally as stressful, leading to poor health and altered psychosocial behaviour (Bartley & Ferrie 2001, McKee et al 2005).

Coping with stress

There are a number of measures that both individuals and organisations can engage in to combat the causes and effects of stress, many of which are linked to the 'playing' element of the AL. In recognition of the problem, employers and governments have been prompted to develop long-term strategies to prevent and reduce the effects of stress (Christiansen & Matuska 2006). In the UK the Health and Safety Executive (HSE 2005) have developed a set of Management Standards to reduce the levels of work-related stress. In recognition of stress in the NHS all health care organisations are expected to achieve targets outlined by the *Improving Working Lives* National Audit Instrument, which sets out a framework of good employment practices (DoH 2001b). At an individual level people can manage their own stress by learning to recognise the signs and adopt healthier lifestyles by acknowledging the importance of balancing work and leisure more effectively.

Effects of the absence of work and play

Absence from work can be caused by a multitude of factors such as illness, injury, retirement, redundancy and unemployment. In all cases there will be an immediate impact upon psychological wellbeing, which may be a loss of self-esteem, confidence and social status. Research has shown that this leads to increased prevalence of a range of physical and mental health problems, including premature death, at all stages of the lifespan (Price et al 2002, Brown et al 2003).

Not all absence from work, however, is viewed negatively. For some people redundancy and retirement provide them with the opportunity to make lifestyle and career changes that they would not have otherwise made. Given support and advice, people can be assisted to make the necessary psychological adjustments to enable them to enjoy this aspect of living (Mein et al 2003, Warr et al 2004).

> **Exercise**
> 1. Consider what lifestyle changes you would have to make if you were to lose your job tomorrow.
>   - How do you think it would affect your health?
>   - What impact would your situation have upon those around you?
> 2. What plans have you made towards your own retirement?
>   - Try to imagine what it might feel like.
>   - What would be your main concern?

Sociocultural factors

The structure and culture of a society has considerable influence upon the type of work that is both available and undertaken, and many differences can be seen throughout the world. For some societies, work remains central to ensuring the self-sufficiency of a whole community of people, such as in remote tribes where there will be long-established traditions governing the nature of work which will have changed little over time. By contrast in the industrialised world, it has

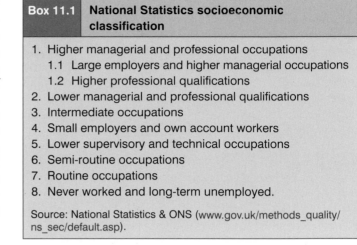

> **Box 11.1**　**National Statistics socioeconomic classification**
>
> 1. Higher managerial and professional occupations
>   - 1.1 Large employers and higher managerial occupations
>   - 1.2 Higher professional qualifications
> 2. Lower managerial and professional qualifications
> 3. Intermediate occupations
> 4. Small employers and own account workers
> 5. Lower supervisory and technical occupations
> 6. Semi-routine occupations
> 7. Routine occupations
> 8. Never worked and long-term unemployed.
>
> Source: National Statistics & ONS (www.gov.uk/methods_quality/ns_sec/default.asp).

become necessary for individuals to constantly learn new skills in order to maintain the supply of goods and services to sustain an established national economy. In the UK the type of work that is undertaken by an individual determines a person's socioeconomic classification (see Box 11.1) The classification enables information to be collected such as employment and health statistics and trends (Office for National Statistics 2006b).

Influence of beliefs upon working and playing

Prevailing beliefs, values and traditions held by individuals or societies can have a strong influence upon the AL of working and playing. For example, in some societies culture will influence the type of work that men and women traditionally undertake and can also influence play, sport and leisure activities. As countries have become more industrialised many traditional values and beliefs, relating particularly to work, have also changed. There are many examples in the Western world of a reversal of traditional roles, where women have become the main earner of the family income and men have taken primary responsibility for caring for the family at home (Crompton 2006). Because sociocultural beliefs can be so strong, many of the changes that have occurred have required support from equal opportunity legislation, to ensure that, for example, women and people with disabilities have access to equal pay and opportunities in the workplace. Despite the gradual social changes that have taken place it is often possible to observe traditional cultural values in the play of children. The different games that boys and girls play are often gender-specific and have the potential to influence work choices in adult life. In adult life the pursuit of leisure activities is generally influenced by the amount of spare time or finance that is available.

Social change and the effects upon work and play

In relation to the activity of working and playing there is a need to understand the significant impact that change can have upon the AL, especially in relation to health and wellbeing. Over the last century, life for many people has changed rapidly, in terms both of pace and technology, and the effects that this has had upon health are widely recognised. So rapid are the changes in the workplace that globally organisations are experiencing many skills shortages, whilst at the same time needing to provide cost-effective services against the backdrop of often fierce business competition. As a result many people are working longer hours and engaging in education and training activities to enhance their employment opportunities, but ultimately this reduces their leisure and relaxation time (HSE 2003). Throughout the world many physical and psychological health problems can now be directly attributed to the work that people undertake. In response both employers and governments are implementing schemes and legislation to ensure that working practices take into consideration the physical and psychological wellbeing of their staff, such as flexible working and reduction in working long hours (Working Time (Amendment) Regulations 2006, Employment Act 2002). However, it is worth pointing out that, in many countries, children and adults are exploited in the workplace and have little to no access to any kind of leisure or play activities, neither are there any laws to help relieve their plight (WHO 2004).

By contrast there is growing concern that where changes in a society's play and leisure activities have occurred, there are also reports of increases in sedentary lifestyles, which may cause health problems for the future such as obesity, diabetes and heart disease (Rollo 2004). In recognition of the growing need to balance work, play and health, there has been substantial growth in the leisure industry, providing activities for people at every stage of the lifespan. The ability to pursue many of the activities available is influenced by many factors such as affordability, availability and physical health and capability (Office for National Statistics 2006a). If safety is to be maintained it is important that individuals are aware of the dangers that some pursuits may have for them and carefully choose activities that meet their individual needs and circumstances (Mullineaux et al 2001). For example, Schnohr et al (2000) highlight the dangers that exist for men who take up jogging in an effort to keep fit, only to find that this may be actually detrimental to their health.

Changes in society are also linked to changes in the behaviour of people, and one of the growing concerns in the UK is the increasing reports of antisocial behaviour affecting people of all ages across the lifespan, notably within the workplace and in schools (Godin 2004, Smith 2004). In the UK and Europe this has prompted the introduction of a number of laws governing the responsibility that employers have to protect their staff, including incident measurement and monitoring.

Whilst crime rates are reported to be generally falling, the fear of crime is still a concern, particularly when there are increasing reports of attacks upon the elderly, antisocial behaviour, gun crime and murders (Office for National Statistics 2006a, Ch. 9). Schools are similarly reporting an increase in antisocial behaviour, exposing teachers as well

as students to attack. Along with advances and availability of new technologies, the incidence of bullying has widened to include on-line bullying and also an emerging trend for the recording of violent attacks on mobile phones which are then circulated via the internet. Increasing incidents and trends have prompted many education authorities and schools to take positive action to combat the rising problems (DfES 2003, 2006). There is recognition that a lack of recreational facilities for young people, combined with boredom and a lack of parental control, are contributing towards the increase in juvenile crime (Caspi et al 2003). Unfortunately many crimes are also associated with an escalating rise in drug, alcohol and substance abuse, causing misery to thousands of people across the lifespan. Over time a combination of government intervention and public pressure often lead to the introduction of new laws, national strategies and initiatives in an attempt to reduce and solve the problems (The Home Office 2006).

> **Exercise**
> 1. Discover how the values and traditions about work and play have changed over time within your own family.
> 2. Try to determine what factors might have influenced these changes.
> 3. How might these values differ from someone of another culture?
> 4. How might values change in the future?

Environmental factors

In the work environment as discussed in Chapter 3, there is an equal responsibility for individuals and organisations to ensure health and safety. To support this many countries have legal requirements for employers to have procedures in place that enable risks to be identified and as far as possible prevented. In the UK the Health and Safety at Work Act 1974 serves to ensure that organisations take steps to assess and identify risks and provide essential information, policies, guidelines, equipment, training, skills, environments and facilities in an attempt to reduce accident rates. To reinforce compliance with the law the Health and Safety Executive (HSE) provides a comprehensive information, audit, research and investigation service that constantly informs good practice in ensuring health and safety. The HSE provides information about the health risks associated with a whole range of industries and occupations that range from physical injury to genetic disorders, infertility, stress, tumours, skin, cardiac and respiratory disorders, through exposure to harmful substances and unsafe environments. The development of new technologies within the workplace means that new risks and hazards are emerging all the time, for example the problems that are now known to be associated with computer work such as the injury to the wrist known as repetitive strain injury (RSI) and headaches and visual problems associated with the use of visual display screens.

It is important to recognise that not all work and play activities are governed by legislation and the individual takes sole or joint responsibility for their own health and safety. For example, people who are self-employed are expected to abide by the health and safety regulations and take personal responsibility to identify risks and secure personal insurance to protect themselves financially in the event of an accident. Under the legislation, employers of homeworkers also have the same duty to protect the health and welfare of their staff.

However, housewives and retired people, whilst just as much at risk from accidents and stress, do not benefit from any form of statutory protection for the work they carry out. For children and young adults, the responsibility for health and safety lies with the parents or guardians and the agencies or organisations that they engage with. Regulations governing the safety of children relate mainly to educational and health and safety legislation. Lessons learned from high-profile incidents often lead to regulations being introduced or amended, such as the introduction of risk assessments for environments and activities. For adults pursuing leisure activities it would be expected that there would be equal responsibility upon the individual and activity provider to consider the risks that might be involved.

To support the needs of disabled people, The Disability Discrimination Act 2005 and the Equality Act 2006 guide the requirements for employers and service providers to make environmental adaptations to reflect the changing nature of work, daily living and leisure activities. Retail and leisure industries such as hotels, leisure clubs, banks, supermarkets and shopping centres are adapting services, for example lowering counters and cash machines, and providing electronic shopping vehicles to improve access and independence for disabled people.

Exercise

Think about the places you visit regularly in your day-to-day life and identify where adaptations have been made or could be made to meet the needs of the following disabilities:

1. mobility difficulties
2. visual difficulties
3. hearing difficulties
4. decision-making and problem-solving difficulties.

A variety of access adaptations, facilities and special services are available, particularly for people with mobility and other commonly known disabilities. You may have recognised that further improvements could be made to reflect the diversity of disabilities.

Politicoeconomic factors
The purpose of work in society
The ability to earn an income has two purposes; firstly, to sustain an individual lifestyle and secondly, to contribute collectively towards the national economy. At a national level, work enables the production of goods and services that can be widely traded (industrialisation) and forms the basis of national wealth. The way in which the national economy is sustained is the business of governments, and concerns ensuring that a country has a sufficiently skilled workforce. This involves recognising the impact that changing working trends may be having upon society such as 24-hour services, or new technologies, and putting in place a range of systems and services to support labour market requirements. The following are examples of initiatives and services which over time have been provided in the UK to support the AL of working and playing:

- minimum age of employment
- minimum wage
- working time regulations
- sickness and maternity pay
- paid holiday leave
- flexible working regulations and schemes
- child, family and incapacity benefits
- unemployment benefits
- retirement age and pensions reviews
- health and social care service policy and review
- education service policy and review.

In an industrialised country those who are in work contribute to the provision of the services through income tax and national insurance payments. These payments contribute to national services such as health and social care, education, unemployment and sickness payments and retirement pensions. When balancing the national economy it is vital that there are enough people in work in order to continue to provide such services.

At an individual level, paid work provides an income to provide for personal and family needs. In the UK a person's wage or salary is generally associated with their occupation and level of responsibility and pay increases are negotiated through trade unions or linked to individual work performance. Nonetheless the link between poverty and ill health is well documented, and developed countries seek to support low pay through a variety of health and social care benefits and schemes.

The changing nature of work
Since the mid 20th century there have been significant changes in the nature of work influenced by some of the following:

- introduction of new electronic technologies
- introduction of information communication technologies and commercial globalisation
- increased workforce migration and diversity
- increase in part-time and flexible working
- increase in early and flexible retirement.

With rapid changes set to continue it will be difficult to predict what the nature of work and the workforce may look like in the future. The ambitious reforms within the NHS are an example of how organisations will be expected to transform themselves in response to changing customer expectations, and the need to provide efficient services within financial constraints (DoH 2000, 2005b). As a result, more than ever before, organisations will need to ensure that employers, employees and trade unions work together to create flexible, innovative and more positive attitudes towards work.

In 2004 ten countries joined the European Union, and the UK opened up its labour market to attract a significant number of migrant workers into areas of work experiencing skills shortages. It is expected that the numbers of migrant workers will continue to rise as more countries join the European Union at a later date, increasing the overall diversity of the population (Office for National Statistics 2005b). The issue of international migration has many challenges throughout the world. Very often migrant workers are vulnerable groups who are exploited in such a way that their personal health and safety are in jeopardy. In the UK, cases such as the 23 Chinese Morecambe Bay cocklepickers who lost their lives and the growing problem of human trafficking testify that even in developed countries individuals are at risk (British Broadcasting Company 2006).

In order to continuously sustain national social and economic health, governments introduce policies and initiatives to influence education and employment, in an attempt to ensure that workforce skills are available. In the UK this has led to the introduction and amendments of employment regulations and initiatives such as:

- The Education Act 2005
- The Employment Act 2002
- Improving Working Lives (DoH 2001b)
- Investors in People (2004)
- The Childcare Act 2006
- The Immigration and Asylum Act 1999.

Support for the activity of working

As discussed earlier in this chapter, health and safety legislation exists to protect individuals at work, but, in addition, there are also a range of other employment laws that have been introduced to reflect changing needs, such as:

- The Employment Rights Act 1996
- The Industrial Tribunal Act 1996
- Disability Discrimination Act 2005
- The Equality Act 2006.

These acts outline the responsibilities of employers to provide good employment environments and working relationships covering issues related to disability, equality and diversity, race, sexual orientation, religion and beliefs and age. By way of additional support the following services and organisations exist.

Trade unions   Trade unions have a responsibility to act in the best interests of their members to negotiate nationally

and locally not only on issues of pay but also to ensure fair employment rights and conditions as follows (Boeri et al 2001):

- worker health and safety education and surveillance
- development of national and local policies
- worker education and training
- support for workers in dispute with employers.

Exercise

1. Find out which trade unions are associated with health care in the UK.
2. What services do they provide for health care staff?
3. What support could a health care worker expect to receive from the trade union regarding a personal health problem due to working conditions?
4. If you are living and working in another country find out what the laws are with regard to trade unions and their activities.

Occupational health services   Occupational health services consist of specifically trained occupational health doctors and nurses and other health specialists and therapists such as stress counsellors who are employed by organisations to provide comprehensive employee health screening and health promotion services to staff. The range of services available include pre-employment screening, prevention and management of occupational/workplace disorders, surveillance and research (Oakley 2005).

Employment services   In the UK there are a wide range of statutory and voluntary services that help people to secure suitable work. The process begins in schools and colleges with careers advice. National services such as *jobcentre plus* and other independent employment and recruitment agencies provide advice and guidance for individuals seeking to change jobs or develop alternative careers (Department for Work and Pensions 2005).

Employment legislation also supports the provision of services to help people seek and secure work. The legislation works to ensure that organisations provide fair and equal opportunities for people who might otherwise have been unequally paid, dismissed, or excluded from employment on the grounds of their gender, race or disability.

Exercise

1. Locate the Department for Work and Pensions website (**www.dwp.gov.uk**) to find out what employment services, schemes and benefits are available for young people and adults.

Support for play in society

The importance of play in society is central to enjoyment and viewed as complementing working life. It is influenced by the standard of living and may be dependent upon the provision of appropriate facilities. Across the lifespan there are a variety of reasons why one individual may have more time for play or leisure than another and this is largely influenced by social class, income, culture and social provision.

During childhood and adolescence, encouraging human growth and development through play has many benefits to society that have been highlighted throughout this chapter. Schools may provide the foundation for introducing sport and leisure activities, but the extent to which these are pursued in later life is influenced by a number of individual, social and economic factors. Just as legislation has improved attitudes and access to work opportunities, so too has it influenced changes in attitudes and improvements for access to play, sport and leisure. This has led to improvements in facilities for disabled people to access local sports facilities to participation in international events such as the paralympic games, which are now held in conjunction with the Olympic games every 4 years. As a result of increased disability awareness there has been an amendment to the Disability Discrimination Act that requires active promotion of disability equality in access all aspects of leisure activities as well as the workplace (Disability Rights Commission 2006).

For families, changing work patterns have led to a growing demand for child care and leisure services such as nurseries, play schemes and out-of-school clubs which in turn have increased the demand for accredited child care and play specialists (Office for National Statistics 2006a). In addition there has also been a rapid increase in the provision of family-orientated recreational services such as holiday play schemes, holiday centres, theme parks, various sporting activities, cinemas and eating out, which only a few years ago would not have been available. Similarly for adults there is a vast array of sport, leisure and recreational activities available, but a lack of finance, time and physical ability remain the main obstacles for not engaging in these activities. As services and opportunities have increased so too has the requirement to ensure public service standards and safety as discussed in Chapter 3. To this extent governments become obligated or pressurised to introduce or amend legislation and services.

A lack of opportunity to engage fully in recreational activities has an impact throughout the lifespan ranging from boredom in children and young adults, the adoption of adverse recreational habits (poor diet, smoking, increased use of alcohol and recreational drugs) to the social deprivation of elderly people (Office for National Statistics 2006a, Ch. 7). Ultimately changes begin to impact upon individual and community health, safety and wellbeing to such an extent that action to remedy situations is required either through political will, pressure groups or high-profile media coverage such as of the sale of drugs and the problem of children as young as 8 years old vandalising housing estates late at night in some of Britain's towns and cities.

CONCLUSION

The framework of the model of living has been used to demonstrate how the model can be used to guide your understanding of how the AL of working and playing in everyday life is influenced and why the AL is important to health and individualised patient care. It is hoped that by engaging in the exercises provided throughout this chapter you began to appreciate the interrelatedness of the other ALs. The following exercises provide you with two mini case studies that will help you begin to apply the model in practice. These exercises will enable you to identify what is influencing a change upon the AL of working and playing and how this is impacting upon the other Activities of Living.

Effects upon the activity of working and playing

Exercise

1. Read through Case study 11.1 and consider how the activity of working and playing is being influenced from a lifespan, dependence/independence and factors affecting health perspective.

Case study 11.1

Individuality in the AL of working and playing

Gill, a former company secretary, is 39 years old and has suffered from a back problem for many years, the result of which is that she is now registered disabled and constantly needs to use a wheelchair. Gill is a single mum bringing up her son aged 17 and daughter aged 19.

The following points may have been considered:

Lifespan

Gill would normally be expecting to live a full and active life, enjoying her family and freedom to pursue leisure time. She would have developed expertise in her job and possibly be looking to increase her income or career aspirations.

Change in dependency

There is potential for loss of financial and personal independence. Gill will need to consider alterations to her environment to promote independent living.

Factors affecting health
Biological

- loss of mobility with the potential to affect other physiological functions such as eliminating, personal cleansing and dressing, expressing sexuality.

Psychological
- risk of depression and stress
- loss of self-esteem and confidence.

Sociocultural
- risk of social isolation and exclusion
- increased dependence upon children, family and friends and support agencies
- may need to give up leisure activities and identify new activities.

Environmental
- may need adjustments to home and work environment
- may have difficulties driving or using public transport.

Politicoeconomic
- may have difficulties continuing in employment
- may have concerns regarding family income
- may have anxieties about securing social benefits
- may have little knowledge about support mechanisms available.

Exercise

Consider for a moment if Gill had been a patient in your care in a general hospital ward.

1. Without the use of the model, how thorough would your assessment of her individual needs have been?
2. How is Gill's problem impacting upon the other ALs?

Exercise

1. Read through Case study 11.2 and identify the impact of a change in health status upon the Activities of Living.

Case study 11.2

How altered working and playing activities may impact upon other ALs

Mike is a 23-year-old man who works as a car mechanic for a small local company. He is due to be married in 6 months. He has sustained a crush injury to his right foot, whilst at work. He is the top striker for his local football team.

Effect on other Activities of Living

1. **MSE**
   - safety issues at work may prevent him returning until he is fully recovered
   - risk of delayed healing through further injury or infection if returns to normal work and play activities.

2. **Communicating**
   - may be angry and upset
   - may feel isolated by altered contact at work or friends
   - may need to discuss financial worries with appropriate people/agencies.

3. **Eating and drinking**
   - may need to ensure diet is conducive to healing and medication
   - may increase weight during period of reduced activity.

4. **Eliminating**
   - may have difficulty due to reduced mobility.

5. **Mobilising**
   - normal activities reduced due to injury
   - may require extensive physiotherapy intervention
   - unable to go to work or take part in football.

6. **Expressing sexuality**
   - may affect relationship with fiancée
   - may feel body image is altered.

7. **Maintaining body temperature**
   - risk of infection may increase body temperature.

8. **Sleep and rest**
   - may be interrupted due to pain and discomfort.

9. **Dying**
   - dependent upon seriousness of injury or recovery complication.

SUMMARY POINTS

The two cases demonstrate the following:
1. Working and playing can be affected by all the factors affecting health.
2. Working and playing can be affected by all the other ALs.
3. The lack of ability to engage fully in this activity can have detrimental effects upon health and the quality of life.
4. Engaging in this activity presents many risks to health and wellbeing.

THE MODEL FOR NURSING

INDIVIDUALISING NURSING FOR THE ACTIVITY OF WORKING AND PLAYING

The application of the model for nursing is based upon integrating the components of the model of living with each of the four phases of the nursing process (assessing, planning, implementing and evaluating) as shown in Figure 11.1.

This part of the chapter will now concentrate upon helping you to understand how the information from the model of living can be applied to nursing practice. In the first part of this chapter, the model of living helped you to understand how the activity of working and playing is usually carried out, a summary of which can be found in Box 11.2.

By systematically integrating the model of living as shown in Box 11.2 to each stage of the nursing process you

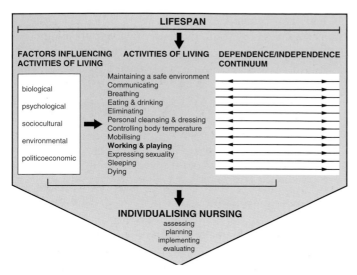

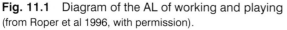

Fig. 11.1   Diagram of the AL of working and playing
(from Roper et al 1996, with permission).

will be able to increase the individuality of the nursing care plan. It is important to remember that when considering the holistic needs of patients, some or all of the other ALs may also be affected, particularly the AL of maintaining a safe environment. You will need to refer to other AL chapters as appropriate. By working through the exercises and case scenarios that follow you will gain an appreciation of the interrelatedness of all of the ALs. Whilst working through this section and when encountering individual patients in practice, you may find it useful to refer back to the information contained within the first part of this chapter, remembering the importance of keeping up to date with related information in order to ensure that patients always receive

a high standard of care. The use of the model also helps to identify nursing interventions that are associated with the activity of working and playing, which in general will be related to the following:

- teaching patients about health and safety at work and at play
- preventing accidents and ill health associated with working and playing
- supporting patients to cope with altered health states
- providing care to support individual needs
- helping patients to adapt to change and adopt healthier lifestyles.

ASSESSMENT OF NEEDS AND PROBLEMS

Assessing the individual using the model for nursing

The application of the model begins by using the components of the model of living to collect the following information:

1. the patient's normal habits and routines within the AL of working and playing
2. the factors that may be causing the activity to be altered
3. identification of actual and potential problems related to the AL.

The initial assessment of individual needs is important, as it provides essential information upon which all other aspects of the nursing care are to be planned. It is important to recognise that whilst the process of nursing begins with an assessment, it is a continuous activity that should be undertaken regularly in order to support the changing needs of patients through their entire care episode.

Box 11.2	Summary of the model of living in health – working and playing

Lifespan
- normal activity expected for age group

Dependence/independence
- expected level of dependence/independence related to lifespan
- identified level of dependence related to other Activities of Living.

Factors affecting working and playing
Biological
- general physical health
- age and general physique/fitness or energy levels.

Psychological
- level of intelligence
- personality, temperament and self-discipline
- emotional stability and ability to cope with stress and changes within the AL
- motivation
- attitudes to work and play.

Sociocultural
- recognition of individual personal attitudes, beliefs and values, religious beliefs
- social class
- gender differences
- attitudes to work and play.

Environmental
- identification of risks and hazards
- provision of adequate protection.

Politicoeconomic
- availability of work/job security
- personal economic status
- access to relevant social systems and legislation
- affordability of leisure activities.

Collection of specific information related to the AL of working and playing

Prior to the assessment

Assessment begins by using the components of the model of living to act as a framework for assessing the patient's normal habits and routines, in order to identify the extent to which ill health is influencing the ability to carry out the activity of working and playing. When conducting an assessment the following points must be considered:

1. The actual or potential problem identified may be more specifically aligned to another AL (demonstrating the interrelatedness with other ALs).
2. Collaboration with other professional groups or agencies may be required in order to fully solve or alleviate the problem.

Identification of health problems associated with working and playing

In order to identify the individual needs of patients, it is important to be able to determine the extent to which the AL has changed. Box 11.3 summarises some common issues that bring about a disruption in the AL.

Exercise

1. What employment and social services are available in your area to support the issues identified in Box 11.3?
2. What recreational activities are available in your area for young people?
3. Identify your learning needs and produce an action plan that you can discuss with your mentor/preceptor.

The patient assessment

The ability to provide individualised nursing care is based upon the knowledge of a person's individuality. As demonstrated in the model of living, the activity of working and playing is extremely complex and highly individualised, requiring careful assessment and support. When assessing the activity it is important to determine the following:

- the extent to which ill health is affecting the activity
- the extent to which a change in the activity is influencing ill health.

For example, patients are not usually admitted to hospital as a result of not being able to undertake the AL of working and playing, but the activity may be seriously disrupted and require adaptation due to a problem associated with another AL. Hence a thorough assessment is vital in order to ensure that the subsequent care plan is relevant to what the patient can realistically achieve and should aim to address the following:

- how actual problems may be solved
- how to prevent potential problems becoming actual ones
- how to prevent solved problems from recurring
- how to alleviate problems which cannot be solved
- how to help the person cope with temporary or permanent altered states.

Data collection

In relation to working and playing you will need to base your assessment on the following:

- What are the individual's experiences or attitudes to work and play?
- In which kind of working and playing activities does the person normally engage?
- How much time does the individual spend working and playing?

| Box 11.3 | Factors which may alter or disrupt the AL of working and playing |

Lifespan
- presence of illness, injury or disability preventing normal expected activity at lifespan stage.

Dependency/independency
- inability to fully undertake activities at any stage of the lifespan caused by a change in personal health, social and financial circumstances.

Factors affecting health
Biological
- presence of physical ill health or injury
- presence of disability (physical or sensory).

Psychological
- stress, inability to cope with changes
- changes in personality, mood and behaviour
- lack of motivation
- lack of knowledge to promote independency
- inability to acquire new knowledge and skills.

Sociocultural
- changes in domestic and employment circumstances
- culture, harassment and violence at work
- antisocial behaviour/disruption
- cultural restrictions.

Environmental
- exposure to risks and hazards
- lack of adequate protection
- change in work environments
- lack of recreational facilities.

Politicoeconomic
- redundancy/retirement
- high unemployment
- restricted access to social support systems
- lack of education and training opportunities.

- What factors are influencing the individual's approach towards work and play (ability, knowledge, experience, resources)?
- Has the individual had to make any previous adjustments to work or play in the past?
- What identifiable problems or difficulties is the individual currently experiencing?
- How are current problems or restrictions impacting upon normal activity?

When undertaking an assessment you will need to utilise the following skills:

- interviewing skills
- observation skills
- listening skills.

Exercise

1. Consider what assessment skills you have and the ones you need to develop when undertaking an assessment of working and playing.

INTERVIEWING

- asking open and closed questions about work and play experiences
- determining the priority of questions to be asked

- giving information and checking understanding
- involving relatives.

OBSERVATION

- verbal and nonverbal responses
- mood and personality
- body language
- physical ability and health for activity
- stress, pain and anxiety.

LISTENING

- act on verbal and nonverbal cues
- use of own body language to reassure and encourage the patient.

By using the components of the model of living with the identified assessment skills, a systematic assessment of the patient can take place. Regular use of the model in this way will help you to develop an effective assessment style and ensure that patients receive a thorough and professional assessment. The components of the model in relation to conducting an assessment of working and playing will now be considered as shown in Box 11.4.

Patient assessment exercise

Using the assessment guide outlined in Box 11.4 consider the information that you might gather from Case study 11.3.

Box 11.4	Working and playing assessment guide

Lifespan
- At what stage of the lifespan is the patient?
- Does the patient have an understanding of the importance of work and play and associated risks/hazards?
- What are the individual's normal occupational/leisure activities?
- How physically demanding are the individual's normal activities?

Dependency/independency
- What constraints are influencing dependency (e.g. age, ill health)?
- How is the individual coping with changes within the AL?
- How might the individual manage the AL in the future?

Factors affecting health
Biological
- Is the patient in good physical health?
- Is there presence of a disability?
- How is the individual's current health status affecting the AL?

Psychological
- Does the individual have sufficient understanding/information to manage the AL safely, i.e. avoid stress and hazards?

- Does the individual have sufficient knowledge to receive and be motivated by appropriate information?
- What is the individual's reaction to current health status, e.g. boredom, agitated, anxiety?
- What are the individual's reactions to other life events, e.g. retirement, redundancy?

Socioeconomic
- Is the individual's social role altered/compromised by current health status?
- To what extent are the individual's family, social or work obligations altered?
- What support does the individual require to maintain the AL?

Environmental
- Does the individual have sufficient knowledge and understanding of safety issues?
- Is the individual aware or able to assess risks/hazards in the environment?
- Does the person need help or advice?

Politicoeconomic
- Does the individual have any economic concerns?
- Does the individual require help or advice from other agencies?
- Is a lack of resources compromising health or recovery?

You can record the information on the Patient Assessment Sheets provided in Appendix 3. This case study will be used as the main scenario for the chapter. Other short case studies will be used to help you transfer your understanding of working and playing to other individual situations and other ALs.

Case study 11.3

Working and playing – main case scenario

John is a 45-year-old sports teacher at a local comprehensive school and was admitted to hospital 4 days ago following an acute myocardial infarction (AMI). He is married with three teenage children. John is highly committed to his work and has been under pressure lately with teaching and team management responsibilities, as well as arranging league games with other schools. He is presently making a good recovery from the MI but is having difficulty identifying how to adopt a healthier lifestyle in order to prevent further health problems. John believes that his interest in sport would enable him to stay healthy particularly as his own father died of a heart attack in his early 60s. John eats a healthy diet, has never smoked cigarettes and only drinks alcohol occasionally.

Exercise

Using your knowledge and experience identify what John's individual working and playing needs are, as follows:

1. Identify the normal lifespan stage/lifestyle expectations, level of dependence and the factors which have led to the health breakdown.
2. Identify the actual and potential needs/problems associated with the AL of working and playing.
3. Identify which other ALs are affected.

Assessment of lifespan, dependency and factors contributing to health breakdown

Using these components of the model will enable you to determine the individual's normal habits and routines and identify where the patient is vulnerable within the AL. This aspect of assessing working and playing focuses upon the following:

- health expectation against stage on the lifespan
- usual routines and habits
- normal dependency capability
- previous coping mechanisms.

By using the components of the model again it becomes possible to also identify the factors that have contributed to John's health breakdown as shown in Box 11.5.

From a working and playing perspective it is possible to determine that as an individual John has the following problems, which have resulted in a health breakdown:

Box 11.5 | Assessment of lifespan, dependency and factors contributing to health breakdown

Lifespan
- AMI is a common medical problem in adult life, exacerbated by a stressful lifestyle.
- Under pressure at work and home. Need to identify why John has not been able to identify or make changes to his current lifestyle.

Dependency
- High degree of dependence currently being experienced
- Dependent upon medical, nursing and pharmacological care
- Normally very independent coping with work, home and social responsibilities.

Factors leading to health breakdown
Physical
- Family history of heart disease
- Lifestyle has exceeded physical health.

Psychological
- Stress from work overload
- Unhealthy work behaviours and inability to reduce or recognise the dangers.

Sociocultural
- Personal health beliefs
- Strong work ethic and family values
- High drive to achieve success.

Environmental
- Able to combine work with leisure interests, but to the detriment of not balancing work and relaxation.

Politicoeconomic
- Pressure to achieve success for school (work) and meet targets
- Pressure to work to provide income for family.

- an acute cardiac problem which will require him to readjust his lifestyle
- a potential predisposition to heart disease
- a health education need in relation to physical activity and stress management
- a health promotion need to adopt a healthier lifestyle.

Identification of actual and potential problems associated with working and playing

Having identified the problems or needs that are individual to John, the next stage is to determine which of the problems are actual and require solving or those which are potential and require prevention. By continuing to use the factors affecting health as a framework, it becomes possible for you to apply your knowledge of health to the patient's individual situation and identify where the patient may need support to carry out the activity in the immediate and long term. Upon identification of the problem(s) it is important to recognise that nursing activities may need to be complemented with a range of other health and social care agencies.

Physical problems

Physical problems associated with the AL of working and playing are generally linked to physical health, strength, mobility and sensory function, resulting in either a temporary or permanent effect upon independence. Broadly speaking physical dependence in the activity is associated with being young, old or unable to carry out aspects of the AL without assistance from other people, equipment or services. An understanding of the issues that alter independence is essential, in order to support the needs of patients in the nursing context. In modern societies there is an increasing emphasis upon helping people to optimise their abilities to engage in work and play activities following an alteration in their normal health state (Storey 2003).

Physical disability There is a tendency to think about disabilities as being associated with familiar chronic ill-health conditions and impairments; however, because the range of conditions is so wide and varied it is difficult to have a single agreed list of classifications. Because of the range of classifications and the various ways in which disabilities are reported and recorded it is also extremely difficult to accurately measure the prevalence. In the UK it is estimated that there are 8.6–11 million people with a disability and it is recommended that specialist surveys should be carried out to improve the accuracy of information (Department for Work and Pensions 2004) Disabled people often face many barriers and discrimination that can have an impact upon their ability to engage fully within the activity of working and playing. In the UK in 1997 the government set up a Disability Rights Taskforce in order to identify the issues and advise upon what action should be taken to promote the rights of disabled people, which also includes the needs of people with learning disabilities (see **www.disability.gov.uk**).

The degree to which disabled people may be restricted within the AL will be dependent upon the particular disability and the provision of appropriate access, equipment and services. Unfortunately in many cases it will be society's attitudes towards disability that create the greatest barrier, which have consequently required a number of acts of parliament to be implemented and reviewed.

After working through the following exercise, you might initially have considered it difficult for the activities to continue, but with some adjustment, very often activities can be pursued but in different ways. As a nurse it is important to have an understanding of how other agencies can help patients achieve the required adjustments.

> **Exercise**
> 1. Identify one work and one play/leisure activity that require physical fitness.
> 2. Could the activities you have identified continue if a person had either of the following:
>   - breathing difficulties
>   - mobility difficulties.
> 3. What adjustments would be required in order to help the person continue with the activities?
> 4. How could you, as a nurse, help the patient to achieve the adjustments?

Sensory loss or impairment The loss of hearing, sight, smell and sensation can be either temporary or permanent, capable of causing a range of minor to serious effects upon the individual's ability to carry out the AL of working and playing. Actual and potential problems with loss of sensation may also impact upon other ALs such as MSE, communication and mobility and these will be further discussed in the appropriate chapters. For most people who encounter problems, a period of adjustment is required, which sometimes involves the use of new equipment and skills. As technology continues to develop, many people with sensory difficulties are able to increase their independence and enjoy new aspects of life and work. Problems with hearing and sight can occur suddenly or gradually, resulting in partial or complete loss of ability, caused from birth through a genetic disorder or throughout life by injury or disease. Problems with speech can range from mild to severe and may be related to development and learning difficulties from childhood to changes caused by injury or disease.

> **Exercise**
> 1. Identify what common diseases, accidents or injuries are associated with the following:
>   - loss of sight
>   - loss of hearing
>   - loss of speech.

Psychological problems

Psychological problems relating to the AL of working and playing have two dimensions. One is that the mental health of patients may become disrupted as a result of changes or demands within the AL and the other is that underlying health problems or learning disabilities may be affecting the ability to carry out the AL effectively. As a result it is likely that any psychological problems identified will influence personal safety and self-motivation that may in turn impact upon other ALs (Davis & Rinaldi 2004, Zijlstra & Vlaskamp 2005).

It is important to recognise that special consideration must be given to those individuals who have intellectual limitations or difficulties, in order to ensure that their needs are accurately identified.

> **Exercise**
> 1. Identify possible psychological differences between the following:
>   - a person who has been made redundant
>   - a person who has been out of work for 2 years
>   - a person who cannot pursue a career choice through disability
>   - a person who recently retired on the ground of ill health
>   - a person who has to cease a lifetime leisure activity through ill health/injury.

You may have identified that whilst the situations are different they may trigger similar kinds of health problems such as stress, depression and loss of confidence and self-esteem. The extent to which patients react to any of the situations will depend upon their individual personalities, experience and motivation, as well as having access to available support mechanisms and services.

Sociocultural problems

The purpose of identifying problems related to sociocultural aspects of living is twofold: firstly to establish an understanding of how the individual normally carries out the AL and secondly to determine how the AL has become affected by ill health or injury. For individuals who may need to adapt their lifestyle either temporarily or permanently there may be considerable anxiety surrounding personal beliefs, values and social status.

Environmental problems

Assessment of environmental problems associated with working and playing involves consideration of the following:

1. That the environment within which the individual carries out their normal activities may have resulted in a problem occurring.
2. That the problem identified may relate to activities being restricted because the environment cannot be adapted to meet their immediate or future needs.

It is also important to recognise that some of the aspects of care related to this AL may extend beyond the scope of nursing. For example, patients may need specialist advice regarding employment, state benefits or environmental adaptations. It is therefore vital that nurses have a good understanding of the roles and functions of other multidisciplinary agencies in order to ensure that appropriate and timely referrals are made.

Politicoeconomic problems

Throughout the world it is well recognised that there are strong links between ill health, poverty and an individual's subsequent ability to fully engage in meaningful work and play, for which many international agencies seek to find resolutions (WHO 2002b). Even in the UK there are wider determinants of ill health across the lifespan that are associated with social and economic inequalities (DoH 2003a) Although not all health problems are directly associated with poverty, the need to maintain economic security can result in health problems occurring and compromise recovery.

Defining actual and potential problems

Returning to Case study 11.3 it is possible to identify what John's actual and potential problems might be, as shown in Box 11.6.

Identification of impact on other ALs

In reality, rarely would one AL be affected in isolation. Whilst this chapter concentrates upon working and playing it is important to consider the impact that a change in activity might have upon the other ALs. Box 11.7 demonstrates how the problems identified from Case study 11.3 may impact upon the remaining ALs.

Box 11.6	Actual and potential problems identified for the main case scenario	
Type of problem	**Actual problems**	**Potential problems**
Physical	Is unable to work or continue leisure pursuits due to having suffered an acute myocardial infarction	May be unable to resume previous work and leisure activities
Psychological	Is anxious about his health and ability to carry out a full and active life	May be agitated and bored by being in hospital
Sociocultural	Concerned about being dependent upon others	May be concerned about career prospects
Environmental	Anxious/frustrated about his health state and the impact upon work and home	Concerned about his ability to change/reduce activities
Politicoeconomic	Concerned about his responsibilities	May be concerned about longer-term financial issues

Exercise

Using the information presented so far in this chapter consider how different your assessment and identification of working and playing might be with the following brief case studies. Check your answers against the information in Boxes 11.8, 11.9 and 11.10.

1. A 46-year-old engineer whose job requires a considerable amount of physical strength, lifting, crouching and climbing, has over the last 4 years begun to develop chronic arthritis (see Box 11.8).
2. A 21-year-old man with a promising career ahead of him is severely brain injured in a motorcycle accident. He has made a good recovery but his speech and left-sided coordination have been permanently affected (see Box 11.9).
3. A patient who is in despair from being unable to secure a job and support his family has attempted to take his own life with an overdose (see Box 11.10).

PLANNING NURSING ACTIVITIES

Planning nursing activities involves the following:

- identifying the priorities
- establishing short- and/or long-term goals
- determining the nursing actions/interventions required
- documenting the nursing care plan.

Planning nursing care accurately and effectively begins with exploring the actual and potential problems that have been identified and determining the nursing interventions that are required to achieve the following:

- to solve actual problems
- to prevent potential problems occurring
- to prevent solved problems from reoccurring
- to develop positive coping strategies for any problem which cannot be solved.

Throughout the planning phase it is important that the nurse remains focused upon the patient's problems and what is appropriate to the patient's recovery in the immediate, short and long term.

Box 11.7	Impact of actual and potential working and playing problems upon other ALs	
Activity of Living	Actual problems	Potential problems
Maintaining a safe environment	Stress at work and family history of heart disease may have contributed towards suffering the AMI	At risk from subsequent cardiac problems if lifestyle not adjusted
Communicating	Will be anxious about current health state and implications for the future work and play activities and require information and reassurance	May be unable to come to terms with future adjustments
Breathing	Pain, altered respirations and oxygen therapy will limit activity in hospital	Concern that work and play activities may cause breathing problems and pain
Eating & drinking	Loss of appetite due to anxiety or reduced activity	May need to alter diet and take regular medication to prevent further problems
Eliminating	May experience problems due to reduced activity and medication	May experience some problems if lifestyle becomes too sedentary
Personal cleansing & dressing	Will require assistance until fully recovered and mobile	May neglect self if becomes depressed about personal situation
Mobilising	Reduced mobility will prevent normal activity	Physical strength may become affected due to change in activities
Sleep & rest	Difficulties in sleeping due to change in environment, pain and/or anxiety	Difficulties in sleeping due to altered activity and worry
Expressing sexuality		May be anxious about body image and self-esteem
Maintaining body temperature	May notice changes in body temperature due to reduced activity	
Dying	Is concerned about dying	Worried about future activity and life expectancy

---

| Box 11.8 | Engineer with chronic arthritis |

Physical
- How limiting are his mobility problems in relation to work and play and other ALs?
- How has he been managing his symptoms?

Psychological
- How has he been coping?
- What is his mood and outlook on life?

Sociological
- How important is work and leisure to him?
- What support is he getting from home, family and work?
- What restrictions are being experienced?

Environmental
- Can any adaptations be made to improve/support activities?
- Is safety compromised?
- Are there any environmental factors that have contributed to the health breakdown?

Politicoeconomic
- What financial pressures exist forcing the need for activities to continue?
- Is the individual aware of resources or agencies which could help?

| Box 11.9 | Motorcyclist with a head injury |

Physical
- What activities will he be able to take part in?
- Are there any other identifiable physical risks?
- How are other ALs being affected?
- How physically fit are his carers?

Psychological
- To what extent can he express his needs?
- How is he able to communicate?
- How is his family coping with the situation?

Sociological
- Is it possible to identify his own current views and expectations?
- What are the views of his family?
- What personal support is there available?
- What social support is available?

Environmental
- What facilities exist for him to engage in work and play activities?
- Do any adjustments need to be made at home, work or for recreation?
- What risks and hazards are there?

Politicoeconomic
- What activities and facilities are there to maximise independence?
- What agencies are available to support employment and independent living?

NB: Additional information would need to be obtained, from the family and other health, social and employment care agencies.

| Box 11.10 | Patient who has taken an overdose |

Physical
- What are the risks to physical wellbeing?
- Are there any side-effects from the overdose?
- What has been the effect of unemployment on his physical health?

Psychological
- What is his current mood?
- What are the risks of a further suicide attempt?
- How long has he been feeling suicidal?
- How are other ALs being affected?
- What have been his coping mechanisms to date?
- Does he have sufficient knowledge of how to get help?

Sociological
- What support has he been getting from family, friends and other agencies?
- How has his social life changed through unemployment?
- What other social risks are there?

Environmental
- What are the risks of being isolated at home?
- What activities are available to improve his situation?

Politicoeconomic
- What is the extent of the financial problems?
- How has he managed financially so far?
- Is he aware of agencies that can help?

Factors influencing the planning stage

It is important to recognise the factors which can influence the planning stage which in relation to working and playing may be as shown in Box 11.11.

Identification of priorities

Having undertaken a comprehensive individualised assessment, the next stage is to plan the nursing care. The initial assessment will have helped to identify a range of actual and

Box 11.11	Factors influencing planning care for the AL of working and playing
Nurses	**Patients/clients**
• Knowledge of normal living and dependency across the lifespan in various cultures • Knowledge of normal physiology required for a range of work and play activities • Knowledge of how the activity of work and play might disrupt normal physiology • Knowledge and skill in required evidence base for nursing interventions • Skill in observation and assessment • Skill in determining priorities • Knowledge of a range of multiagencies to support health and social care including employment services and legislation • Staffing levels, skill mix, supervision and ongoing professional development	• An understanding of the importance of health in relation to work and play • Personal beliefs, values and experiences • Ability to communicate needs and describe expectations and feelings • Anxiety/concern about coping mechanisms • Ability to discuss very private and personal aspects of life

potential problems within the AL and give an indication of the impact this is having on the other ALs. In order to plan effective care focused upon solving actual problems and preventing potential ones from occurring, you will need to determine the priorities for nursing care. Initially life-threatening problems associated with other ALs may take priority over working and playing problems, but as the patient begins to make good progress towards a physical recovery it is important that any problems associated with working and playing are given priority. By using the dependency/independency element of the model it is possible to develop priority criteria to help determine the degree of altered dependency that the patient is experiencing. Box 11.12 shows an example of dependency/independency criteria.

It is important to recognise that dependence/independence can change and this requires continuous assessment.

> **Exercise**
> 1. In relation to Case study 11.3 review the actual and potential problems identified and determine the priority against them (see Box 11.13).

The priorities identified amongst the other ALs are described in Box 11.14.

You will see from this exercise that John's problems in relation to work and play would not, in the immediate phase of his care, take priority over other physical life-threatening problems such as the potential for cardiac arrest and associated psychological needs. As John begins to make a physical recovery and prepare for discharge, concerns about his return to normal living will take on an increasing priority. The information in Boxes 11.12 and 11.13 also illustrates the interrelatedness between the ALs, which is important to recognise in order to ensure that holistic care is provided.

> **Exercise**
> 1. You may wish to return to the brief case studies and identify the actual and potential problems associated with each.

Goal setting

Goal setting in relation to the AL of working and playing is dependent upon the extent to which normal activity is altered and the anticipated timescale for returning to an agreed level of independence. For example, a relatively minor problem may result in a patient being able to resume normal activities within hours, whilst for some patients they may never return to the previous level of activity and require complete readjustments to the AL, which may take many years. The goal statement is important as it describes what the patient is expected to, or has agreed to, achieve. In relation to working and playing, the overall goal(s) may need to be broken down into immediate, short and long term, recognising that optimum dependence within the AL may take place over a period of time. When setting goals, it is important to ensure that information about individual normal habits and routines, identified during the assessment phase, are acknowledged and integrated into the goal statement. This will help to ensure that goals are both realistic and achievable, and, wherever possible, goals should be agreed with the patient (see Chapter 1). The more realistic, measurable and observable the goal(s), the easier it becomes to monitor and evaluate the progress the patient is making. Box 11.15 outlines the short- and long-term goals identified for John that are central to:

Box 11.12	Dependency/independency priority criteria
Priority 1	Completely independent in the AL/independency maintained
Priority 2	Potential problem in the AL/remains mostly independent
Priority 3	Actual problems identified within more than one AL/some dependency noted but remains mostly independent
Priority 4	Existence of actual and potential problems in a number of other ALs with associated increasing dependency
Priority 5	Life-threatening actual and potential problems/total dependency

Box 11.13	Priority of actual and potential working and playing problems related to main case scenario				
Working and playing	Actual problems	Priority	Potential problems	Priority
Physical	Has an excessive workload and social commitments which limit relaxation time	3	At risk from subsequent cardiac problems if lifestyle not adjusted	5
Psychological	Is anxious about his health and ability to carry out a full and active life	3	May be agitated and bored by being in hospital	3
Sociocultural	Concerned about being dependent upon others	3	May be concerned about career prospects	3
Environmental	Anxious/frustrated about his health state and the impact upon work and home	3	Concerned about his ability to change/reduce activities	3
Politicoeconomic	Concerned about financial circumstances and career prospects	3/4	May be concerned about longer-term financial issues	3

Box 11.14	Identification of main case scenario priorities in all other ALs				
Activity of Living	Actual problems	Priority	Potential problems	Priority
Maintaining a safe environment	Overwork has contributed towards suffering an AMI	4	At risk from subsequent cardiac problems if lifestyle not adjusted	4
Communicating	Will be anxious about current health state and implications for the future work and play activities and require information and reassurance	3	May be unable to come to terms with future adjustments	1
Breathing	Pain, altered respirations and oxygen therapy may limit activity in hospital	4	Concern that work and play activities may cause breathing problems and pain	4
Eating & drinking	Loss of appetite due to anxiety or reduced activity	3	May need to alter diet and take regular medication to prevent further problems	3
Eliminating	May experience problems due to reduced activity and medication	3	May experience some problems if lifestyle becomes too sedentary	2
Personal cleansing & dressing	Will require assistance until fully recovered and mobile	2/3	May neglect self if becomes depressed about personal situation	2/3
Mobilising	Reduced mobility will prevent normal activity	3/4	Physical strength may become affected due to change in activities	2/3
Sleep & rest	Difficulties in sleeping due to change in environment, pain and/or anxiety	3/4	Difficulties in sleeping due to altered activity and worry	3/4
Expressing sexuality			May be anxious about body image and self-esteem	2/3
Maintaining body temperature	May notice changes in body temperature due to reduced activity	3		
Dying	Is concerned about dying	3	Worried about future activity and life expectancy	3/4

Box 11.15	Identification of short- and long-term goals for working and playing problems for Case study 11.3		
Problem	Short term	Long term
John is currently unable to work or continue leisure pursuits due to having suffered an acute myocardial infarction	To identify the lifestyle changes that are required to enable recovery and consideration for a safe return to work and play activities	To return to work having recognised own physical safety limits and adopt healthy work and recreational behaviours that limit physical exertion to limit further cardiac problems

- helping him to understand why his AMI occurred
- helping him to recognise what activities may cause further symptoms
- helping him to adopt an altered lifestyle.

Once the short- and long-term goals have been set the appropriate nursing actions can be planned to enable the goals to be achieved.

Exercise

1. You may wish to return to the brief case studies and identify the short- and long-term goals associated with each patient.

IMPLEMENTING CARE TO MEET WORKING AND PLAYING NEEDS AND PROBLEMS

Having identified the actual and potential problems and agreeing where possible with the patient and/or significant carer the desired goals, the next step is to produce and implement a care plan. By using the factors affecting health as framework, a range of nursing interventions, specifically associated with the activity of working and playing can be identified. The aim of the nursing interventions is to help individual patients resume a lifestyle that is as healthy and normal as possible.

This section will outline the most common interventions under the headings of the five factors affecting health, broadly describing the dependency, comforting and preventative aspects of nursing as outlined by the Roper et al model (1996). It is essential that as a nurse you constantly update your knowledge and skills in the areas outlined as follows in order to ensure that patients receive quality care.

Nursing interventions related to physical factors influencing ill health

The object of nursing actions related to the patient's physical problems within the AL of working and playing are central to:

- helping restore optimum physical health and lifestyle
- helping to prevent further complications
- helping the patient to cope with any physical and lifestyle changes.

For every different type of work and play activity, some kind of physical ability is required. Many chronically disabling diseases and common accidents which impact upon the ability to carry out the AL will basically require the cardiopulmonary, nervous and musculoskeletal systems. The many activities that have been identified so far highlight, as with the AL of maintaining a safe environment, that no one single biological system can be aligned to the AL of working and playing. When planning care for individual patients, it is essential that the systems affected are fully identified and that you have sufficient understanding of any associated biological function. To this extent all the other AL chapters will contain information that may be appropriate to the AL of working and playing, demonstrating once again the interrelatedness of the model.

Physical disability

Every day nurses encounter patients with disabilities and altered activity, be this either temporary or permanent, but for the patient this can be a very frightening experience. A physical disability is often defined by the medical diagnosis, which creates an emphasis upon physical and medical needs. In doing so, the potential exists for patients to adopt what is referred to as the *sick role* (Young 2004). This is characterised by an increased dependence upon carers, social withdrawal and a reduction in the ability to adapt to new lifestyles. Whilst it is vital to ensure that the patient's physical and medical needs are met, it is equally important to ensure that working and playing needs are not neglected at the expense of other priorities. The nurse must remember that for patients there may be considerable concern related to this AL and that failure to identify or provide adequate support for needs may ultimately affect recovery. Regaining optimum independence in the AL can take many weeks, months or even years. In the UK it is estimated that over 15 million people are living with long-term conditions which cannot currently be cured, such as heart disease, respiratory disease and diabetes. As a result a 10-year programme of major health reform is currently underway in order to ensure that the future needs of people with long-term conditions can be met (DoH 2005c, 2006). This will require a range of health and social care professionals to work collaboratively in order to provide integrated programmes of care, of which nurses will play a pivotal role in ensuring that timely and accurate patient assessments and referrals are conducted (Ouwens et al 2005). To be effective in supporting patients with disabilities the nurse should concentrate upon the following actions:

- supporting the patient's physical recovery from injury or disease
- making appropriate and timely referrals to other professionals and agencies in order to maximise physical, environmental and socioeconomic support mechanisms
- helping the patient/family come to terms with their disability
- helping patients determine what limitations the disability places upon them
- helping patients/families to make decisions, priorities and identify needs
- providing sufficient and accurate care and discharge information.

For some patients with severe physical problems it may not be possible for them to live independently without the support of family, friends, specialised equipment and/or facilities. Box 11.16 gives an example nursing care plan to meet John's physical needs.

Box 11.16	Nursing care plan to support identified physical needs in relation to the working and playing main case scenario	
Problem	**Goal**	**Nursing intervention**
Has an excessive workload and social commitments which limit relaxation time At risk from subsequent cardiac problems if lifestyle not adjusted	To help the patient identify the lifestyle changes he needs to make in order to promote a full recovery and prevent further complications	Identify short- and medium-term physical limitations Assess lifestyle, make decisions and priorities Identify changes to work and recreational activities to limit physical exertion Plan individualised mobilisation programme Plan recovery programme and identify changes/support at work

Nursing actions associated with psychological factors influencing ill health

Illness and injury within the AL of working and playing can have a radical impact upon the lives of patients and their families, causing extreme stress and anxiety, especially when faced with the prospect of permanent disabilities (Larner 2005). Many patients experience feelings of disbelief, anger, grief and a sense of hopelessness, which they may find difficult to express. The scope of nursing care is to anticipate the patient's feelings and handle situations that arise as sensitively and honestly as possible in order to help patients cope with and manage their conditions. In the UK this has also led to the introduction of Expert Patient Programmes (EPP), designed to help patients develop skills and confidence to better manage their conditions (DoH 2001c, Thomas 2004). At the same time it is also important to encourage as much patient independence as possible in order to prevent adoption of the sick role. Early detection of any signs of depression and immediate referral to the appropriate specialist is essential if the patient's recovery is to be optimised. Patients should be encouraged to balance activity and rest during their recovery period. Some patients, however, may feel agitated and bored during their recovery and will need access to appropriate activities. Introduction to activities such as relaxation techniques can help patients to plan how they might manage necessary lifestyle changes. There should always be a broad range of activities available to meet the patient's physical and individual needs. These are commonly books, board games, television, music and access to telephones/mobile phones and the internet. Providing that health and safety is not compromised the patient can be supported to maintain a limited amount of work and

domestic responsibilities, as often the anxiety of being isolated can cause additional strain. This has the advantage of making some observations about how the patient might cope beyond discharge.

For some people with learning difficulties or mental health problems it may not be possible for them to gain or maintain full independence in the AL. Community living and rehabilitation services exist to help individuals learn how to cope and be valued within society. Many voluntary organisations, training centres and employers provide support and opportunities for even the most profoundly disabled people to gain work, leisure and life skills (see useful disability websites at the end of this chapter.). The psychological care identified for the main case scenario is illustrated in Box 11.17.

Nursing actions associated with sociocultural factors affecting ill health

Nursing care related to sociocultural factors involves supporting patients to maintain as normal a lifestyle as possible, from the onset of illness through to discharge and beyond. For many patients a return to normal activity will take place within a matter of weeks, as soon as healing has taken place and physical strength is regained. Some patients, however, will need to make significant changes to their work and lifestyle. If patients are expected to achieve their recovery goals, it is vital that their individuality within the AL is fully appreciated and that social care as well as health care needs are provided for, by involving a range of professionals such as therapists, social workers and other specialist advisors. The aim of nursing care from the outset is to encourage optimum independence associated with the effects of being isolated and a loss of personal influence and control due to illness or injury. As

Box 11.17	Nursing care plan to support identified psychological needs in relation to the working and playing main case scenario	
Problem	**Goal/aim**	**Nursing intervention**
John is anxious about his health and ability to carry out a full and active life John may be agitated and bored by being in hospital	To minimise anxiety and promote independence	Encourage John to express concerns to staff and family Listen carefully and observe nonverbal communications Deal with issues sensitively and honestly Record progress accurately and report/refer concerns immediately Identify activities to relieve boredom/agitation

previously mentioned, the nurse must acknowledge the risk that patients can become overly dependent upon their carers, be they nurses or family members. To limit this it is important to set independence goals that the patient can work towards that are realistic and achievable. Alternatively some patients may have difficulty in coming to terms with being cared for by someone else and a flexible and creative approach to meeting the patient's needs will be required. By realising the disruption that illness or disability can cause within the AL, it is possible for the nurse to recognise how situations might be adapted. The aim is to help patients maintain their normal, everyday lives, even though they may be restricted by their physical state or environment. In a multicultural society like the UK, individual needs will vary enormously and the nurse must have an understanding of the basic needs and difference reflected within the local community (Hogg & Holland 2001, Henley & Schott 2001).

Providing creative solutions for patients not only promotes independence but also provides the nurse with the opportunity to make some observations about how the patient may cope during recovery and after discharge.

When the AL of working and playing is disturbed through illness or disability, normal day-to-day contact with family, friends and other work and social groups alters. In the family this can create difficulties, particularly if the family members are themselves normally dependent upon the patient, for example a young mother with children or an elderly husband who looks after an infirm wife. By recognising the needs of patients to maintain some control over their responsibilities, a flexible approach to care can be maximised through flexible visiting arrangements. Access to telephones is another important way of helping patients keep in touch with family, friends and work colleagues. Increasingly the use of text messaging and email is used. In some hospitals patients may be able to access email through computers that are sited near the bedside and in general patient areas.

In the home, patients are able to control visitors, but in hospital the activity can be restricted in a number of ways. The nurse must recognise the importance that visiting plays in supporting the psychological and sociocultural needs of the patient, in order to minimise some of the problems that are associated with the experience of isolation and separation. However, it is also important that patients have sufficient periods of rest, and there will be some occasions when the nurse will need to advise the patient and family, particularly if this is having an adverse effect upon the patient's recovery. Overall, visiting arrangements need to take into consideration the need to balance safety and flexibility to benefit both the patient, their families, other patients and the care environment (Plowright 2005, Tanner 2005).

Essentially nursing care associated with the patient's sociocultural needs concentrates upon preparation for discharge and needs to involve the family and significant carers. It is important to bear in mind that standard discharge information needs to be tailored to specific needs, for example men and women often have different needs and support mechanisms which must be taken into consideration. In 2002, the Department of Health introduced the Patient Advisory and Liaison Service (PALS) into every hospital and Primary Care Trust to support and improve the access and information needs of patients and encourage staff to be more responsive to patients' needs. The service acts as a catalyst for improving the care of patients in any health care setting by responding to concerns and complaints expressed by patients and their families and providing feedback to the organisation. Nurses should know where the PALS department is situated within their organisation in order to appropriately signpost patients and families. More importantly nurses should engage with the service so that they may learn how to make often simple improvements that can lead to enhancing the patient's experience (DoH 2003b).

> **Exercise**
>
> What individual recovery differences might there be for the following patients who have undergone abdominal surgery:
>
> 1. A 40-year-old married man with a physical job.
> 2. A 36-year-old single parent with two children under 12 years and a part-time job.
> 3. A 70-year-old lady who lives alone.

It may have been noted that each of the patients in the exercise will have different levels of support available to them. Differences in age, domestic, social and financial circumstances will all influence the extent to which standard discharge guidance will be followed. Discharge information therefore should not only be clear but also relevant to each individual taking into consideration the following:

- individual ability
- age
- gender
- interests/habits and routines
- personality
- previous lifestyle
- work environment
- home environment
- leisure environment.

For some patients, however, a return to a previous lifestyle is not possible and whilst this is daunting there is often the opportunity to gain new skills and interests. The impact of chronic illness or disability can severely restrict social roles and functions, causing patients to withdraw from domestic, social and recreational activities. Patients may also be fearful of social attitudes towards them, causing them to withdraw even further. Often patients can benefit from counselling and psychotherapy to help them develop personal confidence and self-worth, assertive skills and stress management techniques (Bishop 2005). In order to help patients and their families achieve as normal a life as possible, nursing care must be based upon preserving patient individuality and dignity. In addition it is vital that the nursing care plan reflects the interventions that specialists from other agencies can make towards enhancing patient care, helping both patients and their families live as normal a life as possible. Box 11.18 identifies the nursing interventions associated with John's sociocultural needs.

Nursing actions associated with environmental factors affecting ill health

Ill health and disability often limit mobility and subsequently restrict activities, particularly outdoor activities. In hospital it can be difficult to provide patients with a range of activities sufficient to their needs of promoting independence and preventing boredom. The role of the nurse is to help the patient identify a range of activities that can be carried out whilst either confined to bed or the immediate ward area, such as the dayroom. Some patients may be well enough to use other facilities available within the hospital such as shops, cafés, gardens, play areas, library and multi-denominational places of worship. There may also be other activities that are arranged as part of the patient's recovery or rehabilitation programme such as physiotherapy and occupational therapy sessions. The nurse, in conjunction with the appropriate allied health professional, has a responsibility to identify any risks that might be associated with any

activities and ensure that reasonable action has been taken to prevent any accidents or incidents occurring. In hospital a certain amount of equipment and staff will be available to promote activities, but in the home patients may require adaptations to be made, before independent living can be optimised (see Chapter 3). In the workplace employers are encouraged to provide appropriate facilities and flexible approaches to helping people back to work. In order to engage fully in work and play activities, patients may require a range of appliances and adaptations to be available either in the home, at work or in places for play, education or leisure. Without proper support and resources, patients are at risk from being increasingly isolated in their own homes.

For children, admission to hospital can be strange, frightening and even dangerous. The natural curiosity of children in play has the potential for accidents to happen and again the nurse must be able to identify and prevent risks. If necessary an education service can be provided within the hospital and play coordinators and therapists provide specialist support for play in accordance with the individual needs of the child. Paediatric units recognise the importance of supporting family-centred care in order to enhance normality for the child but also support the coping needs of parents (Glasper & Richardson 2005).

Box 11.19 describes the nursing interventions associated with environmental needs for the main case scenario.

Box 11.18	Nursing care plan to support identified sociocultural needs in relation to the working and playing main case scenario	
Problem	Goal/aim	Nursing intervention
John may have concerns about work and home life	To minimise anxiety and encourage contact with family and work colleagues to promote a safe recovery	• Encourage John to express concerns with family and to staff • Encourage family to discuss concerns with staff • Listen carefully and observe nonverbal communications • Support contact with work in conjunction with John and his family in order to reduce anxiety • Ensure financial concerns are properly referred • Agree with John a recovery plan central to his work and recreational activities

Box 11.19	Nursing care plan to support identified environmental needs in relation to the working and playing main case scenario	
Problem	Goal/aim	Nursing intervention
John may feel agitated and constrained by the reduced activity due to confinement to the ward	Ensure safety and promote independence in preparation for discharge	• Familiarise John with the ward and any routines and equipment • Point out safety measures and risks • Show John how to call for assistance if required • Agree types of activities that can be undertaken safely during the recovery period • Discuss with John how he might assess risks within the home or work in preparation for discharge

Nursing actions associated with politicoeconomic factors affecting ill health

When patients become ill or disabled it is important to acknowledge that not all their anxieties will be related to their physical health and that they may have greater concerns about their financial circumstances and ability to return to work. For some people an absence from work may affect promotion or training prospects and a chronic illness or disability may even lead to the patient having to change jobs and possibly retrain. It is important that nurses are aware of the information and agencies that are available to support the patient's individual needs in order to reduce anxiety and promote independence. At the most basic level, patients should be provided with information regarding their recovery and supported to identify how their health status may affect normal working and playing activities. If patients need financial support they should be given accurate information about what they may be entitled to and how to make the claim.

Patients who are likely to be away from work for long periods or unable to return to their original type of work will need specialist advice from a range of agencies. However, navigating the way through the variety of benefit agencies that are available can be very daunting and confusing. In helping patients and their families or carers, it is essential that nurses have a broad understanding about the types of allowances that are available and ensure that referrals are made immediately. For example there are specific allowances available to help patients, their families and carers with hospital travel costs, carer and attendance allowances. As a resource DirectGov is an online service that brings together a wide range of public service information, providing factsheets and web links for further advice and application forms (**www.direct.gov.uk**).

Exercise

Think about some of the legislation and agencies that you have been introduced to within this chapter and consider the following:

1. What other professionals or organisations could you contact to help?
2. How can you keep up to date with legislation and service developments?
3. How might you best provide patients with information?
4. If you live outside the UK consider these questions in relation to your own country.

By understanding the politicoeconomic needs associated with ill health and injury nursing care can focus upon ensuring that the patient has access to accurate information and advice regarding employment and health promotion.

Promoting health

It is important to recognise that when promoting health there may be a cost implication that may prevent the patient from achieving set goals. For example patients who need to purchase special foods or medications may appear to be noncompliant with their treatment when in fact there is an underlying financial implication. In addition nurses need to recognise that ill health may be directly linked to working life. For example it may be difficult for patients to avoid factors which are contributing towards their ill health because they cannot afford to change jobs or learn new skills. Alternatively patients may become ill as a result of being unable to work, and an exploration of this with the patient may reveal that health problems such as increased alcohol intake, increased smoking, drug dependency, poor diet, stress and insomnia may be linked directly to unemployment (Mathers & Schofield 1998, Bartley & Ferrie 2001). It is therefore important that nurses recognise early how the patient's health and lifestyle might have been affected over time by work activities and the need to secure an income.

Access to work and play

Following an episode of ill health or an injury, most patients will return to normal individual activities fairly quickly, without any complications. Patients with long-term health problems or disabilities, however, will need support to find alternative activities and possibly learn new skills. One of the greatest problems facing individuals with disabilities is discrimination and a lack of understanding and opportunity on behalf of employers. In recognition of the rights of disabled people to secure and retain employment and enjoy recreational activities many pieces of legislation have been introduced, including:

- Disability Discrimination Act 2005
- Community Care Act 1990
- Human Rights Act 1998.

The legislation is geared not only to assist disabled people to gain access to work and leisure but also to change public and employer attitudes towards recognising the value and contribution that disabled people can make. In the UK, employers have been actively encouraged through the *Disability Symbol* accreditation scheme to review their recruitment and employment policies in order to recruit and retain people with disabilities (Department for Work and Pensions 2006). In addition there are a variety of government services and agencies that exist to help people find suitable employment, redeployment and access to financial support. In addition a range of specialist living, employment and training centres exist nationally to provide information, education, equipment and support within communities and nurses need to be aware of what services are available within their areas.

Within the nursing care plan it is important not to ignore the play and recreational needs, remembering that these activities provide a balance to the whole AL. For children in the UK most hospitals and other health and social care environments recognise the importance of providing resources either in terms of personnel or equipment to prevent boredom or support continuing developmental and social needs (Mitchell et al 2004). The range of activities therefore needs to cater for babies right through to adolescents. Providing such a range of resources can be expensive and often this depends upon donations and fundraising activities. All equipment requires careful consideration, particularly if they are potentially a safety hazard in relation to falls, ingestion or cross-infection. Other equipment may be expensive and pose security risks, such as handheld electronic games, mobile phones, etc. The nurse will need to assess carefully each particular child's needs in relation to the following:

- age
- physical, psychological and social developmental stage
- length of stay
- safety knowledge and needs.

Upon discharge from hospital, parents and families often require detailed advice about play and return to school. Advice needs to be practical and realistic and related to what is known about family circumstances. For example it may be difficult for a parent to take extended leave from work to look after a child and this may have a financial impact upon the family. The nurse has an important role in ensuring that parents have access to accurate information and other services in order to prevent financial difficulties.

Provision of recreation resources for adults equally requires careful attention, and the nurse should not presume that all patients can have their needs met through watching television, reading or doing jigsaws. Supporting a patient's recreational needs begins with the nurse identifying what the patient's usual recreational activities are and find some way to support individual needs whilst in hospital and if necessary beyond discharge. Often the onset of illness and disability reduces independent access to some of the most basic personal resources such as money to buy newspapers or snacks or make telephone calls. The nurse needs to recognise that this can have detrimental effects upon a patient's recovery, as shown in the following exercise.

Exercise

Eve is an 83-year-old retired school teacher who has no immediate relatives. She has suffered with rheumatoid arthritis for many years and has been admitted to hospital with a fractured femur. Her usual daily recreation is to read the *Times* newspaper. The staff on the ward are concerned that she is becoming increasingly withdrawn.

1. Why do you think Eve is becoming withdrawn?
2. What might be the economic factor influencing her recovery?

You may have discovered one of many things about Eve as follows:

- Eve's preferred daily activity of reading the newspaper enables her to keep in touch with world affairs.
- Her individual need to read a newspaper had not been assessed or met.
- Due to being an emergency admission she does not have any money with her.
- It may be some time before she has a visitor.
- She may not have reading glasses with her.
- She may have been too embarrassed to ask for help or money.
- Observations of withdrawal are in relation to social deprivation.

This exercise demonstrates the importance of acknowledging and assessing the economic factors that can influence health and its recovery. In the home the patient would make more independent choices about the types of activities they could engage in, but in hospital the provision of more individualised resources can be difficult.

Many hospitals now have cash machines available at a central site and are installing individual bedside telephones and pay-per-view televisions. However, not all patients use cash cards and some may not have enough money to spend on such amenities and the issue of security for personal belongings becomes a cause for concern.

The issues raised in this section have highlighted the importance of assessing the politicoeconomic factors

Box 11.20	Nursing care plan to support identified politicoeconomic needs in relation to the working and playing main case scenario	
Problem	Goal/aim	Nursing intervention
John may have concerns about financial issues	To reduce any anxieties	• Discuss any concerns with John and his family • Provide accurate and timely information • Make appropriate and timely referrals to specialist agencies and advisors

affecting health in order to ensure that nursing care is appropriate to individual needs at a variety of stages in the patient's recovery. Box 11.20 describes the issues that John from Case study 11.3 might have in relation to politicoeconomic factors and his current ill-health state.

IMPLEMENTING WORKING AND PLAYING NURSING ACTIVITIES

The delivery of quality care is dependent upon the quality of the information detailed within the nursing care plan. In the care setting a variety of health professionals will need to refer to the nursing care plan and it is essential that the plan is conducive to the delivery of consistency in care standards. Prior to the implementation of nursing activities the following must be in place:

1. A detailed written care plan and verbal handover to ensure that all staff are aware of patient progress, goals to be achieved and skills required to deliver the care.
2. Competent practitioners are identified to safely deliver the planned care.
3. Nursing actions and patient progress are recorded and goals are evaluated.

The nursing plan is a document that guides the required nursing activities to help the patient achieve the identified goals. The plan should be constantly reviewed and updated to record the following:

- when a goal/desired outcome has been achieved
- when nursing intervention has been changed to support goal achievement
- when the goal needs to be modified
- when the evaluation date needs to be changed
- when problems change or develop.

Factors influencing implementation of working and playing nursing actions

To ensure the effectiveness of implementing the working and playing plan it is important to identify the factors that might influence this.

Knowledge
- normal health and the impact of illness on the AL
- psychological health and requirements for engaging in the AL
- social and cultural implications for poor health or recovery
- environmental influences and concerns
- political and economic influences and concerns
- knowledge of care and services outside of the sphere of health (social and employment services).

Skill and competency
- philosophy of care and attitudes to patient care
- communication/interpersonal skills

- observation skills
- problem-solving skills
- technical/caring skills
- management/leadership skills (directing, coaching, delegating, supervising skills)
- teaching skills
- research skills.

Resources
- appropriate skill mix
- sufficient equipment
- sufficient support services
- knowledge of and access to specialist agencies.

Working and playing and medically derived care

In addition to the identified nursing care plan it is also important to consider the impact that medical or other health care intervention can have which requires the nurses to integrate into the plan, as described in Box 11.21.

EVALUATION OF NURSING ACTIVITIES

The evaluation stage provides the basis by which to determine if the patient is making the desired progress and provides the mechanism for judging the effectiveness of the nursing actions. Evaluation activities should be ongoing and take place on a continuous, hourly, daily or shift basis in accordance with the level of disturbance associated within the AL.

To evaluate effectively the following skills are required:

- observing
- interviewing
- listening
- analysing
- measuring.

The steps in evaluating are as follows. It is recommended that where possible the patient is involved in describing the progress/achievement made.

1. Check the identified goals against patient progress:
   - Have the goals been partially or completely met?
2. Is the timescale realistic?
3. Record the progress as follows:
   - goal completely met, state the evidence to support this and discontinue the problem
   - goal partially met, then decide if there is a need to extend the timescale or modify the plan
   - goal not met, then decide if there is a need to extend the timescale, change the plan or reassess the whole problem.

Box 11.22 provides you with an evaluation of John's care and identifies the evidence and nursing skills that would be required to make an accurate evaluation.

Box 11.21	Identification of medical and social care associated with working and playing
Medical and social derived care	**Nursing intervention/support**
Specific medicotechnical intervention	• Knowledge, skill and competency to manage equipment, observe results and report changes • Knowledge and skill to describe to patients the effects upon the AL of working and playing
Specific pharmacological intervention	• Knowledge and skill regarding action and side effects • Knowledge and skill to describe to patients the effects upon the AL of working and playing
Specific nutritional information intervention	• Knowledge and skill to support patient Knowledge and skill to describe to patients the effects upon the AL of working and playing
Specific physiotherapy intervention	• Knowledge and skill to provide 24 hour continuing physiotherapy care Knowledge and skill to describe to patients the effects upon the AL of working and playing
Specific social, occupational and employment service intervention	• Knowledge of available services and professional specialists. Skill in assessment and referral • Knowledge and skill to describe to patients the effects upon the AL of working and playing

Box 11.22	Evaluation skills and evidence related to the main case scenario	
Goals/aims	**Evaluation skills**	**Evaluation evidence**
To help John identify the necessary lifestyle changes that he will need to make in order to continue work, family and recreation activities, that meet his needs and prevent further cardiac problems	Communication skills Interviewing skills Observation skills Information finding skills Assessment skills Negotiation skills Problem-solving skills Creative skills	• John will be able to express some confidence about his recovery and return to independent living • John asks questions freely and demonstrates control over his recovery and return to work and home • John will be able to discuss the information and help he has been given • John will have been able to maintain contact with work and home without this having a detrimental affect upon his health • John's family will express confidence about his discharge from hospital • John is able to identify activities and situations which may create health problems

Box 11.23	Plan review for the main case scenario	
Goal	**Evaluation**	**Plan review**
To help John identify the necessary lifestyle changes that he will need to make, in order to continue work, family and recreation activities that meet his needs and prevent further cardiac problems	John has made a good recovery from his AMI He is confident about his discharge from hospital and is able to describe how he will adapt his lifestyle accordingly John will need to continue medical treatment and cardiac rehabilitation	Care and observation will continue as an out-patient May need referral to appropriate health, social and employment specialists, for example: • Stress counsellor • Practice nurse/GP • Social worker • Cardiac support group • Employment services • Physiotherapist • Occupational health • Dietitian

Plan review

If the goals are achieved, nursing actions effectively become redundant. Where goals are not achieved the following questions need to be asked:

1. Is more information required to determine goal achievement?
2. Should the nursing plan be adapted to enable the goal to be achieved?
3. Has the problem changed?
4. Can the planned nursing care be stopped?
5. Has the problem worsened?
6. Should the goal and intervention be reviewed?
7. Was the goal inappropriate?
8. Does the plan require intervention from other health care professionals?

John's plan recognised that long-term goals could not be realistically met during his hospital stay. Therefore upon discharge information regarding his progress and continuing care needs would need to be accurately forwarded to the appropriate professional who will be involved in John's care, as shown in Box 11.23.

SUMMARY POINTS

1. The model is intrinsically linked to the model of living.
2. The AL of working and playing can be affected by ill health and also be the cause of health-related problems.
3. Individualised nursing care can be accomplished by using the four stages of the nursing process in conjunction with the components of the model.
4. Accurate, continuous assessment is vital as all other stages are dependent upon it.
5. All stages can be influenced by various situational factors relating to the nurse, the patient, relatives and the environment.
6. A variety of skills and other professionals are required to deliver optimum care to patients.

References

Bartley M, Ferrie J 2001 Glossary: unemployment, job insecurity and health. Journal of Epidemiology and Community Health 55(11):776–781

Bishop M 2005 Quality of life and psychosocial adaptation to chronic illness and acquired disability: a conceptual and theoretical synthesis. Journal of Rehabilitation 71(2):5–13

Boeri T, Brugiavni A, Calmfors L 2001 The role of unions in the twenty-first century. Oxford University Press, London

British Broadcasting Company (BBC) 2006 Man guilty of 21 cockling deaths (news.bbc.co.uk/1/hi/england/lancashire/4832454.stm)

Brown DW, Balluz LS, Ford ES et al 2003 Associations between short- and long-term unemployment and frequent mental distress among a national sample of men and women. Journal of Occupational and Environmental Medicine 45(11):1159–1166

Caspi A, Lahey BB, Moffitt TE 2003 Causes of conduct disorder and juvenile delinquency. Guilford Press, East Sussex

Childcare Act 2006. HMSO, London (www.opsi.gov.uk/acts/acts2006/20060021.htm)

Christiansen CH, Matuska KM 2006 Lifestyle balance: a review of the concepts and research. Journal of Occupational Science 13(1):49–61

Community Care Act 1990. HMSO, London (www.opsi.gov.uk/ACTS/acts1990/Ukpga_19900019_en_1.htm)

Cox T, Griffiths A, Rial Gonzalez E 2000 Research on work related stress. European Agency for Safety and Health at Work. Office for Official Publications of the European Communities, Luxembourg (agency.asha.eu.int/publications/reports/stress)

Crompton R 2006 Employment and the family: The reconfiguration of work and family life in contemporary societies. Cambridge University Press, Cambridge

Davis M, Rinaldi M 2004 Using an evidence based approach to enable people with mental health problems to gain and retain employment, education and voluntary work. British Journal of Occupational Therapy 67(7):319–322

Department for Education and Skills 2003 Tackling bullying: Listening to the views of children and young people. DfES, Nottingham (www.dfes.gov.uk/bullying/pdf/Childline%20DP%20Bullying%20(download).pdf)

Department for Education and Skills 2005 Skills: Getting on in business, getting on in work. The Stationery Office, London (ww.dfes.gov.uk/publications/skillsgettingon/)

Department for Education and Skills 2006 Don't suffer in silence. DfES (www.dfes.gov.uk/bullying/index.shtml)

Department of Health 2000 The NHS plan: a plan for investment, a plan for reform. HMSO, London

Department of Health 2001a Working together – learning together a framework for lifelong learning in he NHS. HMSO, London (www.dh.gov.uk/assetRoot/04/05/88/96/04058896.pdf)

Department of Health 2001b Improving working lives standard. DoH Publications, London (www.dh.gov.uk/assetRoot/04/07/40/65/04074065.pdf)

Department of Health 2001c The expert patient: a new approach to chronic disease management for the 21st century. DoH Publications, London (www.dh.gov.uk/assetRoot/04/01/85/78/04018578.pdf)

Department of Health 2003a Tackling health inequalities: a programme for action. DoH Publications, London (www.dh.gov.uk/assetRoot/04/01/93/62/04019362.pdf)

Department of Health 2003b PALS core national standards and evaluation framework. DoH Publications, London (www.dh.gov.uk/assetRoot/04/11/93/15/04119315.pdf)

Department of Health 2005a A national framework to support local workforce strategy development: A guide for HR directors in the NHS and social care. DoH Publications, London (www.dh.gov.uk/assetRoot/04/12/47/47/04124747.pdf)

Department of Health 2005b Commissioning a patient led NHS. DoH Publications, London (www.dh.gov uk/PublicationsAndStatistics/Publications/PublicationsPolicyAndGuidance/PublicationsPolicyAndGuidanceArticle/fs/en?CONTENT_ID=4116716&chk;=/%2Bb2QD)

Department of Health 2005c National service framework for long term conditions. DoH Publications, London (www.dh.gov.uk/assetRoot/04/10/53/69/04105369.pdf)

Department of Health 2006 Our health, our care, our say: making it happen. Health and social care working in partnership. DoH Publications, London (www.dh.gov.uk/assetRoot/04/14/00/65/04140065.pdf)

Department of Trade and Industry 2003 Flexible working – the right to request and the duty to consider: a guide for employers and employees. HMSO, London (www.dti.gov.uk/files/file21364.pdf)

Department for Work and Pensions 2004 Review of disability estimates and definitions. HMSO, London (www.dwp.gov.uk/asd/asd5/ih2003-2004/IH128.pdf)

Department for Work and Pensions 2005 Five year strategy: opportunity and security throughout life. HMSO, London (www.dwp.gov.uk/publications/dwp/2005/5_yr_strat/pdf/report.pdf)

Department for Work and Pensions 2006 Jobcentre plus, disability symbol. DWP (www.jobcentreplus.gov.uk/JCP/Customers/HelpForDisabledPeople/DisabilitySymbol/index.html)

Disability Discrimination Act 2005. HMSO, London (www.opsi.gov.uk/acts/acts2005/20050013.htm)

Disability Rights Commission 2006 Doing the duty. The Stationery Office, London (www.drc-gb.org/PDF/Doing_The_Duty.pdf)

Education Act 2005. HMSO, London (www.opsi.gov.uk/acts/acts2005/20050018.htm)

Employment Act 2002. HMSO, London (www.opsi.gov.uk/acts/en2002/2002en22.htm)

Employment Equality (Age) Regulations 2006. HMSO, London (www.opsi.gov.uk/si/si2006/20061031.htm; last accessed October)

Employment Rights Act 1996. HMSO, London(www.opsi.gov.uk/acts/acts1996/1996018.htm)

Equality Act 2006. HMSO, London (www.opsi.gov.uk/acts/acts2006/ukpga_20060003_en.pdf)

Gabriel Z, Bowling A 2003 Quality of life from the perspective of older people. Ageing and Society, 24:675–691

Glasper EA, Richardson J 2005 A textbook of children's and young people's nursing. Elsevier Health Sciences, Edinburgh

Godin IM 2004 Bullying, workers' health and labour instability. Journal of Epidemiology and Community Health 58(3):258–259

Hall L, Torrington D, Taylor S 2004 Human resource management. Pearson Higher Education, London

Hartnell C, Lyon R 2003 The retirement handbook, 4th rev edn. Age Concern, London

Health and Safety Executive 2003 Working long hours. HSE Publications, Suffolk (www.hse.gov.uk/RESEARCH/hsl_pdf/2003/hsl03-02.pdf#search=%22Effects%20of%20working%20long%20hours%20%22)

Health and Safety Executive 2005 Tackling stress: the management standards approach. HSE Publications, Suffolk (www.hse.gov.uk/pubns/indg406.pdf)

Henley A, Schott J 2001 Culture, religion and patient care in a multi-ethnic society: a handbook for professionals. Age Concern, London

Hogg C, Holland K 2001 Cultural awareness in nursing practice: an introductory text. Arnold, London

Home Office 2006 Respect taskforce. Home Office Publications, London (www.homeoffice.gov.uk/anti-social-behaviour/)

Human Rights Act 1998. HMSO, London (www.opsi.gov.uk/acts/acts1998/19980042.htm)

Immigration and Asylum Act 1999. HMSO, London (www.opsi.gov.uk/ACTS/acts1999/19990033.htm)

Industrial Tribunal Act 1996. HMSO, London (www.opsi.gov.uk/ACTS/acts1996/1996017.htm)

Investors in People 2004 The Investors in People Standard. The Stationery Office, London (www.IIPuk.co.uk)

Khan H, Cuthbertson J 1998 A comparison of the self reported mental and physical stress of working and full-time homemaker mothers – a UK pilot study. Stress Medicine 14(3):149–154

Larner S 2005 Common Psychological challenges for patients with newly acquired disability. Nursing Standard 19(28):33–39

Lindon J 2005 Understanding child development: linking theory to practice. Hodder Arnold, London

Lombardi EL, Ulbrich PM 1997 Work conditions, mastery and psychological distress: are housework and paid contexts conceptually similar? Women and Health 26(2):17–39

Mathers CD, Schofield DJ 1998 The health consequences of employment: the evidence. Medical Journal of Australia 1684:178–182

McKee RF, Song Z, Wanberg C et al 2005 Psychological and physical well-being during unemployment: a meta-analytical study. Journal of Applied Psychology 90(1):53–76

Mein G, Martikainen P, Hemingway 2003 Is retirement good or bad for mental and physical helath functioning? Whitehall II longitudinal study of civil servants. Journal of Edpimiology and Community Health 57(1):46–49

Mitchell M, Johnston L, Keppell M 2004 Preparing children and their families for hospitalization: a review of the literature. Neonatal Paediatric Nursing 7(2):5–15

Mullineaux DR, Barnes CA, Barnes EF 2001 Factors affecting the likelihood to engage in adequate physical activity to promote health. Journal of Sports Sciences 19(4):279–288

Mullins LJ 2004 Management and organisational behaviour, 7th edn. Financial Times Management, London

Oakley K 2005 Occupational health nursing, 2nd edn. Whurr Publishers, London

Office of National Statistics 2005a Life expectancy, more aged 70 and 80 than ever before. HMSO. London (www.statistics.gov.uk/cci/nugget.asp?id=881)

Office for National Statistics 2005b International migration: net inflow rose in 2004. HMSOM, London (www.statistics.gov.uk/cci/nugget.asp?id=1311)

Office for National Statistics 2006a Social trends 2006. HMSO, London (www.statistics.gov.uk/socialtrends36/)

Office of National Statistics 2006b The National Statistics Socio-Economic Classification. HMSO, London (www.statistics.gov.uk/methods_quality/ns_sec/default.asp)

Ouwens M, Wollerscheim H, Hermens R 2005 Integrated care programmes for chronically ill patients: a review of systematic reviews. International Journal of Quality in Health Care 17(2):141–146

Plowright C 2005 Who benefits from restricted visiting hours in hospitals? Nursing Times 101(26):18

Price R, Choi JN, Vinokur AD 2002 Links in the chain of adversity following job loss: how financial strain and loss of personal control lead to depression, impaired functioning and poor health. Journal of Occupational Health Psychology 7(4):302–312

Rollo I 2004 Understanding the role of exercise in health promotion. Nursing Times 100(37):36–38

Roper N, Logan W, Tierney AJ 1996 The elements of nursing. A model for nursing based on a model for living, 4th edn. Churchill Livingstone, Edinburgh

Roper N, Logan W, Tierney AJ 2000 The Roper–Logan–Tierney model for nursing based on activities of living. Churchill Livingstone, Edinburgh

Schnohr P, Parner J, Lange P 2000 Mortality in joggers: population based study of 4,658 men. British Medical Journal 321(7261):602–603

Slater A, Lewis M 2002 Introduction to infant development. Oxford University Press, London

Smith PK 2004 Bullying: recent developments. Child and Adolescent Mental Health 9(3):98–103

Storey K 2003 A review of research on natural support interventions in the workplace for people with disabilities. International Journal of Rehabilitation Research 26(2):79–84

Tanner J 2005 Visiting time preferences of patients, visitors and staff. Nursing Times 101(27):38–42

Thomas S 2004 The role of health professional in supporting expert patient schemes. Professional Nurse 19(8):442–445

Warr P, Butcher V, Robertson I et al 2004 Older People's well-being as a function of employment, retirement, environmental characteristics and role preference. British Journal of Psychology 95(3):297–324

Work and Families Act 2006. HMSO, London (www.opsi.gov.uk/acts/acts2006/20060018.htm)

Working Time (Amendments) Regulations 2006. HMSO, London (www.opsi.gov.uk/si/si2006/20060099.htm)

World Health Organization 2002a Active ageing: a policy framework, WHO, Geneva (whqlibdoc.who.int/hq/2002/WHO_NMH_NPH_02.8.pdf)

World Health Organization 2002b Dying for change, poor peoples experience of health and ill-health. WHO, Geneva (siteresources.worldbank.org/INTPAH/Resources/Publications/Dying-for-Change/dyifull2.pdf)

World Health Organization 2003 Work organisation and stress. Protecting Workers' Health Series No 3, Systematic problem approaches for employers, managers and trade union representatives. WHO, Switzerland (www.who.int/occupational_health/publications/en/oehstress.pdf)

World Health Organization 2004 Child and adolescent rights – an overview of the Convention of the Rights of Children. WHO, Geneva (www.who.int/child-adolescent-health/RIGHTS/crc_over.htm)

Young J 2004 Illness behaviour: a selective review and synthesis. Sociology Health and Illness 26(1):1–31

Zijlstra HP, Vlaskamp C 2005 Leisure provision for persons with profound intellectual and multiple disabilities: quality time or killing time? Journal of Intellectual Disability Research 49(6):434–448

Further reading

Alexander M, Fawcett JN, Runciman PJ 2006 Nursing practice: hospital and home, the adult, 3rd edn. Churchill Livingstone Elsevier, Edinburgh

Brooker C, Nicol M 2003 Nursing adults: the practice of caring, Mosby, Edinburgh

Useful websites

www.cipd.co.uk/subjects/emplaw/general/legaldevs.htm (CIPD Law Update)

www.dfes.gov.uk (Department for Education and Skills)

www.direct.gov.uk (Direct Gov)

www.disabilityalliance.org (Disability Alliance)

www.dlc.org.uk (Disabled Living Centre Council)

www.dlf.org (Disability Living Foundation)

www.dwp.gov.uk (Department for Work and Pensions)

www.eoc.org.uk (Equal Opportunities Commission)

www.eoc.org.uk (Equal Opportunities Commission)

www.hse.gov.uk (Health and Safety Executive)

www.IIP.co.uk (Investors in People UK)

www.opsi.gov.uk (Office of Public Sector Information)

www.rcn.org.uk (Royal College of Nursing)

www.unison.org.uk (UNISON)

www.who (World Health Organization)

Expressing sexuality

Karen Holland

INTRODUCTION

Human beings are sexual beings and how an individual manages their sexuality in health is determined by many factors. Biological differences in sex and sexual development and the influence of society and culture, including sexual behaviour across the lifespan, are fundamental to this management. It is essential if a holistic approach to care is to be adopted that there is also an understanding of how these factors can affect the care given to patients who are ill (see Chapter 1 for further information on the factors).

This chapter will therefore focus on the following:

1. **The model of living**
   - expressing sexuality in health and illness (see model of living – Chapter 1)
   - dependence/independence in the AL of expressing sexuality
   - factors influencing the AL of expressing sexuality.

2. **The model for nursing**
   - nursing care of individuals with health problems affecting the Activity of Living: expressing sexuality (i.e. application of Roper et al (1996, 2000) in practice).

THE MODEL OF LIVING

Before examining the different aspects of expressing sexuality as an activity it is important to define both sexuality and sexual health. Roper et al (1996) view sexuality as more than sex and sexual intercourse, which they see as 'an important component of adult relationships'. Human sexuality they believe is also expressed in personality and behaviour. They state that:

❝ *Femininity and masculinity are reflected not only in physical appearance and strength but also in style of dress; in many forms of verbal and non-verbal communication; in family and social roles and relationships and in choices relating to work and play.* ❞ (Roper et al 1996, p. 22)

How do others view sexuality?

McCann (2000, p. 134) states that 'people are sexual beings all of the time, whether they are healthy, ill or disabled' and offers two quotations from the literature that he believes help us to understand the 'human aspects of a person's sexuality':

Adams (1976, p. 166) for example states that:

❝ *The definition of sexuality can be as narrow as the act of intercourse or as broad as seeing the entire universe. Each individual determines the answer to defining his or her sexuality. Sexuality is a celebration of oneself, a voyage into body, mind and spirit. It is based on one's cognition, emotions and physical functioning.* ❞

Stuart & Sundeen (1979, p. 356) argue that:

❝ *Sexuality is an integral part of the whole person. Human beings are sexual in every way, all the time. To a large extent human sexuality determines who we are. It is an integral factor in the uniqueness of every person.* ❞

Brooker (2005, p. 488) indicates that:

❝ *there is much more to sexuality however than just sexual intercourse – in that it can be considered as being the sum of the physical, functional and psychological attributes that are expressed by one's gender identity and sexual behaviour, whether or not related to the sex organs or to procreation.* ❞

It can be seen from all these possible explanations of sexuality that it is a complex, yet important, part of who we are. An awareness of this is essential when considering patients' or clients' needs in a holistic way. Ensuring sexual health is part of meeting these needs. The World Health Organization defines sexual health in the following broad terms:

❝ *Sexual health is a personal sense of sexual well-being as well as the absence of disease, infections or illness associated with sexual behaviour. As such it includes issues of self-esteem, self-expression, caring for others and cultural values. Sexual health can be described as the positive integration of physical, emotional, intellectual and social aspects of sexuality. Sexuality influences thoughts, feelings, interactions and actions among human beings and motivates people to find love, contact, warmth and intimacy. It can be expressed in many different ways and is closely linked to the environment one finds oneself in, the environment can hinder or enhance sexual expressions.* 99 (WHO 2000)

In January 2002 the World Health Organization convened an international technical consultation on sexual health and as a result of this and further reviews by a group of worldwide experts agreed some working definitions to support 'ongoing discussions about sexual health' (www. who.int/reproductive-health/gender/sexual_health. html) (it must be stated, however, that these are not WHO definitions). These definitions concern sex, sexuality, sexual health and sexual rights (see Table 12.1).

The World Health Organization has now made 'sexual health a separate area of work in its own right' (World Health Organization 2004a).

Exercise

1. Consider the definitions in Table 12.1 and consider what influences these from a cultural, political and personal perspective.
2. Determine the extent to which education about the implications of these definitions are evident in various countries worldwide.

In keeping with World Health Organization guidelines, Jamison (2002, p. 163) states that sexual health can be

66 *largely regarded as:*

- *a capacity to enjoy and control sexual and reproductive behaviour in accordance with a social and personal ethic*

Table 12.1 Working definitions from WHO-convened international technical consultation in January 2002 (*www.who.int/reproductive-health/gender/sexual_health.html*)

Sex

Sex refers to the biological characteristics that define humans as female or male. While these sets of biological characteristics are not mutually exclusive, as there are individuals who possess both, they tend to differentiate humans as males and females. In general use in many languages the term sex is often used to mean sexual activity; but for technical purposes in the context of sexuality and sexual health, the above definition is preferred.

Sexuality

Sexuality is a central aspect of being human throughout life and encompasses sex, gender identities and roles, sexual orientation,eroticism, pleasure, intimacy and reproduction. Sexuality is experienced and expressed in thoughts, fantasies, desires, beliefs, attitudes, values, behaviours, practices, roles and relationships. While sexuality can include all these dimensions not all of them are always experienced or expressed. Sexuality is influenced by the interaction of biological, psychological, social, economic, political, cultural, ethical, legal, historical, religious and spiritual factors.

Sexual health

Sexual health is a state of physical, emotional, mental and social well-being in relation to sexuality; it is not merely the absence of disease, dysfunction or infirmity. Sexual health requires a positive and respectful approach to sexuality and sexual relationships, as well as the possibility of having pleasurable and safe seual experiences, free of coercion, discrimination and violence. For sexual health to be maintained the sexual health rights of all persons must be respected, protected and fulfilled.

Sexual rights

Sexual rights embrace human rights that are already recognised in national laws, international human rights documents and other consensus statements. They include the right of all persons, free of coercion, discrimination and violence, to:

- the highest attainable standard of sexual health, including access to sexual and reproductive health care services
- seek, receive and impart information related to sexuality
- respect for bodily integrity
- choose their partner
- decide to be sexually active or not
- consensual sexual relations
- consensual marriage
- decide whether or not, and when to have children
- pursue a satisfying, safe and pleasurable sexual life

The responsible exercise of human rights requires that all persons respect the rights of others.

| Box 12.1 | Reproductive health: WHO goals |

People should be able to exercise their sexual and reproductive rights in order to:

- experience healthy sexual development and maturation and have the capacity for equitable and responsible relationships and sexual fulfilment
- achieve their desired number of children safely and healthily when and if they decide to have them
- avoid illness, disease and disability related to sexuality and reproduction and receive appropriate care when needed
- be free from violence and other harmful practices related to sexuality and reproduction.

From World Health Organization (1998).

- *freedom from psychological factors such as fear, shame, guilt and false beliefs inhibiting the sexual response and impairing sexual relationships*
- *freedom from organic disease, disorders and deficiencies that impair sexual and reproductive functioning.* **""**

The World Health Organization has also adopted the term 'reproductive health' to encompass a whole range of goals which include those related to sexuality and sexual behaviour (see Box 12.1). Expressing sexuality as an Activity of Living is therefore an essential part of existence as a human being.

EXPRESSING SEXUALITY IN HEALTH AND ILLNESS – ACROSS THE LIFESPAN

Childhood

Sexual identity begins at birth, i.e. boy or girl, and many societies attach great importance to this. Boys, for example, may be more welcome in societies where men are considered to be more important than women. Understanding the differences between cultures and their views and behaviour regarding sexuality is essential for ensuring that the needs of patients are considered holistically.

How sexuality is expressed will depend in a large part on experiences at different ages. Babies will have enjoyed being cuddled and young children may have enjoyed playing games such as mothers and fathers, where gender roles are imitated and acted out. However, given that in many countries children are now being brought up in a single-parent household the image of two parents living together is no longer always the norm.

There are also other problems with children coming to realise the complexities of human sexuality and the different ways in which men and women behave; these will often have major repercussions later on in life and during illness. Sexual abuse of children is an example and the trauma of such an experience may seriously affect their personality and their sexual development.

Exercise
1. Reflect on your own childhood. How did you learn about the gender and sex differences between men and women?
2. Find out what children in different cultures learn about how men and women are supposed to act.

In some South Asian communities, for example, there are very strict codes of behaviour for men and women (Henley & Schott 1999, p. 454). They may not mix with each other in public, and often visit ill relatives or go shopping separately. Children may therefore very rarely see their parents touching each other in public. Children brought up in an Orthodox Jewish home will come to know that men and women do not touch each other whilst the woman is menstruating as it is considered unclean or 'polluting'. This belief is also to be found in Muslim, Hindu, Sikh and Traveller-Gypsy cultures (Holland & Hogg 2001).

An area where it is also possible to see the effect of adult sexual behaviour on the child is that of HIV/AIDS where it is estimated that '13 million children currently under the age of 15 have lost one or both parents to AIDS, most of them in sub-Saharan Africa' (UNAIDS 2002). It is also estimated by UNAIDS that at the end of 2000 '1.3 million children were living with HIV/AIDS and that 4.3 million had already died of the disease' (UNAIDS 2002). Many of these children will have become infected through their mothers as HIV may be transferred from an infected mother to her infant before or during birth, or afterwards through breast milk (Atkinson 2006) The other modes of transmission for HIV can be seen in Box 12.2.

Exercise
1. Using the worldwide web as a resource, find out how caring for children with AIDS is taking place in different countries.
2. Share and discuss your findings with colleagues.

This will enable you to see how very often the politico-economic and environmental factors have a major influence on how AIDS is managed and how sexuality is perceived in the country in which you live.

Adolescence

Most societies have a way of defining age groups as part of the social organisation of people. This is often linked to groupings based on gender. In Western society one such group is adolescents. Adolescence is heralded by the onset of puberty (in young men) and the menarche (in young women) resulting in the capability for fertilisation/conception.

Box 12.2	Mother to child transmission

This form of transmission is known as 'vertical transmission' i.e. down 'from' an infected mother to her child in the womb or during delivery, when the mother's blood and the child's blood become mixed. There is a possibility that transmission through amniotic fluid and ('horizontally') through breast milk can also take place (Gibb et al 2003).

From birth until 11–18 months, the baby will carry the mother's HIV and other antibodies. Therefore, all babies born to HIV-infected mothers are found to be HIV antibody-positive. At about 11–18 months, the baby will lose the mother's antibodies and go on either to being HIV antibody-negative (not carrying the virus) or to developing his or her own antibodies (being infected in their own right). A few of these babies go on to become HIV antibody-negative but positive to another test which isolates antigen (particles of the actual virus) so that they are carrying the virus but not the antibodies.

At the beginning of the HIV epidemic it appeared that approximately 50% of children born to HIV antibody-positive mothers became infected in their own right.

In countries where there are good antenatal facilities and the mother remains well throughout pregnancy, the rate of transmission from mother to child is dramatically lower. If the mother's immune system is robust, if she is treated in the last trimester and has an early elective caesarian section, transmission is reduced to less than 1% (De Cock et al 2000, WHO 2000).

From Atkinson (2006), p. 1172.

Exercise

1. Consider your own adolescent years. How did you learn about what was happening to your body at this time. Who explained what was happening to you?
2. Discuss with colleagues what it was like to be 12 or 14 years of age.

Sex education for young people is of paramount importance given the increase in sexually transmitted disease (STD) and a rise in teenage pregnancy (DoH 2006) (www.doh.gov.uk). For example in the UK:

66 *In 1997 the conception rate for girls under the age of 16 was 8.9% per 1000. For girls aged 15–19 the rate was 62.3 per thousand. These are the highest rates of teenage pregnancy in Western Europe.*

Half of under-16 conceptions and more than a third of conception to 16–19 year olds end in abortion.

Virtually all the sexually transmitted diseases are increasing. The commonest conditions are genital warts (some types of which can be associated with the subsequent development of carcinoma of the cervix), chlamydia and gonorrhoea, which if untreated can result in ectopic pregnancy and infertility. Chlamydial infection seen in clinics has risen by 21% between 1996 and 1997 and a further 135% from 1997 to 1998 (latest figures). Population surveys have reported rates of chlamydia as high as 20%, particularly in young women.

There has been no reduction in the annual number of new diagnoses of HIV made and the latest annual figures (1999) saw the highest number of new HIV diagnoses ever recorded. 99 (DoH 2000)

In response to this the Government is committed to developing a National Sexual Health and HIV Strategy (DoH 2000) and the strategy group has been set up to address HIV, teenage pregnancy and sexual health issues. This is an example of how political and social factors influence daily living and tries to ensure that combating health problems in the early years will prevent further breakdown in adulthood and old age.

Adolescent health generally, as well as sexual health, has become a key target for many organisations worldwide (WHO 2003). A study in Croatia (WHO 2004b) for example found that 'adolescents find it difficult to communicate on sexual matters with their partners' and recommended that 'they needed information and advice in matters of reproductive health and sexuality'. This would include 'school based education programmes for sexual and reproductive health, with an emphasis on communication with parents and peers, questioning stereotypical gender based sexual expectations and negotiation skills for safe sex'.

It is interesting to note that the WHO in 2004 published a report on adolescent health and development in nursing and midwifery education. This included a set of core competencies for adolescent health and development, curricular content examples and a curriculum assessment tool for the same topic (WHO 2004a). Domain five of the competency statements focuses on gender development: identity and family life/reproductive health. Examples of competencies are:

- knowledge of normal development of sexuality (physiology and socialisation)
- assessment of prevalent values and practices associated with sexual activity
- knowledge of prevalent sexually transmitted infections, prevention strategies and sequelae
- knowledge of family planning concepts and interventions.

Exercise

1. Consider the education on sexual and reproductive health that you had in school and during your nursing programme.
2. What were you taught and how has that influenced your ability to discuss sexual health with the patients in your care?

Adulthood

Adulthood in Western society can be described as having three stages following the end of the adolescent period (see Table 12.2).

Table 12.2 Summary of aspects of the development of sexuality throughout the lifespan

	Prenatal	Infancy (0–5 years)	Childhood (6–12 years)	Adolescence (13–18 years)	Young adulthood (19–30 years)	Middle years (31–44 years)	Late adulthood (45–64 years)	Old age (65+)
PHYSICAL SEXUAL DEVELOPMENT		Growth of sex organs		♂ PUBERTY ♀ MENARCHE	Continuing sex differences in body build and strength **Completion of development of secondary sex characteristics**	**Changes of pregnancy ♀**	MENOPAUSE ♀	Physical and hormonal changes may cause decline in libido and potency
PSYCHOSEXUAL DEVELOPMENT		Establishment of sexual orientation (masculine/feminine)	Establishment of sexual	Consolidation of sexual self-image	Development and modification of sexual self-image and attitudes towards sex, sexual relationships, sexual behaviour and sex-related roles and functions			Decreasing differentiation of role and function according to sex
SEXUALITY AND SOCIAL ROLES			Sex differences in roles and functions within family, school and community settings	Problem of unwanted teenage pregnancy	Sex differences in family roles ♂ **as FATHER** Sex differences in social roles ♀ **as MOTHER** Sex differences in occupational roles			
INTERPERSONAL/ SEXUAL RELATIONSHIPS		Mainly confined to FAMILY relationships	Friendships with same and opposite sex	Homosexual liaisons Heterosexual friendship and partnerships	**ESTABLISHMENT AND DEVELOPMENT OF ADULT SEXUAL PARTNERSHIPS:** Temporary liaisons or long-term mateship/marriage (heterosexual or homosexual)			Possible loss of sexual partner through death
SEXUAL BEHAVIOUR		**EARLY SELF-STIMULATORY SEX PLAY**		**MASTURBATION** Various forms of noncoital behaviour with same and opposite sex	**ADULT SEXUAL BEHAVIOUR PATTERNS** Attracting/courting behaviours Self-stimulatory activities Sexual intercourse			Possible decline in sexual behaviour and in libido
SEXUAL REPRODUCTION				**CAPABILITY FOR EJACULATION AND FERTILISATION** **CAPABILITY TO CONCEIVE ♀**	♂ **EJACULATION AND FERTILISATION OF FEMALE** ♀ **CAPABILITY FOR CONCEPTION AND REPRODUCTION (i.e. FERTILE)**		♀ **OF FEMALE** Incapable of conception after menopause	

From Roper et al (1996).

Box 12.12	Methods of contraception

Spermicidal agents
- Foam, gels, jelly, pessaries suitable for use with barrier methods. Not adequate when used alone.

Barrier methods
- Condom
- Femidom (female condom)
- Cervical cap
- Diaphragm.

Hormonal contraception
- Oral contraceptive pills
- Depo-Provera injections
- Norplant system – discontinued but some women may have had the system in place until 2004.

Intrauterine devices (IUDs)
- Mirena intrauterine system (progestogen-only intrauterine contraceptive device)
- Gyne T Slimline.

Surgical methods
- Tubal ligation
- Vasectomy.

Emergency contraception (EC)
- Yuzpe regime EC
- Progestogen-only EC
- IUD insertion.

From Walsh (2002), p. 811.

Box 12.13	Assessing the Individual for the AL of expressing sexuality

Lifespan
- Consider the effect of age on sexuality and sexual behaviour.

Dependence/independence
- Dependence is linked to lifespan and age, e.g. childhood
- Dependence is linked to specific needs, e.g. learning difficulties
- Ill health affects the dependence/independence balance, e.g. trauma, paralysis.

Factors affecting expressing sexuality
Biological
- Stage of physical sexual development
- Gender differences in body structure and function.

Psychological
- Attitudes to sexuality
- Emotional state
- Sexual orientation, e.g. homosexuality

Sociocultural
- Sociocultural similarities/differences
- Society views
- Media portrayal
- Sexual practices.

Environmental
- Home circumstances.

Politicoeconomic
- Legal factors, e.g. age of consent for sex
- Effects of work on sexual behaviour.

Adapted from Roper et al (1996).

THE MODEL FOR NURSING

USING THE MODEL TO INDIVIDUALISE NURSING FOR THE ACTIVITY OF LIVING – EXPRESSING SEXUALITY

In order to enhance your understanding of how health and illness affects this Activity of Living the next section will focus on specific case studies, and will utilise the Roper et al (1996, 2000) model for nursing as a framework to assess, plan, implement and evaluate nursing care (see Chapter 1 for full explanation of the nursing process).

ASSESSING THE INDIVIDUAL IN THE AL OF EXPRESSING SEXUALITY

It is important to remember that every individual must be considered 'holistically' and that expressing sexuality will be affected by health problems specific to other Activities of Living. For example, if a patient is unable to move due to an accident causing paralysis then they may be unable to be dependent in expressing their sexuality. The summary of lifespan, dependence/independence and factors affecting expressing sexuality can be seen in Box 12.13.

Assessing the individual

Assessment involves three phases:

- collection of data when taking a nursing history
- interpretation of the data collected
- identification of the individual's actual and potential health problems.

Collection of data when taking a nursing history

The nursing history will involve all Activities of Living and, as seen in Chapter 1, all must be taken into account in the holistic assessment of individuals.

If patients' expectations are to be understood and their problems (whether actual or potential) with this AL are to be addressed then assessment must be undertaken. A resumé of topics addressed in relation to each of the

Box 12.14	Health problems affecting the AL of expressing sexuality

Lifespan
Childhood congenital abnormalities, e.g. spina bifida.

Dependenceindependence
For example rheumatoid arthritis, multiple sclerosis, paraplegia and tetraplegia, trauma.

Factors affecting health
For example breast cancer; surgery – leading to colostomy/ileostomy formation; HIV/AIDS; sexually transmitted infections, e.g. chlamydia; surgery – leading to hysterectomy; cervical cancer; testicular cancer; abortion/ miscarriage; prostate problems.

components of the model is provided in Box 12.13 and will serve as a reminder of the many dimensions of the AL of expressing sexuality, which underpin nursing assessment. Examples of health problems which could affect the AL of expressing sexuality can be seen in Box 12.14.

Assessment of the AL of expressing sexuality

When assessing the AL of expressing sexuality the following questions can be considered, which also take account of the whole life of the individual.

Lifespan
- How old is the person?
- Do they have a life history of health problems?
- Is there anything in their life history that may affect the way in which they view their present health problems?

Independence/dependence
- Has the individual experienced any difficulties in relation to independent living?
- Are they able to go out and meet other people or are they dependent on others to transport them?
- Will they experience difficulties in the future as a result of their current health problems?

Factors affecting the AL of expressing sexuality
- What specific health problem are they suffering from?
- What do they understand about their present health status?
- What effect is this having on their other Activities of Living?
- What effect is their health problem having on their emotional wellbeing?
- Are there any cultural needs to be taken into account prior to assessment?
- Are there any specific spiritual or religious needs that the patient may have?
- Does the individual have any environmental needs which will affect future care?

- What resources could be required to help the individual manage their health problems both in hospital and at home?

Exercise
1. Reflect on how you have undertaken to assess individual needs in relation to the above questions in your practice to date.
2. Identify specific situations where you could include these in your assessment of the AL of expressing sexuality for individuals in your care.

Consider the following case study and using the same approach decide which questions would be appropriate in the assessment of his needs. Given the sensitive nature of his health problem these questions will have to be asked sensitively and with understanding.

Case study 12.2

Assessment focusing on the AL expressing sexuality

A young man, aged 24, arrives at the Accident and Emergency Department with painful micturition and a urethral discharge.

You may have decided to ask the following questions in relation to the ALs.

Questions as part of the assessment
- How long has he had the problem?
- Has he experienced anything like it before?
- What kind of pain is he experiencing?
- What helps the pain?
- What makes it worse?
- When did the problem start?
- Did the pain start at the same time as the discharge?
- Does the discharge smell?
- What does he think the problem is?

The above questions should highlight issues that may be an indication of whether he has experienced anything like this before and if it could be due to other health problems. From this a decision can then be made about his history, whether to continue with more sensitive questions around the young man's sexual behaviour that will be essential if the care he is to receive is appropriate.

Additional sensitive questions
- Has he had any sexual relations recently?
- If yes, when?

- Was this with a regular partner or not?
- Did they take precautions (e.g. condoms)?
- Would he be willing for you take a swab for identification of any infection?

The following information may be helpful in caring for this young man and will indicate why these questions have been identified as relevant to his care.

Sexually transmitted diseases

Despite the increased availability of health education and protection during sexual activity the number of people with sexually transmitted diseases (STDs) is not decreasing. For example the Health Protection Agency in the UK (2006) reported that:

- An overall rise in the number of new diagnoses seen in genitourinary medicine (GUM) clinics of 3% in 2005 compared to 2004 (from 767 785 in 2004 to 790 443 in 2005).
- Genital chlamydia remains the most commonly diagnosed STD in GUM clinics with an increase in diagnoses of 5% (from 104 733 in 2004 to 109 958 in 2005).
- Genital herpes increased by 4% (from 19 073 in 2004 to 19 837 in 2005).

Examples of sexually transmitted diseases, their signs and symptoms can be seen in Box 12.15.

Undertaking a health history is an essential part of any nursing assessment, and an understanding of the

---

Box 12.15	Sexually transmitted diseases

Gonorrhoea

Cause of infection: *Neisseria gonorrhoea*. Transmitted almost exclusively by sexual intercourse.

- Symptoms appear 3–7 days after initial content.
- Men may experience inflammation of the urethra (urethritis) and a purulent discharge. Some itching and burning around meatus is present, and urethral meatus is red and oedematous. Can be asymptomatic in 2% of men.
- If untreated an ascending infection of prostate, seminal vesicles, bladder and epididymis may occur.
- Diagnosis confirmed from smear taken from site of infection, e.g. endocervical, pharyngeal, rectal and urethra
- The female vagina is resistant to gonococcus, therefore vulnerable areas are vestibular glands, the urethra and endocervix. The glands become red, swollen and sore. A purulent discharge may drain from the urethra and ducts of the glands. Dysuria and frequency can occur. Fifty per cent of women may have vague and mild symptoms.
- Treatment: Penicillin or, for drug-resistant strain, spectinomycin or a cephalosporin, e.g. ceftriaxone.
- Partner notification and treatment are required.

Chlamydia trachomatis

Cause of infection is a parasitic sexually transmitted infection of the reproductive tract.

- The woman may present with symptoms of increased vaginal discharge, intermenstrual spotting and vague pelvic pain. Unfortunately the woman is often asymptomatic and the infection may go unnoticed and untreated for several years.
- Chlamydia is a common cause of pelvic inflammatory disease as well as an increasing cause of infertility.
- Diagnosis is confirmed via an endocervical swab for cells using a Chlamydia-specific antigen swab.
- Doxycycline 100 mg twice daily for 7 days is an effective treatment. Azithromycin, one 1 mg tablet by mouth

provides an equally effective cure and significantly reduces patient error regarding compliance.
- Sexual partners of the woman require treatment as well.

Human papillomavirus infection (HPV)

Cause of infection is condylomata acuminata or genital warts. Previously thought to be benign but recently associated with several genital cancers in both men and women.

- Risk factors for acquiring the virus are early age at first intercourse (less than 17 years old), multiple sex partners, a history of sexually transmitted diseases, poor personal and sexual hygiene, a sexual partner with similar history, a history of anal intercourse, and immunosuppressive drugs or immunodeficiency for any reason. Sexual intercourse is the method of transmission.
- The infection may be silent.
- Those presenting with external warts will be screened for other sexually transmitted diseases and if present they will be treated.
- A colposcopy examination and smear tests will be done and the partners of infected patients should also be examined and treated if necessary.
- Treatment: external warts are treated with podophyllin 10–25% in tincture of bezoin. This caustic agent is applied with a cotton applicator and washed off in 4 hours. The surrounding skin is coated with petroleum jelly before application of the podophyllin. It is not used on internal warts. Cervical and vaginal warts may be bathed in an 85% solution of trichloracetic acid. This produces a stinging sensation; a vaginal discharge follows for about 1 week as the tissue sloughs away.

Syphilis

Cause of infection is the spirochaete *Treponema pallidum*. It is a serious disease – less common than gonorrhoea.

- Incubation varies between 10 and 90 days. In most cases the disease is spread by sexual intercourse. It does not survive outside the host.

(continued)

Box 12.15	Sexually transmitted diseases *(continued)*

- In the untreated condition three stages are distinguished:
  - Primary lesion – small painless chancre or ulcer. It is deep and has indurated edges. Usually this heals spontaneously giving the false impression that the disease is cured. It appears most commonly on the penis of the male and the labia, vagina or cervix in the female.
  - Secondary stage – usually characterised by a rash appearing all over the body. This may be accompanied by condylomata lata on the female vulva. This is a cauliflower-appearing collection of flat grey vulval warts. As are all lesions of syphilis they are teeming with spirochaetes and are highly infectious. The rash is usually accompanied by fever and malaise. This soon regresses and patient enters latent stage (absence of symptoms). Three outcomes now possible: patient enters third stage immediately or after delay of 10–30 years; the disease remains latent for the rest of person's life; or a spontaneous cure occurs.
  - In the tertiary stage, bones, heart and central nervous system, including the brain, can be affected. Personality disorders arise and typical ataxic gait of the tertiary syphilitic appears. A large ulcerating necrotic lesion known as a gumma now occurs.
- Treatment: penicillin is drug of choice (usually by injection as oral medication is not effective).

Human immunosuppressive virus infection (HIV)
Cause of infection (can occur through non-sexual contact) is human immunodeficiency virus, which causes damage to the immune system. It is associated with a spectrum of disease ultimately presenting as acquired immune deficiency syndrome (AIDS).

- The virus infects the cells – primary target is T4 or T helper cells of the immune system – and destroys them. The body's immune system is weakened making the individual prone to a variety of opportunistic infections, malignant diseases and neuropsychiatric complications.
- HIV is transmitted by sexual intercourse, inoculation of infected body fluids through skin or onto mucous membranes, transplantation of tissues and transfusion of contaminated blood. HIV may also be transmitted from mother to baby either through the placenta or during delivery. Transmission of HIV has occurred through blood, semen, vaginal fluids and occasionally breast milk.
- Symptoms: some people may develop an acute illness 2–6 weeks after infection. Symptoms include fever, myalgia, arthralgia, headache, diarrhoea, sore throat, lymphadenopathy and a maculopapular rash.
- It is estimated that 40% of HIV-infected individuals will have developed AIDS 8 years after antibodies to the virus in the blood are found (seroconversion), 95% after 15 years.
- The most common opportunistic infection in individuals with AIDS is *Pneumocystis carinii*. The most common neoplasm is Kaposi's sarcoma, which is most likely to develop in homosexual or bisexual men.
- Treatment: antiviral drugs can work at several points in the life cycle of the virus. Azidothymidine (AZT) is the most widely used. The development of a vaccine to prevent HIV infection remains to be achieved.

Adapted from Walsh (2002), pp. 790–791.

elements of the nursing model that comprise the living aspects will enable you to ensure that the questions directly affecting the young man's sexuality and sexual behaviour will be relevant. However, what is not possible within this example is to identify how his other Activities of Living are affected by what is happening, due to the fact that we have no further information about his life and health. If it does indicate that he has a sexually transmitted disease then we can only surmise how his life could be affected.

For example, his symptoms may prevent him from going to work or going out socially (working and playing), he has painful micturition (eliminating), he has a urethral discharge and will need to bathe more frequently than usual (personal cleansing and dressing). Understanding the physiological factors affecting sexual health will enable you to explain to him why he has painful micturition and a urethral discharge; understanding about the psychological factors will enable you to give him support to cope with having a sexually transmitted disease.

Exercise
1. Given the information about the young man's health problem and taking into consideration the above issues, identify a plan of action for his care, both during and after being seen by the doctor in the Accident and Emergency department.
2. What confidentiality issues will you need to consider when planning any care or treatment for this man?

SUMMARY POINTS

1. Expressing sexuality is affected by lifespan, dependence/independence and biological, psychological, sociocultural, environmental and politicoeconomic factors.
2. Assessment of patient/client in the daily activity of expressing sexuality needs a holistic approach.
3. Sensitive questioning is essential in caring for patients with health problems related to expressing sexuality.

APPLICATION OF THE ROPER, LOGAN AND TIERNEY MODEL IN PRACTICE

Using the information in the previous section of this chapter we will now explore how the model can be used in the care of two patients who have a health problem which affects the AL of expressing sexuality (Casestudies 12.3 and 12.4).

Case study 12.3

Focus on health problem in the AL of expressing sexuality (an evidence-based total care approach)

Razia Bibi, a 40-year-old woman, is admitted to the gynaecology ward for a hysterectomy.

Health history
Following attendance at an Asian Well Women's Clinic a cervical smear revealed that she had cervical cancer, which had invaded the upper vaginal wall (Stage IIa carcinoma – see Box 12.16 for classification). She had been complaining of irregular vaginal bleeding, associated with sexual intercourse, and a vaginal examination by a woman doctor had also revealed an ulcerated area on the cervix. A vaginal discharge was also present and this was now offensive. She was very upset by her symptoms and she had found it very difficult to tell her husband about her problems, especially as it affected her ability to help out in the family shop. This was her first cervical smear.

Her oldest daughter Nafisa, aged 22, had noticed her mother was not well and had advised her to go to the clinic for help. She had attended with her. Razia had five other children aged 20, 16, 14, 9 and 4. All were boys except the oldest and the youngest. She had tried to use the intrauterine contraceptive device (IUCD) after her fifth child but had to have it removed due to it causing increased bleeding at menstruation. Since her last child she had also begun to experience some urinary incontinence – when coughing or sneezing. This added to her stress about the cancer and need for surgery.

On admission
Razia Bibi was visibly distressed on arrival on the ward with her eldest daughter. Although her mother did not speak much English Nafisa offered to translate. She was a trainee interpreter at another hospital, but also worked in her father's clothes shop. She was interested in health care. She explained that her mother was worried about her children and who would take care of them whilst she was in hospital, and also if anything should happen to her.

Box 12.16	International classification of carcinoma of the cervix
Stage 0	Pre-invasive carcinoma, also known as carcinoma in situ (CIN3)
Stage IA	Microinvasive carcinoma; less than 5 mm in depth
Stage IB	Neoplasm confined to the cervix
Stage IIA	Neoplasm has infiltrated adjacent parametrial tissue or upper vagina; if the carcinoma is endocervical then it has extended up into the uterus at this stage
Stage IIB	Tumour extending to the parametrium but not to the pelvic wall
Stage IIIA	Lower third of the vagina is involved or the parametrium
Stage IIIB	Involves lymph nodes as far as the pelvic wall or there are isolated metastases in the pelvis, often obstructing a ureter
Stage IV	Spread of growth to adjacent organs
Stage IVB	Spread of growth of distant organs

From McQueen (2006).

Exercise

1. Before assessing Razia Bibi's needs on admission, identify what issues would need to be considered in relation to:
   - lifespan
   - dependence/independence
   - factors affecting sexuality.

Refer to the model of living section for examples.

The following may have been considered.

Lifespan
Razia Bibi is a Muslim woman and as such will have been subject to the beliefs and expectations of her culture. In certain Muslim communities men and women are segregated (purdah) but the degree of segregation varies. Henley & Schott (1999, p. 513) state that:

> *In some Muslim families and communities in Britain, though not all, strict purdah is regarded by both men and women as the right way to live, and is a matter of pride and family honour. A good husband is expected to try to enable his wife to live in purdah. Many women in these families rarely leave their homes, going out only to visit other family members, either on foot or by car (rarely by public transport). Family visits are often a very important part of their role, and at certain times – illness, a death, a birth, a wedding – visiting is an absolute obligation.*

This need for male–female segregation will affect her communication with the wider social community, in particular the health service. We have seen that she has attended an Asian

Well Woman's clinic rather than a general one but not all Asian women will be able to do this. This service may not be available in other local communities. We have also seen that her eldest daughter does not stay home all the time, preferring instead to work in the interpreting service, which will bring her into contact with men and women from other cultures.

Beliefs about menstruation will have a major impact in relation to her care needs and nurses need to be aware of these in order to be able to explain the outcomes of having a hysterectomy on her daily life. For example, Dhami & Sheikh (2000, p. 51) point out that:

> " *Whilst menstruating, women are exempt from some of the important religious rites, such as ritual prayer, fasting and Hajj. Sexual intercourse is prohibited at such times. All other forms of physical contact between husband and wife, for example hugging and kissing, are allowed. A period therefore may have a number of social and psychological ramifications. There are also a number of possible implications for clinical care. Women may be reluctant to attend for gynaecological symptoms, cervical smear tests or coil checks for fear of bleeding following pelvic examination. Many Muslim women are unaware that traumatic bleeding of this kind is quite distinct from menstrual bleeding and hence the same religious constraints do not apply.* "

The impact of no longer having menstrual periods will therefore be very significant to Razia Bibi's daily life as a Muslim woman.

Dependence/independence

Razia Bibi is obviously very dependent on her daughter in relation to health problems and communication with health professionals. She needs to have a good relationship with her daughter to ensure that her feelings and concerns are respected and that these are translated to the health care team. Any matter relating to sex is normally taboo to anyone other than between husband and wife (Dhami & Sheikh 2000). She will become dependent on her carers once she is admitted to hospital and this dependency will vary during the perioperative period until her discharge home and post discharge.

Factors affecting sexuality

Beliefs about how her body works will be an important aspect for the nurse to determine as this will in turn influence how the intended surgery and its outcomes will be understood by Razia Bibi. We have already seen (p. 396) that the beliefs of Asian women in regard to the menopause and undergoing a hysterectomy will expose her to potentially stressful situations in many areas or daily living activities, for example personal cleansing and dressing and elimination.

The psychological impact of having a hysterectomy on her as a woman who could still have more children will need to be considered as well as her understanding of the short- and long-term impact of cervical cancer. Her home circumstances (environmental factors) will need to be considered in order to be able to plan effective discharge. How she will manage when she leaves hospital will be an important issue to consider. Her religious and cultural beliefs will also be an important factor in her care.

ASSESSMENT OF RAZIA BIBI'S NEEDS

Using this knowledge of her background and potential influencing factors you can now assess her individual needs on admission to hospital (use the questions on pp. 403–404 as a framework).

Collection of data on admission

> **Exercise**
> 1. Using the 12 Activities of Living as a framework, identify Razia Bibi's actual problems on admission to the ward.

Ensuring a safe environment in which to carry out the initial assessment of Razia Bibi's needs will be an important aspect of the nurse's role. You will need to ensure that privacy is maintained as well as ensuring comfortable seating for both Razia Bibi, her daughter and the nurse. Ensuring confidentiality during the assessment interview is also an essential aspect of care (see NMC 2004, Ch. 2). The assessment of her needs at various stages of her care will now be explored using an evidence-based approach.

Activities of Living – evidence-based approach
Expressing sexuality
It is important that the date of the last menstrual period is determined as Razia Bibi could be pregnant. She has tried to use an intrauterine coil and may no longer be taking precautions. Sensitive questioning will be required in relation to sexual activity between her and her husband. Her daughter who has been interpreting may not wish to know about this aspect of her parents' lives and it may be that another interpreter unconnected with the family might be recommended. It is also important to know what kind of vaginal discharge she has been having and how she has been managing to cope with it. This can be either physiological (i.e. normal) or pathological (Sutherland 2001). Physiological discharge can increase in certain circumstances, such as during pregnancy (leucorrhoea), sexual arousal or premenstrually. Pathological discharge is caused by either infective (e.g. chlamydia, *Candida albicans* (thrush) or gonorrhoea) or noninfective causes (e.g. cervical polyp, cervical cancer, 'lost tampon' or condom).

Sutherland (2001, p. 323) suggests the following questions might be asked of a woman to determine its origins.

- How is it different from normal?
- Why is she worried about it?
- Are there any other associated symptoms (dysuria, soreness, intermenstrual bleeding, pelvic discomfort)?

- Has anything happened to make her vagina less acidic (is she overwashing with strong soaps, using disinfectant in the bath, douching, is she menopausal)?
- Does it have a characteristic smell?
- Does she have any reason to be worried about sexually transmitted infection?
- Has she treated herself unsuccessfully with an over-the-counter preparation?

It is apparent from these possible questions that not all of them will be applicable to Razia Bibi, given her overall history and her personal circumstances and cultural background. Sensitivity will be required in both the questioning approach taken and the phrasing of the questions themselves.

Most importantly will be Razia Bibi's understanding of the surgery to be undertaken, i.e. the hysterectomy, and its outcome. This is essential for consent to surgery and for postoperative care. Rodgers (2000, p. 804) states that:

> 66 *The nurse has an important role to play in obtaining consent prior to surgery. For a patient to give valid consent she must comprehend fully what she is consenting to, i.e. her consent must be informed. The nurse can provide the team with knowledge of the patient's individual need for information and her comprehension of the information given. The nurse will also provide the patient with information about the procedure and the recovery period and may be able to clarify points previously discussed between the patient and the doctor. However the nurse cannot and must not be the provider of information in order for the doctor to obtain informed consent for surgery. This is a medical staff responsibility.* 99

Actual problem   Razia Bibi has cervical cancer and requires surgery for its removal.

Communication

From the case study information it can be seen that Razia Bibi does not speak much English and needs her daughter to interpret for her. She will, however, not be able to interpret throughout Razia Bibi's stay in hospital as she has her own commitments. Other alternatives will have to be found to ensure her communication needs are met. It can also be seen that she has been unable to talk to her husband about her health problems and their effect on herself and her family. It is important that nurses do not rely on families interpreting for their relatives, as this can cause both embarrassment for the patient and also can lead to misinterpretation (Gerrish et al 1996). Trained interpreters/translators, familiar with medical terminology and the health service as well as language, should be available in these circumstances. However, these are not always available when needed (Robinson 2002).

Actual problem

- She is unable to communicate her self-concerns.
- She is unable to converse in English with the nurse and other members of the health care team.
- She is unable to talk to her husband about her problems.
- She is visibly distressed on her admission to the ward.

Working and playing

She normally works in her husband's shop but as her illness has become problematic she is no longer able to do this. This may have caused an increase in her stress, especially following the diagnosis of cervical cancer and its implications for the future. Her health problems, especially the offensive vaginal discharge, may also have affected her going out and meeting with other women in her community. These have also begun to affect how she takes care of her family. An understanding of how important all these are to women in an Asian culture is essential if care is to be individualised and culture specific.

Actual problem

- She is unable to play an active part in her family's care.
- She is unable to take an active part in her husband's business.

Personal cleansing and dressing

Razia may be dressed in traditional Muslim clothes – either a shalwar (trousers), kameez (long shirt) and a chuni or dupatta (long scarf) which covers her head, mouth and nose (Holland & Hogg 2001), or if a Bangladeshi woman, a 'sari worn over a waist-length blouse and a long underskirt' (Karmi 1996, p. 56). She will need to be reassured that she can continue to wear these during her stay in hospital. She may be very concerned that she will have to wear a hospital gown that exposes parts of her body that she normally keeps hidden. Again reassurance on admission is crucial.

Razia is very upset by her symptoms, in particular the offensive vaginal discharge. As a Muslim woman she will already have a washing and cleansing routine, and will need to be assured that there will be running water available for her daily needs. Alternatives will have to be found when she is recovering postoperatively.

Actual problem

- Razia has concerns regarding removal of her clothes for examination and going to theatre.
- Razia has an offensive vaginal discharge.

Dying

It is important to determine on admission what she has been told about her illness and what she understands about it. Even though death is seen as marking 'the transition from one state of existence to the next' and inevitable as part of our acts of living (Sheikh & Gatrad 2000), Razia may still be fearful for her family and her children – as she is a relatively young woman. She will need to maintain her daily prayers and may also wish to do this in the company of her family.

Actual problem   Razia is anxious regarding opportunities and facilities for daily prayers.

Elimination

Razia has recently begun to experience urinary incontinence problems, which have added to her distress and concerns she has for the impending surgery. An explanation that she may well have a catheter in place may be necessary, exposing her to further personal distress due to invasion of her body and dignity.

Actual problem

Razia has urinary incontinence when she sneezes or coughs.

SUMMARY

> The above problems in some Activities of Living can be determined from the information offered in the case study. However, during the admission assessment and obtaining further information from Razia Bibi and her daughter, other actual problems may become apparent in the other activities.
> The kind of questions which will highlight these can be found in the other specific chapters, e.g. breathing. It is also important to acknowledge the involvement of the multidisciplinary team in her care, and how an integrated care approach would be an appropriate way of managing her stay in hospital and post discharge. Following the assessment stage, care planning would be undertaken, along with the setting of patient and nurse goals (see Chapter 1). Priority for the nurse will be to prepare Razia for theatre (see Chapter 3 for a more detailed account of preoperative preparation of a patient).

PREOPERATIVE CARE OF RAZIA BIBI

> **Exercise**
> 1. Using the 12 Activities of Living as a framework identify Razia Bibi's needs and potential problems prior to going to theatre.

NB: We cannot predict her actual problems as she is an individual with her own life history – reality would be different – we can only offer some potential problems that she may experience.

Potential problems in the preoperative period will take account of the actual problems already identified on admission and will focus mainly on physiological and psychological needs.

Razia will:

- need to know what the surgery is going to mean to her afterwards in order to ensure that her consent to the surgery is based on all the facts (informed consent)
- need to know that removing her uterus will mean that she is no longer able to have children
- need to be reassured about her privacy and dignity during the operation
- need to be physically prepared for going to the operating theatre for surgery.

> **Exercise**
> 1. Using the model for nursing and the Activities of Living identify the physical preparation Razia Bibi will require prior to surgery.

The following may have to be considered.

- preoperative fasting
- skin preparation, e.g. shaving (as above)
- elimination – suppositories/bladder
- personal care
- medication – writing in notes
- baseline observations – temperature, blood pressure, pulse, urinalysis and weight.

> **Exercise**
> 1. Determine what care Razia will receive during the intraoperative period – from her leaving the ward to returning. You need to consider the following stages: operating theatre transfer; receiving the patient in the anaesthetic room; anaesthesia; patient care in the main theatre; patient care in the recovery area; immediate postoperative management and transfer back to the ward.
> 2. Using the 12 Activities of Living framework identify the potential problems Razia Bibi is likely to experience following an abdominal hysterectomy (again it is difficult to predict actual problems – but we can offer all potential problems in the postoperative period).

The following may also have been considered.

CONTINUING POSTOPERATIVE CARE

Razia will have had major abdominal surgery with all that it entails (Table 12.3 indicates the types of patient problems that could occur in the postoperative period).

1. **Maintaining a safe environment**
   - postoperative observations
   - pain relief
   - handover from theatre nurse
   - wound care.

Table 12.3 Potential problems common to the patient after operation

Problem	Causative factors	Goals
Pain	Surgical intervention Nausea and vomiting Abdominal distension Anxiety	The patient will state he or she is free from pain
Dehydration and electrolyte imbalance	Decreased oral intake Fluid loss during surgery via drainage tubes Altered gastrointestinal activity	Minimum fluid intake of 2.4 litres per day Electrolytes within normal limits
Alternation in patterns of elimination	Decreased fluid volume Immobility Pain	Patient will return to normal pattern of elimination once bowel function returns
Reduced mobility	Surgical intervention Altered sensation Pain and discomfort Weakness Immobility	Short term. Patient will sit out of bed within 4–12 h; will not develop complications of immobility (deep vein thrombosis, pressure sores, chest infection); will walk to the bathroom within 4–12 h (with assistance)
Potential for infection	Decreased level of consciousness Inadequate airway clearance Decreased sensations Impaired skin integrity Decreased mobility	No infection will occur and wound will heal without complications
Inadequate respiration	Respiratory irritation from anaesthesia Pain and discomfort Decreased mobility	Respiratory rate 12–20 per minute; breathing to be of normal depth and pattern
Inadequate circulation	Effects of anaesthetic Surgical intervention Increased fluid loss Decreased mobility	BP systolic 90 mmHg; pulse regular, within range 60–90 bpm
Anxiety	Fear of unknown Lack of knowledge Pain and discomfort Diagnosis	The patient is able to talk about concerns and fears
Insufficient knowledge about health care	Lack of knowledge and skill	The patient will verbalise an understanding of the factors involved in improving health after discharge

From Walsh (2002), p. 183

2. **Communication**
   - reduce anxiety
   - interpreter service
   - talk to relatives.

3. **Elimination**
   - urine output (catheterised for 1–2 days)
   - bowel movement.

4. **Breathing**
   - maintaining clear airway
   - deep breathing exercises – physiotherapy
   - pulmonary embolism, etc.

5. **Personal cleansing and dressing**
   - oral hygiene and inability to meet own hygiene needs
   - pressure area care.

6. **Mobility**
   - restricted mobility.

7. **Sleeping**
   - interrupted sleep pattern due to surgery.

8. **Controlling body temperature**
   - postoperative stress
   - risk of infection.

9. **Dying**
   - concerns regarding the cervical cancer and its removal
   - need to take account of religious/spiritual practices.

10. **Working and playing**
    - concerns regarding her inability to be at home helping the family.

11. **Expressing sexuality**
    - concerns re: future sex life, inability to have children, perceptions of her womanhood, etc.
    - body image.

12. **Eating and drinking**
    - fluid intake/output
    - bowel action
    - dietary needs – cultural preferences.

Nursing interventions during this period can be summarised as follows:

1. 'promote comfort and control pain
2. maintain fluid and electrolyte balance and adequate nutrition
3. assist a return to normal patterns of elimination
4. encourage increasing levels of activity
5. promote wound healing
6. maintain ventilation
7. maintain circulation
8. decrease patient anxiety
9. prepare patient for discharge and self management' (Brown 2002, p. 182).

Evaluation of postoperative care

Brown (2002, p. 190) suggests the following criteria may be included in determining successful outcomes of care:

1. The patient is free from pain and discomfort, as shown by verbal expression and participation in physical activities and ability to rest and sleep.
2. The fluid intake and electrolyte concentrations are normal for the patient.
3. The patient is taking a nutritionally balanced diet.
4. Urinary and bowel elimination are re-established and normal for the patient.
5. The patient is ambulatory, active and participating in care.
6. The incision is clean, dry and intact.
7. Vital signs are normal for the patient.
8. No manifestations of complications are present.
9. The patient and family demonstrate an understanding of the required care during convalescence and the resources available.

It is important to remember, however, that every patient is an individual and Razia Bibi's pathway following a hysterectomy, and any potential problems she might experience, will be unique to her.

Discharge home and follow up

Well-planned and effective discharge planning will be essential in ensuring Razia Bibi's postoperative recovery and wellbeing (Rodgers 2000, p. 827). Patients who have had major surgery no longer have a prolonged stay in hospital. A referral may need to be made to the district nurse team and she will need a follow-up appointment to return to the outpatient clinic, e.g. 6 weeks following discharge home from hospital.

Exercise

1. Consider your clinical practice experience to date. How many of the health problems seen in Box 12.14 have you come across?
2. How did you assess, plan, implement and evaluate care in the AL of expressing sexuality for individuals who were experiencing these health problems?
3. Focus on one of these and identify what you did well and what you found difficult to deal with in your care of the patient.

SUMMARY POINTS

1. An awareness and understanding of cultural needs is essential in ensuring culturally appropriate care in relation to expressing sexuality and sexual health.
2. Health problems affecting the Activity of Living expressing sexuality can be seen to be interdependent on other Activities of Living.
3. The nurse needs effective assessment and communication skills to be able to plan care and implement care that is evidence based.

Case study 12.4

Myocardial infarction and expressing sexuality

This will focus on a health problem not directly connected to the AL of expressing sexuality – but one which has major implications for assessment of need in relation to the individual's specific sexual functioning: a patient who has experienced a myocardial infarction.

Case study

Mr John Eaves is a 55-year-old man, recovering from a myocardial infarction and he is transferred to a ward from the Coronary Care Unit (CCU) where he has been a patient for 3 days.

Health history

He is overweight and has smoked 20 cigarettes a day prior to admission. His wife is 40 years of age and they have three children – aged 18, 14 and 12. His wife uses

(Continued)

Myocardial infarction and expressing sexuality

the contraceptive pill but she now wants to stop and to use other means instead. He is worried that she could get pregnant again and this together with worrying about not having sex in case he puts more strain on his heart is already creating some tensions between them. He has been transferred to the ward after spending 3 days in the CCU. During his stay there he had one cardiac arrest but was successfully resuscitated. He has a vague memory of the event but realises he is vulnerable to further cardiac arrests.

Exercise

1. Before assessing his needs on admission to the ward consider what knowledge you will need with regard to myocardial infarction (MI) and the care of patients following MI.

The following may have been considered.

- knowledge of the anatomy and physiology of the heart
- knowledge of what happens when a myocardial infarction occurs – to the heart itself and to the rest of the patient's physiological systems
- current evidence-based practice in caring for patients who have had an MI
- current medication and treatments for MI
- knowledge of care from admission to discharge home and rehabilitation programmes post MI.

FACTORS AFFECTING EXPRESSING SEXUALITY FOLLOWING AN MI

Rutter (2000c, p. 216) points out that:

> *Myocardial infarction (MI) is often thought of as a male illness but more post-menopausal women die each year from MI than from breast cancer. Sudden death during sexual intercourse is often a great anxiety for men and women with a diagnosis of heart disease or hypertension, but such death is very rare. However many people who survive MI suffer psychological damage that affects the quality of their lives by affecting self-confidence and their sexuality. Some patients are still anxious and depressed and have sexual problems 1 year following the heart attack. They feel fragile and vulnerable and this dampens sexual arousal and contributes to a fear of resumption of sexual intercourse which will have an impact on the partner and may lead to frustration.*

Mr Eaves may well experience similar feelings and thoughts as he begins to recover from his MI. Other factors such as his beliefs about his age and his wife's

may add to his concerns – she no longer wants to take precautions by taking the contraceptive pill which means that he has to take more responsibility to prevent further pregnancies. Given his illness and the need for a period of rehabilitation following his MI the added fear of becoming dependent on his wife could add to the tensions, i.e. there will be a period of time when he is unable to go to work. Worries about this together with when to safely resume sexual activity will need sensitive discussion with Mr Eaves, and his wife, before he is discharged home from hospital. Muller et al (1996) undertook a major study examining the sexual activity of post-MI patients and concluded that 'although baseline risk of MI is increased, sexual activity has now been documented to have a low likelihood of triggering an MI' (see Box 12.17 on next page for details of study).

ASSESSMENT OF NEEDS ON TRANSFER FROM CCU – DIRECTLY RELATED TO THE AL OF EXPRESSING SEXUALITY

Expressing sexuality may not be the priority problem that Mr Eaves identifies – he has been near to death in the CCU and suffered a cardiac arrest – although he does not remember much about the event. His main problems may arise from a realisation that he could have prevented the onset of the MI, by not being so overweight and not smoking. The nurses will have to cope with withdrawal symptoms of not being able to smoke, resulting in further tension and stress because he is unable to smoke.

As can be seen in his health history, Mr Eaves has already expressed some concerns regarding sexual activity post MI which could be linked to concerns that his wife is much younger than him and that he should still be sexually active.

Exercise

1. What are the nursing priorities in caring for Mr Eaves with regard to his wellbeing and his concerns regarding sexual activities?

In order to consolidate learning to use the model for nursing as a framework for care undertake the following exercise.

Exercise

1. Identify a patient/client with a health problem directly related to the AL of expressing sexuality.
2. Devise a care plan for this patient – using the documentation found in the appendices or one that is familiar to you.

| Box 12.17 | Sexual activity and myocardial infarction (an abstract) |

Synopsis

A total of 1774 patients with myocardial infarction (MI) served as the basis for this study. In this group 858 (48%) were sexually active in the year prior to their MI. Nine percent reported sexual activity in the 24 hours preceding the MI and 3% reported sexual activity in the 2 hours preceding the MI. The relative risks of an MI occurring in the 2 hours after sexual activity were 2.5. That risk decreased from 3.0 for those who did not exercise heavily and to 1.2 for those who exercised heavily three or more times a week. There were too few women who reported sexual activity in the 2-hour hazard period preceding MI to determine if the relative risk varied by sex.

The authors concluded that sexual activity can trigger the onset of an MI. The relative risk is low. The absolute risk caused by sexual activity is also extremely low (one chance in a million for a healthy individual).

Commentary

The present study provides information of great value for counselling more than 500 000 patients who survive an MI each year and the 11 million patients with existing cardiac disease. Counselling has often been ineffective in decreasing the fear of triggering a cardiac event. With these data, health care professionals counselling patients can reassure them that although their baseline risk of MI is increased, sexual activity has now been documented to have a low likelihood of triggering an MI. The risk is particularly low for patients who engage in regular exercise. Based on these data physicians should encourage patients with known coronary heart disease to participate in a cardiac rehabilitation programme and perform regular exercises. Such exercise can decrease the cardiac work required for sexual activity and reduce the risk of triggering the onset of an MI.

From Muller et al (1996), p. 10 (www.ingenta.com).

CONCLUSION

Expressing sexuality and sexual health is essential for wellbeing, but how this is managed will depend on the culture and society in which we live. The case studies in this chapter have demonstrated some of the issues and problems facing patients who have illnesses that have either a direct or indirect impact on sexuality and sexual behaviour. Using a framework for care, such as the Roper et al (1996, 2000) model of living and model for nursing, has ensured that a holistic approach has been taken to identifying actual and potential problems in a systematic way.

SUMMARY POINTS

1. Sexual activity can be affected by indirect health problems in other Activities of Living, e.g. myocardial infarction.
2. Professional counselling might be necessary for some patients who experience either short- or long-term problems in expressing sexuality as a result of illness.
3. It is important to remember that partners need support in coping with illnesses that affect their sexual relationships.

References

Abernathy K 1997 The menopause. In: Andrews G (ed) Women's sexual health. Baillière Tindall, London, pp 336–364

Adams G 1976 Recognising the range of human sexual needs and behaviour. American Journal of Maternal Child Nursing 6: 166–169

Alexander MF, Fawcett JN, Runciman PJ (eds) 2006 Nursing practice: hospital and home – the adult, 2nd edn. Churchill Livingstone, Edinburgh

Atkinson J 2006 The person with HIV/AIDS. In: Alexander MF, Fawcett JN, Runciman PJ (eds) Nursing practice – hospital and home (the adult). Churchill Livingstone, Edinburgh, pp 1169–1190

Baltes PB, Staudinger UM, Lindenburger U 1999 Lifespan psychology: theory and application to intellectual functioning. Annual Review of Psychology 50:471–507

Barlow H 2003 Breast disorders. In: Brooker C, Nichol M (eds) Nursing adults: the practice of caring, Mosby, Edinburgh, pp. 771–792

Brooker C, Nicol M 2003 Nursing adults: the practice of caring. Mosby, Edinburgh

Brooker C 2005 Mini encyclopaedia of nursing. Churchill Livingstone, Edinburgh

Brown A 2002 The patient undergoing surgery. In: Walsh M (ed) Watson's clinical nursing and related sciences, 6th edn. Baillière Tindall/Royal College of Nursing, London, pp 65–192

Burnet KL 2006 The reproductive systems and the breast: Part 2 The breast. In: Alexander MF, Fawcett JN, Runciman PJ (eds) Nursing practice – hospital and home (the adult). Churchill Livingstone, Edinburgh, pp 253–356

Cancer Research UK 2004 (www.cancerresearchuk.org/cancerstats/incidence)

Carlisle D 1998 HIV and breast feeding: a global issue for midwives. RMC Midwives Journal 1(3):78–80

Clifford D 2000 Professional awareness in psychosexual care. In: Wells D (ed) Caring for sexuality in health and illness. Churchill Livingstone, Edinburgh

Cottton J, Jones M, Steggall M 2003 Nursing patients with sexual health and reproductive problems. In: Brooker C, Nichol M (eds) Nursing adults: the practice of caring. Mosby, Edinburgh, pp. 705–769

Davis DL 1986 The meaning of menopause in a Newfoundland fishing village. In: Morse JM (ed) Qualitative health research. Sage, London

De Cock KM, Fowler MG, Mercier E 2000 Prevention of mother to child HIV transmission in resource poor countries:

translating research into policy and practice. Journal of the American Medical Association 283(9):1175–1182

Department of Health 2000 National sexual health and HIV strategy. DoH, London (www.doh.giv.uk/nshs)

Department of Health 2006 Sexual Health Quarterly Bulletin, issue 14. DoH, London (www.cph.org.uk/sexualhealth)

Dhami S, Sheikh A 2000 The family: predicament and promise. In: Gatrad AR, Sheikh A (eds) Caring for Muslim patients. Radcliffe Medical Press, Oxford

Forte D, Cotter A, Wells D 2006 Sexuality and relationships in later life. In: Redfern SJ, Ross FM (eds) Nursing older people, 4th edn. Churchill Livingstone, Edinburgh

Gerrish K, Husband C, Mackenzie J 1996 Nursing for a multi-ethnic society. Open University Press, Buckingham

Gibb DM, Duong T, Tookey PA et al 2003 Decline in mortality, AIDS and hospital admissions in perinatally HIV-1 infected children in the United Kingdom and Ireland. British Medical Journal 327:1019–1023

Gibson C E 2006 The patient facing surgery. In: Alexander MF, Fawcett JN, Runciman PJ (eds) Nursing practice – hospital and home (the adult). Churchill Livingstone, Edinburgh, pp 901–943

Golub S 1992 Periods: from menarch to menopause. Sage, London

Greer G 1991 The change, women, ageing and the menopause. Hamish Hamilton, London

Health Protection Agency 2006 Sexually transmitted infection statistics (www.hpa.org.uk/infections)

Henley A, Schott J 1999 Culture, religion and patient care in a multi-ethnic society. Age Concern England, London

Herbert RA, Walker R 2005 Reproduction. In: Montague SE, Watson R, Herbert RA (eds) Physiology for nursing practice. Elsevier: Edinburgh, pp 725–775

Holland K, Hogg C 2001 Cultural awareness in nursing and health care. Arnold, London

Jamison JR 2002 Maintaining health in primary care – a guide for wellness in the 21st century. Churchill Livingstone, Edinburgh

Karmi G 1996 The ethnic health handbook. Blackwell Science, Oxford

La Fontaine JS 1985 Initiation. Penguin Books, Harmondsworth

Mayor V 1996 Asian women and the menopause. In: Webb C (ed) Living sexuality – issues for nursing and health. Baillière Tindall, London

McCann E 2000 The expression of sexuality in people with psychosis: breaking the taboos. Journal of Advanced Nursing 32(1):132–138

McQueen ACH 2006 The reproductive systems and the breast: Part 1 the reproductive system. In: Alexander MF, Fawcett JN, Runciman PJ (eds) Nursing practice – hospital and home (the adult). Churchill Livingstone, Edinburgh, pp 253–356

Mok J 1993 HIV-1 infection, breast milk and HIV-1 transmission. Lancet 341:941

Montague SE, Watson R, Hubert RA 2005 Physiology for nursing practice. Baillière Tindall, London

Muller J, Mittleman M, Maclure M, et al 1996 Sexual activity and myocardial infarction. ACOG Clinical Review 1(5):10

Nursing and Midwifery Council 2004 Code of professional conduct. NMC, London

Robinson M 2002 Communication and health in a multi-ethnic society. The Policy Press, Bristol

Rodgers SE 2000 The patient facing surgery. In: Alexander MF, Fawcett JN, Runciman PJ (eds) Nursing practice: hospital and home – the adult. Churchill Livingstone, Edinburgh, pp 799–831

Roper N, Logan W, Tierney A 1996 The elements of nursing, 4th edn. Churchill Livingstone, Edinburgh

Roper N, Logan W, Tierney A 2000 The Roper, Logan, Tierney model of nursing. Churchill Livingstone, Edinburgh

Rutter M 2000a Becoming a sexual person. In: Wells D (ed) Caring for sexuality in health and illness. Churchill Livingstone, Edinburgh, pp 151–170

Rutter M 2000b Life experiences and transitions in adolescence and adulthood. In: Wells D (ed) Caring for sexuality in health and illness. Churchill Livingstone, Edinburgh, pp 189–206

Rutter M 2000c The impact on illness on sexuality. In: Wells D (ed) Caring for sexuality in health and illness. Churchill Livingstone, Edinburgh

Schott J, Henley A 1996 Culture, religion and childbearing in a multi-cultural society. Butterworth-Heinemann, Oxford

Selfe L 2006 The urinary system. In: Alexander MF, Fawcett JN, Runciman PJ (eds) Nursing practice – hospital and home (the adult). Churchill Livingstone, Edinburgh, pp 357–393

Sheikh A, Gatrad AR 2000 Caring for Muslim patients. Radcliffe Medical Press, Oxford

Stewart D 1999 The attitudes and attributions of student nurses: do they alter according to a person's diagnosis or sexuality and what is the effect of nurse training? Journal of Advanced Nursing 30(3):740–748

Stuart GW, Sundeen SJ 1979 Principles and practice of psychiatric nursing. Mosby, St Louis

Sutherland C 2001 Women's health – a handbook for nurses, Churchill Livingstone, Edinburgh

United Nations Programme on HIV/AIDS 2002 Children on the brink 2002, UNAIDS (www.unaids.org/youngpeople/index.html)

Walsh M 2002 (ed) Watson's clinical nursing and related sciences, 6th edn. Baillière Tindall/Royal College of Nursing, London

Waugh A, Grant A 2006 Ross and Wilson anatomy and physiology in health and illness. Churchill Livingstone, Edinburgh

Wells D 1999 Transitions: healthy ageing – nursing older people. In: Health H, Schofield H (eds), Healthy ageing: nursing older people. Churchill Livingstone, Edinburgh

Wilson EW, Rennie PIC 1976 The menstrual cycle. Lloyd-Luke, London

World Health Organization 1998 Reproductive health: meeting people's needs. WHO/RHT/98.17

World Health Organization 2000 Working with street children – module 4 – understanding sexual and reproductive health including HIV/AIDS and STDs among street children. World Health Organization, Geneva (www.who.int/substance_abuse/PDFfiles/module4.pdf)

World Health Organization 2003 Progress in reproductive health research, No. 64. WHO, Geneva

World Health Organization 2004a Adolescent health and development in nursing and midwifery education. WHO, Geneva

World Health Organization 2004b How do perceptions of gender roles shape the sexual behaviour of Croatian adolescents? Social Science Research Policy Briefs. WHO, Geneva

Further reading

Andrews G 2001 Women's sexual health. Baillière Tindall, London

Davidson N 2000 Promoting men's health – a guide for practitioners. Baillière Tindall, London

Sutherland C 2001 Women's health – a handbook for nurses. Churchill Livingstone, Edinburgh

Useful websites

www.bbc.co.uk/health/sex
www.doh.gov.uk/sexualhealthandhiv/index
www.who.int/reproductive-health

Family planning association sites (examples)

www.brain.net.pk/~fpapak (Pakistan)
www.fpaindia.com (India)
www.fpa.org.uk (United Kingdom)
www.ifpa.ie (Ireland)

Sleeping

Jane Jenkins

INTRODUCTION

Roper et al (1996, 2000) highlight that sleeping is vital for everyone and is therefore an important Activity of Living. All human beings have periods of activity and inactivity and adults spend up to a third of their lives asleep. These periods of activity and inactivity are regulated by a sleep–wakefulness cycle controlled by the hypothalamus. A 24-hour sleep–wake cycle is learnt through experience and is called the 'circadian' rhythm and is produced by the 'biological' clock (Kindlen 2003). Babies learn this sleep–wake pattern over the first few months of life and mothers are always overjoyed when their baby has 'learnt' to sleep through the night and be awake in the daytime with short periods of rest and sleep throughout the day. The greatest amount of rest is produced when the person is asleep but body functions do still continue during this time but at a reduced level. Roper et al (2000, p. 48) define sleep as a 'recurrent state of inertia and unresponsiveness, a state in which a person does not respond to what is going on in the surrounding environment'.

Sleeping is very different to stages of unconsciousness leading to a coma, and unconsciousness produced by anaesthesia, as although consciousness is lost during sleep, it is for a short time only and new stimuli will wake the person. According to Roper et al (2000), sleep can be recognised by a person closing their eyes, lying still for some of the time, moving at intervals, and relaxing so that the mouth opens and breathing is noticeably slower.

However, the quantity and quality of sleep may be affected by a person's health status and the quantity and quality of sleep that a person has may affect their health and wellbeing. Sleeping can, certainly, be affected by health problems which relate to other Activities of Living, such as suffering from acute or chronic pain linked to minor or major health problems, being stressed, anxious or depressed, or suffering from a marked loss of weight linked to anorexia, bulimia or cancer. It is important to remember that we are all individuals with life activities that are interlinked and when illness causes one or more activity to be affected then most of the activities can

become compromised. This may then result in physical, emotional or social problems.

To enable an insight to be gained into both the normal and abnormal patterns of sleep, exercises and case studies have been introduced, as previously noted, which will incorporate evidence-based practice and cultural issues.

The aspects to be covered in this chapter are:

1. **The model of living**
   - sleeping activity in health and illness across the lifespan
   - dependence and independence in relation to the activity of sleeping
   - factors which influence the activity of sleeping.

2. **The model for nursing**
   - nursing care of individuals with health problems which affect their activity of sleeping.

It is important to be able to answer the question: Why do we need to sleep? Roper et al (1996, p. 375) state that the function of sleep 'is still not fully understood'. Lavie et al (2002) identify theories but le May (2006) considers that sleep's major role is in the maintenance and/or restoration of physical and cerebral functioning, centring around the body's ability to restore itself, grow and conserve energy. Restoration and growth of all body cells are promoted by sleep. This is based on the fact that adrenaline, noradrenaline and corticosteroids are produced during wakefulness and they inhibit the formation of protein in tissues, whereas, in sleep, all of these are produced in small quantities only, therefore allowing protein to be formed, aided by the production of human growth hormone during the night. This may be the reason that children go to bed and appear to have grown overnight. Conservation theory is identified as energy used during the day must be balanced by a sleeping/resting phase to recuperate energy used up (Roper et al 1996).

It may be necessary to review knowledge of the normal anatomy and physiology of the central nervous system (CNS) and sleep patterns before continuing with this chapter.

MODEL OF LIVING

ACTIVITY OF SLEEPING IN HEALTH AND ILLNESS, ACROSS THE LIFESPAN

Howard (2004) identifies that the need for sleep varies through life according to the person's age, but generalities can be made and these will be discussed in relation to the lifespan. (It is important to note that the need for sleep can differ from these ranges.)

Birth and childhood

Babies usually sleep for 18 hours in any 24 hours and have up to 6–8 periods of sleep during this time and these periods tend to be between feeds. At about the age of 3, they will have about 13 hours of sleep per night and a short nap in the daytime, decreasing at the age of 10 to about 8–10 hours (Howard 2004).

Adolescence

The need for sleep temporarily increases during teenage years and at least 10 hours of sleep per night is needed; still teenagers may be sleepy in the daytime. By the time the child is 17, they will usually sleep for 7–8 hours and very little will wake them during this time (Lavery 1997).

Adulthood

Adults have developed their pattern of sleeping and resting by now and sleep between 7 and 8 hours per night. From the age of 30 onwards sleep becomes shallower and doesn't last as long and individuals may wake up far more easily. Sleep patterns begin to change from the age of 40 to 45 in men and 50 to 55 in women.

Women sleep longer than men but tend to complain more of insufficient sleep. Hormonal levels affect women's sleep and those who suffer from premenstrual tension do have less sleep at this time than those who do not. Pregnancy can affect sleep patterns for a variety of reasons, such as movements of the baby and needing to micturate more frequently due to increased pressure on the bladder, particularly in the later stages of pregnancy. Daytime naps may be taken to try to overcome this disturbed sleep pattern. The menopause can also be a time for sleep disruption as a result of hot flushes and night sweats; however, the amount of deep sleep is higher and this may provide some rationale for the fact that women live longer than men (Reet 2003, Lavery 1997).

The elderly

Older people tend to sleep for shorter periods at night, maybe only 5 hours and tend to wake up more frequently, are wakeful during the night and feel less refreshed in the morning. This lack of night-time sleep is complemented by daytime naps (Howard 2004). Many factors have been identified to explain why elderly people appear to sleep less. Physical factors may be influential, e.g. needing to go to the toilet as their bladder function changes, disordered breathing, pain and discomforts. Psychological factors may also be responsible, such as after the death of a spouse, the concerns of living and sleeping alone, or changes in mental states, e.g. in depression and dementia. Environmental and economic factors relating to safety and possible inability to heat their houses properly can also affect their sleeping habits (Reet 2003). It is important to be alert to the reasons for changes in the sleep pattern of older people and consider how sleep can be promoted.

> **Exercise**
> 1. Observe the sleeping patterns of different age groups, if possible, for example a baby or child, an adult or an older person (aged 65 and above) during the daytime.
> 2. What did you notice about their pattern of sleeping?
> 3. Ask individuals about the sleeping patterns of a baby or child, an adult and an older person during the night.
> 4. Are they able to identify changes in their sleeping patterns or needs in relation to sleep?
> 5. Did they have any health problems which may have affected their sleeping. If so, what did they notice as different?

Some differences in observations of people may have been noted. This may depend on the level of activity (mental or physical) they have been involved in during the day. People who exercise more tend to sleep for longer times, which may be due to the rise in temperature produced by exercise, which seems to promote sleep (Lavery 1997). Montgomery & Dennis (2002) concluded that physical exercise can promote sleep in the over 60 age group. Food may affect sleep in different ways, keep a person awake with heartburn, indigestion or hunger or can promote sleep (Reet 2003). Drinks such as tea, coffee and cola contain caffeine, which is a stimulant and, as le May 2006 points out, this will affect the individual's sleep pattern. The environment may have an effect on whether they take daytime naps, particularly in the afternoon or evening. Mothers will have been overjoyed when their babies sleep through the night but don't seem to be as pleased when their offspring sleeps for hours as a teenager and will not get out of bed. Sleep may have been affected by colds, coughing, snoring of partners or transient pain such as toothache and people may well have complained of broken sleep. When individuals go on holiday they frequently complain of poor sleep on the first night, but with a change in daily routine this problem is usually short-lived.

DEPENDENCE AND INDEPENDENCE IN RELATION TO THE ACTIVITY OF SLEEP

Each individual is, according to Roper et al (1996), independent for the activity of sleeping and their independence level is related to their position on the lifespan.

Babies are dependent on others for the maintenance of their environment and their safety, but spend most of their time asleep, while the older person may spend a lot of time in bed, although not always asleep (Roper et al 1996). Children and adolescents can also be dependent on others for sleep, for they are affected by tension and noise. Childhood sleep problems, such as nightmares, night terrors and disturbed sleep, may need specialised support. Adults can become dependent on others to ensure that the noise levels are low, for instance when they work shifts.

The main issue of dependency in adults relates to the use of hypnotic drugs, as Roper et al (1996) identify. Drugs may be used when other remedies have not been successful in aiding sleeping problems. Morin et al (1999) concluded that temazepam (a hypnotic drug), on its own or combined with cognitive-behavioural therapy, improved short-term outcomes for older adults with persistent insomnia. However, these hypnotic drugs produce a different form of sleep to natural sleep and can create dependency. The drugs reduce the amount of restorative sleep but can aid the onset of sleep, reduce wakenings and increase the overall amount of time spent asleep and, for these reasons, individuals take sleeping pills.

Different drugs can be prescribed such as hypnotics (benzodiazepines or anxiolytics or tranquillisers) which act on the central nervous system by depressing brain function to induce sleep (e.g. nitrazepam, temazepam, lorazepam and diazepam) or barbiturates, which depress nervous system activity (e.g. amylobarbitone). Barbiturates are no longer prescribed due to their addictive and overdose risks as well as the high risk of depressing respiration rates (Morgan & Closs 1999, Reet 2003, Howard 2004, le May 2006). Holbrook et al (2000) concluded that benzodiazepines do improve sleep duration but can lead to adverse effects in adults with insomnia. The pharmacological effect of hypnotics wears off after 2 weeks as the body learns to tolerate them and they produce physical and psychological dependence. Withdrawal from these pills may result in even worse insomnia.

According to the National Institute for Health and Clinical Excellence (NICE) (2004), 10–30% of individuals who take benzodiazepines are physically dependent upon them and some 50% suffer from withdrawal symptoms. NICE (2004) recommends that their use is restricted to severe insomnia sufferers, prescribed in the lowest dose possible and for up to 4 weeks only. New non-benzodiazepine hypnotic drugs, zopiclone, zolpidem and zaleplon (known as Z drugs), have been shown to have lower dependency levels. For further information see the latest edition of the British National Formulary at www.bnf.org and NICE (2004).

Exercise
1. Ask some patients who have been taking sleeping tablets why they started to do so.
2. Find out if any of them have tried to quit and, if so, how successful they have been.
3. Ask patients who have taken sleeping tablets for the first time, whilst in hospital, what effect they had upon their sleeping habits and how they felt the next day.

There are many reasons why individuals start taking sleeping tablets. This may have been as a result of bereavement, hospitalisation, illness, or worry over unemployment, financial, domestic or work problems. They may well have described problems when they tried to stop taking sleeping tablets, depending on the length of time they had been taking these medications. They may also describe different coping strategies used, support they had and whether the initial sleep problem had been alleviated. The 'hangover' feeling, insomnia and nightmares may well have been described.

A 'hangover' feeling on the next day is based on the residual effects of the drugs taken. Rebound effects can occur, when the person tries to stop taking the sleeping tablets, such as insomnia which may last for 3–7 nights after just a 3-week course; nightmares may occur as the person often wakes up in the part of the sleep cycle when vivid dreams take place and anxiety levels can be raised. Impaired judgement, poor coordination and memory, reduced work performance, road traffic accidents and falls may occur when the individual stops taking the sleeping tablets. All of these effects are increased by the use of alcohol (Morgan & Closs 1999, le May 2006).

Depending on the absorption, distribution and elimination rates of the drugs used, drug accumulation and dependency can occur. Halfens et al (1994) consider that dependency can result from a short exposure to these drugs, e.g. short hospitalisation when sleeping tablets are offered as a routine measure.

For these reasons, it is better to promote nonpharmacological aids to sleep, such as a quiet dark room with a comfortable bed, mattress and appropriate pillows, reading, relaxation therapy, taking food and drink which aid restful sleep, and ensuring correct temperature to provide sufficient warmth yet be cool enough to allow sleep (Reet 2003).

Exercise
1. Ask adults what they do if they are unable to sleep.
2. Go to a health food store, and find out what nonpharmacological remedies are available for individuals with sleeping difficulties.

Adults may have developed their own remedies for sleep problems. Reite et al (2002) and Lavie et al (2002) identify that good sleep hygiene (habits) should be emphasised with individuals who have difficulty sleeping. Some solutions that may be offered are: ensuring that the room temperature is suitable; wearing comfortable night clothes; being in familiar, secure, quiet surroundings; avoiding consumption of a large meal, coffee, or alcohol and refraining from physical exercise or smoking before going to bed; reading a book and having warm milky drinks. Counting sheep is always laughed at but this does provide the person with a task to focus on, which is monotonous and not stressful, and may work for some people.

Natural alternatives are considered by Lavery (1997) and Reite et al (2002) and nonaddictive sleep remedies, such as tryptophan, can be used. Tryptophan is an amino acid which is good for protein repair and converts to melatonin which aids sleep. Although available on prescription only it is found in milk and carbohydrates, so a hot milky drink with a biscuit may help. Melatonin, the sleep hormone produced by the pineal gland, is beneficial for improving sleep, but it is not fully understood and therefore is not recommended for anyone who is pregnant or below the age of 35. Another herbal product, kava kava root, can depress the central nervous system and relax muscles, so it can help to relax the individual and if taken before bedtime it can allow the individual to initiate sleep. Valerian and St John's wort are two other non-prescribed drugs that are reported to have sedative or antidepressant properties. Bent et al (2006) concluded that there was evidence to suggest that valerian might improve sleep quality without producing side-effects.

There are different levels of consciousness – from being fully alert and awake through to being unconscious and comatosed with natural sleep somewhere in between. Temporary loss of consciousness may occur due to fainting or syncope. Montague et al (2005) points out that this occurs when there is a temporary reduction in blood flow to the brain, which is quickly rectified by ensuring that the head is lower or is at the same level as the heart. Heat syncope is caused due to pooling of blood in the periphery and the extremities especially in hot climates in an attempt to lose heat. Consciousness is restored when the individual is moved to cooler areas.

Unconscious states, however, are not as easy to rectify and can lead to death. Coma states may result from brain tumours, head injuries, overdoses or metabolic disorders. The outcomes vary because of the differing causes but it is essential that you are able to assess levels of consciousness accurately and this will be discussed in the model for nursing section. General anaesthetics will also render the individual unconscious but, when the anaesthetic is reversed, their conscious levels will be restored to normal. Individuals can be frightened at the thought of surgery because they are aware that their conscious level will be compromised and that they will not be able to control this.

FACTORS INFLUENCING THE ACTIVITY OF SLEEP

Roper et al (1996, 2000) state that sleeping is influenced by many factors. In a healthy individual such things as exercise, food, drink, mood, noise, housing and work practices can affect the quantity and quality of sleep. These factors will be explored individually but include:

1. anatomy and physiology related to sleep (biological factors)
2. emotional issues related to sleep (psychological factors)
3. practices, associated health beliefs and habits in different cultures related to sleep (sociocultural factors)
4. environmental factors and how these relate to sleep (environmental factors)
5. policies, laws and economics related to sleep (politicoeconomic factors).

Anatomy and physiology related to sleep (biological factors)

In order to promote health and to care for people who have sleeping problems it is necessary to understand certain body rhythms, the normal cycles of sleep and the anatomy and physiology of relevant parts of the nervous system.

Sleeping is influenced by circadian rhythms. These rhythms are influenced by external factors or zeitgebers (exogenous) such as meal times, light, dark, noise, silence, sleep and rest patterns and internal factors (endogenous) such as cell function. These two sets of factors usually coincide if a normal routine is maintained, i.e. go to bed at a regular time, eat at regular times, respond by waking when it is light and sleeping when it is dark. However, air travel and shift work can upset this rhythm and can cause health problems (Reet 2003, Howard 2004).

> **Exercise**
> 1. Ask different people what they consider may happen to sleep patterns when individuals: fly to and from Australia or stay in Iceland or Greenland or work shifts.
> 2. Find out how these changes may affect their daily lives.

Individuals who have visited Australia may complain of 'jet lag'. This only occurs when people fly in an easterly or westerly direction and occurs because the circadian rhythm is affected. Flying from the UK to Australia takes 24 hours but, due to the time difference between the two places, it makes arrival time 36 hours later than departure time; there is therefore a 12-hour difference. For example, when a person leaves the UK at 8 p.m., i.e. night time, they will arrive in Australia at 6 a.m., i.e. morning. The person will be ready for bed as his 'internal body clock' says it is evening whereas people around him will be ready to go to work and it is daylight (see Fig. 13.1). So the external clues (zeitgebers) are confusing, resulting in the symptoms of 'jet lag'. These symptoms last a few days, whilst the circadian rhythm readjusts itself, and include difficulties with sleeping, decreased alertness and ability to concentrate, gastrointestinal upsets and general fatigue. When the internal clock resets to its new schedule then the symptoms disappear (Rutishauser 1994).

The amount of light also affects the sleep–wake cycle, so in Iceland or Greenland the external clues in relation to daylight and darkness are different to those in the United Kingdom. In Iceland and Greenland, there are long periods of darkness every day in winter with very short periods of daylight and long periods of daylight and short periods of darkness in the summer (Roper et al 1996). As darkness indicates to the body it is time to retire to bed and sleep,

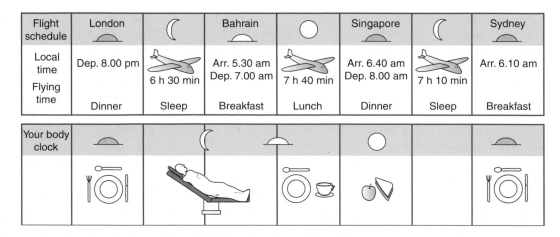

Flight schedule	London		Bahrain		Singapore		Sydney
Local time	Dep. 8.00 pm	6 h 30 min	Arr. 5.30 am Dep. 7.00 am	7 h 40 min	Arr. 6.40 am Dep. 8.00 am	7 h 10 min	Arr. 6.10 am
Flying time	Dinner	Sleep	Breakfast	Lunch	Dinner	Sleep	Breakfast
Your body clock							

Fig. 13.1   Changes in circadian rhythms when flying from London to Australia (from Rutishauser 1994, with permission).

problems arise if the time is actually still daytime and the individual is at work. Equally, when daylight is predominant, then the clues of needing to go to bed are lost. Yet people living in these countries still sleep at 'night' and work during the 'day' and learn to use other external clues, such as meal times to ensure their sleeping and waking cycle is in keeping with their lifestyle.

Practice nurses working in travel clinics need to give appropriate advice to individuals to minimise these problems, such as taking a night-time flight, trying to sleep during the flight, eating only a small amount, avoiding alcohol and drinking plenty of water. It is then advisable to take on the routine of the new time zone as soon as possible and to do some exercise rather than sleeping on arrival. Herxheimer & Petrie (2006) reviewed evidence assessing the effectiveness of oral melatonin for alleviating jet lag. Nine out of the ten trials reviewed found that melatonin can prevent or reduce jet lag and may be used as part of a sleep education programme for adult travellers, flying through five or more time zones in an easterly direction. However, Buscemi et al (2006) disagree and consider that there is no evidence to support the use of melatonin for jet lag but occasional short-term use appears to be safe.

Individuals who work shifts also complain of problems and again this is due to disturbances in their circadian rhythm. Sometimes this may not be resolved and may lead to illness. When individuals work days then nights, their sleep–wake patterns are reversed, so they are active at night and asleep in the day. Outside influences, e.g. daylight and noise, affect the ability to change the 'internal body clock' so the person may present with the same symptoms of jet lag but of a long-term nature.

It is probable that when a person works nights, they will lose some sleep. If they are unable to make up this sleep loss, then various problems can occur, such as poor concentration, reduced efficiency and poor decision making, thereby increasing the risk of accidents and errors. Individuals themselves may become very irritable and 'touchy' (Reet 2003).

Being on permanent days or nights is better than swapping from one pattern to the other as the body can develop a regular sleep–wake pattern. Muecke (2005) concluded that there are adverse psychological and physiological effects of night rotation, particularly in the over 40 age group and that the effects of tiredness on nurse performance may affect the quality of patient care in a negative manner. Berger & Hobbs (2006) identified that nurses can adopt counter measures such as power napping and ensure they complete challenging tasks before 4 a.m. to reduce patient care errors. Brooks (1997) debates the future of permanent night shifts for health care personnel and concludes that choice and ability to adapt circadian rhythms influence the person's likelihood of developing health problems, absenteeism, job satisfaction, social and domestic disruption. It appears generally, from an employee's perspective, that working permanent nights is preferable to working internal rotation. However, internal rotation gives greater flexibility of rostering and there may be a conflict between these two different facets in the National Health Service (NHS). Bendak (2003) identified that working 12-hour shifts in various occupations is becoming a popular shift pattern allowing staff to have an increased numbers of days off by working 3 or 4 long days. Staff were positive in relation to social benefits but there were inconsistent results with regard to health, sleep problems, fatigue and effect on care.

Legal action may be faced by organisations, such as hospitals and nursing homes, if they fail to take steps to combat the ill effects of disrupted sleep patterns as a result of employees working irregular shift patterns. Learthart (2000) concluded that internal rotation is the reason given for many staff leaving the profession and that studies indicate that shift work can cause health problems. Employers should minimise the potential effects of poor health when working nights (Rajaratnam & Arendt 2001). The use of a risk assessment tool, before introducing internal rotation, is advocated by Martell (2001). Horrocks & Pounder (2006) consider that it is advisable to have a long lie in, take an afternoon nap before beginning a night shift, take regular exercise, abstain from drinking alcohol and eat a proper meal before commencing the shift, and work in bright light. This may help to promote a good sleep routine, but the latter element may affect the patient's sleep routine.

The circadian rhythm is greatly influenced by internal factors, such as the sleep–wake cycle, body temperature and cortisol secretion. Various physiological changes occur when individuals go to sleep and wake up which they are generally unaware of. When lying down and resting, metabolic rate is lowered, cardiovascular and renal systems are affected, resulting in temperature, pulse and blood pressure being lowered and the rate of urine formation slowed. When going to sleep, further changes occur, noticeably the secretion of blood cortisol decreases and growth hormone increases. When getting up again the growth hormone levels fall, cortisol levels rise, blood pressure and urine formation increase and heat is generated thereby increasing body temperature (Reet 2003). It is important to note that these changes are normal and therefore when on night duty it must be considered whether changes in vital sign measurements are due to normal changes related to sleep.

These internal or endogenous factors (cell functions) are set by an internal clock. This internal clock is set by cells in the hypothalamus which provide the impetus for the sleep–wake cycle. The biological clock within the hypothalamus and specifically in the suprachiasmatic nucleus drives special cells in the reticular formation within the brain stem, known as the raphe nuclei and nucleus locus coeruleus to determine the level of consciousness (see Fig. 13.2).

If individuals were left without any outside clues to time, then this sleep–wake cycle would occur every 25 hours but social habits, meal times, alarm clocks keep this cycle to a 24-hour time span. Sensory impulses enter the cells in the reticular formation and this triggers the person to wake up. It is then difficult to get back to sleep as sensory information reaches the brain easily now. Conversely when stimuli are low then sleep is easy (Kindlen 2003).

Certain hormonal levels, such as adrenaline and corticosteroids, are responsible for wakefulness and activity. Individuals go to sleep in the late evening when adrenaline and corticosteroid levels are at their lowest. The growth hormone level rises during the night and, at about 5 a.m., the temperature level starts to rise, as does adrenaline and corticosteroid levels which initiate waking. The pineal gland secretes a hormone called melatonin during darkness. Levels of melatonin, the sleep hormone, fluctuate daily, depending on the amount of light entering the eye. When it is dark, or the individual closes their eyes, there is a lack of light entering the eye and so melatonin is released, which tells the body it is time to prepare for sleep (Lavery 1997). A report in the clinical research highlights in *Nursing Times* (1998) has identified that people with myalgic encephalomyelitis (ME) have unusually high levels of melatonin which may be a reason for their chronic fatigue problems.

There are two different types of sleep, namely non-REM (non-rapid eye movements) and REM (rapid eye movements), and these types of sleep combine to form a sleep cycle which lasts for about 90–100 minutes. According to Roper et al (1996) an adult has 4–6 cycles per night (see Fig. 13.3).

Non-REM sleep is sometimes classed as orthodox sleep and comprises 70% of adult sleep. Non-REM sleep can be noted by the use of an electroencephalogram (EEG) because when an individual falls asleep the electrical activity in the brain changes and these changes may be recorded on a graph. Alpha waves can be seen on an EEG when the

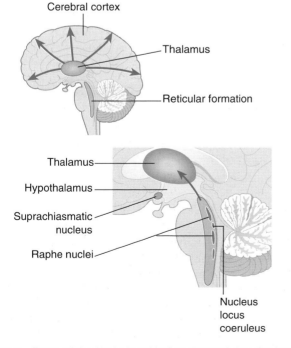

Fig. 13.2 Parts of the brain involved in determining the level of consciousness (from Kindlen 2003, with permission).

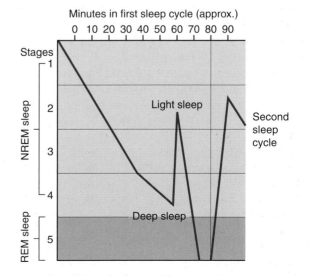

Fig. 13.3 One sleep cycle (from Roper et al 1996, with permission).

individual relaxes but remains awake, the beta waves which are associated with waking and being alert disappear and delta waves of inactivity appear. Many body systems take a rest and therefore the heart rate and blood pressure fall and the body relaxes. There are four stages of non-REM sleep, with Stages 1 and 2 being classed as light sleep and Stages 3 and 4 as deep sleep or slow-wave sleep with REM sleep having just one stage, Stage 5 (le May 2006, Kindlen 2003, Reet 2003, Roper et al 1996).

Exercise

1. Ask individuals what they think happens and how they feel when they are falling asleep.
2. Ask individuals what they remember about being asleep and what they remember when they wake up.
3. Compare your experiences of sleep with that of colleagues.

Individuals will recollect different experiences. Individuals may have described a feeling of floating, falling, drowsiness, disturbed sleep, being woken up, dreaming, not being able to remember a dream, talking in their sleep or grinding their teeth, and others may talk about someone snoring.

All of these recollections are part of sleep and the different stages of the sleep cycle. Each stage has certain characteristics. Stage 1 or 'just dropping off' stage can be noted by the fact that eyes close and roll, the person feels relaxed and drowsy, a drifting or floating sensation may be felt, especially falling, and individuals can sometimes hear voices or see pictures. They are easy to wake during this stage. However, if they are woken up at this time they cannot remember being asleep. This stage only lasts for 15 minutes and only occurs on the first cycle of the night's sleep. Stage 2 lasts for about 15 minutes, and is characterised by greater relaxation, dream-like thoughts, and individuals may remember dreams if they wake up now. They can still be woken easily.

Stage 3 lasts for about 20 minutes and is a period when there is complete relaxation of muscles, the pulse slows and the temperature falls. Individuals are not easy to wake during this stage and have no conscious thoughts. Although they may dream, they do not remember dreams if they wake up now. The growth hormone is released during this stage and it is therefore a time when blood cells and body tissues, especially skin, can be rebuilt. Energy levels can be restored at this time. The final Stage 4 in non-REM sleep is when the individual is completely relaxed, rarely moves and is difficult to wake. Growth hormone continues to be released (le May 2006, Montague et al 2005, Kindlen 2003, Reet 2003, Roper et al 2000).

Stage 5 is REM (rapid eye movement) or paradoxical sleep and is characterised by light sleep, dreaming, eyes move rapidly from side to side, with little body movements. Vivid dreams are recalled if an individual is woken up during this stage. It is thought that this stage is used to update memories and integrate experiences with the past. Physiologically there is an increase in the blood pressure, pulse and respiration rate, with an increased blood flow, whereby protein levels can be renewed in the brain. Hormonally, there is an increase in the levels of testosterone and women have increased blood flow to vagina, whilst men can have erections. Individuals are easily woken at this time. The first episode of REM sleep lasts for only a few minutes, but as the night progresses, this time increases. Individuals change position in bed when they move from REM sleep to non-REM sleep (le May 2006, Montague et al 2005, Kindlen 2003, Reet 2003, Roper et al 2000).

Non-REM sleep is thought to be restorative for the body whereas REM sleep is thought to restore the mind. Within the cycles, there is a pattern throughout the night. The non-REM sleep becomes shorter and the periods of REM sleep become longer. Babies have more REM sleep than non-REM sleep, whereas adults generally have more non-REM sleep than REM sleep (Montague et al 2005, Roper et al 1996).

The electroencephalogram (EEG) and the recordings of eye movements or electroculography (EOG) and chin muscle tone by electromyography (EMG) have provided the means to explore sleep. The five stages of sleep are shown in Figure 13.4 as noted on an EEG recording (le May 2006, Morgan & Closs 1999).

Different sleep problems are associated with the different stages of the sleep cycle. For example, Stage 1 problems may be enuresis (bed wetting) or teeth grinding, whereas Stage 2 problems often present as talking during sleep, Stage 3 and 4 problems involve sleepwalking, night terrors, as well as sleep talking and bedwetting. Stage 5 problems are mainly related to nightmares.

The amount of sleep needed varies with each individual. Individuals can need anything between 2 and 15 hours of sleep a day; if they have more than that, it can cause the same problems as if they have too little. Individuals need to find a balance which suits them. Sleep deficits can build up over time but these deficits can be compensated if the individual takes a longer than normal sleep. Stage 3 and 4 non-REM sleep deficit is made up first, then REM sleep.

Hodgson (1991), Hoffman (2003), Honkus (2003) and Béphage (2005) identify numerous effects of sleep deprivation, some physiological, e.g. falling body temperature, and slight changes in cardiovascular, respiratory and hormonal levels. Behavioural changes occur, such as restlessness, irritability, aggressiveness and depression, and anti-social behaviour may be displayed, but there do not appear to be any serious, lasting neurological problems. Care with driving and working whilst short of sleep is vital as there is an increased risk of being involved in a road traffic accident or having an accident at work. Individuals only need to lose 2 hours sleep to be tired enough to fall asleep whilst driving. Extra sleep does not appear to improve performance and may even make things worse. The Think Road Safety website runs UK road safety campaigns and the 2006

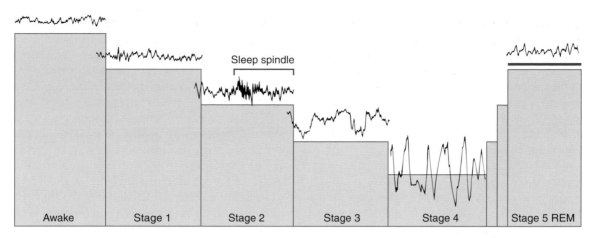

Fig. 13.4 Progressive changes in the electroencephalogram (EEG) following the onset of sleep, showing the patterns characteristic of each stage of sleep, non-REM (Stages 1–4) and REM (stage 5) (from Hobson 1995, with permission).

campaign targeted young men under 30 as they are more likely to have a sleep-related accident. Falling asleep at the wheel is the cause of around 20% of accidents on long journeys on trunk roads and motorways and this commonly occurs between midnight and 6 a.m. (see www.thinkroadsafety.gov.uk).

Lavery (1997) and Honkus (2003) suggest that lack of sleep will not only present with poor concentration, lack of judgement, irritability, depression, stress, dark circles under eyes, but fewer white blood cells are circulating and so there is a lowered resistance to infection. Recovery from surgery or illness is noted to be better if the individual is a good sleeper. Morgan & Closs (1999) consider that lack of sleep will impair tissue restoration. Equally, when patients are fasted or lacking in nutrition for other reasons, they may be tired as the metabolic rate falls in the night.

Apart from the external and internal factors influencing sleep patterns the lifestyle of an individual can affect sleep also. Bedtime routines appear to be useful in training the individual to sleep well.

> **Exercise**
> 1. Ask different people what their routine is at bedtime.
> 2. Ask them if they can identify what aids or disrupts their sleep.
> 3. Discuss with colleagues the findings of these investigations.

Individuals may discuss their eating, drinking, smoking and/or reading activities before bedtime. Caffeine is a stimulant as it increases the amount of circulating adrenaline and its effects can last for 14 hours, so coffee is not advised prior to retiring to bed. Likewise, smoking stimulates the nervous system which raises the blood pressure and adrenaline and so should be avoided. Alcohol tends to send individuals to sleep quickly but they wake early in the morning. A lack of

exercise or too much exercise late at night can delay sleep as can too much mental stimulation just prior to retiring to bed (Reet 2003, le May 2006). It is, however, the routine that is important to the individual and not particularly the components of that routine.

Psychological factors

In everyday life, individuals talk about having a good night's sleep and equate this to feeling well. Equally, after what the individual considers to be a poor night's sleep, there is a feeling of not being on top form, not ill but not their usual self. It may well be a topic of conversation when in a strange place. It may be that certain individuals are more suited to employment involving shift work because of their individual personalities and their ability to adapt to sleep changes. Humm (1996) did identify that toleration of night duty in 46 nurses was related to certain personality factors, in particular their 'rigidity and flexibility of sleeping habits'.

> **Exercise**
> 1. Ask individuals what affects their sleep in relation to their mood.
> 2. Ask them what effect different moods have on the amount and type of sleep they have.
> 3. What are their bedtime routines which they use to aid sleep?

Individuals recount many different moods which affect their sleep. They may be excited about a holiday or getting married and this nervous excitement may result in transient insomnia, but the person is happy and generally feels well and is using the time of rest for reflecting on the preparations and thinking forward with anticipation to the events. They may also talk about times when life situations have not been good, for example work difficulties, unemployment, family tensions or divorce. This may have interrupted their sleep patterns, where they experience difficulty getting to sleep, waking frequently and ultimately they feel worse on waking than they did before retiring to bed. A planned admission to hospital for investigations or surgery may affect the individual's sleeping habits even prior to admission.

Following bereavement, sleep patterns may be disrupted for several reasons, e.g. due to worry over safety, not being used to sleeping alone, as well as the grieving process itself. It is important that people get back to their normal sleep routines as soon as possible to avoid long-term problems.

Insomnia is strongly related to depressive and anxiety-type illnesses. Depressed individuals may suffer from severe insomnia for several weeks where they complain of being awake for hours, difficulty in getting off to sleep, waking early and having disturbed sleep with frequent dreams (le May 2006). People who suffer from anxiety states also complain of tension and this affects sleep. They may present with difficulty getting off to sleep and maintaining sleep throughout the night.

As it would appear that moods affect sleep, then individuals need to consider healthy living choices which include effective sleep routines. Simple measures may be all that is needed, especially going to bed when they feel tired and avoiding the temptation to sleep downstairs in a comfortable armchair. Some people may choose to listen to relaxation tapes, listen to their own favourite music, read a book or watch TV, go for a short walk, take a bath, or eat a snack or take a warm milky drink as it contains an amino acid which forms melatonin, to help soothe the mind and prepare the body for sleep (Lavery 1997).

However, some may consider the use of meditation to relax the whole body, or yoga which can provide a relaxing sequence ready for sleep, involving simple stretching and relaxation exercises suitable for all ages and levels of ability or biofeedback mechanisms whereby the visualisation of a relaxing place, perhaps on a beach or by a stream, is conjured up in the mind and the individual concentrates on this picture (Bray 2001, Hoffman 2003).

Traditional Chinese medicine may be used, such as shiatsu massage, hypnosis or t'ai'chi which can relieve muscular tension and mental stress. Certain herbal remedies, e.g. passion flower or hops are good for general insomnia; St John's wort is used for depression; dill for jet lag; lettuce for restless and excitable people. The use of aromatherapy oils is increasing, whether they are inhaled or absorbed through the skin, e.g. jasmine, rose and lavender are found to be relaxing and soothing. Reflexology therapeutic foot massage is said to suit some individuals, whereas homeopathic remedies are available for a variety of sleep problems, e.g. for acute insomnia aconite can be used, arsenicum album is useful for early waking between 1 and 3 a.m. due to overactive mind, nightmares may be lessened by nux vomica, whereas sepia can be used for individuals who find it difficult to fall asleep (Lavery 1997).

Sociocultural factors

Sociocultural beliefs and practices can influence sleeping and resting as these determine when, where, in what and with whom individuals sleep. Bedtime routines such as adopting a regular bedtime, where the individual has had a period of relaxation before bedtime and the avoidance of daytime naps, caffeine, alcohol and nicotine late at night may be socially orientated. On a simple level, there are individuals who are classed as the 'larks', these are morning people, who go to bed early, rise early and work best in a morning; whereas the 'owls' are evening people, who go to bed late, get up late and work best in an evening (Howard 2004). Rutishauser (1994) considers that some people are better suited to shift work than others. The 'larks' seem to have more difficulty in adjusting to shift work, whereas the 'owls' seem to adjust better. Consider personal experience and whether this is the same for other family members. Are there conflicts between the 'larks and the owls' and when is your best time to study and work?

Roper et al (1996) identify that different cultures adopt different patterns of sleep. North European countries, predominately, sleep at night but Mediterranean cultures take a siesta in the afternoon and then retire for night-time sleep at a later time to the North Europeans. Siestas can improve the individual's mood, their concentration and productivity and do not affect sleep at night. Equally, the place in which people sleep is linked to their cultural roots. For example, Westerners sleep in a bed, whereas Japanese sleep on a bed roll on the floor and there are the 'cardboard cities' where the homeless sleep rough under and on cardboard. Sleeping alone or with a partner, in nightwear or nude is the norm for Westerners whereas people from Eastern countries often sleep with several people in the same place. Eskimos apparently sleep in the same clothes day and night, presumably linked to maintaining body temperature (Roper et al 1996).

Lavery (1997) discusses the influence Indian culture has on sleeping patterns. Indians believe in an Ayurvedic system which has three energy systems or doshas, namely 'pitta, vata and kaphas'. Individuals are seen as a mixture of all three energy systems but two predominate. 'Vata' people are thin, excitable, tire easily and are light sleepers with irregular sleeping habits and are prone to sleep problems. On the other hand, 'pitta' individuals are of medium build, get angry or irritable when stressed, and tend to wake during the night feeling hot or thirsty but wake feeling alert. 'Kapha' people are calm, confident and slow moving. They love to sleep and sleep long periods and wake up slowly. Also, these energy phases occur at different times of the day, e.g. 'vata' occurs early morning, 'pitta' in the afternoon and 'kapha' in the late evening. Ayurveda advises people to go to sleep when it is 'kapha' time (6–10 p.m.) as sleep will be slow and then wake up in 'vata' time, before 6 a.m. which is the active phase. To sleep well these doshas need to be balanced. If they become imbalanced by illness then sleep is affected.

Dreams are also linked to these three doshas, as 'pitta' types usually have action and adventure dreams but if they are not balanced then these dreams can turn into anger and conflict. 'Vata' types have imaginative and action dreams but again if they are not balanced then become dreams of anxiety where the person is falling, running away or being chased. 'Kapha' types have tranquil dreams of lakes and oceans but unfortunately they are rarely remembered (Lavery 1997).

Chinese philosophy is different as they believe that individuals live between heaven and earth and the energies of these two provide the energy for life. If the energies are balanced then they are in good health. 'Yin' and 'yang' energies are governed by three different forces, namely the spirit or 'shen', which is responsible for consciousness; energy or 'qi', which moves, warms and protects and essence; or 'jing', which is responsible for growth and development. When a person is well, then all of these forces are in harmony and sleep is peaceful, growth and development takes place. If ill, then there are problems with 'shen' and 'jing' and growth and renewal cannot take place (Lavery 1997).

Sleep and dreaming are also influenced by the ethereal soul or 'hun' and this is stored in the liver at night. If the person develops liver problems, then the 'hun' wanders, causing restlessness and exhausting dreams. If the person sleeps well then the 'hun' collects images and these images keep the person mentally and spiritually happy and creative (Lavery 1997).

Dreams that don't upset the person's sleeping pattern are normal but if they do affect the sleeping pattern, then these are related to some pathology. The type of dream is governed by balance of energy, and when it occurs, as each hour of the day and night relates to different organs and emotions, e.g. 3–5 a.m. is the start of the spiritual day and relates to lungs, sadness and grief, so dreams at this time may cause breathing problems, or feelings of loss and be of a spiritual nature (Lavery 1997).

These different aspects are important for you to consider when nursing patients from these cultural backgrounds.

> **Exercise**
> 1. If possible, speak to people who have lived in very different parts of the world, e.g. Australia, Alaska, Iceland or India, and find out about their sleeping habits.
> 2. Ask them what kind of sleep patterns they have and what affects them.

Environmental factors

For most people, sleep takes place in a specific room designed for sleep as environmental factors do influence sleep. Sleep is usually easier when individuals are in familiar surroundings, which are cool, dark, private and quiet. Roper et al (1996) and Howard (2004) identify that having their own belongings and being somewhere safe and quiet is important in aiding sleep.

However, these surroundings can change in life, e.g. following bereavement, moving to a smaller house or bungalow or changes in health which necessitate sleeping in a chair. Shift workers have to consider their environment and use thicker curtains to block out sunlight, and lessen noise in the household. Homeless people have a very different environment to those who sleep in a house, as well as those who sleep in bed-and-breakfast houses or where multiple individuals share rooms and even beds and, therefore, their sleeping habits may well be affected.

The Government set up a Rough Sleepers Unit in 1999 (Communities and Local Government 2006) and set a target to reduce rough sleeping by at least two-thirds by 2002 and this figure was met in December 2001. The number of those individuals sleeping rough fell from 1850 in 1998 to 532 in 2002 and this is being maintained and improved; in June 2006 the number stood at 502, with some dramatic reductions, such as in Birmingham where 56 people slept rough in 1998, falling to just 7 in 2005, and in Westminister, London in the same timespan the figure fell from 237 to 133. This had been achieved by a variety of measures and the health and wellbeing of these individuals, including their sleeping habits, would hopefully have improved (www. communities.gov.uk/index.asp?id=1150131).

> **Exercise**
> 1. Ask individuals what type of environment they sleep in.
> 2. Ask them what environmental factors affect their sleeping habits.
> 3. Consider the differences and discuss findings with colleagues.

They may well describe a variety of settings but familiarity and safety issues may be prominent. They may say that the mattress and pillows are important yet some prefer a firm or soft mattress and pillow. According to Howard (2004), noise affects progression through the stages of sleep and increases the frequency of waking and body movements. Women and older people are more prone to waking due to noise, but it appears to be the significance of the noise and not the volume of noise which wakes them up. Le May (2006) discusses research that supports the link between age and noise, demonstrating a decline in the intensity of noise required to wake an older person. Traffic and aircraft noise is a problem for some yet others sleep well in this type of environment but wake easily when a baby cries or when they hear the sound of breaking glass. The temperature of the room is important and 18°C or 65°F is ideal, if above or below these temperatures then this affects sleep. It is for the same reason that fever affects sleeping. Exposure to bright sunlight in the day seems to promote sleep at night. Latitude does not seem to affect sleep, i.e. in Iceland where there is little night in summer and little light in winter individuals still sleep.

Home design takes particular note of the bedroom environment and feng shui, a traditional Chinese art and science of home design, can be used to position furniture, rooms and buildings so that they are in harmony with individuals and lines of energy in the Earth. It is thought that, by placing the head of the bed against a wall, this will give the feeling of security and allow individuals to relax. The colour scheme may also be important and pinks, peach, pale yellow, blue or green, and lilac are seen as restful (Lavery 1997).

Snoring (the noise produced from the soft palate and other parts of the upper respiratory tract) is another 'environmental' problem as the peace and quiet of a household can be disrupted by someone who snores and it can have major effects on the sleeping partners. Snoring is most common in middle-aged, older and obese men, although 40% of all adults snore (Morgan & Closs 1999).

Politicoeconomic factors

The link to politicoeconomic factors that affect sleep may not be immediately obvious as Roper et al (1996) identify. However, the type of housing and the number of bedrooms and siblings has a link to economic factors which may impinge on sleeping habits. Employment practices may also link to economic forces and therefore shift workers may have a link to sleep. The Hours and Employment Act of 1936 controls the number of hours a person can work, in particular that of women and young people.

Exercise

1. Look on the Department of Trade and Industry website (www.dti.gov.uk).
2. Identify policies in relation to working time regulations and issues relating to hours of work and night duty.

You may have accessed a document entitled 'Your guide to the working time regulations: sections 1–4′ formulated in 2000, amended in 2003, by the Department of Trade and Industry. This document states that the working time limit is for a 48-hour week and sets out what constitutes working time, which includes working lunches, travel as part of the job, training related to job and working abroad. These regulations have applied to junior doctors since August 2004. A phased approach has been taken to achieving a 48-hour week, by starting at 58 hours per week from August 2004, reducing to 52 hours by July 2009 and then reducing to 48 hours from August 2009 to August 2012 (Working Times Regulations, at www.dti. gov/employment/employment-legislation/working-time regs/index). This issue has had vast implications to the roles of junior doctors and nurses and has resulted in blurring of these roles.

The average weekly working time is calculated over a 17-week period usually. The document states that the 'average weekly working time is calculated by dividing the number of hours worked by the number of weeks over which the average working week is being calculated'. So a worker working 40 hours per week for 17 weeks and 12 hours overtime in the first 10 weeks, with no annual leave would have an average working limit of $(40 \times 17) + (12 \times 10) = 800$ divided by 17 = 47.1 hours per week, so the limit of the 48-hour week is complied with. Workers can agree to work longer than a 48-hour week but they need to sign an opt-out agreement with their employer.

There are specific regulations in relation to working at night and these are outlined in this document. For example, a night worker is someone who works at least 3 hours a night and night-time is between 11 p.m. and 6 a.m. Night workers should not normally work more than 8 hours a night and night working time is calculated over 17 weeks. Average hours worked at night need to be calculated and these are worked out as follows:

- Number of hours worked in the 17 weeks divided by the number of days in the period (after rest days have been deducted), e.g. a night worker works 4×12-hour night shifts per week over 17 weeks. $17 \times (4 \times 12) = 816$.
- 119 days in 17 weeks minus 17 rest days = $119 - 17 = 102$.
- 816 divided by 102 = 8 hours per day, as the average hours of work, which is within the normal working time allowed.

It may be interesting to review a qualified nurse's duty rota in the 1950s and compare it to today (with their permission). These are the rules for individuals working in the UK. In other countries these regulations may well be different and stories of 'sweat shops' where young people work long hours, in appalling conditions, with little time off are frequently retold.

In addition to ensuring working times are within the average limits, employers must offer night workers a free health assessment before they work on nights and on a regular basis whilst they remain on nights. It is, however, unusual that individuals are unable to work nights due to medical disorders. The employee does not have to take up this offer but if they do then they would need to complete a health questionnaire and undergo a medical examination if there are any doubts about the employee's ability to work at night.

Workers are also entitled to have a period of 11 hours uninterrupted rest per working day and at least one full day a week off work. Whilst at work, workers are entitled to a 20-minute rest break, during the shift, if they work more than 6 hours at a stretch. Young workers have different rules regarding rest on a daily, weekly and shift basis. However, the night work limits, rights to rest periods and rest breaks don't apply in certain circumstances, for example where the job requires round-the-clock staffing, such as in hospitals. It is therefore interesting to consider the effect of shift patterns and working hours on nurses.

Fitzpatrick et al (1999) investigated shift work and its impact on qualified nurses' performance and outcomes. They found that nurses working an 8-hour shift performed better than those working a 12.5-hour shift. They considered that mental and physical tiredness may well have affected the nurses and working several 12.5-hour shifts compounded the problems. Dingley (1996) attempted to define the optimum shift pattern for hospital night staff by comparing staff who worked permanent nights and those who worked internal rotation. The mental alertness of both groups was assessed at the beginning and end of each shift. Nurses felt they were more alert at the beginning of the shift and at the beginning of a span of nights than at the end. Yet, when tested, their performances were worse at the beginning than at the end of the shift and peaked after 4 nights. The need to conduct a risk assessment was also identified, by Dingley (1996), before any rotational system was put in place. Martell (2001, p. 7) quotes research in the *Lancet* and says that irregular shift patterns and night working 'outstrip our biological adaptation to the 24-hour cycle of light and darkness … sleep loss results in performance deficits, … slowed physical and mental reaction time, increased errors, decreased vigilance …'. To ensure that optimum and effective work patterns are maintained, it is necessary for employers to consider the length of a shift (8 or 12.5 hours) and the number of consecutive night duty shifts (4 or 8 nights). Wilson (2002) concluded that forward rotation should be used, i.e. mornings, afternoon, nights; a maximum of 3 nights should be worked consecutively, and early shifts to start no earlier than 8 a.m., night shift should be shorter than day shift, minimum of two consecutive nights off, regular shift patterns, 12-hour shifts, choice and flexibility in rostering. It would be useful to consider how these findings relate to your work patterns.

Apart from employment regulations which relate to sleep and rest, there are driving regulations which link to sleep as, unfortunately, accidents whilst driving have occurred when the individual is tired or has fallen asleep. Drivers need to comply with certain rules and alert the Driver and Vehicle Licensing Agency (DVLA) of any problems they may have which may affect their driving, e.g. epilepsy. Brugne (1994) identifies that road safety is dependent upon drivers being awake and vigilant at all times. A microsleep of 1–3 seconds could result in a driver missing a bend or going through a red light. Brugne (1994) identifies that, in the USA, 13% of road traffic accident fatalities were caused by people falling asleep at the wheel. It is, therefore, advisable that individuals are well rested before they set out on a long drive and that they don't drive on a motorway for longer than 2 hours before taking a break. Driving on motorways is monotonous and a long drive may be split up with some main road driving to lessen the monotony. If sleep apnoea is suspected then an individual must not drive and they must be aware that it is a criminal offence to fall asleep at the wheel. They must inform the DVLA once the diagnosis is confirmed. Once symptoms are under satisfactory control then driving can be permitted but confirmation by a specialist is needed if the individual drives a heavy goods vehicle (SIGN 2003).

Exercise

1. Look at the Department for Transport websites (www.dft.gov.uk, www.thinkroadsafety.gov.uk).
2. Identify documents in relation to driving hours, road safety research, driver sleepiness and medication issues.
3. If possible, discuss these findings with an individual who drives a goods vehicle privately or commercially, and older drivers.

Numerous documents relating to drivers' hours and tachograph rules for goods vehicles in the UK and Europe may have been found. The rules are complex due to the nature of commercial driving in this country and overseas and are subject to change. However, the daily driving limit is 9 hours taken between two consecutive daily rest periods or between a daily rest period and a weekly rest period. The weekly driving limit in 2007 is 56 hours and a 90-hour driving limit per fortnight. In the 9-hour daily driving limit, the individual must take a 45-minute break after 4.5 hours driving. It is the responsibility of the driver and employer to ensure that they comply with the drivers' hours and tachograph rules and records are made of both the driving and rest hours. There is a fine of up to £2500 for breach of drivers' hours and £5000 for failing to use a tachograph and if records are falsified, then the £5000 fine is accompanied with 2 years imprisonment (Department for Transport 2006).

The reason why these regulations have been drawn up is that out of a total of 3200 road accident fatalities per year in the UK, it is estimated that between 800 and 1000 involve vehicles being driven for work purposes with another 80 000 nonfatal injuries. In addition to this, studies of the causes of road traffic accidents have demonstrated that tiredness and sleepiness are contributing factors in 20% of accidents overall, particularly on motorways. (www.thinkroadsafety.gov.uk). Specific data have been collated to ascertain relationships between sleep-related accidents on sections of selected trunk roads and motorways in the UK and measures needed to combat driver fatigue.

It was identified by Horne (2001) that sleep-related accidents peak at 2 a.m. to 7 a.m. and 2 p.m. to 4 p.m. when daily sleepiness is higher. These accidents typically involve running off the road or into the back of another vehicle, with no braking beforehand, and many of the accidents are work-related. These accidents are more evident in young male drivers in the early morning and older male drivers in the afternoon. Sleep is preceded by feelings of increasing sleepiness of which drivers are quite aware, although driving impairment is usually worse than is realised by the sleepy driver. They may open the window, stretch at the wheel and turn on the radio. These remedies are only effective for a few minutes and individuals should use the signs to prepare themselves for a break and a period of rest, preferably a short nap combined with a caffeinated drink.

The Department for Transport is also conducting research relating to daytime fatigue linked with over-the-counter medications, alcohol consumption and elderly drivers, and noting the effects on road safety. Horne & Barrett (2001) identify over-the-counter medicines which potentially cause drowsiness and may be hazardous to drivers and other road users. Over 100 medicines may cause drowsiness, namely those belonging to the antihistamines, opioids and muscarinic antagonist groups. Older people are particularly vulnerable to the sedative effects of these drugs and the effects are enhanced when combined with alcohol.

Road safety research reports Nos 25 and 39, produced for the Department for Transport (2001 and 2003 respectively), present the findings in relation to older drivers, illness and medication. Older drivers are increasing in number and particularly female drivers. The risk of an elderly person being killed or suffering serious injuries resulting from a road traffic accident is greater than a younger person because of their increased frailty. Some illnesses are associated with higher road accident risks, e.g. epilepsy, diabetes, heart disease, dementia, sleep apnoea, anxiety and depression, and these may be more prevalent in older people. These findings, combined with the effects of drugs in older people, such as anxiolytics and hypnotics, need to be considered from a health promotion perspective.

Another problem related to sleep and political issues is that of sudden infant death syndrome (SIDS) or cot death. SIDS claims seemingly healthy babies every hour in all countries of the world. The USA death rate from cot deaths is 5000–6000 per year, about one-third of all deaths in the newborn period, whereas four babies in 1000 die from cot death in New Zealand. According to Montague et al (2005) there were about 1400 cot deaths in the UK in 1990 (1.7 per 1000) but this figure fell to 0.7 per 1000 by 1994. This trend has continued and the Office for National Statistics (2004) reported that this fell to 0.48 per 1000 deaths (i.e. 313) in 2004. Infants who die from cot death are usually born with a chronic abnormality with undetected symptoms. However, infant, maternal and environmental characteristics are associated with an increased risk of cot death and the following exercise will help you to identify these characteristics.

Exercise

1. Look at the Department of Health's website (www. dh.gov.uk) or other references on cot deaths such as Foundation for the Study of Infant Deaths (www.fsid. org.uk).
2. Find out what the risk factors are in relation to cot deaths.
3. Consider what advice would be given to Elizabeth to reduce the risk of cot death. Elizabeth is a young unmarried mother, who is living with her parents. They all smoke and she is experiencing problems with breast feeding her 1-month-old son.

There are numerous risk factors. Mitchell et al (1997) identified that many cot deaths in New Zealand occurred when babies were lying on their stomachs, were of babies of mothers who smoked, that babies were three times as likely to die if they slept in their parents' bed as opposed to sleeping in their own cot, and many were not breast fed. Other risk factors such as being born to an unmarried young mother and a greater number of previous pregnancies were also identified. Henderson-Smart et al (1998) identified three main recommendations relating to babies

sleeping on their backs, the baby's head to remain uncovered during sleep and being in a smoke free environment before and after birth. The *New Zealand Herald* (2006) reports that researchers in New Zealand are investigating the possible link with an abnormality in the brain that may prevent babies realising that their bodies are short of oxygen and this is linked with disturbances with the use of serotonin. Serotonin influences breathing, body temperature and arousal from sleep and it may be that some babies don't wake up when they are short of oxygen as the serotonin system is not functioning properly.

There are various measures that can be discussed with Elizabeth to reduce the risk of cot death, for example placing her baby on his back to sleep as he is less likely to choke; reducing smoking in the house and certainly not smoking in the baby's bedroom; ensuring the baby's room is kept at the correct temperature (about 18°C or 65°F); leaving the baby's head uncovered; and ensuring that the baby sleeps on a firm, flat, well-fitting clean mattress (Department of Health 2005 leaflet available at www.dh.gov.uk). It was estimated that the UK cot death rate of 2000 per year could be cut to 500 a year if parents were informed of risk factors. Fortunately, this advice seems to have been successful with fatalities falling steadily.

CONCLUSION

The framework for the model of living has been used to demonstrate how the model can be used to guide understanding of health and everyday life in relation to the activity of sleeping. The final exercise will concentrate on the interrelatedness to the other Activities of Living and the factors which affect sleeping specifically through the use of a mini case scenario to demonstrate how individuality in living occurs.

Exercise

1. Read through the family scenario in Box 13.1.
2. Consider how the activity of sleeping may be affected in each of the family members.
3. Consider the effect on the other Activities of Living.

The following points may have been considered.

1. **Maintaining a safe environment**
   - safety of baby, position in bed at night, security of house.

2. **Communicating**
   - all family members need to be aware of the others' sleep needs and shift patterns.

3. **Breathing**
   - snoring and its effects on household.

4. **Eating and drinking**
   - warm milky drinks and small snacks at night
   - avoidance of caffeine and alcohol at bed time.

Mark, a policeman, and Patsy, a supply teacher, live in a four-bedroom house, with their two children. Their 20-year-old daughter has a 4-month-old baby and their son is working in the local supermarket, over the summer, until he goes back to college to study music (plays the guitar). Patsy's mother is recently bereaved and is living with them for a short time until she can move into a bungalow. She is depressed after the death of her husband and snores loudly. The baby is developing well but cries at night and still needs feeding. The daughter is breast feeding and has the baby in her room. Mark does not always sleep well when on nights and his son practises his guitar at any time of the day or night. Mark's sister is planning to visit the family, during the summer, flying from New York to London.

5. **Eliminating**
   - noise at night with regard to flushing toilets.

6. **Mobilising**
   - driving following night shifts
   - moving house issues
   - exercise habits during the day and prior to retiring at night.

7. **Expressing sexuality**
   - sexual activity of parents in this busy household.

8. **Maintaining body temperature**
   - temperature of the house at night and particularly the baby's room.

9. **Working and playing**
   - music practice needs to be organised around shifts.

10. **Sleep and rest**
    - sleeping habits, jet lag, sleep deprivation of family members such as Mark or the daughter.

11. **Dying**
    - coping with bereavement.

SUMMARY POINTS

1. Individuals spend one-third of their lives asleep.
2. Sleep is an essential part of health and wellbeing.
3. Individuals can learn to adopt a healthy sleep routine.

THE MODEL FOR NURSING

INTRODUCTION

This part of the chapter will link the components of the model of living (lifespan, dependency/independency and

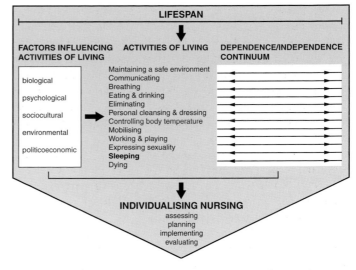

Fig. 13.5 Activity of sleeping within the model for nursing (from Roper et al 1996, with permission).

factors affecting sleeping) with the model for nursing in health and ill health in relation to sleeping. Exercises, mini case scenarios and one major case scenario will be used to allow you to apply the knowledge gained from the model of living section. The application of the model for nursing is based upon the integration of the model of living components and the four stages of the nursing process, as shown in Figure 13.5 (Roper et al 1996). (See Chapter 1 for further details relating to the nursing process.)

The initial stage of this process, assessing, begins with the point of contact of the nurse and the patient and is the start of the nurse–patient relationship. The aim of the assessment stage in relation to sleeping is to collect information about how the individual relates to this Activity of Living when they are well and when they are ill.

Sleeping in health

In order to make this assessment, all the other aspects of the model should be integrated into the sleeping Activity of Living as shown in Box 13.2.

This Activity of Living in health is complex and the nurse needs to be aware of the normal health states of individuals before considering the activity of sleeping in ill health. This information needs to be integrated at each stage of the nursing process to identify individual patient's needs and problems.

Sleeping in ill health

The components of the model will be used to show how a variety of ill-health issues affect the activity of sleeping. It is estimated that 14–40% of the population of Europe and USA has sleep problems with 17% of these being serious problems (Roper et al 1996). In the 'Sleep in America' poll by the National Sleep Foundation (2002), 58% reported experiencing insomnia symptoms, waking feeling unrefreshed (40%),

Box 13.2	Summary of the model for nursing with the activity of sleeping in health

Lifespan
- Consider effect of age and gender on sleeping.

Dependence
- Dependency is linked to changes in the lifespan and health changes, e.g. security, environment, hypnotic drugs.
- Dependency is also linked to changes in health, e.g. fever, bereavement, pain, stress, conscious state.

Independence
- Independence linked to age and health.

Factors affecting sleeping

Biological
- Circadian rhythms, zeitgebers and cell function.
- Intact biological clock.
- Sleep–wake cycle.
- Degree of physical activity.
- Sleep hygiene/habits.
- Body's physiological responses to changes to circadian rhythms.

- Intact nervous system to enable effective sleep–wake cycles.
- Noted by observations of normal sleeping – stages, time asleep, dreaming, activity whilst asleep.
- Note any abnormal sleeping – snoring, insomnia, sleepwalking or talking, nightmares, night terrors.

Psychological
- Effects of emotional state on sleeping such as depression, anxiety, mood swings, excitement, bereavement.

Sociocultural
- Social issues relating to place of sleeping.
- Cultural aspects and beliefs may influence sleeping.

Environmental
- Surroundings, noise, temperature, safety, bedroom design.

Politicoeconomic
- Mechanisms to control working hours, shifts and accidents at work and on the roads.

---

being awake a lot during the night (36%), difficulty falling asleep (25%) and waking up early and not being able to get back to sleep (24%). Insomnia is the most problematic disorder but the International Classification of Sleep Disorders, as set by the Diagnostic Classification Steering Committee, American Academy of Sleep Medicine (2001), identified four different classes of sleep disorders with some 88 distinct sleep and wake patterns. The four classes are namely: dyssomnias (e.g. insomnias, sleep apnoea, and circadian sleep disorders), parasomnias (e.g. abnormal events which occur during sleep, e.g. sleepwalking, nightmares), mental/psychiatric disorders (psychoses, anxiety, dementia, parkinsonism) and sleep disorders (www.absm.org/PDF/ICSD.pdf). Ill health, according to Lavery (1997) is one of the main causes of disrupted sleep as various disorders can affect sleep onset, quantity and quality of sleep.

Reflect on these conditions and identify learning needs following this exercise. It may be useful to discuss these learning needs with a qualified nurse and formulate action plans to address them.

Exercise
1. Using the components of the model (lifespan, dependency/independency continuum, factors affecting health – physical/biological, psychological, sociocultural, environmental, politicoeconomic) and your clinical experience to date, consider what illnesses patients may have which affect sleeping.
2. Check Box 13.3 for some examples.

ASSESSING THE INDIVIDUAL

The aim of this section is to demonstrate how to utilise the components of the model of living to carry out the following three phases involved in assessment in relation to sleeping:

1. Collection of data when taking a nursing history in relation to the activity of sleeping and other related activities.
2. Interpretation of data collected to assess the degree of alteration in the activity of sleeping and the effect on other Activities of Living.
3. Identification of individuals' actual and potential problems related to the activity of sleeping and other related activities.

It is noted that assessment is a continuous activity but a thorough initial assessment is vital and this part of the chapter will describe how the components of the model can be integrated to support the assessment process. (For further details relating to assessment refer to Chapter 1.)

Collection of data when taking a nursing history in relation to the activity of sleeping and other related activities

The assessment stage is vital as all the other stages of individualising nursing are dependent upon it. Therefore, it is important to plan this activity and consider what may affect the collection of data, its interpretation and the identification of patient's problems.

After undertaking the next exercise, reflect on how nurses can ensure that the collection of data is accurate and how

Box 13.3	Summary of illnesses affecting sleep patterns

Lifespan
- Childhood, e.g. difficulty establishing sleep routines in particular sleep onset, nightmares, night terrors, bedwetting, sleepwalking and talking.
- Adult, e.g. insomnia.
- Older person, e.g. difficulties staying asleep and complaint of more disturbed sleep with early morning waking.

Dependence/independence
- Sleeping difficulties will affect many of the other Activities of Living and therefore the individual may become dependent on others, e.g. working and playing.

Factors affecting sleeping

1. Biological
  a. Disturbance with sleep–wake cycles, e.g.
- Insomnia – dissatisfaction with sleep quantity or quality.
- Hypersomnia – excessive daytime sleepiness or difficulty in waking.
- Sleep apnoea – cessation of breathing during sleep due to obstruction of upper airway or loss of respiratory effort.
- Narcolepsy – neurological syndrome, abnormal need to sleep.
- Cataplexy – sudden temporary paralysis due to fright.
- Sleep walking – somnambulism.
- Nightmares/night terrors.
- Night-time attacks of migraine and asthma linked to REM sleep.
- ME (myalgic encephalomyelitis) a debilitating condition which presents with flu-like fatigue, depression and poor sleep. Fibromyalgia is similar but presents with muscle fatigue and multiple tender

body parts. Alpha waves continue to be produced in their sleep so causing them to wake up.
  b. Damage to nervous tract
- Brain damage, e.g. coma/head injuries.
- Overdose of drugs.
- Epileptic fits occur during NREM sleep and can be induced by sleep deprivation.
- Parkinson's disease gives fragmented sleep and sleep apnoea can occur.
- Neuromuscular disorders can affect sleep.
  c. Respiratory/cardiovascular disorders
- Respiratory and heart problems can occur after dreams, especially if emotional dreams such as death and dying in men and separation in women.
- Angina and myocardial infarctions are associated with REM sleep.
- Asthma attacks due to bronchoconstriction occur frequently at night, between 4 and 6 a.m.
  d. Disorders where pain is present
- Duodenal ulcers secrete more gastric juice during sleep so wake up with pain.
- Fibrositis syndrome may be responsible for the generalised pain and stiffness in patients with rheumatoid/osteoarthritis who have sleep disrupted with joint pains.
  e. Disorders involving renal and endocrine systems
- Diabetes mellitus
- Myxoedema patient suffer from snoring and obstructive sleep apnoea.

2. Psychological
- Link with depression and anxiety, e.g. insomnia.

Lavery (1997), Morgan & Closs (1999), Lavie et al (2002), Reite et al (2002).

Exercise

You have been asked to assess a patient who has been admitted to your clinical area and who has been awake all night at home prior to admission in the afternoon.

1. Identify what physical, psychological, sociocultural, environmental and politicoeconomic factors may influence the collection of the data required.
2. Refer to Box 13.4 and consider how these influencing factors can be minimised.

Exercise

1. What skills will you need to develop to enable you to obtain a comprehensive nursing history with a patient who has difficulty sleeping?
2. Check in Box 13.5 with regard to these skills.
3. Reflect on these skills and consider why they are important. Then identify the skills which you may need to improve upon and consider how you can do this. Discuss this with your mentor or preceptor and write an action plan for this learning need.

---

these factors can be minimised so as not to influence the information collected. As noted, there are many factors that may affect the collection of the data and therefore there is a need to use a variety of skills when collecting data. Consider the skills needed in the following exercise.

Having identified that various factors may affect the ability to collect information and that a variety of skills are equally required, it may be useful to consider what data needs to be collected and for what purpose this will be used.

Box 13.4	Factors influencing the activity of sleeping

Physical
- Actual physical state of person and energy levels.
- Actual conscious level of person.
- May be in pain which will affect their ability to sleep and rest.
- Facial expressions/behavioural characteristics such as swollen eyelids, yawning, slow speech.

Psychological
- Actual mental state due to sleep deprivation.
- Actual mental state due to fear and anxiety relating to illness and lack of sleep.
- Actual knowledge of disease and past experiences.

Sociocultural
- Different social/cultural backgrounds of patient and nurse which may affect their ability to communicate.
- Level of interpersonal skills of the patient and the nurse.
- Presence, attitudes and reactions of others.

Environmental
- Ward environment noisy and not very private causing distractions and repetition of answers.

Politicoeconomic
- Quality of the environment.
- Time available to conduct the interview.

Box 13.5	Assessment skills

Interviewing skills
- Asking open and closed questions as appropriate so as not to tire the individual.
- Consider the length of the initial interview.
- Return and complete the interview when the patient has rested.
- Explain issues in lay terms and check understanding.
- Use of silence to allow individual to rest or think.
- Prioritise questions.
- Involve relatives.

Observation skills
- Verbal and nonverbal cues.
- Physical signs, e.g. desire to sleep, yawning, temperature, pulse rate, respiratory rate.
- Psychological cues, e.g. anxiety.

Writing skills
- Completion of accurate and specific report on patient's individual sleep routines, patterns and problems.

Listening skills
- Therapeutic relationship skills.
- Use own body language appropriately.

Box 13.6	Questions for assessing the activity of sleeping

Lifespan and independence
- Does the individual sleep normally in relation to the expectations of the time of the lifespan?

Dependence
- Has the individual experienced any difficulties with sleeping in the past or do they have a longstanding difficulty with sleeping?
- How has the individual coped with these sleeping difficulties?
- How is the individual coping with these sleeping difficulties now?
- Could the individual experience difficulties with sleeping in the future?

Factors affecting sleeping
Physical
- What are the individual's normal presleeping, sleeping and waking routines?
- What time does the individual go to sleep?
- How long does it take to get off to sleep?
- What time does the individual wake up in the morning?
- How long does the individual sleep for?
- How many times does the individual wake up during the night?
- What wakes the individual?
- Does the individual take naps in the daytime?

- Does the individual snore, talk or walk in their sleep, fall out of bed, or have dreams or nightmares?
- What is the individual's usual sleeping position?
- Does the individual take any medication to aid sleep?
- Are there any signs of sleep deficits on admission?
- What specific difficulties is the individual experiencing in relation to sleeping and what are the causes?
- What specific problems are noted in the individual's sleeping pattern or habit?
- What other Activities of Living affect the individual's sleeping problems?
- What effect does the individual's sleeping difficulties have on the other Activities of Living?

Psychological
- What emotional responses affect sleeping?
- What is the individual's attitude to sleep, i.e. quantity and quality needed?
- Does the individual feel refreshed in the morning?
- Does the individual feel sleepy in the daytime?
- Is the individual able to concentrate on tasks in the day?

Sociocultural
- Does the individual normally share a bed or sleep alone?
- What type of clothing does the individual wear in bed?

(continued)

Box 13.6	Questions for assessing the activity of sleeping (continued)

- How many pillows, sheets, blankets does the individual normally use?
- Does the individual's work or lifestyle affect their sleeping habits (e.g. shift worker)?

Environmental

- What factors may alter/inhibit the individual's sleeping pattern at home or hospital?
- Is the individual used to noise, lights or other disturbances during the night at home?

Politicoeconomic

- Are there any difficulties which may have long-term effects on sleep?
- What information and resources does the individual have or need to have in order to assist them in promoting sleep and healthy living?

Exercise

1. Reflect upon a recent admission you have been involved with and identify potential questions that would help you collect specific data.
2. You may wish to check Box 13.6 for possible questions.
3. Reflect on how you feel about asking these questions and how you would ask them in a conversational manner.

Exercise

1. Consider the brief case studies in Box 13.7.
2. Identify specific questions relating to the following patients with specific sleeping problems in ill health.

Box 13.7	**Three brief case studies to explore assessment in the AL sleeping**

A. A 22-year-old woman, who has recently been made redundant and has recently separated from her partner, is admitted with anxiety and depression. This is resulting in the woman complaining of insomnia and early morning wakening. She recently took a drugs overdose and was admitted to hospital.

B. A 40-year-old businesswoman has been complaining of excessive amount of tiredness, fatigue, depression and poor sleep and has been diagnosed, after some time, as having myalgic encephalomyelitis (ME).

C. A 66-year-old retired schoolteacher has been diagnosed with Parkinson's disease. He has been complaining of difficulty getting off to sleep, waking up frequently through the night as the activation of muscle tone affects his ability to sleep. He is generally sleeping less than he did before, therefore making him feel tired through the day.

Case study A questions

- What is your pattern of sleep like now?
- Do you have difficulty falling asleep?
- How long does it take for you to get off to sleep?
- When do you wake up in the morning?

- What do you think keeps you awake or stops you from going back to sleep?
- When did all these problems start?
- What helps you to get to sleep or rest?
- Do you fall asleep in the daytime?
- Have the problems got worse?
- How do you feel in the morning?

Case study B questions

- What did you sleep like before you started being ill?
- When did the problems with sleep start?
- Where do you sleep?
- What level of activity do you have in the daytime?
- What is your pattern of sleep like now in the day and the night?
- What preceded these problems?
- What helps or makes the problems worse?
- What are you able to do in your everyday life?
- How are you coping at work and at home?
- Have the problems got worse?

Case study C questions

- What did you sleep like before you started being ill?
- When did the problems with sleep start?
- What is your pattern of sleep like now in the day and the night?
- Do you have difficulty rolling over in bed or getting in and out of bed?
- What level of physical activity do you have in the day?
- What helps or makes the problems worse?
- Have the problems improved since you have started treatment?
- Have you noticed an improvement in yourself in the daytime if you have a good night's sleep?

It is impossible to cover all feasible adult health problems and their associated sleeping difficulties in this chapter, but it is important to consider that the objective is to collect information to identify:

- the individual's usual habits when they are well
- whether there are any difficulties now in relation to their independence in sleeping
- previous coping strategies with sleeping and associated Activities of Living
- specific problems now.

However, there are common difficulties experienced by individuals with sleeping problems such as:

1. changes in sleep due to hospitalisation
2. changes in sleep patterns
3. changes in conscious levels.

It is useful to consider how each of these difficulties can be assessed and what observations would be required.

Changes in sleep due to hospitalisation

Research identified that hospitalisation does affect people's sleep habits and routines. Closs (1988) interviewed 200 patients on eight surgical wards to elicit their normal sleep patterns at home and then in hospital, along with nurses' recordings of patients' sleep patterns. The majority of patients thought that their sleep was worse in hospital than at home. The length of time taken to get to sleep was longer, they woke earlier and slept for less time during the night as they woke up more frequently. There were many factors which affected their sleep, e.g. gender (women slept better than men), ward design (slept better in small wards) and the type of mattresses (slept better on foam mattresses than horsehair ones). Pain or discomfort, noise, temperature and dissatisfaction with the beds disturbed their sleep.

Tranmer et al (2003) compared the sleep experience of 110 medical and surgical patients during their hospital stay over three consecutive nights and concluded that both groups identified moderate to high levels of sleep disturbance. Surgical patients received more procedural care on the first night, less sedation, more sleep disturbances and reported less sleep effectiveness. Honkus (2003) explores the reasons why patients in critical care units have difficulty sleeping such as noise, lights, discomfort, pain, medications, stress of being unable to sleep. Dogan et al (2005) compared the sleep quality of 150 psychiatric, surgical and medicine patients with 50 healthy non-hospitalised persons. Hospitalised patients' sleep quality was worse than healthy individuals and patients within the psychiatric ward experienced the worst sleep quality. Over a period of time the research findings in different settings and countries have remained the same, identifying that it is difficult to sleep in hospital yet sleep is important in relation to conserving energy, fighting infection and a general sense of wellbeing. It is therefore important that information is collected from the patients in relation to their sleeping habits and routines, and that the nurse considers ways in which sleep can be enhanced.

Interviewing patients is the main method of collecting data to identify changes in sleep due to hospitalisation. The nurse needs to consider what may affect the sleep of the patient due to them being in a strange environment and what may upset their usual sleep routines.

However, there are other subjective assessment methods which can be used to assess sleep. Sleep charts or diaries can be maintained, visual analogue scales can be completed on a daily basis, or rating scales can be completed throughout the day. Visual analogue scales (see Fig. 13.6) involve asking a patient

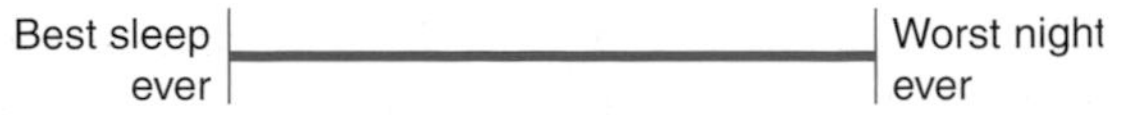

Fig. 13.6   Visual analogue scale for monitoring sleep (from Morgan & Closs 1999, with permission).

to mark on a line which runs from 'best sleep ever' to 'worst night ever' and this can give a visual impression of the type of sleep the individual thinks they have had. On the other hand, rating scales involve asking the patient to rate numerically how they feel at that time, with 1 being 'very alert' to 7 being 'excessively sleepy'. These are discussed fully by Morgan & Closs (1999). Sleepiness assessment scales have been developed, e.g. Stanford Sleepiness Scale (SSS) and Epworth Sleepiness Scale (ESS) as discussed by Lavie et al (2002) (see www.stanford.edu/~dement/sss.html and en.wikepdia.org/wiki/Epworth_Sleepiness_Scale). A pictorial sleepiness scale based on cartoon faces has been devised by Maldonado et al (2004) for use with children or those experiencing cognitive disorders which affect their ability to use other scales.

The nurse needs to develop skills, such as observation, questioning and listening as these are the main ways in which reliable data can be collected. However, Morgan & Closs (1999, p. 72) consider that 'nurses' written records of sleep tend to lack validity and accuracy'. The need to ask open questions, such as 'How did you sleep last night?' or 'Did you experience any problems with sleeping last night?' will elicit better information than if a closed question, such as 'Did you sleep well last night?' is asked. Although patients appear to underestimate the length of time spent asleep and overestimate the time taken to get to sleep, there appears to be a correlation between the patients' reports and their problems even if the estimation of time is inaccurate (Morgan & Closs 1999). Therefore, the accurate collection of data from patients is essential to identify the changes in sleep since their hospitalisation.

Issues relating to environmental aspects need to be clearly delineated, e.g. noise, mattress, bed, temperature and light, from illness issues, e.g. pain, confusion and sleep problems which stem from the actual illness. Reactions to being ill in hospital, such as anxiety, must be differentiated from anxiety as an illness. Changes in the patient's normal circadian rhythms and presleep routines should be identified as separate issues also.

Changes in sleep patterns

Apart from the subjective measures noted previously, there are further objective methods which can be used to assess the associated physiological and psychological events related to sleep. However, this data collection involves expensive and specialised equipment, for example polysomnography and electroencephalogram (EEG) and these are usually only used in specialised sleep clinics. If there is a sleep clinic within the clinical area, it would be useful to discuss these objective measurements.

Changes in conscious levels

It is important that the nurse is able to differentiate between sleep and changes in conscious levels. Altered consciousness can be considered from what may be described as 'normal conscious level through (to) impaired attention, loss of alertness, drowsiness, sleep, stupor and finally coma' as Roper et al (1996, p. 389) identify.

Although the terms drowsy, stupor and coma are used, they aren't really helpful in identifying whether the patient's condition is improving or deteriorating, especially if different nurses undertake these assessments. Nurses need to be alert to any change in a patient's conscious level, as recognising this change, however small it may be, could be lifesaving and possibly prevent brain damage, if it is reported and acted upon appropriately. In an attempt to standardise the assessment of conscious levels the Glasgow Coma Scale (GSC) is commonly used throughout the UK and the world (see Pemberton & Waterhouse 2006, Montague et al 2005, Bowie & Woodward 2003, Jamieson et al 2002, p. 369 and Ch. 3). This allows all health care professionals to utilise the same questions and the same stimuli in the same way and for these responses to be charted in a clear manner so that an accurate picture of the patient's condition can be easily seen.

Three aspects of the patient's behaviour are monitored independently, namely eye opening, verbal response and motor response, and are scored according to the best response. There are two versions of the Glasgow Coma Scale which can cause some confusion (see Fig. 13.7, Roper et al 1996). There is an original 14-point and a revised 15-point version. It is essential that all health professionals using this scale identify which scale they are using (see Roper et al 1996, Bowie & Woodward 2003, Pemberton

GLASGOW COMA SCALE	Eyes open	spontaneously to speech to pain none
	Best verbal response	orientated disorientated monosyllabic response incomprehensible sounds none
	Best motor response	obey commands local pain flexion to pain extension to pain

A

	Eyes opening Score	Motor response Score	Verbal response Score
High score ↑		6 If command such as 'lift up your hands' is obeyed	
		5 If purposeful movements to remove painful stimulus such as pressure over eyebrow	5 If oriented to person, place and time
	4 If eyes open spontaneously to approach of nurse to bedside	4 If finger withdrawn after application of a painful stimulus to it	4 If conversation confused
	3 If eyes open in response to speech	3 If painful stimulation at finger tip flexes the elbow	3 If inappropriate words are used
	2 If eyes open in response to pain at finger tip	2 If the patient's arms are flexed and finger tip stimulation results in extension of elbow	2 If only incomprehensibe sounds are uttered
Low score ↓	1 If eyes do not open in response to pain at finger tip	1 If there is no detectable response to repeated and various stimuli	1 If no verbal response

A normal person would score 15 on the scale; the lowest possible score is 3 which is compatible with, but does not necessarily indicate, brain death. A score of 7 is used as a definition of coma.

B

Fig. 13.7 The Glasgow Coma Scale: (A) 14-point version; (B) 15-point version (from Roper et al 1996, with permission).

& Waterhouse 2006 for further details on these variations). NICE (2003) has published clinical guidelines relating to head injuries which include the use of the Glasgow Coma Scale and advocate the use of the 15-point scale. Good practice is noted, e.g. if a Glasgow Coma Scale score is below 15 then a neck collar and an X-ray or scan of the neck is advocated, if less than 13 or 14 then a CT scan of the head is required within 1 hour of assessment.

Depending on which point version is used, the best response for 'eye opening' is 4, the best response for 'verbal response' is 5 and the best response for 'motor response' is 5 or 6, with 1 being the lowest score for all three areas. The scores are charted and when the scores are combined this indicates the conscious level. The score can therefore range from 3 to 14 or 15. A score of 7 and below indicates a coma, whereas a higher score indicates a higher level of consciousness.

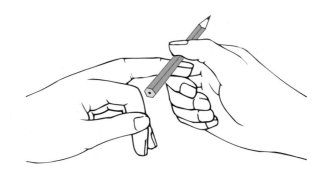

Fig. 13.8 Pressure on finger nail bed (from Teasdale et al 1975, with permission).

> **Exercise**
> 1. Observe other health care professionals carrying out these observations.
> 2. What kind of charts were used to record the observation findings? Are they similar to the Glasgow Coma Scale chart? (See also Fig. 3.15 on p. 84.)
> 3. How do they identify the best response for eye opening, verbal and motor responses?

It may have been possible to observe health care professionals using the Glasgow Coma Scale in Accident and Emergency Departments, Intensive Care Units, High Dependency Units, Neurological Units or general medical or surgical wards. The charts used may have been single Glasgow Coma Scale charts only or they may have been modified to include observations such as temperature, pulse and blood pressure, pupil sizes and reactions.

To monitor the patient's response to the spoken word and the 'eye opening' activity, the health care professional may have been observed noting whether the patient opened their eyes spontaneously because they felt the presence of someone at their bedside (score 4) or if they opened their eyes when the health care professional spoke to them without touching them or by shouting or shaking them gently (score 3). If no response is gained from talking to the patient in this way then the health care professional may have been observed applying a painful stimulus, such as exerting pressure on the patient's finger nail bed by rolling a pen over the nail bed (see Fig. 13.8) (Roper et al 1996).

This is done to the third or fourth digits as they are the most sensitive but care must be taken to avoid pressure on the cuticle. If the patient opens their eyes at this point then 2 is scored but if the eyes don't open then a score of 1 is given. Difficulties may have arisen for the health care professional when monitoring the patient's response to the spoken word if the patient had impaired hearing. If the eyelids are swollen then the patient may not be able to open their eyes and C should be recorded for 'closed'; equally the eyes may remain open and therefore are recorded as not responding to the painful stimulus.

Any damage to the brain stem from trauma or raised intracranial pressure will affect the patient's ability to open their eyes as this ability is linked to being alert and awake. It must be remembered, however, that the patient may not be aware of their surroundings and therefore there is the need to continue with the assessment of the verbal and motor responses.

To assess the best verbal response, the health care professional will have asked the patient various questions and on the basis of their responses will attach a score to the appropriate level achieved. To score 5 on the scale, i.e. orientation, the patient must be able to state their name, say where they are, i.e. which hospital and in which town it is and what month and year it is. The order in which these questions are asked may be altered but if answered correctly the person is said to be orientated to time, people and place.

If the person answers these questions incorrectly or inappropriately then the person is not orientated to time, people or place and is said to be confused and scores 4. The patient may be able to converse, in sentences, with the health care professional but it is a rambling conversation and this must be differentiated between being 'confused' and using 'inappropriate words', which scores 3. Inappropriate words are identified by the individual answering in one or two words only, quite often after painful stimuli have been exerted to assess the eye-opening section of the scale. The words will probably have made little sense and may have been obscene. Incomprehensible sounds score 2 and this should have been noted if the patient only makes a noise but no words can be identified and they moan, mumble or scream. If the patient didn't utter any noise, even with painful stimuli, then they would be said to have no verbal response and would score 1. However, there may be reasons why patients cannot answer questions or make noises, e.g. they don't speak English, are deaf, have a speech defect or have an endotracheal or tracheostomy tube in situ. The health care professional should document these issues to clarify any of them, e.g. put E or T if the patient has an endotracheal or tracheostomy tube in situ.

If the scores obtained for verbal responses are decreasing then the patient's condition is worsening and this may be due to trauma to brain tissue, hypoxia, or raised intracranial pressure. These tests indicate whether the patient is able to receive and understand a variety of inputs (sensory, verbal or physical) and then their ability to respond verbally. The final area to be assessed is that of motor responses, in the upper limbs only, which tests the patient's abilities to receive and understand any of these inputs and then to coordinate a motor response (see Fig. 13.9 for the tests and the responses noted; Pemberton & Waterhouse 2006).

The best motor response is scored at either 6 or 5 (depending on whether using the 15- or 14-point version) and is when the patient is able to respond to a command given by the health care professional, such as, 'Lift up your arms', or 'Stick out your tongue'. If the patient doesn't respond to these commands then the health care professional must assess the patient's motor response to painful stimuli. The trapezium pinch is the safest method to use as the shoulders are easily exposed and the muscle can be grasped and pinched easily. If the patient lifts the arm purposefully towards the area being pinched, then the patient is said to be 'localising to pain' and scores 5 or 4 (depending on the scale used). If using the 15-point scale, then the score of 4 is given if the patient withdraws the finger after the painful stimulus has been applied but they don't try to remove the stimulus. Rubbing of the sternum and pressure applied to the supraorbital ridge is no longer advocated due to the bruises left on the chest and the possibility of damage to the orbital structure. If the patient doesn't appear to localise to the painful stimulus then you should have observed the health care professional apply pressure to the nail bed again and if the patient flexes or bends the elbow and withdraws their hand but does not localise to the finger itself then they would score 3, as they have demonstrated their ability to flex to pain. If the elbows are straightened after the painful stimulus has been applied, then the patient scores 2, as they have shown their ability to extend to pain. If no movement occurs, then the health care professional will score 1 on the chart (see Fig. 3.15 on p. 84).

It is vital that the nurse understands how to conduct a coma assessment using the Glasgow Coma Scale and that the findings are interpreted correctly and actions taken appropriately. There are other reasons, apart from head injuries, why a patient may experience changes in their conscious levels, e.g. fainting or syncope, during a convulsion or fit and when undergoing general anaesthesia. Therefore, it is important for you to consider the possible cause of any alterations in conscious levels (see Montague et al 2005).

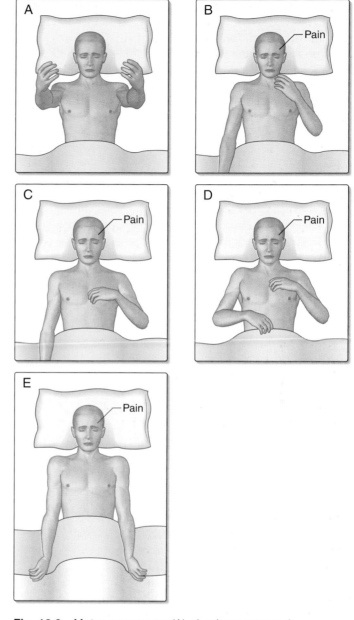

Fig. 13.9 Motor responses: (A) obeying commands, (B) localising to pain, (C) flexing to pain, (D) abnormal flexion (E) extending to pain (from Alexander et al 2006, with permission).

Interpretation of data collected

Once the data have been collected it is necessary to utilise knowledge and decision-making skills to interpret the information prior to the identification of the individual's actual and potential problems. Using the assessment questions outlined in Box 13.6, consider the information that may be gathered from Case study 13.1 by considering the components of the model.

It is now necessary to utilise the components of the model to interpret the information collected with Case study 3.1 relating to chronic systemic joint disease problems which are affecting her sleep patterns.

Emma Simmons

Emma Simmons is a 45-year-old married lady who has rheumatoid arthritis which is currently affecting her hands, wrists, knees and feet. She lives with her husband and two sons aged 13 and 17 years, and is a secretary at the local school. She has been admitted because she is having pain when she types and when normal movement of the hands and feet is attempted. The joints are swollen, tender and warm to touch; she is aware that there is a loss of function in her hands and she is experiencing some stiffness, especially in the morning. The pain in the joints is now affecting her ability to sleep at night with frequent awakenings, which is causing more difficulties for her. She has noticed that she has lost weight over the last year and feels tired. She is currently taking aspirin as an analgesic and a non-steroidal anti-inflammatory agent (NSAID). An assessment of her treatment regime is being carried out with a view to improving her quality of life. The possibility of surgery has been discussed with Emma.

Exercise

1. Consider the factors which may have led to Emma's health breakdown.
2. Identify the effect on other Activities of Living.
3. Check your answers with those in Box 13.8.

From this exercise it can be seen that Emma has:

- a longstanding chronic systemic joint disease
- an exacerbation of this disease which is affecting other Activities of Living
- an occupational problem
- a problem with completing housework
- alterations in socialisation and possible sexual relationships due to disease, pain, difficulty to mobilise and tiredness.

Following this interpretation of the data, it is then necessary to complete the final stage of the assessment process and identify actual and potential problems.

Identification of actual and potential problems

Actual and potential sleep problems will be specific to the individual's sleep difficulty and their health breakdown problem but common sleep problems can be identified in relation to:

1. changes in sleep due to hospitalisation
2. changes in sleep patterns
3. changes in conscious levels.

Changes in sleep due to hospitalisation

Sleep deprivation can occur due to hospitalisation affecting the amount, consistency and quality of sleep. The

---

Box 13.8   **Health breakdown and its effects on other ALs**

Factors leading to health breakdown

- Age and gender – usually affects women in 40–50 age range.
- Dependency continuum may be affected now as work and home activities are proving to be a problem.
- No known cause although:
  - infections, hormones and autoimmune factors (physical) and
  - familial factors (sociocultural) are being investigated.

Other activities being affected

Communilcating

- Pain, in joints and on movement, is affecting her ability to socialise.
- Emma is anxious and depressed over the current exacerbation of her disease and the effects it is having on her life.

Eating and drinking

- Loss of appetite and weight loss due to pain, medications and systemic disease, difficulty using utensils.

Eliminating

- Finding it difficult to sit down on the toilet, especially in the morning when her knees are stiff. Constipating effect of medications.

Personal cleansing and dressing

- Skin is fragile and stretched over the joint surfaces.

Mobilising

- Fatigued easily, warm, painful, swollen stiff joints, especially in the morning. Loss of function in the hands and wrists.

Sleep and rest

- Wakes frequently during the night, feels tired and not rested.

Expressing sexuality

- Pain and impaired mobility may be affecting her sexual relationships with her husband.

Maintaining body temperature

- Mildly pyrexial.

Working and playing

- Tired, difficult to type at work and carrying out some of the household jobs, especially in the morning.

---

strange environment of the hospital ward, the numerous disturbances, discomfort, pain and worry, medications, illnesses and the need for nursing care all contribute to sleep deprivation in the patient. A variety of illnesses affect sleep, such as arthritis which disturbs a person's sleep due to joint pains and asthma which affects sufferers by increasing bronchoconstriction at night, especially around 4–6 a.m., which affects sleep at this time. The quality of life of Parkinson sufferers and their carers is often made worse, according to Crabb (2001), by impaired sleep. This is due to many reasons, such as the ageing process, the medications used and the disease itself.

Through the use of diaries, Schaefer (1997) identified the sleep problems of eight women who suffered with fibromyalgia and found that there was a relationship between muscle aches and pains with sleep and other issues such as the weather. Brostrom et al (2001) identified that sleep was affected in 20 patients suffering from congestive cardiac failure by their daily activities, the disease itself and the cardiac symptoms. The sleep disturbances then gave rise to fatigue, listlessness, loss of concentration and loss of temper. These effects then led on to the need for daytime sleep and seclusion.

Whatever the disease, the resulting sleep deprivation may result in lack of concentration, irritability and fatigue, and may pose safety risks. In addition to these psychological effects, sleep deprivation may have a negative influence on healing. Caution is necessary, according to Closs (1990), in making the direct link of healing and sleep deprivation as the studies to support this link are confined to animals. The promotion of sleep is, however, an essential factor to consider in the management of surgical patients, especially if this link was supported by research conducted on human subjects.

A pilot study conducted by Ersser et al (1999) identified that a marked proportion of older people reported sleeping well in nursing care settings and those in nursing homes slept better than those in a community hospital. However, disturbances in both settings were related to personal needs for micturition during the night, noise, discomfort and pain. Whereas, Hoffman (2003) reported that more than half of adults living at home, 65 and above, two-thirds of those in long-term care facilites and a range of 22% to 61% in acute settings had some difficulty with sleep.

Snoring can also be a major problem for the snorer and those near to them, therefore this may cause other patients in a ward environment to have disturbed sleep patterns. Snoring is caused by an obstruction in the upper airways (nose or throat) and is found to be more common in men, those who are overweight, suffering from hypothyroidism or who have a nasal or tonsil problem. Snoring rarely causes serious health problems.

Night wandering, especially elderly people with Alzheimer's, may cause problems in a hospital or nursing home environment. Whilst night wandering is not sleep-walking (somnambulism), as the person is awake, they are confused about whether it is day or night and a change of environment can often trigger this wandering. The safety of the individual is of utmost importance and it is also important that they don't disturb the other patients around them.

A potential problem is that patients may be at risk of injury if they are restless in bed due to a variety of reasons. The patient may be dreaming, not used to sleeping in a single bed or alone, or may wish to go to the toilet, or the restlessness may be due to medications taken or brain stem irritation. Hospital beds tend to be much higher than ordinary beds and therefore the risk of injury is greater than at home if the patient was to fall out of bed. Cot sides are sometimes used to prevent restless patients from falling out of bed but the use of cot sides does raise ethical and legal issues, as they are classed as a form of physical restraint, and injuries can still occur.

In the UK, the use of physical restraints with older people is classed as a form of abuse and could be in breach of their human rights (Royal College of Nursing 2004). Dimond (2005) considers that to impede a person's freedom by the use of physical restraint is unlawful. The Royal College of Nursing (2004) argues that nurses who use restraints with patients must be able to justify their actions and that restraints should only be used when other interventions have failed and their use should be carefully monitored. The use of restraints doesn't guarantee safety and can cause physical and psychological problems. However, patients may choose to have cot sides or side rails in situ to stop them rolling out of bed or to help them sit up and if so the cot sides are not noted as restraints. Gallinagh et al (2002) concluded that specific protocols are needed in relation to the use of physical restraints. An assessment would be needed to ascertain if restraints are necessary and to decide on which type is the best to use. If they are necessary, the restraint needs to be discussed with the patient and their relatives and if agreed upon, as short-term safety measures only, then the restraints need to be ordered by the medical team and documented fully.

Gallinagh et al (2002) investigated the prevalence and type of physical restraints used with older people on four rehabilitation wards in Northern Ireland. Most of the patients (68%) were subjected to some form of physical restraint and cot sides were the most commonly observed method of restraint. Those who were restrained were dependent on nursing care but no links to staffing levels or incidence of falls were found, even though nurses often cite the risk of injury from falls as the reason for using restraints. In this study, wandering and patient protection were the reasons why nurses used restraints. In a study by Karlsson et al (2000), they identified that nurses' decisions to use restraints in two nursing homes were affected by a variety of issues and although the patient's best interests were considered, the working conditions and the nurses' willingness to take risks when not restraining a patient were also factors used in deciding to use a form of restraint or not.

Another potential problem is that there is a risk that the patient may become dependent on night sedation medication or analgesia and this should be avoided at all costs. Halfens et al (1994) concluded, from a study of 233 patients who used sleep medication in Dutch hospitals, that the administration of sleep medication is not without danger. This medication was given to the patients for the first time and for at least 5 days. After discharge from the hospital, these patients continued to use sleep medication at home. On the other hand, those patients who did not receive sleep medication in hospital did not use it at home following discharge. An alternative to night sedation is needed to discourage patients from being given sleep medication for the first time in hospital and then finding it difficult to stop taking this when they are at home.

Changes in sleep patterns

Actual sleep problems include insomnia, sleep apnoea and narcolepsy and the nurse needs to have an understanding of these problems. Insomnia is the best known actual sleep problem but it can be divided into three types, namely sleep-onset problems, sleep maintenance problems and early-wakening problems. The main cause is often being worried over a particular problem but it is also associated with depressive illness (Irwin 1992).

Sleep apnoea refers to the temporary cessation of breathing during sleep, in between snoring episodes. Obstructive sleep apnoea occurs when the pharynx closes during sleep and is accompanied by loud snoring as the person tries to breathe through a narrowed space. Eventually the space closes and respiration stops for up to 1 minute. The patient then clears the airway with a snort and is aroused and starts to breathe again. This cycle can occur many times each night. It is estimated that nearly 4% of the UK population suffer from sleep apnoea with corresponding excessive daytime sleepiness and complaints of insomnia. Breathing disorders and hypothyroidism can give rise to sleep apnoea. It is more prevalent in males, older people, the obese, smokers, drinkers and those who take sedatives according to Scottish Intercollegiate Guidelines Network (SIGN) (2003). SIGN produced guidelines for the management of obstructive sleep apnoea/hyponoea (OSAHS) in 2003, advocating the use of continuous positive airway pressure (CPAP) (see Chapter 5 for further details). CPAP has been shown to reduce daytime sleepiness. Central apnoea occurs when the drive to breathe is abnormally reduced during sleep, as opposed to obstructed, but this again leads to asphyxia and arousal. According to Montague et al (2005), it is associated with neuromuscular disorders, respiratory and brain stem disorders.

Narcolepsy is a serious but rare sleep disorder occurring in 0.04% of the population. It occurs between the ages of 15 and 25 and varies between being a mild inconvenience to being a severe, debilitating disease with excessive sleepiness and daytime sleep attacks. The overwhelming need to sleep, even in the middle of the day, is the main complaint. Narcolepsy sufferers may fall asleep when standing up, whilst talking, driving a car or whilst swimming. It can be accompanied by cataplexy, where the individual is unable to move, or the person may have hallucinations (Morgan & Closs 1999, Lavie et al 2002).

Problems related to waking behaviours (parasomnias) can cause actual sleep problems such as sleepwalking (somnambulism), grinding of teeth (bruxism) and bed wetting (enuresis). These problems tend to be found in children only and further information can be found in Morgan & Closs (1999) and Lavie et al (2002).

Changes in conscious levels

Any alteration in the conscious level of a person indicates that there is a problem, some of which are extremely serious. Roper et al (1996, p. 389) identify that the stages of altered consciousness can be described as a 'gradual change from a normal conscious level through impaired attention, loss of alertness, drowsiness, sleep, stupor and finally coma'. The latter two descriptors are abnormal states compared to the others and the nurse would need to utilise observational skills to differentiate between the normal and abnormal states and act appropriately.

Exercise
1. Reread Case study 13.1 on p. 438.
2. Using the Activities of Living as a framework, identify Emma's actual and potential problems.
3. Check your identified actual and potential problems with those in Box 13.9.

In this section, how to collect data when taking a nursing history in relation to the activity of sleeping and other related activities will have been considered. In addition, how to interpret the data collected in order to assess the degree of alteration in the activity of sleeping and the effect on other Activities of Living. It is also important to have identified how an individual's actual and potential problems related to the activity of sleeping affect other related activities.

PLANNING NURSING ACTIVITIES

Planning nursing activities involves the following:

- identifying priorities
- establishing short- and/or long-term goals
- determining nursing actions/interventions required
- documenting the plan (refer to Chapter 1 for further information).

To ensure that the nursing activities are planned appropriately, it is necessary to review the individual's actual and potential problems and then consider the level to which the activity of sleeping can be helped. There are different levels of helping, such as:

- to solve or alleviate actual problems
- to prevent potential problems becoming actual ones

Box 13.9	Actual and potential problems that Emma may experience	
Activity of Living	**Actual problems**	**Potential problems**
Communicating	Emma is experiencing pain in her joints and on movement due to the arthritis/inflammation and this is shown by limited mobility, some loss of function in the hands and wrists, facial expression and verbal complaints of pain. Emma is anxious and depressed over the current exacerbation of her disease and the effects it is having on her life.	
Eating and drinking	Emma is experiencing loss of appetite and weight loss due to pain, medications and systemic disease which make it difficult for Emma to hold and use utensils due to the painful swollen joints.	
Eliminating	Emma has difficulty with sitting down on the toilet, in the morning due to her knees being stiff.	Emma is at risk of developing constipation especially due to her restricted mobility and the medications she is taking.
Personal cleansing		Emma may have difficulty in meeting her dressing and hygiene needs due to the pain, tiredness, loss of function in her hands and morning stiffness.
Mobilising	Emma has difficulties mobilising because she tires easily, and the joints in her hands, knees and feet are warm, painful, swollen and stiff, especially in the morning. Emma is experiencing some loss of function in the hands and wrists.	
Sleep and rest	Emma is having difficulty sleeping due to the joint pains and this is shown by waking frequently in the night, and that she feels tired and not rested.	
Expressing sexuality		Emma may be experiencing difficulties in her sexual relationship with her husband due to the constant joint pains and sleep deprivation.
Maintaining body temperature	Emma may feel warm due to her being mildly pyrexial.	
Working and playing	Emma is having difficulty working (at home and school) and socialising due to the pain and her tiredness.	

- to prevent solved problems from reoccurring
- to develop positive strategies for any problems which cannot be solved.

Exercise

1. Reread the three brief case studies in Box 13.7 (p. 433).
2. Identify the levels of helping that may be achieved in relation to these case studies.

The following levels of care may have been considered appropriate:

Case study A

- to develop positive coping strategies for lifestyle changes to alleviate anxiety and depression
- to alleviate insomnia and early morning wakenings by developing positive coping strategies to alleviate anxiety and depression.

Case study B
- to develop positive coping strategies for lifestyle changes to alleviate fatigue, tiredness, poor sleep and depression.

Case Study C
- to develop positive coping strategies for lifestyle changes to alleviate sleep problems and difficulties directly related to Parkinson's disease.

The focus must be on the individual's problems and wishes as opposed to the nurse's ideas. Therefore, involvement of the patient is crucial at this stage. However, this may be affected by the problems that the patient may have, e.g. pain, altered conscious levels, inability to communicate verbally, as noted previously.

Many factors may influence the nurse and the patient in the planning stage of nursing activities with a patient with sleeping difficulties. Consider this in relation to a patient with sleeping difficulties and check these in Box 13.10.

Identifying priorities

Following the assessment, the next stage is to plan the care. Determine priorities of care as this skill is a vital component of any nurse's repertoire. Determine which problem is the most important and grade it as follows:

Box 13.10	Factors which influence planning care for a patient with sleeping difficulties

From the nurse's perspective
- Knowledge of normal physiology and specific pathophysiological processes in relation to sleeping disorders and disorders which affect sleeping habits of individuals.
- Knowledge of normal living and dependency across the lifespan in various cultures in relation to sleeping.
- Knowledge of sleeping difficulties specific to the patient's problem.
- Knowledge of nursing interventions available and evidenced-based practices.
- Knowledge of assessment methods and the accuracy of these methods.
- Skills in observing, assessment, interpreting and prioritising.
- Staffing levels and skill mix on night duty.
- Own sleep habits and sleep hygiene routines.

From the patient's perspective
- Ability and degree of involvement of the patient in the decisions related to care to be planned.
- Knowledge of sleeping difficulties specific to the patient's problem.
- Personal beliefs, attitudes, experiences and coping strategies.
- Enactment of the sick role.

- life-threatening – totally dependent
- urgent – mainly dependent but some ability to be independent
- semi-urgent – some dependency but mainly independent
- non-urgent – totally independent.

This priority status may change day by day, shift by shift or hour by hour and therefore the assessment stage must be a continuous activity to ensure that the nurse remains alert to possible changes.

Exercise
1. Reread the actual and potential problems that have been identified for Emma Simmons in Case study 13.1.
2. Identify which problems are life-threatening, urgent, semi-urgent and non-urgent.
3. Decide which would be the first three problems that need to be addressed, giving a rationale for this choice.
4. Check your decisions with those found in Box 13.11.

It can be seen that Emma's problems are varied in relation to their priorities and involve many of the Activities of Living. A suggested priority order is:

1. Emma is experiencing pain in her joints and on movement due to the arthritis/inflammation and this is shown by limited mobility, some loss of function in the hands and wrists, facial expression and verbal complaints of pain.
2. Emma is having difficulty sleeping due to the joint pains and this is shown by waking frequently in the night, and that she feels tired and not rested.
3. Emma is experiencing loss of appetite and weight loss due to pain, medications and systemic disease which made it difficult for Emma to hold and use utensils due to the painful swollen joints.

The rationale for the priority order is that the pain is the main difficulty which is directly affecting her ability to mobilise, sleep, work and socialise. If nursing actions are not planned then the pain will become worse. If, however, nursing actions are planned to alleviate the pain then the problems with mobilising, sleeping, working and socialising will be diminished if not solved.

The sleeping problems will be better if the pain is relieved but the change in routine and hospitalisation may also have an effect on Emma's sleeping habits and, if sleep deprivation occurs, then more problems arise which can affect her physical and mental wellbeing. Nutritional problems are very important to Emma's wellbeing. There are problems with the medications used for arthritis as they can cause gastrointestinal problems and Emma may be reluctant to take them because of this, which, in turn, will affect her pain levels and subsequently her mobility, sleep, work and socialisation

Box 13.11	Priority status of actual problems experienced by Emma	
Activity of Living	**Actual problems**	**Problem status**
Communicating	Emma is experiencing pain in her joints and on movement due to the arthritis/inflammation and this is shown by limited mobility, facial expression and verbal complaints of pain.	Semi-urgent
	Emma is anxious and depressed over the current exacerbation of her disease and the effects it is having on her life.	Semi-urgent
Eating and drinking	Emma is experiencing loss of appetite and weight loss due to pain, medications and systemic disease which make it difficult for Emma to hold and use utensils due to the painful swollen joints.	Semi-urgent
Eliminating	Emma has difficulty with sitting down on the toilet, especially in the morning due to her knees being stiff.	Non-urgent
	Emma is at risk of developing constipation due to her restricted mobility and the medications she is taking.	Non-urgent
Mobilising	Emma has difficulties mobilising because she tires easily, and the joints in her hands, knees and feet are warm, painful, swollen and stiff, especially in the morning.	Semi-urgent
	Emma is experiencing some loss of function in the hands and wrists.	Semi-urgent
Sleep and rest	Emma is having difficulty sleeping due to the joint pains and this is shown by waking frequently in the night, and that she feels tired and not rested.	Semi-urgent
Maintaining body temperature	Emma may feel warm due to her being mildly pyrexial.	Non-urgent
Working and playing	Emma is having difficulty working (at home and school) and socialising due to the pain and her tiredness.	Semi-urgent
Personal cleansing and dressing	Emma may have difficulty in meeting her hygiene needs due to the pain, tiredness, loss of function in her hands and morning stiffness.	Non-urgent
Expressing sexuality	Emma may be experiencing difficulties in her sexual relationship with her husband due to the constant joint pains and sleep deprivation.	Non-urgent

patterns. (See Taibi et al 2004, Bourguignon et al 2003, Davis 2003 for further information on sleep disturbances with rheumatoid arthritis.)

Goal setting

Goal setting is based upon sound assessment and the identification of problems and priorities. Goals can be short term (hourly to generally less than a week) or long term (for a longer period). Many short-term goals may be needed to achieve long-term goals.

The goal statement is essential so that the process of evaluation can take place. It is therefore important that the goal is written in the terms of what the patient ought to be able or has agreed to achieve. The goals should be written in

observable, realistic and measurable behavioural terms so that it is easier to monitor and evaluate the patient's progress (refer to Chapter 1 for further details on goal setting). This may be a skill that needs to be developed and practised.

Exercise

1. Reread Emma Simmons' actual and potential problems related to Case study 13.1, listed in Box 13.9 on p. 441 in the assessment section.
2. Choose three of these problems and set short- and long-term goals.
3. Check the example given in Box 13.12.

Box 13.12	Short- and long-term goals

Problem
Emma is experiencing pain in her joints and on movement due to the arthritis/inflammation and this is shown by limited mobility, facial expression and verbal complaints of pain.

Short-term goal
Emma will be able to verbalise her pain to nursing staff and assess the effect of medications given for the pain.

Long-term goal
Emma will be able to mobilise, sleep, work and socialise within the pain limits and be able to adapt her lifestyle to cope with the pain.

Once the short-term and long-term goals have been set it will be necessary to determine the appropriate nursing actions which will aid the alleviation of problems and the achievement of the short- and long-term goals.

Determining nursing actions

It is vital that the appropriate nursing actions are chosen to alleviate patient's problems. To be able to do this, the nurse must constantly update their knowledge and skills to ensure that care given is evidence-based and delivered in a safe, competent and professional manner. Nursing actions will be considered in relation to the factors which affect ill health (physical, psychological, sociocultural, environmental and politicoeconomic) and with patients who have 'difficulty with sleeping'. There is a need for the nurse to act as a health educator in relation to all of these nursing actions to ensure that the patient and their significant others are apprised of the problem, treatments and ways in which problems can be minimised and prevented.

Nursing actions associated with physical factors affecting ill health

The purpose of the nursing actions, associated with the physical factors related to sleeping difficulties, is that the nurse provides specific care to individuals who are not able to provide for themselves to promote and maintain health and prevent disease. The place on the lifespan, the level of dependency and biological factors identified in the model of living will need to be considered when the nursing actions are planned.

There are many nursing actions, related to physical care, which affect sleeping but some of the main actions are described below.

Nursing observations of vital signs, conscious levels and sleeping habits

These observations have been noted earlier in this chapter and in Chapters 3, 5 and 9. However, it is important that you consider when and how often these observations should be carried out. This will depend on the severity of the patient's condition and whether the problems are acute or chronic. The initial assessment of vital signs, conscious levels (where appropriate) and sleeping habits can be used as a baseline for future evaluations. It may be that these observations are carried out continuously as the patient is in a critical care environment or a specialised sleep clinic, or they are carried out hourly, 4-hourly or daily.

Once the observations have been made, they must be recorded accurately and the significance of the observations identified and reported to senior members of the health care team. Any alterations in the patient's conscious level must be reported immediately.

Sleep may well be affected by taking these observations and you need to plan the care so that patients are not disturbed during the night to have observations recorded, wherever possible. The timing of some treatments, such as blood transfusions and the observations needed with these, may need to be considered. It may be that the blood transfusion can be completed during the day so that the observations are not needed during the night to ensure that the patient's sleep patterns are not unduly disturbed (Cawthorn & Hope 1992).

Administration of drug therapies The administration of any medications is an important aspect of the nurse's role and professional, legal and local policies govern these actions. The professional practice of the nurse, in relation to the administration of medicines, is guided by the Nursing and Midwifery Council document *Standards for Medicines Management* (NMC 2007a) and further details can be found in Chapter 3 and on the Nursing and Midwifery Council website at www.nmc-uk.org. The nurse needs to have an up-to-date knowledge of pharmacology and needs to consider any ritualistic practices that may occur with 'drug administration rounds', such as the practice of a 6 a.m. drug round.

In relation to sleep issues, the nurse must be aware of certain hypnotics and tranquillisers (benzodiazepines) which act on the central nervous system to promote sleep and reduce anxiety, such as nitrazepam (Mogadon), diazepam (Valium), temazepam (Normison), chloral hydrate (Welldorm), chlordiazepoxide (Librium) and the more recent nonbenzodiazepine hypnotics which have fewer side-effects. As all of these drugs can affect the activity of the central nervous system and breathing system, they must be monitored carefully as the patient is at risk from these medications.

Various problems have been identified when patients take hypnotics and tranquillisers. For example, the sleep is very different to normal sleep, patients may suffer from a hangover feeling, but the risk of dependency is the major problem, with drug accumulation and residual sedation adding to safety issues as mobility and coordination can be affected, and all of these are compounded with withdrawal problems (Morgan & Closs 1999, Reite et al 2002).

These types of drugs are often prescribed as 'prn' (*pro re nata*) medications, i.e. 'when necessary'. The nurse, therefore, is charged with making the decision of when it is necessary to give the medication prescribed by another health care professional who is not present at the time. It is vital that the nurse discusses these issues with the patient and ensures that the appropriate treatment regime is maintained. The nurse and patient, therefore, need to have knowledge of the medication's action, side-effects, patient's condition and other medications. Duxbury (1994) identified that nurses who delivered care via a team nursing approach gave three times as much 'prn night sedation' as nurses who delivered care via a primary nursing approach. This difference may have been related to the beliefs held as the team nurses' views were more consistent with a medical approach of the advantages of night sedation and its continuing use.

Administration of complementary therapies   There are many different forms of complementary therapies which may be useful for the patient with sleeping difficulties, such as aromatherapy, massage, reflexology and pet therapy. The Royal College of Nursing (2003) reports on three categories of complementary and alternative medicine disciplines, namely professionally organised alternative therapies, e.g. acupuncture; complementary therapies, e.g. aromatherapy, reflexology, massage (most frequently used by nurses); and alternative disciplines, e.g. traditional Chinese medicine. There is some evidence to support the effectiveness of these therapies. Ryman & Rankin-Box (2001) discuss relaxation and visualisation and consider they have few side-effects and are cost-effective and encourage patients to develop a sense of wellbeing and self-awareness. Dunn et al (1995) identified that massage, rest and aromatherapy, when used in an Intensive Therapy Unit, proved to be beneficial to most patients and Thorgrimsen et al (2003) identified one study that supported the use of aromatherapy with patients with dementia. Soden et al (2004) found that sleep was improved in cancer patients who were given 4-week courses of aromatherapy massage or massage on its own. Brownfield (1998) also used complementary therapies with patients suffering with rheumatoid arthritis. Relaxation, heat, therapeutic touch, light massage and acupuncture were found to be effective for the eight women in Schaefer's study in 1997. In this study, the writing of a diary was noted as a useful tool as it empowered the women. They were able to predict times when muscle aches and pains may be worse and therefore adapt their lifestyles accordingly. Davis (2003) discusses the use of cognitive-behavioural approaches, massage, exercise, thermal methods of heat application or hydrotherapy for arthritic patients and considers the link of pain and sleep.

The controlled use of essential oils to produce health and relaxation is offered and lavender and sandalwood have been found to be relaxing and promote sleep, whether put in a bath or inhaled in a burner. However, care is needed as this may affect other patients in a ward setting. Massage, with or without oils, is said to reduce anxiety and help sleep and that it is the touch that is important (Lavery 1997).

As the use of complementary therapy has grown, the Royal College of Nursing has formed a specialist interest group for complementary therapies. Trevelyan & Booth (1994), when discussing this specialist interest group, reported that, providing nurses were appropriately trained, there were 'potentially acceptable therapies' that they could use. Acupuncture, reflexology, massage and aromatherapy were amongst those therapies identified. NHS Trusts are developing policies to clarify roles and responsibilities and to ensure good practice. Trevelyan & Booth (1994) discuss that nurses seem to be more aware of possible legal repercussions of their actions and highlight one District Health Authority's action in drawing up a local policy to cover the use of complementary therapies by nurses. Four criteria were set by them, namely consent by the patient, consultation with medical staff, authorisation as agreed between the nurse and the nurse manager and documentation in the patient's notes. Trevelyan & Booth (1994) saw that this type of policy could help to protect the nurse, patient and the organisation.

When nurses are involved in delivering complementary therapies, they are accountable under the Code of Professional Conduct (NMC 2004a, Sect. 3.11) and answerable for their actions. Training is needed in relation to the use of these therapies or the patient may be put at risk due to lack of competence. The Code of Professional Conduct (NMC 2004a, Sect. 1.4) clearly states that the nurse has a duty of care and the patients are entitled to receive safe and competent care. It is, therefore, important for the nurse to ensure that these therapies are in the patient's best interest and that the patient is safe. It must also be remembered that these therapies are 'complementary' and therefore will work along with other treatments, so the total package of care and therapy needs to be considered. Discussion with all members of the multidisciplinary team must take place and the patient must give informed consent prior to their use (NMC 2004a, Code of Professional Conduct, Sect. 3.11). (See Rankin-Box 2001 and RCN 2003.)

The British Medical Association (1993) discusses the variations in the regulations governing nonconventional therapies in Europe. The Netherlands are liberal in their approach, whereas France, Belgium and Italy are more restrictive. In the UK, which is midway between these liberal and restrictive approaches, the Medical Act of 1858 allows qualified doctors to administer unconventional medical treatments to patients as long as they adhere to professional standards of care. Qualified doctors can also delegate the administration of complementary therapies to a non-medically qualified practitioner, as long as certain criteria are satisfied. Non-medically qualified practitioners of nonconventional medicine are free to practice, whatever their level of training, as long as they do not infringe the Medicines Act 1983, by implying that they are registered medical practitioners. They are also prevented from advertising treatments or remedies for a number of conditions (diabetes, glaucoma and epilepsy) but they are allowed to treat these patients.

Consumers of complementary medicine are protected under UK law in relation to the tort-based common law of negligence which protects people under the category of breach of duty of care. Other legislation relating to Trades Description Act 1968, Health and Safety at Work Act 1974, Control of Substances Hazardous to Health (COSHH) Regulations 1988, and Supply of Goods and Services Act 1982 may be used. At present there are no registering bodies to which complaints may be lodged for users of non-conventional therapies.

Use of cognitive-behavioural therapy   There is evidence to support the use of cognitive-behavioural therapy (CBT) with patients complaining of insomnia. Jacobs et al (2004) used CBT, traditional drug therapy or a combination with 63 young and middle-aged adults with chronic insomnia. CBT was the most effective sleep intervention. Sivertsen et al (2006) also found that CBT was superior to using zopiclone treatment for short and long term management of insomnia with 46 older adults. Edinger et al (2001) identified that CBT had lasting effects when used with 75 adults with chronic insomnia. It has also been found to be effective in the treatment of patients suffering from chronic fatigue syndrome and/or myalgic encephalomyelitis according to Bagnall et al (2002).

Exercise

If you are able to experience a night duty shift consider:

1. What actions were taken to ensure that the patients were able to rest and sleep during the night.
2. What disturbed patients' rest and sleep and could it have been prevented?
3. What drugs were used to aid sleep?
4. Were alternative, complementary or cognitive-behavioural therapies considered?
5. What did patients say in the morning in relation to their sleep?

If you have not been able to experience a night duty shift then discuss this with your mentor, preceptor or clinical supervisor.

Specific actions related to the disease process   Nasal clips or strips can be used for snorers. These clips or strips are fixed to the outside of the nose to open nostrils and improve breathing. Patients who suffer from sleep apnoea problems can use a continuous positive airway pressure (CPAP) device. This is when a nasal mask is strapped to the face to deliver air at a slightly higher pressure than normal and so keep the airway open (Lavery 1997). Antisnoring surgery is available (uvulopalatopharyngoplasty, UPPP), where the soft palate is cauterised so that it is less likely to flap. However, the SIGN (2003) guidelines concluded that there was no evidence to support the use of UPPP and that it was not a recommended treatment.

In disorders where sleep is affected, e.g. arthritis, the therapeutic regime may include the use of anti-inflammatory medication, rest, use of heat, appropriately planned exercise and night resting splints in order to reduce the inflammation and pain, preservation of joint function and prevent joint deformities (Walsh 2002).

Nursing actions associated with psychological factors affecting ill health

Stress and worry can affect the patient whilst in hospital and therefore the nurse needs to consider ways in which stress and worry can be minimised. This may simply be the provision of a call bell so that the patient feels safe, provision of a warm bath to help them relax, provision of light food and warm milky drinks at night and the use of relaxation tapes or reading; all of these can help to minimise stress, fear of the unknown, their own worries and the death of others (Howard 2004, Béphage 2005).

Specific relaxation therapies may include guided imagery, yoga, t'ai chi, or meditation, where the patients are shown how to use their mind and body to let go of tension which in turn can help to relieve muscle tension. When there is a need to reduce the tension in muscles and relieve pain, then progressive muscular relaxation techniques can be used. This is done by tensing each set of muscles then relaxing them, working up from the toe to the head (Lavery 1997).

Nursing actions associated with sociocultural factors affecting ill health

In a multicultural society, the nurse will be faced with patient's individual sleep routines and the need to maintain the patient's individual social, cultural, spiritual and religious beliefs is vital. The nurse will need to discuss these issues with the patient and consider how their needs can be met. It is unlikely that the patient will be used to sleeping with so many people in close proximity and they may not be used to sleeping on their own. Béphage (2005) discusses the impact that spiritual comfort or discomfort can have on individuals and the effect it can have on their sleep patterns.

Nursing actions associated with environmental factors affecting ill health

The nurse will need to manage the ward environment to promote a therapeutic environment which enables patients not only to get off to sleep but one which allows them to remain asleep. The main environmental threat in hospitals is from noise (from the nurses, equipment and patients themselves). Nurses need to wear soft-soled shoes, ensure trolleys are well maintained, keep talking down to a minimum and ensure that the patients have a call light which is less noisy than a call buzzer (Howard 2004, Béphage 2005).

Equally the nurse must ensure that patients are comfortable in the bed or chair when they are sleeping or resting. This relates to the pillows, bedclothes, mattresses as all should be appropriate for the patient and their condition. The temperature of the ward, the use of dim lights or blindfolds and the use of ear plugs need to be considered also (Morgan & Closs 1999, Howard 2004, Béphage 2005).

Hogg (1998) discusses the problems of sleep deprivation and disturbances in a High Dependency Unit (HDU) setting and stresses that nurses have a key role to play in preventing these disturbances and ensuring quality sleep to promote recovery. Various strategies are put forward to limit or prevent sleep deprivation by Hogg (1998), such as limiting noise, ensuring that the environment is conducive to sleep and the patient is comfortable, free from pain and anxiety.

Exercise

1. Consider the practice environment and what aspects could disturb your patient's sleep.
2. Consider ways in which these could be minimised.

Nursing actions associated with politicoeconomic factors affecting ill health

The nurse must be alert to the financial hardships hospitalisation and illness can bring to the patient and their immediate family. The ill-health state may affect their ability to work, e.g. narcolepsy or exacerbation of the disease process as in arthritis. This may be a short-term problem and sickness benefits may cover the period of illness. However, patients may have to come to terms with changes in their employment status, need to retrain for different jobs or retire completely. The nurse will need to discuss the economic repercussions of the illness with the family and consider the support needed from health and social care professionals. Worry and anxiety over their illness and the effects this may have on the patient and their family can affect the sleep pattern of the patient at home and in hospital.

Documenting the nursing care plan

Once the nursing actions have been identified then the nursing care plan needs to be written. Nursing care plans should abide by the Nursing and Midwifery Council (2007b) document *Record Keeping Guidance* and identify individualised actions and specify:

- who should be involved in the care planned
- what care should be given
- why that care should be given
- when the care should be given
- where the care should be given
- how the care should be given.

Exercise

1. Write the nursing care plan for the three priority problems identified on p. 443 in the previous exercise relating to Emma Simmons.
2. Check your answers with one of the problems as shown in Box 13.13.

Box 13.13	Nursing care plan – Emma Simmons

Problem

Emma is experiencing pain in her joints and on movement due to the arthritis/inflammation and this is shown by limited mobility, some loss of function in the hands and wrists, facial expression and verbal complaints of pain.

Short-term goal

Emma will be able to verbalise her pain to nursing staff and assess the effect of medications.

Long-term goal

Emma will be able to mobilise, sleep, work and socialise within the pain limits and be able to adapt her lifestyle to cope with the pain.

Care plan

- Observe pain levels and the link to treatment and mobility.
- Administer the prescribed anti-inflammatory medications.
- Ensure Emma's joints are rested and place supportive night splints on affected hands and wrists.
- Assist in the investigations ordered by the medical staff, e.g. full blood count and ESR levels, joint X-ray examination.
- Apply moist heat to joints affected.
- Encourage a planned range of movement exercises.
- Schedule daily care once morning stiffness has subsided, use of a warm bath may help movement initially.
- Listen to patient's worries and concerns about work, home life, etc.
- Plan a health education strategy with Emma when she is ready to participate in the activity.
- Discuss possible adjustments in relation to her lifestyle.

It may be useful to consider the five factors (physical, psychological, sociocultural, environmental and politico-economic) when writing the nursing care plan also. Reread the care plans and decide if all the factors are utilised. Once the nursing care plan has been written then this must be communicated to other health care professionals by verbal handover ready for the next stage – implementation.

IMPLEMENTING NURSING ACTIVITIES

Implementation of nursing activities involves three stages:

1. Preparatory stage of reading the nursing care plan, receiving handover report and ensuring that staff know what is required to accomplish the goals and decide on the skill mix needed.
2. Implementation, where safe, competent practice is the key to successful care. The plan is then put into action and shows both the artistic and scientific side of nursing.
3. Postimplementation stage when nursing activities are communicated to health care professionals (written and verbally) via progress notes.

Success of the implementation depends on the initial assessment, quality of the care plan, organisation of care delivery and the competence of the care given. The written nursing care plan guides the implementation phase to help the patient achieve the goals set but the plan must be reviewed and updated according to changes in the patient's condition (see Chapter 1 for further information on implementation).

To ensure that this stage is both effective and efficient, there are numerous factors which can influence the care given. It is necessary to consider what influences care, what knowledge is needed and what skills are required to ensure that patients receive the best care.

Exercise
1. Reread Case study 13.1.
2. Consider what may influence the implementation of nursing activities planned.
3. Consider what knowledge you would need to implement this care.
4. Consider what skills you would also need.

You may have considered some of the factors in Box 13.14 and it would be useful for you to reflect upon your own level of knowledge and skills. The factors which influence care may differ in practice areas.

Four domains were identified by the Nursing and Midwifery Council (2004b) document *Standards of Proficiency for Pre Registration Nursing Education*. Standard 7 in this document identifies the specific areas of proficiency required to enter the register and these can be linked to the implementation stage. The four domains are:

Box 13.14	Implementing nursing activities

Factors influencing the implementation of nursing activities
- Philosophy of care
- Nursing model used
- Assessment and planning stage
- Care delivery system used
- Resources available – skill mix, sufficient equipment and support services.

Knowledge required when implementing nursing activities
- Normal and abnormal anatomy and physiology of sleep cycles
- Related psychological effects associated with sleeping
- Social and cultural issues relating to poor sleeping, health or recovery
- Environmental influences and concerns
- Political and economic concerns.

Skills required when implementing nursing activities
- Caring skills
- Interpersonal skills
- Clinical psychomotor skills
- Management skills – supervision, delegation, organising team/individuals
- Counselling skills
- Teaching skills
- Research skills
- Problem-solving skills
- Leadership skills.

- professional and ethical practice
- care delivery
- care management
- personal and professional development (see Chapter 2 for further details).

These will be explored in relation to sleeping difficulties and the three scenarios used previously in this chapter.

Exercise
1. Reread the three mini case studies in Box 13.7.
2. Identify issues, from these mini case scenarios, which relate to each of the four domains.

Professional and ethical practice
- *Scenario A:* Confidentiality regarding recently separated partner. Attitudes regarding overdose admission.
- *Scenario B:* Counselling regarding difficulty with diagnosis.
- *Scenario C:* Dopamine used from fetus.

Care delivery

- *Scenario A:* Key worker system.
- *Scenario B:* Empowerment approach.
- *Scenario C:* Multidisciplinary team approach, care delivered on a holistic basis, adaptations needed.

Care management

- *Scenario A:* Close observation due to previous overdose.
- *Scenario B:* Symptom controlled.
- *Scenario C:* Tertiary health promotion, community management, family involvement, Parkinson's Disease Society.

Personal and professional development

- *Scenario A:* Treatment of anxiety and depression, overdose care.
- *Scenario B:* Differences with fibromyalgia and ME.
- *Scenario C:* Action of dopamine, anti-Parkinson's drug therapy, parkinsonian crisis.

Having identified the potential aspects within these domains, it may be necessary to increase your knowledge and skills relating to the aspects identified.

EVALUATION OF NURSING ACTIVITIES

Evaluation of nursing care is integral to the professional accountability of nurses to their clients and is an essential stage of the process, yet, according to the Clothier Report (Clothier et al 1994), it is unfortunately a neglected part. The evaluation stage involves reflection on the degree of goal achievement, so that feedback on care can be gained. Evaluation should be ongoing to gain an insight into the patient's progress and effectiveness of nursing activities. Evaluation can be continuous, hourly, daily, on a shift basis or longer depending on the individual patient's problem and the goals set (for further information on evaluation see Chapter 1). It is important that the nurse asks the patient how they feel they have slept and compare this with the nurse's evaluation.

> **Exercise**
> 1. Reread Case study 13.1.
> 2. Consider the influencing factors which may affect the evaluation of nursing activities.
> 3. Consider the skills needed to evaluate nursing activities.
> 4. Check your answers in Box 13.15.

Again, various factors can influence this evaluation stage and the number of skills which are required.

There are various steps which need to be followed when evaluating care:

1. Check goals against the patient's progress (discuss with patient if possible).
   - Have the goals been completely or partially met?
   - Have they been met at all?

> **Box 13.15** | **Factors and skills influencing the evaluation of care**
>
> **Factors which influence the evaluation stage**
> - Abilities of nurse and patient
> - Standards and quality assurance mechanisms
> - Assessment, planning and implementation stages
> - Goals set
> - Timing of evaluation.
>
> **Skills required in the evaluation stage**
> - Reassessment to include:
>   - observation
>   - interviewing
>   - listening
>   - identification of plan
>   - time scale
>   - plan of action.
> - Analysis of patient's response to care
> - Auditing.

2. Is the time scale realistic?
3. Record the findings and plan accordingly:
   - Goal completely met, then state evidence for this and discontinue the problem
   - Goal partially met, then decide if need to extend the evaluation time or modify the plan
   - Goal not met at all, then decide if need to extend the evaluation time, modify the plan or reassess the problem.

> **Exercise**
> 1. Read the information in Box 13.16 and review the goals set for Emma's problems and evaluate her progress.
> 2. Consider what needs to be done in the next few days and write a revised plan of action if needed.
> 3. Discuss your plan with a colleague and agree its evidence base.

It can be noted that part of the long-term goal has been met, i.e. she is able to mobilise and is sleeping better and feels able to go home which may mean socialising more. However, part of the long-term goal relating to returning to work has not been met.

Where goals have not been met then the following questions may need to be asked:

- Is more information required?
- Should the plan be modified?
- Has the problem changed?
- Has the problem worsened?
- Should the goal be reviewed?
- Was the goal appropriate?
- Does the nursing plan need interventions from other health care professionals?

Box 13.16	Long-term goal review

Long-term goal previously set
- Emma will be able to mobilise, sleep, work and socialise within the pain limits and be able to adapt her lifestyle to cope with the pain.

Evidence available
- Emma is able to walk around the ward area; her joints are still slightly swollen and tender but the morning stiffness and pain is less.
- Emma does not feel able to return to work as yet but feels able to go home and continue with her exercises.
- She is sleeping better and she has woken up less frequently with the aid of the night resting splints. If she does wake up then it is not due to the pain but due to a disturbance on the ward itself.

In Emma's case it may be that the plan needs to be continued for a short time after discharge and be reviewed at a later date in the Outpatients Department and by her GP.

SUMMARY POINTS

> 1. A variety of skills are needed to deliver care to patients with sleeping difficulties.
> 2. Accurate, continuous assessment is vital as all other stages are dependent upon it.
> 3. Ensuring adequate sleep is essential for patient wellbeing.

References

Alexander MF, Fawcett JN, Runciman PJ 2006 Nursing practice hospital and home, 3rd edn. Churchill Livingstone, Edinburgh

American Academy of Sleep Medicine 2001 The international classification of sleep disorders, revised (ICSD-R) Diagnostic and Coding Manual American Academy of Sleep Medicine (www.absm.org/PDF/ICSD.pdf)

Bagnall AM, Whiting P, Wright K et al 2002 The effectiveness of interventions used in the treatment/management of chronic fatigue syndrome and/or myalgic encephalomyelitis in adults and children. NHS Centre for Reviews and Dissemination, University of York

Bendak S 2003 12-h workdays: current knowledge and future directions. Work and Stress 17(4):321–336

Bent S, Padula A, Moore D et al 2006 Valerian for sleep: A systematic review and meta-analysis. American Journal of Medicine 119(12):1005–1012

Béphage G 2005 Promoting quality sleep in older people: the nursing care role. British Journal of Nursing 14(4):205–210

Berger AM, Hobbs BB 2006 Impact of shift work on the health and safety of nurses and patients. Clinical Journal of Oncology Nursing 10(4):465–471

Bourguignon C, Labyak SE, Taibi D 2003 Investigating sleep disturbances in adults with rheumatoid arthritis. Holistic Nursing Practice 17(5):241–249

Bowie I, Woodward S 2003 Nursing patients with neurological problems. In: Brooker C, Nichol M (eds) Nursing adults: the practice of caring, 14. Mosby, Edinburgh

Bray D 2001 Biofeedback. In: Rankin-Box D (ed) The nurses' handbook of complementary therapies, 2nd edn, Chapter 9. Baillière Tindall, Edinburgh

British Medical Association 1993 Complementary medicine: new approaches to good practice. Oxford University Press, Oxford

Brooks I 1997 The lights are bright? Debating the future of the permanent night shift. Journal of Management in Medicine 11(2):58–70

Brostrom A, Stromberg A, Dahlstrom U et al 2001 Patients with congestive cardiac failure and their conceptions of their sleep problems. Journal of Advanced Nursing 34(4):520–529

Brownfield A 1998 Aromatherapy in arthritis: a study. Nursing Standard 13(5):34–35

Brugne J-F 1994 Sleep, wakefulness and the nurse. British Journal of Nursing 3(2):68–71

Buscemi N, Vandermeer B, Hooton N et al 2006 Efficacy and safety of exogenous melatonin for secondary sleep disorders and sleep disorders accompanying sleep restriction: meta-analysis. BMJ 332(7538):385–393

Cawthorn A, Hope 1992 Nursing intervention at night. In: McMahon R (ed) Nursing at night. A professional approach, Chapter 4. Scutari Press, London

Closs SJ 1988 A nursing study of sleep on surgical wards. Report prepared for the Scottish Home and Health Department. Nursing Research Unit. Department of Nursing Studies, Edinburgh

Closs SJ 1990 Influences on patients' sleep on surgical wards. Surgical Nurse 3(2):12–14

Clothier C, MacDonald C, Shaw D 1994 Independent enquiry into deaths and injuries on the children's ward at Grantham and Kestevan General Hospital during the period February to April 1991 (Allitt Inquiry). HMSO, London

Communities and Local Government 2006 Rough sleeping statistics (www.communities.gov.uk/index.asp?id=1150131)

Crabb L 2001 Clinical sleep disorders in Parkinson's disease: the nursing role. British Journal of Nursing 10(1):42–47

Davis GC 2003 Improved sleep may reduce arthritis pain. Holistic Nursing Practice 17(3):128–139

Department of Health 2005 Reduce the risk of cot death. (leaflet available at www.dh.gov.uk)

Department of Trade and Industry 2003 Your guide to the working time regulations. (www.dti.gov.uk/employment/employment-legislation/working-time-regs/index.html)

Department for Transport 2001 Older drivers: a literature review. Road Safety Research Report No 25 (www.dft.gov.uk)

Department for Transport, 2003 Older drivers, illness and medication. Road Safety Research Report No 39 (www.dft.gov.uk)

Department for Transport 2006 Drivers' hours and tachograph rules for goods vehicles in the UK and Europe (GV262), 2nd edn (www.dft.gov.uk)

Dimond B 2005 Legal aspects of nursing, 4th edn. Prentice Hall, London

Dingley J 1996 A computer-aided comparative study of progressive alertness changes in nurses working two different night-shift rotas. Journal of Advanced Nursing 23:1247–1253

Dogan O, Ertekin S, Dogan S 2005 Sleep quality in hospitalized patients. Journal of Clinical Nursing 14(1):107–111

Dougherty L, Lister S 2004 The Royal Marsden manual of clinical nursing procedures, 6th edn. Blackwell Publishing, Oxford

Dunn C, Sleep J, Collett D 1995 Sensing an improvement: an experimental study to evaluate the use of aromatherapy, massage and periods of rest in an intensive care unit. Journal of Advanced Nursing 21:34–40

Duxbury J 1994 An investigation into primary nursing and its effects upon the nursing attitudes about and administration of prn night sedation. Journal of Advanced Nursing 192:3–931

Edinger JD, Wohlegemuth WK, Radtke RA et al 2001 Cognitive behavoioural therapy for treatment of chronic primary insomnia: a randomized controlled trial. JAMA 285(14):1856–1864

Ersser S, Wiles A, Taylor H et al 1999 The sleep of older people in hospital and nursing homes. Journal of Clinical Nursing 8:360–368

Fitzpatrick J, While A, Roberts J 1999 Shift work and its impact upon nurse performance: current knowledge and research issues. Journal of Advanced Nursing 29(1):18–27

Gallinagh R, Nevin R, McIlroy D et al 2002 The use of physical restraints as a safety measure in the care of older people in four rehabilitation wards: findings from an exploratory study. International Journal of Nursing Studies 39:147–156

Halfens R, Cox K, Kuppen-Van Merwijk A 1994 Effect of the use of sleep medication in Dutch hospitals on the use of sleep medication at home. Journal of Advanced Nursing 19:66–70

Henderson-Smart DJ, Ponsonby A-L, Murphy E 1998 Reducing the risk of sudden infant death syndrome: A review of scientific literature. Journal of Paediatric and Child Health 34(3):213–219

Herxheimer A, Petrie KJ 2006 Melatonin for the prevention and treatment of jet lag (Cochrane Review). In: The Cochrane Library, Issue 4. Oxford, Update Software

Hobson JA 1995 Sleep. Scientific American Library, New York

Hodgson LA 1991 Why do we need sleep? Relating theory to nursing practice. Journal of Advanced Nursing 16:1503–1510

Hoffman S 2003 Sleep in the older adult: implications for nurses. Geriatric Nursing 24(4):210–216

Hogg G 1998 Sleep deprivation in a high dependency unit. Professional Nurse 13(10):693–696

Holbrook AM, Crowther R, Lotter A et al 2000 Meta-analysis of benzodiozepine use in the treatment of insomnia. Canadian Medical Association Journal 162(2):225–233

Honkus V 2003 Sleep deprivation in critical care units. Critical Care Nursing Quarterly 26(3):179–189

Horne JA 2001 Sleep-related vehicle accidents: some guidelines for road safety policies (www.lboro.ac.uk/departments/hu/groups/sleep/)

Horne JA, 2001 Barrett PR Over the counter medicines and the potential for unwanted sleepiness in drivers: a review. Department for Transport, Local Government and the Regions (www.roads.dtlr.gov.uk/roadsafety/research24/01.htm)

Horrocks N, Pounder R 2006 Working the night shift: preparation, survival and recovery. A guide for junior doctors. Royal College of Physicians, London

Howard D 2004 Stress, relaxation and rest. In: Mallik M, Hall C, Howard D (eds) Nursing knowledge and practice: Foundations for decision making, 2nd edn, Chapter 8. Baillière Tindall, Edinburgh

Humm C 1996 The relationship between night duty tolerance and personality. Nursing Standard 10(51):34–39

Irwin P 1992 The physiology of sleep. In: McMahon R (ed) Nursing at night. A professional approach, Chapter 3. Scutari Press, London

Jacobs GD, Pace-Scholl EF, Stickgold R et al 2004 Cognitive behavioural therapy and pharmacotherapy for insomnia: a randomized controlled trial and direct comparison. Archives of Internal Medicine 164(17):1888–1896

Jamieson EM, McCall JM, Whyte LA 2002 Clinical nursing practices, 4th edn. Churchill Livingstone, Edinburgh

Karlsson S, Bucht G, Rasmussen B et al 2000 Restraint use in elder care: decision making among registered nurses. Journal of Clinical Nursing 9:842–850

Kindlen S 2003 Physiology for health care and nursing, 2nd edn. Churchill Livingstone, Edinburgh

Lavery S 1997 The healing powers of sleep. How to achieve restorative sleep naturally. Gaia, London

Lavie P, Pillar G, Malhotra A 2002 Sleep disorders: Diagnosis, management and treatment. A handbook for clinicians. Martin Dunitz, London

Learthart S 2000 Health effects of internal rotation of shifts. Nursing Standard 14(47):34–36

le May A 2006 Sleep. In: Alexander MF, Fawcett JN, Runciman PJ 2006 (eds) Nursing practice hospital and home, 3rd edn, Chapter 25. Churchill Livingstone, Edinburgh

Maldonado CC, Bentley AJ, Mitchell D 2004 A pictorial sleepiness scale based on cartoon faces. Sleep 27(3):541–548

Martell R 2001 Research shows dangers of rotational shift patterns. Nursing Standard 16(2):7

Mitchell EA, Tuohy PG, Brunt JM et al 1997 Risk factors for sudden infant death syndrome following the prevention campaign in New Zealand: A prospective study. Pediatrics 100(5):835–840

Montague SE, Watson R, Herbert RA 2005 Physiology for nursing practice, 3rd edn. Elsevier, Edinburgh

Montgomery P, Dennis J 2002 Physical exercise for sleep problems in adults aged 60+. Cochrane Database of Systematic Reviews, Issue 4. Art No: CD003404. DOI:10.1002/14651858. CD003404

Morgan K, Closs SJ 1999 Sleep management in nursing practice. Churchill Livingstone, Edinburgh

Morin CM, Colecchi C, Stone J et al 1999 Behavioural and pharmacological therapies for late-life insomnia. A randomised controlled trial. Journal of the American Medical Association 281(11):991–999

Muecke S 2005 Effects of rotating night shifts: literature review. Journal of Advanced Nursing 50(4):433–439

National Sleep Foundation 2002 '2002 Sleep in America Poll' (www.sleepfoundation.org)

New Zealand Herald 2006 Scientists 'discover cause of cot death', (www.nzherald.co.nz/section/1/story.cfm?c_id=1&objectid=10408803)

NICE 2003 Head injury: triage, assessment, investigation and early management of head injury in infants, children and adults. Clinical Guideline CG004. NICE, London

NICE 2004 Guidance on the use of zaleplon, zolpidem and zopiclone for the short-term management of insomnia. Technology Appraisal 77. NICE, London

Nursing and Midwifery Council 2004a NMC code of professional conduct: standards for conduct, performance and ethics. Nursing and Midwifery Council, London

Nursing and Midwifery Council 2004b Standards of proficiency for preregistration nursing education. Nursing and Midwifery Council, London

Nursing and Midwifery Council 2007a Standards for medicine management. NMC, London

Nursing and Midwifery Council 2007b NMC Record keeping guidance (www.nmc-uk.org) Nursing and Midwifery Council, London

Nursing Times, News Clinical Research Highlights 1998 Melatonin could be the key to ME generation. Nursing Times 94(26):57

Office for National Statistics 2004 All unexplained infant deaths by Government Office Region, 2000–2004 (England and Wales). Health Statistics Quarterly 27 (www.statistics.gov.uk)

Pemberton L, Waterhouse C 2006 The unconscious patient. In: Alexander MF, Fawcett JN, Runciman PJ (eds) Nursing practice hospital and home, 3rd edn, Chapter 28. Churchill Livingstone, Edinburgh

Rajaratnam SMW, Arendt J 2001 Health in a 24-hour society. Lancet 358:999–1005

Rankin-Box D 2001 The nurses' handbook of complementary therapies, 2nd edn. Baillière Tindall, Edinburgh

Reet M 2003 Circadian rhythms and sleep paterns. In: Brooker C, Nichol M (eds) Nursing adults the practice of caring, Chapter 4. Mosby, Edinburgh

Reite M, Ruddy J, Nagel K 2002 Concise guide to evaluation and management of sleep disorders, 3rd edn. American Psychiatric Publishing, Washington

Roper N, Logan W, Tierney AJ 1996 The elements of nursing. A model for nursing based on a model of living, 4th edn. Churchill Livingstone, Edinburgh

Roper N, Logan W, Tierney AJ 2000 The Roper–Logan–Tierney model of nursing based on activities of living. Churchill Livingstone, Edinburgh

Royal College of Nursing 2003 Complementary therapies in nursing, midwifery and health visiting practice. RCN, London

Royal College of Nursing 2004 Restraint revisited – rights, risk and responsibility. Guidance for nursing staff. RCN, London

Rutishauser S 1994 Physiology and anatomy a basis for nursing and health care. Churchill Livingstone, Edinburgh

Ryman L, Rankin-Box D 2001 Relaxation and visualization. In: Rankin-Box D (ed) The nurses' handbook of complementary therapies, 2nd edn, Chapter 18. Baillière Tindall, Edinburgh

Schaefer KM 1997 Health patterns of women with fibromyalgia. Journal of Advanced Nursing 26:565–571

Scottish Intercollegiate Guidelines Network (SIGN) 2003 Management of obstructive sleep apnoea/hypopnoea syndrome in adults, No 73. SIGN, Edinburgh

Sivertsen B, Omvik S, Pallesen S et al 2006 Cognitive behavoioural therapy vs zopiclone for treatment of chronic primary insomnia in older adults: a randomized controlled trial. JAMA 295(24):2851–2858

Soden K, Vincent K, Craske S et al 2004 A randomised controlled trial of aromatherapy massage in a hospice setting. Palliative Medicine 18(2):87–92

Taibi D, Bourguignon C, Taylor AG 2004 Valerian use for sleep disturbances related to rheumatoid arthritis. Holistic Nursing Practice 18(3):120–126

Teasdale G, Galbraith S, Clarke K 1975 Observation record chart. Nursing Times 71(19):972–973

Thorgrimsen L, Spector A, Wiles A et al 2003 Aroma therapy for dementia. Cochrane Database of Systematic Reviews, Issue 3. Art No: CD003150

Tranmer JE, Minard J, Fox LA et al 2003 The sleep experience of medical and surgical patients. Clinical Nursing Research 12(2):159–173

Trevelyan J, Booth B 1994 Complementary medicine for nurses, midwives and health visitors. Macmillan, Basingstoke

Walsh M 2002 Caring for the patient with a disorder of the musculoskeletal system. In: Walsh M (ed) Watson's clinical nursing and related sciences, 6th edn, Chapter 24. Baillière Tindall, London

Wilson JL 2002 The impact of shift patterns on healthcare professionals. Journal of Nursing Management 10(4):211–219

Further reading

Alexander MF, Fawcett JN, Runciman PJ 2006 Nursing practice hospital and home, 3rd edn. Churchill Livingstone, Edinburgh (Allan D, Disorders of the nervous system, Chapter 9; Lucas B, Disorders of the musculoskeletal system, Chapter 10; Pemberton L, Waterhouse C, The unconscious patient, Chapter 28)

British National Formulary (www.bnf.org)

McMahon R (ed) 1992 Nursing at night. A professional approach. Scutari Press, London

Rankin-Box D 2001 The nurses' handbook of complementary therapies, 2nd edn. Baillière Tindall, Edinburgh

Walsh M (ed) 2002 Watson's clinical nursing and related sciences, 6th edn. Baillière Tindall, London (Allan D, Caring for the patient with a disorder of the nervous system, Chapter 20; Walsh M, Caring for the patient with a disorder of the muskulo-skeletal system, Chapter 24)

Useful websites

besttreatments.co.uk/btuk/conditions (Clinical evidence for patients from the BMJ Best Treatments – insomnia in adults, sleep problems in children)

www.bnf.org (British National Formulary)

www.clinicalevidence.com (Clinical evidence relating to insomnia and sleep apnoea)

www.dft.gov.uk and www.thinkroad safety.gov.uk (Department for Transport)

www.journalsleep.org (On-line journal of sleep)

www.nmc-uk.org (Nursing and Midwifery Council (NMC))

www.sleepfoundation.org (National Sleep Foundation (NSF))

Dying

Debbie Roberts

INTRODUCTION

According to Roper et al (1996, p. 395) 'Dying is the final Activity of Living and is normally (unless it is sudden and unexpected) preceded by a process (i.e. the process of dying) in which the individual actively participates'. It is because of this that dying is included as an Activity of Living. An understanding of death, dying and bereavement is essential if nurses are to undertake care that is holistic and takes account of individual beliefs and religious practice.

This chapter will therefore focus on the following:

1. **The model of living**
   - death and dying as an Activity of Living
   - lifespan and death and dying
   - factors influencing the AL of dying.

2. **The model for nursing**
   - nursing care of individuals with health problems affecting the Activity of Living: dying.

THE MODEL OF LIVING

DEATH AND DYING AS AN AL

What is death? Rutishauser (1994, p. 625) states that 'people die as a result of the failure of one or more body systems through injury, disease or ageing'. Death then is 'the stage when a person ceases to exist in their previous physical form' (Holland & Hogg 2001, p. 154). Other types of death are 'clinical death' (the appearance of death signs upon examination) and 'social death' (when the individual is treated essentially as a corpse although still clinically and biologically alive) (Bond & Bond 1997). Death can occur at any age, and may occur suddenly, e.g. in an accident or suicide, or gradually, e.g. from cancer. How people cope with the aftermath of death will vary according to their cultural, religious and spiritual beliefs. They are often said to be 'bereaved'. 'Grief' or the feelings and emotion that 'may follow a bereavement' is also expressed in 'different ways according to the culture to which they belong' (Holland & Hogg 2001, p. 156).

DYING IN HEALTH AND ILLNESS – ACROSS THE LIFESPAN

Childhood

Hindmarch (2000) argues that the death of a child is different from other forms of bereavement, and although a comparatively rare event in the Western world, the impact of child death is out of all proportion to its incidence. The death of a child is upsetting because it does not fit into our perception of 'the natural order of things'. This is true even when the child who dies is an adult with elderly parents. Roper et al (1996) highlight other issues associated with death in early childhood such as sudden infant death syndrome. In industrialised countries sudden infant death syndrome has become one of the major causes of infant mortality. However, Roper et al (1996) explain that if infants survive the first year, their life expectancy increases. Extensive research and subsequent education of the public has reduced the numbers of sudden infant deaths in the United Kingdom, but for a variety of reasons, infant mortality remains high in some developing countries (Roper et al 1996). The impact of childhood death is made evident to us in the number of children that die as a result of environmental and other health hazards. The World Health Organization (2002) states that 'seven out of ten childhood deaths in developing countries can be attributed to just five main causes, or a combination of them: pneumonia, diarrhoea, measles, malaria and malnutrition' and that 'around the world, three out of every four children who seek healthcare are suffering from at least one of these conditions'. Prevention of death in children due to these illnesses is therefore a priority for the World Health Organization.

The bereaved child

Children are perceptive, will often know when something is wrong and will want information. People often worry about how and when to tell children about an impending death. Ideally, when someone the child is close to dies, news of the death should be delivered by a parent or a close family member. If the death is expected, parents will often forewarn children. However, often these people are also bereaved themselves and may require the support of nursing staff.

Initially, the information given to children should be short, clear and unambiguous. The words 'died' and 'dead' are easily understood. The age of the child will affect the child's perception of the event. Wright (1996) explains the impact of chronological age of the child on their perceptions of death (see Box 14.1). In order to develop an understanding of the reactions of children to the news of a death undertake the following exercise.

Exercise

1. Examine Box 14.1 and consider how the nursing interventions could be adapted for children of various ages and stages of development.

Children will dictate the amount of information they need by the questions they ask. Questions should always be answered truthfully. Children should be allowed to cry rather than being told to be brave, to scream, be angry or be silent. Wright (1996) explains that many children will be unable to remain still when discussing death and may find it comforting to walk around or continue to play with toys, or want food. Wright (1996) goes on to suggest that children should be encouraged to see, and if they wish, touch the person who has died. This process should not be forced or hurried, and similarly, the child should not be made to feel guilty for not wishing to do anything. When seeing the dead person, the child will require careful explanation of what they see and be helped to reach meaning and understanding (Wright 1996).

Box 14.1	Chronological age and perceptions of death

Below 5 years
- Lack of understanding about the finality of death.
- An inability to run through the events and arrive at a logical conclusion, 'Going round in circles'.
- A belief that they can cause what happens to them and around them (egocentricity).

5–10 years
- Concrete thinking, literal understanding.
- Understanding the physical causes of death, both internal and external.
- Concern with other people's feelings (empathy).
- An interest in the tangible expressions of grief: rituals, pictures, gravestones.

10 years and older
- A more abstract understanding.
- A great sense of justice/injustice, fate.
- Reflection on belief systems.
- Strong emotional reaction.

From Wright (1996), p. 67.

Adolescence

As in childhood, death in adolescence can take place for many different reasons. However, Roper et al (1996) highlight the increasing suicide rates amongst adolescents within industrialised societies. In the UK the Government set out to reduce the numbers of people who commit suicide in the plan known as *Saving Lives: Our Healthier Nation* (Department of Health 1999). However, the document does not distinguish between suicides at any particular age group. Death from suicide amongst adolescents may be more likely to be induced by drugs and/or alcohol. King (2001) demonstrates a number of key characteristics which are present in adolescents who attempt suicide. These include: experiencing stressful life events, being sexually active, poor family environment, low parental monitoring, marijuana use, recent drunkenness, current smoking and physical fighting (King 2001). The World Health Organization (2002) reports that at least 100 000 annual deaths in young people worldwide are attributed to suicide, whilst 'every year, almost 1.5 million adolescents die from substance abuse, reproductive ill health, suicide, injuries and violence' (WHO 2002).

Exercise

1. Access the World Health Organization website (www.who.int/en) and find the latest policies and recommendations on adolescent health and deaths.
2. Consider the implications for adolescents in your country.

Adulthood

Death in early adulthood is still likely to be perceived as untimely, i.e. happening before it should, especially in view of the fact that people are living longer (Roper et al 1996). The National Statistics site (official UK statistics) reports that 'in 1997 life expectancy at birth in the United Kingdom was approaching 75 years for men and 80 years for women compared with just 50 years for males and 54 years for females in 1911' (Office for National Statistics 2000). Death in adulthood is caused by a number of illnesses or traumatic events and the incidence of deaths between the ages of 45 and 75 is higher for men than women in the United Kingdom (Roper et al 1996). Roper et al (1996) suggest that death in later adulthood often serves to remind mankind of its mortality, making the possibility of death, and the process of dying, more of a reality.

Exercise

1. Access the World Health Organization website (www.who.int/en) and find the latest information on life expectancy in different countries.
2. Consider the implications for health care of adults in various countries.
3. Discuss with colleagues.

Old age

Perceptions about death in old age are often different to those concerning death at other times across the lifespan; death may be viewed as a natural event in old age. People tend to live longer and may have higher expectations of health in old age. Helman (1996) explains the concept of social death in old age whereby the person, although physically alive, will be seen as less alive socially in the eyes of society or even family members. Helman (1996) cites examples of social death as including those who have been confined to institutions for the rest of their lives, such as prisons, nursing homes, homes for the mentally handicapped and hospices. In some cases, during this transition between old age and death older people will lose the will to live and this concept is examined later in this chapter.

The maximum lifespan for humans seems to be approximately 100–115 years with the number of people exceeding 100 set to rise. According to the Health Education Authority (1998) the number of people aged 65 will increase by 30% between 1996 and 2021 and the numbers of over-90s will double in the same period; centenarians will quadruple by 2016. Further to this, Costello (2001) explains that the majority of patients who die in hospital are over the age of 65. Findings from Costello's study show that nurses working in elderly care wards demonstrate a lack of what he terms 'emotional engagement'; that is to say, nurses provide individual care to older patients who are dying, but the care is aimed at meeting physical needs (Costello 2001).

Before thinking about how to care for others it is important to understand the range of views associated with death and dying. Consider the following.

Exercise

Reflect on your personal experiences with people who are dying.

1. Do you feel differently about incidents involving children, adolescents, or people who try or succeed in taking their own lives?
2. Where do you think these personal ideas may have originated from?

The major causes of death differ in various parts of the world, and different stages of life. In the case of death in childhood it is not unusual for nurses to experience a sense of guilt and even failure following the death of a child. Costello & Trinder-Brook (2000) conducted a retrospective study of children's nurses and found that often the nurses could not provide any rational explanation for these feelings of guilt and failure. The study also showed that nurses experience great conflict when trying to foster hope with parents who are struggling to come to terms with preparing for the death of a child (Costello & Trinder-Brook 2000).

Brysiewicz (2002) explains that in South Africa, violent death due to interpersonal violence is a huge problem, with the majority of those involved being young adults 'in the prime of their lives'. Emergency nurses interviewed in Brysiewicz's study saw themselves as being engaged in a battle with death, fighting for victory. In this study violent and sudden loss of life resulted in the nurses feeling that they had failed the client when the battle was lost (Brysiewicz 2002). Feelings which are not dissimilar to those of the paediatric nurses in Costello and Trinder-Brook's study.

The origins of views on death and dying may be difficult to trace. Undertaking the reflective exercise may have been difficult to pinpoint feelings about particular life events. We inherit or learn certain guidelines through which we come to know how to live in our own social group or society. These guidelines are termed culture (Holland & Hogg 2001). Holland & Hogg (2001) suggest that our culture determines the pattern in which we undertake a variety of roles and responsibilities. In particular the beliefs, rituals and customs which we associate with death are deeply embedded. Personal experiences associated with death and dying may have a profound impact on how an individual nurse is able to support patients' families and colleagues in future situations.

DEPENDENCE/INDEPENDENCE IN THE AL OF DYING

As in previous chapters the activity of dying sees people moving along a continuum between dependence and independence. Ultimately, throughout the activity of dying the person will move towards dependence; however, independence should be promoted for as long as possible or desirable by the person. Indeed having and maintaining control during the terminal stages of life seems to be crucially important (Carter et al 2004, Johnston & Smith 2006). Taking charge and maintaining control is concerned with people's ability to define and describe their needs and includes the patient's right to delegate control to others (Carter et al 2004). Being in control is seen as a mechanism for maintaining independence and therefore quality of life (Johnston & Smith 2006). The ability of individuals to maintain control during the terminal stages of an illness may depend on the nurse's ability help the patient to exercise autonomy (deAraujo et al 2004). deAraujo et al provide some examples such as letting the patient decide what time they wish to take a bath, and helping and coaxing them to take part in some activity that they are becoming increasingly unable to do all by themselves (deAraujo et al 2004). Transition towards dependence may be a gradual or rapid process and is sometimes referred to as a dying trajectory. Each day may bring fluctuations along the independence/dependence continuum. Individuals may be aware of the gradual decline in the ability for self-care. Not all dying people will want or need nursing care. Roper et al (1996) suggest that, for those who do want or need care, it is the role of the nurse to help the dying person to balance the degree of dependence/independence in the Activities of Living up until death.

The onset of the process of dying is difficult to diagnose (see Biological factors). When medical treatment cannot halt the course of a disease and can only alleviate the symptoms of the fatal illness, the illness is referred to as terminal. However, there may be a considerable length of time between terminal diagnosis and the rapid physical decline associated with the event of death; for example when someone who is HIV-positive develops AIDS, the illness may last many months or years. The dying trajectory is long. During the intervening period symptomatic relief becomes paramount and is known as palliative care (Roper et al 1996). Palliative care is the active total care offered to a patient with a progressive illness and their family, when it is recognised that the illness is no longer curable, in order to concentrate on the quality of life and the alleviation of distressing symptoms within the framework of a coordinated service (World Health Organization 1990). Dougan & Colquhoun (2000, p. 963) state that the term palliative care 'is given to the approach adopted when cure is unlikely and it is expected that the patient will die in the foreseeable future'. They state that 'palliative care has been developed to help those who are dying slowly, or as is often said, living with dying' (Dougan & Colquhoun 2000, p. 963). They offer a model for palliative care which supports the view of the patient on a dependence/independence continuum, whilst recognising the interdependence of the Activities of Living and holistic care.

SUMMARY POINTS

1. Death can occur at any time along the lifespan.
2. Attitudes towards death are often shaped by our personal experiences and cultural background.
3. Death may be expected, sudden, peaceful or violent. Bereavement may be affected accordingly.

FACTORS AFFECTING THE ACTIVITY OF DYING

According to Roper et al (1996) there are core factors which have an impact on all the Activities of Living, and the activity of dying is no different. In the following sections each of the factors will be explored in relation to the activity of dying.

Biological factors

For most purposes it can be assumed that death has occurred when a person's pulse and respiration have ceased. However, throughout adulthood, cells throughout the body are dying. Kennedy (2003) explains that cells die because they have come to the end of their natural lifespan, or because they have been fatally injured. For example, red blood cells are continually replaced, whereas other cells cannot be replaced if they become injured, as in the case of cells in the spinal cord. Kennedy (2003) also states that death is a process which begins with the failure of one part of the body, thus altering the internal environment of the body, impairing the function of other organs and tissues. This leads to failure of the life of the body as a whole. But Roper et al (1996) suggest that sometimes a more elaborate diagnosis of death is required, especially if there has been admission to hospital and sophisticated, artificial, 'life-support' systems are being used to maintain vital body functions. The concepts of 'clinical death' (death of the person), 'biological death' (death of the tissues) and 'brain death' (irreversible brain damage) reflect the different interpretations (Roper et al 1996, p. 404). Therefore, diagnosing the point at which a person is dying is difficult and problematic. The nervous system is often used as an indicator of status along the dying trajectory. Table 14.1 demonstrates the role of different parts of the nervous system and the consequences of loss of functions.

Table 14.1 Role of different parts of the nervous system (CNS) in different behaviours and the consequences of loss of functions

Part of CNS	Role	Consequences of loss		
		State		Features
Cerebral cortex	Awareness Understanding Purposeful behaviour		Vegetative state	Eyes open and move Breathes spontaneously May grimace, gasp and groan No voluntary movement
Brain stem	Maintains consciousness Controls breathing, swallowing Reflex control of muscles (e.g. eyes, face; larynx limbs) Autonomic control of circulation	Brain death		Coma Breathing stops Involuntary limb movement Incontinence
Spinal cord	Reflex control of muscles (e.g. limbs) Autonomic reflexes	Death		

Adapted from Kennedy (2003).

Loss of cerebral function (whilst the brain stem is intact) results in total loss of personality and absence of purposeful activity. The person may exist in this 'vegetative state' for many years; breathing occurs spontaneously, the heart beats, blood circulates and reflex movements occur. Kennedy (2003) explains that the *person* has died even though the body remains alive and sometimes this may give the false impression that conscious awareness still exists.

Complete and irreversible brain death

There is medical agreement about the criteria indicating complete and irreversible brain death, requiring confirmation by at least two experienced doctors. A series of criteria is applied by the two experienced doctors on two separate occasions. The doctors will not be those assigned to care for the patient and have not usually met the patient prior to undertaking the tests. Roper et al (1996, p. 404) suggest that the criteria include:

- fixation of pupils
- absence of corneal and vestibulooccular reflexes
- absence of response within the cranial nerve distribution to sensory stimuli
- no response to bronchial stimulation when a catheter is passed into the trachea
- no spontaneous breathing movement when the patient is disconnected from a mechanical ventilator.

In order to understand the application of the brain stem death criteria it is useful to revise the anatomy and physiology of the brain.

The brain   The brain lies within the cranial cavity and constitutes approximately one-fiftieth of the body weight (Waugh & Grant 2006). The brain is divided into five areas:

1. the cerebrum (the largest part of the brain)
2. the midbrain
3. the pons
4. the medulla oblongata
5. the cerebellum (situated at the back of the head; coordinates activities associated with the maintenance of balance and equilibrium of the body).

Together the midbrain, the pons and the medulla oblongata form the brain stem (see Fig. 14.1).

Vital centres lie deep within the medulla oblongata. These centres consist of groups of cells associated with autonomic reflex activity and their activities are seen in Box 14.2.

Having revised the anatomy and physiology of the brain you should have a better understanding of the brain stem death tests. Each of the tests relates to one of the vital centres inside the medulla oblongata. If no response is gained when the test is carried out it indicates that no autonomic nervous response is present, and the person is pronounced brain stem dead (see Table 14.1 on left).

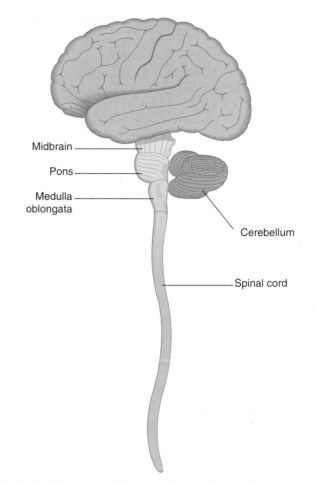

Fig. 14.1   The parts of the central nervous system (from Waugh & Grant 2006, with permission).

According to Gill (2000) death is not perceived by all as being merely a biological event. Brain stem death, in particular, is not universally accepted; this is largely due to social, cultural and philosophical issues and values which are mostly Western in nature. In many societies Gill (2000) suggests that concepts such as intelligence and the soul extend beyond the brain. The common issues as to why brain death is rejected are complex and intermingled. Here are some examples.

- *Personhood:* Belief that a person is a unity of mind and body. From a Western philosophical perspective it is suggested that rationality is located in the brain, so when the brain is destroyed, so is the person. However, in some cultures such as Japanese, personhood is seen as more than rationality. The Japanese view the body and spirit as being connected, so whilst cardiorespiratory function persists the person is not seen as dead. The death of an individual's brain is not necessarily equated with the actual death of that individual. Death is seen as a long process, rather than as a single event. Helman (1996) explains that in Japan a death may sometimes only be recognised as final following a series of rituals conducted by the family and the community in which the person lived.

Box 14.2	Vital centres in the medulla oblongata

Cardiac centre

Controls the rate and force of cardiac contraction. Sympathetic and parasympathetic nerve fibres originating in the medulla pass to the heart. Sympathetic stimulation increases the rate and force of the heartbeat and parasympathetic stimulation has the opposite effect.

Respiratory centre

Controls the rate and depth of respiration. From this centre nerve impulses pass to the phrenic and intercostal nerves which stimulate contraction of the diaphragm and intercostal muscles, thus initiating inspiration. The respiratory centre is stimulated by excess carbon dioxide, and, to a lesser extent, by deficiency of oxygen in its blood supply and by nerve impulses from the chemoreceptors in the carotid bodies.

Vasomotor centre

Controls the diameter of the blood vessels, especially the small arteries and arterioles which have a large proportion of smooth muscle fibres in their walls. Vasomotor impulses reach the blood vessels through the autonomic nervous system. Stimulation may cause either constriction or dilation of the blood vessels depending on the site.

Reflex centres of vomiting, coughing, sneezing and swallowing

When irritating substances are present in the stomach or the respiratory tract, nerve impulses pass to the medulla oblongata, stimulating the reflex centres to initiate the reflex action of vomiting, coughing or sneezing to expel the irritant.

From Waugh & Grant (2006, p. 155)

- *Death and the soul:* Many cultures, such as Muslims, have firm beliefs about the existence of the soul or spiritual element of a person. Gill (2000) points out that it is medically impossible to establish the existence and location of the soul, although it is not perceived to be within the brain.
- *The significance of other organs:* There are cultural differences about which organs are most important. In particular the heart function seems crucial. Gill (2000) explains that for Jewish people, for example, it is the heart not the brain which is the 'seat of life'; therefore whilst the heart is beating (as in brain stem death) the person is still seen as alive (Gill 2000).

This Western concept of brain stem death may have particular significance when cadaveric organ donation is concerned. It would not be acceptable to remove organs from someone who is perceived to be alive by the family.

In order to explore the concept of brain stem death further read Case study 14.1. In cases where brain stem death is diagnosed, families have little time to prepare; timespan from injury to diagnosis can be hours as opposed to days or months when someone is diagnosed as terminally ill. Whilst reading the case study consider the impact of this death on the family involved.

Exercise

1. What kind of support will the family need?
2. Develop some strategies to use in the clinical setting.
3. Will your support be different for different cultural groups?
4. How will you support a family during the decision to donate organs and beyond?

Case study 14.1

To illustrate and discuss brain stem death

20.00: John and Jane are 14-year-old twins who are out with a group of friends playing around the site of a disused factory. The football ended up on the roof and appeared to be easily accessible to both of them. Encouraged by his friends, John goes up to get the ball; he falls through the roof and falls awkwardly on his side some 3 metres below. John answers his name when one of his mates calls out to him. John gets up and is helped out back through the roof. John is sure he is OK and swears Jane to secrecy, saying 'Mum will kill us if she finds out we were up on the roof!'.

21.00: John and Jane arrive home. John says that he feels tired and feels like an early night, so he goes to bed. Shortly after, Jane also goes to bed, keeping their secret safe.

23.00: John's parents, Madge and Reg are preparing to go to bed. As she had done for the past 14 years Madge puts

her head around Jane's door to make sure she is asleep. As she walks towards John's room she hears a strange noise which she later describes as 'John sounded like he did when he had a cold as a baby; all snuffly, like he couldn't get his breath'. Madge goes into the room to see if he is all right and gives him a nudge but she cannot rouse him.

'His breathing sounded really strange … I called Reg … we couldn't wake him … we didn't know what to do … it was like it was happening in slow motion, not real somehow … Reg must have called the ambulance'.

23.15: Ambulance arrives; John's right pupil is fixed and his left pupil is sluggish to react; the crew say something about a Glasgow Coma scale of 5, his pulse is 26 beats per minute, respirations shallow at a rate of 14 per minute; blood pressure is 160/40. John is intubated in the ambulance.

Case study 14.1 (continued)

23.25: John is seen in Accident and Emergency and taken for a CT scan, Madge and Reg follow John's trolley but they feel almost invisible. The CT scan reveals massive extradural haematoma. John's left pupil becomes fixed. Madge and Reg sign something for John to have an operation, the words on the paper are long and technical, they hear what the consultant is saying but don't really understand. They can tell by the look on the doctor's face that John is in a very serious condition. They wait in a small room with no windows for what seems like an eternity for some news of their son, the nurses do pop in from time to time but they are frightened to go outside in case they miss the doctor.

During the operation John undergoes a craniotomy and removal of the extradural haematoma, he is paralysed and sedated with drugs.

01.00: John is then transferred to another department (a neurological high dependency unit). Both pupils are fixed and dilated. Glasgow coma scale now 3. His intracranial pressure is monitored; the reading is 46 (normal is 10–15). Madge and Reg finally get to see John and watch the nurses come and go every few minutes. The neurosurgeon and the consultant anaesthetist visit John and review his neurological state at 09.00.

09.00: Decision made to carry out brain stem criteria tests. The coroner is informed and the first set of tests is carried out at 09.30.

14.00: Second doctor performs the second set of brain stem tests and John is declared dead. Madge, Reg and Jane are there with John; each with their own feelings of loss, anger, guilt and love.

Transplant Law – United Kingdom

Wilkinson (2000) explains the legislation surrounding transplant surgery in the United Kingdom. The Human Tissue Act (1961) describes the circumstances in which organs may be removed. Only a designated person may authorise removal of organs once there is no reason to believe that the person had expressed an objection to their body being used in this way; or a surviving partner or relative objects; or there are religious objections. The Human Organ Transplant Act (1989) prohibits the sale of human organs and stipulates that living organ donors are genetically related to the recipient. Wilkinson (2000) goes on to say that unrelated live donation can take place if the Unrelated Live Transplant Authority approves the case.

Cultural and religious objections to transplant are explained by Holland & Hogg (2001). Jehovah's Witnesses do not receive blood transfusions and believe that human life should not be prolonged with another creature's blood. The view of Muslims towards brain stem death is that it is accepted for the purpose of organ transplant. Holland & Hogg (2001) further explain the Muslim Law Council's view that organ donation is supported as a means of alleviating pain or saving life on the basis of the rules of Shariah (Holland & Hogg 2001, p. 155).

Exercise

1. Find out about the legislation concerning organ donation and transplant in your own and one other country, and make some comparisons.
2. Is there an organ donor register, and how do people make it known that they wish to donate their organs after their death?
3. Discuss your findings with tutors and colleagues.

Organ donation

Seriously ill or injured people will often be attached to a ventilator to allow the heart and lungs to continue to function, and for oxygenated blood to perfuse all the organs and tissues. However, when the person's condition is incurable a diagnosis of brain stem death is made and the time recorded for the death certificate. According to the British Organ Donor Society (BODY) there is no definite age limit for potential organ and tissue donors, the condition of the organs being a more significant consideration. However, generally donors may be up to 65 years old for heart, liver and lungs and 75 years old for kidneys. There is no age limit for corneas (BODY 2001). Organs used for transplant include kidneys, heart, lungs, liver, pancreas and bowel. Usually one organ is transplanted, sometimes two, very occasionally three. Tissues used include corneas, heart valves, bone, skin and connective tissue. (When skin is retrieved it is removed from discrete areas of the body resulting in a barely noticeable mark as only a thin sliver of skin is required. In the case of corneas, the eyes are retrieved and replaced with either cotton wool and plastic caps or glass eyes.)

All internal organs must be retrieved from what is known as a 'beating heart donor' (although kidneys can be retrieved after up to 1 hour of heart death). Currently there is a National Organ Donor Register within the UK, a national database of people who wish to donate their organs to help someone else when they die. Transplant coordinators are able to access information on a 24-hour basis to see if their potential donor has already expressed a wish to donate. However, BODY (2001) suggests that when medically and legally practical, families, or in some cases friends, should be approached concerning the possibility of internal organ and tissue donation. It is necessary to maintain artificial breathing and a beating heart until the donated organs are retrieved in the operating theatre (a beating heart donor).

Transplant coordinators will often meet donor families and explain what will happen over the next few hours and answer any questions or concerns a family may have. Some families are keen to have information about the outcome of the organ retrieval, often wanting information about the recipient's progress.

Exercise

1. Where dedicated transplant services exist try to find out about the role of transplant coordinators with donor families and recipients.
2. If you were caring for someone who is seriously ill and the family asked you about possible donation of organs, what would happen where you work? Who would be contacted?

For further information about UK transplant law and becoming an organ donor see the British Organ Donor Society website at www.argonet.co.uk/body/DoH.html.

Psychological factors

According to Ross (1994) the importance of hope to life can be seen not only in death caused by its absence, but also in healing produced by its abundance. Ross (1994) describes the work of Limandri & Boyle (1978) in examining hope or will to live. In her classic work Ross explains that often once an individual loses the will to live, a sense of hopelessness and helplessness prevails which can result in the rapid decline of the individual and subsequent death. This is sometimes termed 'passive suicide'. Case study 14.2 helps to illustrate what Ross (1994) is describing.

Exercise

Reflect on the scenario between Marie and the nurse. Has anything like this ever happened to you?

1. Describe the situation.
2. Think about your own feelings.
3. What are/were the possible courses of action?

The following may have been considered.

There may have been feelings of conflict between wanting to do something to help the patient, but being aware that in the United Kingdom, nurses may not shorten life. Just as there are psychological factors which affect patients with regard to death and dying, it is important to recognise that nurses also have psychological attitudes towards death and dying. The culture of the nurses also plays an important part in terminal care provision in hospital; or rather the enculturation or socialisation that the nurses have undergone.

Case study 14.2

Marie

I had looked after Marie since she had been admitted to our medical ward with advanced carcinoma of her left breast; she had multiple metastases and was fully alert and aware of her diagnosis. Her carcinoma was now terminal. Marie knew she was dying and often remarked how lucky she was to be pain-free. One lunchtime I was caring for Marie and two other ladies in the same bay so I went to check if any of them needed any medication, in particular any analgesia. This is the conversation that took place:

Marie: 'How long am I going to be here Nurse?'

Nurse: 'I'm not sure Marie, why are you thinking about going home?'

Marie: 'Oh, no, I wouldn't manage at home … I want to be here … But there must be something you can do to help me. I want to go to sleep.'

Nurse: 'Are you tired Marie? Aren't you sleeping very well?'

Marie: 'No, I'm not talking about being tired, I just feel so dreadful … the waiting is terrible … wondering if it will be today … I don't want to go on feeling like this, there must be something you could do? Can't you give me a pill? Please give me a pill; let me go to sleep.'

In this case study Marie is using the euphemism of sleep. The nurse seeks clarification from Marie by asking whether she is tired or having difficulty in sleeping, but in fact Marie is asking the nurse to help her to die. Marie is aware of her diagnosis and has reached the stage of accepting her imminent death. She has lost the will to live.

In the case study Marie used the euphemism of sleep to convey her view of dying. It is very important to use words which the patient is able to understand. The impact of using medical terminology and/or jargon is outlined in Case study 14.3.

Case study 14.3

Pavel

Student nurse Lloyd had been told in report that the consultant had just finished his ward round and had told Pavel (a Polish national) about his diagnosis of lung cancer. Lloyd could see Pavel sitting up in bed smiling and chatting with the other men in his bay. As Lloyd approached Pavel he called over to Lloyd and said: 'Oh, I'm so relieved, I can't tell you how glad I am. The doctor has just told me I have a neoplasm; I can't wait to see my wife to give her the good news.'

Here Pavel has clearly heard the word neoplasm and has misunderstood what this word means. Many people may assume that because they do not hear the word cancer, that everything must be fine. Pavel is unaware that neoplasm is a medical word meaning new growth; however, this often refers to a cancerous tumour. In Pavel's case he has lung cancer, but has focused on the word neoplasm.

The following section examines some attitudes towards death and dying demonstrated by nurses, in particular some of the beliefs and rituals employed by nurses when someone is terminally ill or dies in hospital.

Attitudes to death and dying amongst nurses

Smith (1992) states that the emotional climate of a ward may be attributed to nurses' perceptions of whether death and dying are explicit components of the work. According to Smith's research study, nurses are able to manage their emotions by distancing themselves from the patient, particularly on wards where nurses encounter death more often. It seems that nurses become socialised into becoming hard or blasé about death, although it is not clear from Smith's study how this change comes about. The study demonstrates that nurses employ certain strategies in order to manage the death, for example nurses who know the patient well are allocated to care for the patient. The patient is also often removed from the main ward area to a side room.

> **Exercise**
> 1. Reflect on your experiences of death in hospitals.
> 2. How was the death managed with respect to the strategies which Smith (1992) outlines?

It should be acknowledged that not all nurses have the opportunity to choose regarding whether or not to care for a dying person; this is particularly true of student nurses. Smith (1992) demonstrates that qualified staff and student nurses develop a separate set of social relations with dying patients. The qualified staff are more likely to get to know dying patients and therefore invest in the deaths of patients whom they knew. The staff hierarchy also serves to separate technical from emotional nursing by assuming that at certain stages of nurse education students should be able to perform specific technical tasks surrounding death and dying.

It is generally assumed that the more experienced you are, the better you are able to cope with upsetting situations (Smith 1992). Experience shows that, in practice, feelings are rarely acknowledged amongst nurses. Therefore, staff are likely to develop distancing strategies outlined by Smith (1992) which prevent nurses from personal involvement. Nurses package care, dividing the emotional from the technical labour. The process of dying is more difficult to define than the act of death; death requires clearly identified skills and tasks, whereas the point at which patients are recognised as dying, and the skills required to care for them during their transition from life to death are less definable.

However, according to Smith (1992), nurses feel that being present at a death enables them to conclude care. For many staff, performing last offices attains closure. Therefore, it seems that, for nurses, learning about the emotional aspects of death is largely experiential.

Dealing with death and dying in the clinical setting is difficult. In a study exploring the perspective of newly qualified nurses within the UK whilst caring for dying people in hospital, Hopkinson et al (2003) outline several important themes. Firstly, the study describes how we all hold a personal view of how dying people should be cared for and that as nurses we assign value to giving time to care for our patients' needs. However, we sometimes feel that our care is compromised due to lack of time. Hopkinson et al also suggest that nurses can be placed in conflict as things are hidden from view. For example, there may be things which it is impossible for us to know (how long will the patient live?), or things which are outside our personal knowledge and experience. This may be particularly important for student nurses. Similarly nurses may also experience feelings of helplessness, guilt, uncertainty, frustration or anger, particularly when the reality of death fails to meet our personal ideal (Hopkinson et al 2003). Other areas which cause tension and conflict amongst nurses are explained by Nordgren & Olsson (2004) who describe nurses' perceptions of caring for patients dying from congestive heart failure within a cornary care unit. The study shows that informants reasoned that if patients and relatives felt safe, comfortable and cared for, this would help to increase wellbeing. According to the informants, effective symptom control is a prerequisite for a dignified death. Informants felt unsatisfied if they could not allieviate patients' suffering. Symptoms which were thought to be particularly difficult to control in patients with end stage congestive heart failure were those of breathlessness and anxiety. Indeed, Nordgren & Olsson go on to say that informants felt that they sometimes had to perform procedures that they felt were extremely painful, or that tests, treatments and investigations sometimes caused patients to suffer unnecessarily.

Holland & Hogg (2001) suggest that sometimes experiencing death and dying are part of an initiation into nursing for student nurses. They also state that after encountering death-related experiences student nurses' perceptions begin to change; and rather than worrying about how they will cope, student nurses speak of caring for and communicating with dying patients. In clinical practice, nurses are encouraged to reflect upon their experiences with a mentor or supervisor in order to make sense of what they have experienced in practice. Hopkinson et al (2003) suggest that we all hold a personal view of how dying people ought to be cared for. Importantly for nurses they go on to say that the make up of our personal ideal is not constant; rather it is an evolving entity influenced by personal and professional experiences.

> **Exercise**
> 1. Think about your own personal ideal; try to write down how you think dying people should be cared for.

As previously illustrated, brain stem death can occur within a matter of hours and thus can have a devastating effect on the family. The following section will review sudden death from a different perspective. In particular, the role of the nurse in breaking bad news is discussed.

Sudden death

Sudden or unexpected death is always traumatic for those who are left behind. Families will not have time to prepare for the death and will often be shocked, angry or in a state of disbelief. It is suggested that experiences at the time of a sudden death have a powerful effect on the whole process of grieving (Wright 1996). Wright offers some valuable advice for staff who are faced with the situation of having to tell families that there has been a sudden death. In particular Wright (1996) examines the role of the nurse in making a telephone call to relatives and suggests that this kind of telephone call will often cause acute distress to both the receiver of the call and the worker who makes the call.

Language used at the time of the call by the member of staff must be considered as it plays an important role. There should be an agreed and concise definition of words which are used to describe the condition of an acutely ill relative who arrives in an Accident and Emergency Department, words which will be clearly understood by most people. Wright (1996) suggests the examples of Critical, Serious, Fair and Good. He goes on to suggest that if the patient has already died, it may be preferable to tell the relatives at the hospital rather than over the phone because this allows relatives to actualise the information by seeing the deceased:

> 66 *A dilemma will occur if the informer is asked over the phone if the patient has died, or is uncertain about whether to disclose over the phone that the patient has died …. If the hospital is quickly accessible it is better to tell people at the hospital. If they have a long distance to travel, and believe that by rushing they can be with their loved one before death or at the time of death, then it is essential to be honest over the phone.* 99
> (Wright 1996, p. 14)

Wright (1996) goes on to offer some guidelines concerning how to conduct such a telephone call (see Box 14.3).

Case study 14.4 demonstrates the impact of sudden death when the news of the death is not delivered well.

Breaking bad news is difficult for those who have to deliver it and is often unpleasant and difficult to hear. Therefore, information given needs to be delivered in a sensitive manner whilst being correct and honest. Nurses will often play a crucial role in delivering such news; they will often accompany doctors whilst the news is delivered. Use of euphemisms for death should be avoided; words such as dead or died are unequivocal (Wright 1996). In the case study whilst the information may have been correct, the doctor did not display any sensitivity. You may have questioned whether the setting was right. Many

---

Box 14.3	Giving information over the telephone

- Clear, concise information must be given.
- Say who you are and from which hospital.
- Be clear about who you are speaking to.
- If it is not the most significant relative, where can he/she be found.
- Give the name of the ill/injured person and their condition.
- If there is doubt as to the identification, tell them you believe it is the person.
- After telling them all this, check they are clear about which hospital, how to get there, what you have said.
- Then advise them to get someone to come with them, to drive carefully or get someone else to drive for them, to inform other close relatives or friends where they are heading.
- Records of the time of the call, who responded and how are important. After a death some relatives will want to clarify details.

From Wright (1996), p. 15.

Case study 14.4

Your father has died

Catherine is a student nurse in the second year of her course; she is on a placement in a large Accident and Emergency Department. She arrives on duty and is asked to accompany a doctor while he tells a woman that her father has died whilst in the department.

Doctor: 'Has your Father been ill recently?'

Woman: 'Well, he's old, and you know what old people are like … they always like to moan about something! But of course he's suffered with high blood pressure for years; and last year he did have a small stroke.'

Doctor: 'Your Father has had another stroke today: I'm afraid there was nothing we could do … he died pretty quickly.'

At this the woman screamed at the top of her voice, over and over again. The doctor sat and watched her scream and said nothing. Catherine didn't know what to do. She didn't know whether to hold the woman, to try and talk to her, or to watch; just like the doctor. After several minutes of screaming the doctor stood up and said: 'I'm very sorry'. He then left.

Exercise

1. Reflect on previous situations where bad news has been broken to you both in your personal and professional life.
2. How was the news delivered and received?
3. Can you identify any of the elements of good practice suggested in this chapter?

Accident and Emergency Departments have specific relatives' rooms, away from the bustle of the department and with comfortable furniture, so that the room appears less clinical. Other factors to consider include establishing what the relative already knows about the health of the patient. In this case the doctor did seek clarification by asking the woman if her father had been unwell recently. He did not allow the woman time for reflection. Catherine did not know what to do because she did not know what to expect and she had not anticipated the woman's response. Breaking bad news requires great skill and practice (Holland & Hogg 2001).

Sociocultural factors

Culture plays an important part in how a person reacts to and behaves during the terminal phase of an illness. A person's culture may have a direct impact on their nursing care. For example, Neuberger (1994) explains that Jews have strict laws about not shortening a dying person's life. This may limit the use of opiate-type pain control that depresses respiratory function. Jews 'grip on to life' whereas Hindus regard their death as insignificant. Holland & Hogg (2001) suggest that for Hindus and Muslims fasting is not uncommon even during the terminal stage of a disease. Devout Muslims do not take anything into their bodies by mouth, nose, injection or suppository during daylight hours for the holy time of Ramadan (Holland & Hogg 2001). This means that providing effective pain relief may be extremely problematic. Indeed, people observing a faith in hospital may have daily religious rituals which should be maintained in order to promote wellbeing. Obstruction in executing such rituals may serve to further compound feelings of anxiety and isolation.

Hindus and Muslims bathe many times a day often before prayer and will want to continue to practise this even when very ill and will require a lot of help in order to achieve this need. However, it should be remembered that modesty is crucial to Muslims: men remain covered from waist to knee and women from head to foot. Women must be treated by women and men by men, to do otherwise renders the person 'unclean' (Holland & Hogg 2001).

Attitudes towards health and illness then will have a subsequent impact on the meaning of death and bereavement which the individual experiences. Consider the following brief case study (Case study 14.5).

Case study 14.5

Cultural needs of the dying

Rifat Begum is a 68-year-old woman in the terminal stages of cancer and is aware of her condition. Staff on the ward want to move her to a side ward later because her condition is deteriorating. Her husband Mohammed Hafiz is unhappy about this.

Exercise

1. What knowledge of Rifat's culture would help you to communicate with her and her husband concerning the move into a side ward?
2. Are there any specific cultural needs which must be met?
3. Find out how other cultures view death and dying and consider how you could ensure that other colleagues are made aware of these.

Rifat is a Muslim. It will be important to her and her family that her privacy and dignity are not compromised, e.g. that her body is not exposed unnecessarily, and that she may find it impossible to be nursed by male members of the health care team. Prayer will also be important to Rifat (Holland & Hogg 2001) and her family may read the Holy Qur'an to her (Holland & Hogg 2001). It is vital to maintain effective communication with the family and to ensure that visiting is facilitated. Nurses can enhance their care by talking to the family and the patient so as to provide individualised care (Holland & Hogg 2001).

Sociocultural factors can also extend beyond the patient themselves as families play an important role in supporting the patient; and in turn, the family may require support from the nurse. For example, participants in a study by Aldred et al (2005) revealed that heart failure had a significant negative effect on the lives of both patients and their families. As patients were increasingly less able to leave the house so partners adopted an increasingly important supportive role, both emotionally and in terms of doing household tasks and providing physical care. Because of the fatigue and breathlessness caused by the heart failure, patients stated that they spent much of their time in the house, being unable to socialise with friends, resulting in feelings of isolation and loneliness. The participants also reported that hobbies like gardening or walking had also been lost to the disease, and partners had also had their activities curtailed. Aldred et al (2005) go on to explain that roles within the partners' relationship had changed as a result of the heart failure. Female patients reported that male partners had to assume responsibility for traditionally feminine household tasks (and vice versa).

Mourning and grief

Following a death, bereavement and the expression of grief is important. How people grieve is dependent upon the society in which they live and the culture in which they spent their formative years. Mourning and grief are surrounded in ritual and some of these will now be explored. One major theory which attempts to explain the emotional stages which people go through when facing death or during bereavement is that of Kubler-Ross (1969) and she identified five stages of grief (see Box 14.4).

Box 14.4	Kubler-Ross's five stages of grief

1. Denial
2. Anger
3. Guilt
4. Depression
5. Acceptance.

The terms bereavement, grief and mourning are often used interchangeably, but Costello (1995) explains that they have distinct definitions:

- bereavement being the fact of death which may result in grief
- grief being the feelings associated with loss
- mourning being the social expression of grief.

However, individual responses to grief may vary tremendously and according to Costello (1995) are dependent on a number of factors which include the strength of the relationship, timing of the death, cause of death and the age of the dead person.

The role of ritual in mourning is expounded by Helman (1996) as a standardised and socially acceptable mode of behaviour which helps to relieve the sense of uncertainty and loss. Excessive or pathological mourning is prevented by mourning rituals which encourage emotional display of grief and providing the mourner with a defined timeframe of mourning (Helman 1996). Therefore, mourning ritual provides a socially valid way of expressing and relieving unpleasant emotions. Cowles (1996) carried out an expanded concept analysis of cultural perspectives of grief and found that although cultural differences are perceived to exist in mourning rituals, traditions and behavioural expressions of grief, in fact there are no particular differences in the individual, intrapersonal experiences of grief that can be attributed to cultural heritage or ethnicity alone. Cowles' findings indicate that the intrapersonal experience of grief is similar across cultural groups. Participants in the research study described grief consistently as being a process that occurs over time and does not follow any established linear pattern. The experience of grief is unique to every individual, and according to Cowles (1996) to assume that a client is experiencing grief in a certain manner, or to attribute that behaviour solely to ethnic or cultural heritage, precludes any attempt to understand the very individual.

SUMMARY POINTS

1. Culture plays an important role in how individuals react to death, grief and loss. The nurse should have an understanding of a variety of cultural approaches to the activity of dying.
2. Nurses should remember to assess everyone as an individual and not allow labels of Christian or Muslim or other religion to dictate how to care for someone.
3. Effective communication is the key to supporting people during the grieving process.

Environmental factors

Roper et al (1996) reported in 1991 that, in England and Wales between 1975 and 1987, most people died in hospital. However, within England, Wales and Northern Ireland, the National Survey of patient activity data for specialist palliative care services reports that for the year 2004–2005, 36% of deaths occurred in hospital; 27% occurred at home and a further 31% were reported as occurring in a palliative care unit. However, given the choice it could be argued that most people would wish to die at home. There has been a steady decline in home deaths in the Western world. People are less exposed to death and dying than in years gone by and Laungani & Young (1997) suggest that in Western society, when death occurs most of the time in hospital, it is medicalised rather than viewed as a natural event. In the United Kingdom some specialist services have been developed to enable people to remain at home for as long as possible, and to provide an alternative environment to that of a hospital for terminal care.

Huda Abu-Saad & Courtens (2001) provide a useful chapter on the history of palliative care which includes the development and philosophy of the hospice movement. They suggest that the hospice can be seen as a place for care (as in the United Kingdom) or as a philosophy of care (as in the USA). In both cases the notion of the hospice is focused on an integrated, patient-centred approach to care. A hospice provides multidisciplinary team care that aims to meet the complex and changing needs of people with life-threatening disease, and their family, and offers a wide range of care including symptom relief, rehabilitation, terminal care, outpatient support, family counselling, day care and bereavement follow-up (Huda Abu-Saad & Courtens 2001, p. 17).

Models of palliative care (see Dougan & Colquhoun 2000) that include domiciliary services where the primary health care team plays a major role are of major importance to helping people to remain at home. The general practitioner has overall responsibility for the medical care of patients and coordinates the care; the district nurses play a key role in nursing care. Nursing care in the United Kingdom is also provided by Marie Curie Cancer Nurses and Macmillan Nurses, who are specialists in cancer care and are responsible for providing symptom relief, psychosocial support, information and support in bereavement (Huda Abu-Saad & Courtens 2001, p. 15).

Different clinical settings have been demonstrated as having an impact on the levels of support offered to families. A study by Street et al (2005) conducted in Australia showed that there are key factors contributing to the level of support offered to families. In particular within palliative care settings patients were described as having a high symptom burden, often complicated by social and emotional issues. The study demonstrated that the in-patient palliative care settings provided newer facilities and involved both patients and their families in care activities and decision making. The staff were required to deal with both constant changes in the patients' condition and the need to communicate changes with families. Interestingly, as family members handed over the responsibility to staff for physical care, they became vigilant over how the care was delivered (Street et al 2005).

Exercise

If hospice facilities exist near to where you live or work you may find it useful to try and negotiate an informal visit to discuss the services it offers patients, their families and friends.

1. Following your visit reflect on whether the hospice matched up to your expectations. Where did your preconceived ideas about the hospice originate?
2. Are there any support services existing in your locality which would enable someone to remain at home throughout terminal illness?

SUMMARY POINTS

1. In the United Kingdom most people die in hospital but would rather die elsewhere.
2. Specialist services exist which may help individuals to remain at home during a terminal illness.

Politicoeconomic factors

Roper et al (1996) highlight that the economic status of a country is reflected in the causes of death and the life expectancy of the population. In the UK the National Statistics Office produces data concerning infant mortality rates and causes of death. The major cause of death for men and women is circulatory diseases. It is known that cardiovascular disease is linked to a high intake of saturated fat and low intake of dietary fibre (Rutishauser 1994), so-called Western disease, because the disease is not prevalent in developing countries. Furthermore, cardiovascular disease is environmentally determined as immigrant groups take on the incidence of their host country (Rutishauser 1994).

The death of a family member can also have economic consequences for those who are left behind. For example, in the UK on the death of a spouse the State pension falls. The Government also provides some financial assistance in the form of death grants, widows' pensions and widowed mothers' allowance. During the terminal phase of illness other monies may also be available but these may vary depending on where you live.

At the time of death and shortly after

Student nurses may worry about how they will cope with seeing for the first time someone who has died and are unsure about what to expect. Carrying out care of the deceased person (last offices) not having met before is difficult and does not allow the person to be placed in context. Therefore, if carrying out last offices is problematic, discuss concerns with a mentor or someone in practice who may be able to help with a therapeutic relationship with the person during their illness. Continuing to care for that person after they have died will seem a more natural thing to do, and will help ensure closure on the relationship.

In order to prepare for 'last offices' the following section of the chapter will examine some physical changes that occur at the time of death and offers some suggestions for carrying out care of the deceased person (see Jamieson et al 2002, Ch. 12 for further details). Nurses are sometimes unsure of the family's needs at the time of death, and again some suggestions are offered.

Physical changes at the time of death

After death circulation ceases and the internal environment of the body deteriorates rapidly, the body cools, the tissues and muscles lose their tone and rigor mortis (stiffening of the body) sets in after 2 or 3 hours (Roper et al 1996). The face will stiffen before the hands and feet. The body is at its stiffest between 12 and 48 hours after death (depending on the environmental temperature), but then wears off over the next day or two. The skin may change colour and become purplish and mottled in appearance, blood drains from the surface structures of the body. Initially after death the person should be laid flat on his back with arms placed against his sides. False teeth must be correctly positioned and the mouth closed. If the lower jaw falls, it may be supported with a pillow or small sandbag whilst rigor mortis sets in. Likewise, the eyes should be closed; eyelids can be held shut with damp cotton wool or gauze. Sometimes the body is then left for up to an hour before being washed. The body is also usually screened from view during this time.

The body is usually washed. Some relatives may wish to be involved in this procedure. In particular, Muslims will expect to wash their relatives themselves, Jewish people may also prefer the nurse not to take part if they are not Jewish themselves. Remember that sometimes when the body is turned, air is sometimes forced out of the lungs and over the larynx, resulting in a groan coming from the deceased. Tubes, catheters and infusions are usually removed unless they are required for postmortem requirements. If leakage is apparent from wounds or orifices, use packing or padding according to your local policy. Permission to remove jewellery must be sought. Many cultures will wear jewellery which is of great importance, for example Sikhs will often wear a steel bangle or Kara which should not be removed (Holland & Hogg 2001). Jewellery which remains on the body is usually secured with tape. The body should be appropriately dressed (some areas will use special shrouds, others encourage the use of nightwear) and a legible nameband is worn (some hospitals require a second nameband at the ankle). Policy may also require documentation to be placed on the chest. The body is then wrapped in a sheet. If there is a risk of infection, the body is placed in a cadaver bag, which is sealed and labelled 'Danger of infection', together with the name of the infection (Dougherty & Lister 2004).

When someone dies in hospital relatives can often feel that they have given part of the deceased person to the organization and as a result may be reluctant to state their own needs. Wright (1996) suggests that it is the role of the nurse to facilitate and encourage normal requests. Furthermore, Wright's research demonstrates that it is important for relatives to see the deceased where they died, even if this is the resuscitation or treatment room. Seeing the deceased where they died appears to allow the bereaved person to become closer to the event, which they have a strong need to feel part of. Therefore, nurses should actively encourage the bereaved to see the body, and make it a perfectly natural thing to want to do. More regrets and problems arise from not seeing the body and later, of course, the decision cannot be rectified, for example Wright (1996, p. 27) states that:

> 66 *We have to state clearly what is possible in explicit terms:*
> - *You can hold his hand if you want to.*
> - *Feel free to talk if you have things to say.*
> - *I am sure you want to say goodbye.* 99

It is important to remember that the need to hold the person is normal and should be encouraged. It is also suggested that after a death the relatives will often appear to be reluctant to leave the deceased and the hospital. After saying goodbye and being asked if there are any unanswered questions, people will need permission to leave (Wright 1996). However, relatives should be given adequate time and should not feel that they are being rushed out.

It should be acknowledged that not everyone wants or needs to view or touch the body. The need to do so will depend on the beliefs and attitudes associated with death and dying. Muslims believe that death is not the end of life but rather as the time when an individual departs from this earthly realm to be closer to God. Burial practices are also affected by culture. Roper et al (1996) points out that in some instances ritual prior to burial or cremation carries great importance. Holland & Hogg (2001) explore this concept further and explain that for some cultures, such as Chinese, death is seen as a transition whereby the person moves from one social status to another. During this time, rituals, or rites of passage, take place. The rituals help those who are dying or bereaved to know what is expected of them (Holland & Hogg 2001). The nurse should also be aware of local information regarding registering a death. You may need to provide directions to your nearest Registrar's Office,

| Box 14.5 | What to do after a death |

Registering a death

- It is important that what is written on the death certificate is explained to the next of kin, and that he/she knows how to register the death.
- Deaths must be registered within 5 days at the offices of the Registrar of Births, Marriages and Deaths for the district where the death occurred or the body was found.
- The informant must take the notice given by the doctor and also, unless forwarded by the doctor, the medical certificate of cause of death.
- The Registrar will need to know the deceased person's full name, maiden name (if applicable), sex, date and place of birth, last employment and marital status. For this reason, the deceased's birth and marriage certificates are useful to have to hand.
- The Registrar issues a certificate of registration of death (free) and death certificate (charged) and these are needed later for various purposes (e.g. claiming benefits).

Arranging the funeral

- A Funeral Director will make all the arrangements although the decisions (e.g. cremation or burial) are made by the family.
- Costs are determined by the choice of coffin and headstone (if required) the venue and form of the ceremony, the distances involved, notification, procedures and any gathering after the funeral. Relatives should request an estimate of the costs before agreeing arrangements.

From Farrell (1990).

together with times when the Registrar will be present. Therefore, it may be useful to find out these details in advance so that relatives can be provided with this information (see Box 14.5 for responsibilities of the informant and the Registrar following a death in the United Kingdom).

Exercise

1. Access different registries of births, deaths and marriages via their websites.
2. Consider the similarities and differences between different cultural practices in relation to registration of death (examples of useful websites can be found at the end of this chapter).
3. Consider how a person's religion would influence the arrangements mapped out by Farrell (1990).
4. Discuss the different practices with tutors and colleagues.

THE MODEL FOR NURSING

In this section of the chapter the model is applied to a case study and will examine the processes of assessment, planning, implementation and evaluation of the activity of dying. Reflect on the case study and consider the impact of the activity of dying on nursing practice. In addition reflect on some personal experiences throughout the section in order to consider beliefs and values in relation to the activity of dying. Engaging in the reflective exercises may also help to assimilate learning. This section will explore:

- issues associated with assessing the individual for the activity of dying
- identifying problems
- planning care in partnership
- some nursing interventions associated with Bobs' story
- evaluation: the good death.

ASSESSING THE INDIVIDUAL FOR THE ACTIVITY OF DYING

As with all the other Activities of Living outlined in this book, assessment has three phases (see Chapter 1). Knowledge about the person and his family or carers is gained through the process of assessment and the nurse aims to come to understand the person and his beliefs and values about the activity of dying. It is not possible to plan individualised nursing care without first having undertaken a careful assessment (Roper et al 1996). Roper et al (1996) remind us that assessment is not a once-only activity, assessment may take place on admission to hospital for terminal care, or be a reassessment of a patient whose condition has worsened and for whom terminal care is now required. Assessment takes place as the person's condition changes and new problems emerge, or identified problems are resolved. When assessing an individual for the activity of dying the following questions in relation to the model should be considered:

Lifespan
- How old is the person?
- Has a terminal diagnosis been made?
- Are there any previous experiences which have affected the person's view of death and dying?

Dependence/independence
- Is the person experiencing any difficulties in relation to independent living?
- What future problems are they or you concerned about?

Factors affecting the activity of dying
- What specific health problem is the individual suffering from? Remember this is not the same as the 'medical diagnosis'.

- What does the person understand about their medical diagnosis and prognosis?
- What effect is their health problem having on their emotional wellbeing?
- Are there any cultural needs to be considered prior to undertaking assessment?
- Does the individual have any spiritual or religious needs?
- Are there any environmental needs which the person may have which will affect future care?

> **Exercise**
> 1. Reflect on occasions where you have observed or participated in assessing the needs of a dying person.
> 2. Were all these areas given consideration prior to undertaking the assessment? Was each area considered with equal importance or value?
> 3. Identify how these areas could be used to inform your nursing practice next time you have to undertake such an assessment.

In some cases nurses may feel that the activity of dying is not appropriate to their clinical area and may decide to omit this Activity of Living from an individual's assessment. However, many people are frightened of dying when they come into hospital. For example, a general anaesthetic is not without risk and even if the surgery is 'minor', someone might still be scared when faced with a general anaesthetic. Similarly, some older people may view hospitals as places where people go to die. There may be any number of reasons why someone might feel worried about dying and these need to be explored, in order to help the person feel at ease. Nurses may also omit this Activity of Living from the assessment process because they feel ill-prepared to deal with any fears which the person may present.

> **Exercise**
> 1. Read Case study 14.6 – up to Visit one – and consider which of the factors (which have just been highlighted) are important in relation to Bob's story.
> 2. Write down the areas which will need to be given consideration before the nurse can undertake the initial assessment. You may find it beneficial to use Box 14.6.

Assessing biological factors
The following may have been considered. The nurse will need to be aware of Bob's underlying disease: that of HIV and subsequent development of AIDS. In Bob's case he has been aware of his diagnosis for some time and has lived with his disease for many months. However, it is only over the past 12 months that his disease has been at the terminal stage, where he has been dying from, rather

Case study 14.6

Bob's story

Bob and Kevin have been partners for 4 years and they live together in an urban area. Bob is 28; Kevin is in his early 30s. Bob contracted HIV as a result of unprotected sex. Bob has a good job in the travel industry and feels that he has everything to live for; a caring partner in Kevin, they own their home and have an active social life. Bob has a younger brother and an older sister who live near their mother some 150 miles away, Bob keeps in touch with his siblings. However, Bob's mother had not spoken to him since he declared his homosexual lifestyle to her when he was 17. Bob had lived with HIV for 6 years before developing AIDS.

Bob found that he was unable to continue working once his condition worsened. Bob is allocated a carer through Social Services. Bob has had the same carer since he was diagnosed with AIDS and Jean spends about 30 hours a week with Bob, taking him to hospital for appointments and supporting him through his low days. Bob had built up an excellent rapport with Jean. He did not like strangers to call on him at home and if his District Nurse was not on duty, Bob would instruct Jean not to let anyone else visit. Bob had been a patient on the District Nurses' caseload for about 12 months.

As time went on, Bob was feeling dreadful, he developed a chest infection and a sarcoma affected most of the right side of his face, his right arm and leg. As a result the District Nurse visits increased from weekly to daily, and by Friday of this particular week, the district nurse said that she would visit twice a day from now.

Visit one

Two nurses visited Bob on Friday evening to see if he would agree to them visiting in turns over the weekend. Bob, although embarrassed, agreed that he needed care over the weekend and would allow them to call. In particular he was coughing, especially at night. Jean was spending much longer periods with Bob, and Kevin was there as much as his own work would allow. Bob spent most of his time in bed, which had been moved downstairs into the lounge to allow Bob to watch TV and for friends to call and talk. Bob was fully aware of how ill he was, and would remind Kevin constantly about the arrangements for his funeral. Everything had been arranged some 2 years earlier, when Bob was well. Bob had not eaten for 3 days and despite Jean's best efforts to tempt him to eat, he refused. Jean felt sure that Bob must eat and was very worried that he wasn't eating. Bob was also complaining of feeling bloated and said that his bowels appeared to have stopped working.

Visit two

On Saturday morning Bob was in a great deal of pain. Jean managed to sit Bob in a chair to have a wash and Bob saw himself in the mirror. He was shocked by his own appearance and asked Jean to remove the mirror. The sarcoma was increasing rapidly especially over his face and Bob was becoming very frightened. He asked the District Nurse questions about his future and desperately wanted Kevin to hurry home from work. The nurse assessed Bob's pain and felt that his regime of analgesia needed to be reviewed by the doctor (which she arranged). Bob liked to take a very low dose of his pain killers and took them at irregular intervals which often resulted in his pain not being controlled. However, Bob felt that at least this way he remained in control.

Jean was worried that she wasn't coping very well and felt responsible for the deterioration in Bob's condition. Jean had never been involved with anyone who was so ill and likely to die.

The District Nurse helped Jean to make sense of what was happening. The nurse also advised Jean to contact Bob's family and encourage them to visit as it was likely that Bob would die within 24 hours. The nurse talked to Jean about what to expect when Bob's condition got worse and who to contact should he die; or if she felt Bob was in pain. The nurse explained that the funeral director must be advised when a person dies from HIV or AIDS as not all undertakers will accept 'infected bodies'; any family or friends who wanted to pay their last respects would need to do so before the undertakers arrived because they would seal Bob's body in a body bag and this would not be reopened. Jean was not aware of this and was visibly shaken and distressed by the information.

Visit three

The District Nurse called again on Saturday evening. Bob and Kevin were lying on the bed, drinking whisky and chatting about past times. They were both cheerful and reminiscing about their life together. Jean was more relaxed with Kevin around. Kevin helped the District Nurse to wash Bob and change the sheets because Bob had been incontinent. The District Nurse talked to Kevin about whether the family would be visiting and reiterated that they should see Bob before the undertakers arrived, while Bob was still in the house.

Visit four

The District Nurse called on Sunday morning to find Bob dead in the bed. Jean and Kevin had followed Bob's instructions to the letter. He was dressed in his Scottish national costume and wearing Kevin's favourite aftershave. Bob's brother, sister and mother had all visited before Bob died and said their goodbyes. Kevin and Jean stayed with Bob but couldn't bring themselves to call the undertakers. Kevin looked numb but needed to talk, but Jean was inconsolably racked with guilt that she could have done more, and feeling that all her effort was to no avail.

Box 14.6	Assessing the individual for the AL of dying

Lifespan: relationship to dying
- Age group of dying person and family/friends.

Dependence/independence in dying
- Status in relation to all ALs.
- Status during grieving and bereavement.

Factors influencing dying
Biological
- terminal illness/cause of death
- diagnosis of death
- effects on other ALs
- effect on physical and mental health of family/friends.

Psychological
- beliefs about death and dying
- knowledge and awareness of approaching death

- whether or not significant others know prognosis
- fears, anxieties and feelings
- effect of loss on family/friends.

Sociocultural
- social customs surrounding death and dying
- religious/cultural rights.

Environmental
- home/hospital/hospice

Politicoeconomic
- causes of death and life expectancy as indicators of socioeconomic status
- state support for the dying and the bereaved.

From Roper et al (1996), p. 410.

than living with, AIDS. According to Waugh & Grant (2006) there are several key characteristics associated with the physical factor of dying associated with AIDS (see Box 14.7).

Assessing psychological factors

It is through an effective therapeutic relationship that assessment becomes possible. The emotional factors will vary, as will the nature of the problems experienced (Roper et al 1996). In order to assess Bob psychologically the nurse will need to establish a relationship. According to Peplau (1992) the nurse–patient relationship is the central feature of nursing practice, in that the nurse and patient act together to solve the patient's problems. Other therapeutic activities include the creation of partnership, intimacy and reciprocity; manipulation of the environment to include care delivery systems, familiarity (similarities to home, or previous experiences); teaching; providing comfort; use of complementary therapies and utilising tested physical interventions (McMahon & Pearson 1998).

The relationship between patient and nurse is particularly important when providing care in the latter stages of life. Perhaps unlike other stages on the life–death continuum the nature of the nurse–patient relationship changes. According to Mok & Chiu (2004) trusting and connected relationships are dependent on the nurse's ability to be caring in both action and attitude. Mok & Chiu demonstrate that using a holistic approach with patients means not only attending to the patient's physical, psychosocial and spiritual needs but also includes the skill of being aware of the

Box 14.7	Complications of living with acquired immune deficiency syndrome (AIDS)

When AIDS develops the main complications are widespread recurrent opportunistic infections and tumours. Outstanding features include:

- Pneumonia may be present, commonly caused by *Pneumocystis carinii,* but many other microbes may be involved.
- There may be persistent nausea, diarrhoea and loss of weight due to recurrent infections of the alimentary tract by a wide variety of microbes.
- Meningitis, encephalitis and brain abscesses may be recurrent, either caused by opportunistic microbes or possibly HIV.
- There may be deterioration in neurological function characterised by forgetfulness, loss of concentration, confusion, apathy, dementia, limb weakness, ataxia and incontinence.
- Skin eruptions, often widespread, may be seen, e.g. eczema, psoriasis, cellulitis, impetigo, warts, shingles and cold sores.
- Generalised lymphadenopathy may occur, i.e. noninfective enlargement of lymph nodes.

- There may be malignant tumours: lymphomas, i.e. tumours of lymph nodes, Kaposi's sarcoma, consisting of tumours under the skin and in internal organs.

From Waugh & Grant (2006), p. 382.

patient's unvoiced needs; providing comfort without actually being asked. The patients in Mok & Chiu's study considered nurses to be reliable, available and present, and that they listened to the patients' deeper feelings. The nurses were able to intercede on behalf of patients with family members and medical staff and were able to provide care according to the patients' unique needs. Indeed the patients considered that the nurses who did this had 'gone the extra mile' and were perceived by patients as part of their family. For the dying patients in the study the relationship with the nurses gave the patients incentive to continue to live; the relationship was described as going to the refueling station and being refilled with fuel in order to keep going, enabling the patients to find peace and security (Mok & Chiu 2004).

According to Sundeen et al (1998) there are four stages to a therapeutic relationship.

Preinteraction   This begins before face-to-face interaction whereby the nurse will begin to formulate ideas about the patient. It is suggested that planning is required for the first interaction. Before the first visit the nurse will be aware that Bob is reluctant to be seen by strangers and therefore she will have to plan a careful introduction.

Orientation   The first meeting is said to influence the whole relationship. There is a need for careful introductions and explanations. During this meeting a contract can be developed which may be formal (the nursing care plan) or informal (a verbal agreement), which shapes the future of the relationship. The nurse must try to ensure that a good foundation is laid for their relationship so that she may continue to visit over the weekend and support Bob, Kevin and Jean.

Maintenance or working phase   Here the relationship develops, nurse and patient can work together towards agreed goals. The relationship allows each party to express their feelings. The nurse is able to respond to feelings during this phase.

Termination phase   Ending the relationship may be emotionally painful for both patient and nurse.

Exercise
Read Visit one in Bob's story. Here a new District Nurse is going to meet Bob for the first time. The nurse has to ensure that this first meeting results in a positive outcome so that Bob will allow her to visit over the weekend.

1. How should the nurse conduct this first interview?
2. What special considerations need to be made?

Consideration may have been given to how the nurse will start to develop the therapeutic relationship with Bob, Kevin and Jean. It will be important for the nurse to adopt an open posture and try to get to Bob's eye level, rather than standing over him. All questions should be directed to Bob, and he should be encouraged to answer for himself, rather than allowing Jean to respond on his behalf.

Buckman (1988) outlines some practical tips on talking to someone who is dying.

Getting started with assessment: talking to someone who is dying
Assessment is essentially concerned with the collection of data, but traditionally nurses find it extremely difficult to discuss and document information related to the activity of dying. Indeed, some nurses who use the model ignore this section of the model suggesting that it is inappropriate to their clinical area.

Buckman (1988, p. xiii) suggests:

> 66 *Most of us don't know what to say because nobody has told us …. Most people don't know how to help, not because of their own failings but because serious illness and the threat of death are very powerful forces. They can – and often do – tear relationships apart, separating and isolating the patient from family and friends and making everybody confused and embarrassed.* 99

Buckman (1988) provides some practical advice on how to support someone who is dying. He argues that as health care professionals we must learn how to improve our communication with individuals in difficult situations because talking about distress will ultimately help to relieve distress. According to Buckman (1988) the key to communication is effective listening.

- The setting is important, so you should ensure privacy, or try to engender an air of privacy by closing curtains around the bed.
- You need to establish if the patient wants to talk. Don't be afraid to ask the obvious question: 'Do you feel like talking?' and don't worry if the patient says 'No', but be prepared to ask again later.
- Remember to be an effective listener, don't interrupt but stop what you are saying if the patient interrupts.
- Use nodding and paraphrasing to encourage the person to talk. Reflect things back, 'Yes, I see, tell me more …'.
- Don't be afraid to say nothing. Just being with someone can be valuable in its own right.
- Remember you can be honest about how you feel in this situation: 'I find this difficult to talk about …. I'm not very good at talking about', or even, 'I don't know what to say'.
- Seek clarification to make sure you haven't misunderstood what the person is saying, but be careful not to change the subject.
- Avoid 'if I were you I'd …'. You are *not* him. Ideally you should not be giving advice at all.
- Encourage the person to look back on their life. Reminiscences serve as reassurance that life has meaning. You may both end up crying, but that's OK.
- Respond to humour. Humour serves as an important factor in our way of coping with major threats and fears, it allows us to ventilate, to get rid of intense feelings and to get things into perspective.

During the assessment process it is important to establish what the patient (and his family or carers) knows in terms of diagnosis and prognosis. Classic work undertaken by Glaser & Strauss (1965) identified four awareness contexts in terminal illness, each with its own difficulties (see Box 14.8).

It is important to establish the needs and wishes of the patient. However, this may not be as straightforward as it sounds. Hughes & Neal (2000) point out that needs and wishes are not necessarily synonymous as need may be identified by the health care professional on the basis of technical knowledge (normative need) or by the person on the basis of their subjective knowledge or experience (felt or expressed need). Furthermore it is suggested that family members will also have a view of the dying person's need which may not be easily separated from their own perceived needs. Establishing the patient's needs and wishes may be particularly problematic if the awareness context is one of closed awareness, suspicion awareness or mutual pretence.

Exercise

1. Reflect on your clinical experiences with regard to assessing the activity of dying.
2. How would each of the awareness contexts outlined in Box 14.8 impact on your assessment of someone who is dying?

Assessing the needs of dying patients: other tools which may be used during assessment

Dying patients have multiple needs and therefore it is argued that palliative care needs assessment should cover a broad range to include psychosocial, spiritual, emotional and cultural needs, in addition to physical needs. Any assessment should also include input from patients and carers (Llamas et al 2001). It should be acknowledged that a number of tools exist which may be a useful aid in assessing the needs of dying patients. Llamas et al (2001) review a number of these tools which may be used in tandem with the Activities of Living (Roper et al 1996).

Consider if any of these tools are used in clinical practice. Discuss the tools with nurses and patients who use them to develop some conclusions about their effectiveness.

Actual and potential problems: identification and planning

This section will explore the problems experienced by Bob, Kevin and Jean. At each visit the nurse will undertake an assessment to identify new problems or to ascertain if known problems have been resolved (reassessment). In order to identify and plan nursing needs and apply the model, the case study will be used to provide structure to ideas.

Actual and potential problems are assessed by the District Nurse each time she visits Bob. The Activities of Living are used as a framework to aid the assessment process. The actual problems could be things that Bob, Kevin or Jean tell the nurse, or they may be things which the nurse observes or can anticipate (potential problems). It is important to remember who has the problem. For example:

Visit one

Activity of Living: eating and drinking (see Chapter 6)
Bob has not eaten for 3 days. The problem here is that Jean is worried about Bob, not that Bob is not eating. However, if Bob had said that he was hungry, or felt sick, or had a sore mouth then Bob would be expressing a need.

Food refusal can often be a source of conflict between patients and their carers. Hughes & Neal (2000) suggest that if the seeking of food is a biological imperative, the giving of food also takes on a social imperative. They suggest that nutritional support may be justified if symptoms which diminish the quality of life, such as pressure sores, develop. Limited food intake should not necessarily be viewed as a problem to be rectified (Hughes & Neal 2000). Hughes & Neal (2000) explain that in many cases patients with terminal illness can experience comfort despite minimal, if any, food or fluid intake. They also point out that, for some, a decision not to eat may be a direct attempt to hasten death, or acceptance of the inevitability of death. Food may also have a cultural significance at the end of life (Hughes & Neal 2000). As already discussed in this chapter, many people will want to continue to observe cultural or religious rituals even during the terminal stages of an illness.

Box 14.8	**Four awareness contexts in terminal illness**

Closed awareness
- Similar to denial whereby the patient does not recognise his impending death, even though everyone else does.

Suspected/suspicion awareness
- The patients suspects what others know and tries to confirm or refute his suspicion.

Mutual pretence awareness
- All parties realise that the person is dying but everyone pretends that the other does not know.

Open awareness
- Patient, family and staff recognise and accept that the person is dying and they act on this awareness relatively openly.

From Glaser & Strauss (1965).

Nursing intervention
- to establish if not eating is a problem for Bob through careful interviewing
- to support Jean whilst Bob is not eating.

Activity of living: elimination (see Chapter 7)
Actual problem   Bob has stated that he feels bloated and that his bowels appear to have stopped working.

Nursing intervention
- for Bob to state that he does not feel bloated and uncomfortable.
- to help Bob maintain his normal pattern of bowel movements.

Friedrichsen & Erichsen (2004) investigated the lived experience of constipation in cancer patients. They demonstrate that constipation causes intense bodily and psychological suffering and patients in the study often found their symptoms difficult to describe in words. The physical discomfort also resulted in feelings of worry and desperation. Patients also described how the symptoms would consume all their mental energy; it totally engaged them, often putting them in a bad mood with everyone (Friedrichsen & Erichsen 2004). Whilst Bob does not have cancer it is important for the nurse to be able to use information like this to help Bob. The nurse transfers knowledge gained from one situation and is able to use and apply it in similar cases. Whilst diarrhoea is more common in people with HIV who are terminally ill, constipation can also be experienced and so it is vital to assess the patient carefully in an holistic manner.

Activity of Living: sleeping (see Chapter 13)
Actual problem   Bob is not sleeping well due to a cough caused by a chest infection.

Nursing intervention
- to help Bob and Jean adopt the position of most comfort which facilitates Bob's breathing.

In consultation with the general practitioner and Bob and Kevin, consideration may be given to obtaining a sputum specimen which may be sent to the laboratory for culture. Appropriate antibiotics may then be prescribed. However, Bob may decide to decline such treatment.

Visit two
Activity of Living: communication (see Chapter 4)
Actual problem 1   Bob has an altered body image which he is having difficulty accepting.

Actual problem 2   Bob is frightened about his future.

Actual problem 3   Bob has stated that he is in pain.

> **Exercise**
> 1. From what you have read in this chapter write down some suggestions as to how you would address Bob's communication needs in relation to the first two problems he has expressed.
> 2. What would Jean's needs be in relation to these areas.

Nursing interventions   Consideration may have been given to the elements suggested by Buckman (1988) earlier in the chapter; in addition the effects of fatigue and altered concentration span, as Bob may get tired very quickly and need to rest. Through careful dialogue, it may be discovered that Bob is frightened of being in pain, or that the pain will worsen and become unbearable. Of course, Bob may just be frightened of the unknown, and may ask you questions to which there is no answer. Do not be afraid to be honest, and tell the person what you are feeling; for example: 'I wish there was something I could tell you about that, so that you would be less frightened'. Remember that just being with an individual who is dying can be therapeutic in its own right. Some people may find it beneficial to speak with a priest or appropriate holy person.

Pain   Pain is something which many nurses are concerned that their patients will suffer from. Symptoms of pain irrespective of their prevalence, seem to impact on daily functioning and quality of life (Huda Abu-Saad & Courtens 2001). Bob has expressed that he is in pain, therefore the nurse must make an accurate assessment of his pain. The following section will review some principles of pain management.

Pain management   Huda Abu-Saad & Courtens (2001) suggest that the primary aim of symptom management in palliative care is to control the symptoms which are distressing to the patient, tailoring all therapy to the patient's needs. Huda Abu-Saad & Courtens (2001) also state that that treatment should be based on a logical approach, starting at the level most appropriate for the patient and progressing to the next step if the pain cannot be controlled. This system is often referred to as a pain ladder. The World Health Organization (1998) developed the three-step analgesic ladder which is summarised in Table 14.2.

Roper et al (1996) suggest that the basic principle of pain management is that sufficiently potent analgesics are given regularly so that pain is not only relieved, but prevented and if pain does occur, then the dose should be increased or the drug changed. *It should be remembered that increasing drug dosages or changing drugs is the responsibility of the doctor.* However, the doctor often relies on the nurse's assessment of the patient's pain (see Roper et al 1996 for information on tools for pain assessment and discussion of the physical and psychological aspects of pain).

According to Benner et al (1996) nurses influence medical decision making by the way in which they present information to the doctor. Experienced, expert nurses cue doctors as to what is important. Doctors also appear to

Table 14.2 Three-step analgesic ladder

Level one		Level two		Level three	
Non-opioid +/− Adjuvant	Pain increasing	Opioid for mild to moderate pain +/− Non-opioid +/− Adjuvant	Pain persisting or increasing	Opioid for moderate to severe pain +/− Non-opioid +/− Adjuvant	Freedom from cancer pain

WHO (1998) Working Party on Clinical Guidelines in Palliative Care Guidelines for Managing Cancer Pain in Adults. National Council for Hospice and Specialist Palliative Services. London.

get used to a nurse's reporting style and are able to utilise the expert nurse's judgements and are more likely to listen. Moreover, experienced nurses can read when the doctor has understood their report of the salient facts whereas inexperienced nurses can not tell if the doctor has missed the relevant points. Therefore, developing a therapeutic relationship is vital in order for the nurse to assess the patient's pain and his response to it. Fear of pain should also be considered and acknowledged; such fear can be distressing and psychologically painful in itself.

Nurses will also need to understand the action of the drugs which they administer and be able to notice any undesirable side-effects. In particular, the action and side-effects of opiates need to be considered. Huda Abu-Saad & Courtens (2001) provide a useful account of pain and symptom management across the lifespan.

Visit three

Activity of Living: personal cleansing and dressing (see Chapter 8)
Actual problem   Bob is no longer independent in washing and dressing himself and requires assistance.

Nursing intervention
- to keep Bob's skin clean and dry at all times
- to educate Kevin and Jean of the importance of keeping Bob's skin clean and dry
- to demonstrate to Bob's carers how to care for Bob's skin, and how to help Bob to get dressed.

The interventions may require greater care to prevent causing pain and anxiety, and may take longer as a result. It should also be recognised that the activity of personal cleansing and dressing in particular gives the nurse the opportunity to utilise expertise in communication in order to further develop the therapeutic relationship.

Activity of Living: elimination (see Chapter 7)
Actual problem   Bob is not able to control the flow of urine.

Nursing intervention
- to minimise the harmful effects of urine on Bob's skin by keeping the skin clean and dry
- use barrier cream in groins to prevent excoriation of the skin
- promote Bob's dignity by allowing him to do as much as he wants or is able for himself.

Visit four

During visit four the nurse must focus her attention to caring for Kevin and Jean. Providing care at home to someone who is dying places great strain on the carers. Roper et al (1996) acknowledge that in the first few days after a death, the family and/or carers will be physically and emotionally exhausted; particularly when the death has been protracted. At this time the nurse must offer practical comfort and support. The next section examines emotional support in relation to Bob's story.

Activity of Living: communication (see Chapter 4)
Actual problem   Kevin and Jean require support following Bob's death.

> ### Exercise
> 1. How would the nurse support Kevin and Jean?

Nursing intervention   Think about the practical advice that Kevin might require, for example where and when he might register Bob's death. The nurse will need to encourage Kevin and Jean to talk, and be there to listen.

PLANNING CARE

According to Webster (1998) the patient is often identified by nurses as the key person in planning care; however, in practice patients play little or no part in this activity. Truly involving the patient in nursing care planning may be a skill which requires practice. One of the mechanisms suggested by Webster (1998) is to only document 'patient-centred information'; however, in order to do this it is vital for the nurse to 'know the patient'. The concept of knowing the patient is relevant to therapeutic decision making and has two elements: the nurse's understanding of the patient and the selection of individualised interventions (Radwin 1996). Nurses appear to value treating each person as an individual and this concept appears to enable nurses to actualise a cherished value (Radwin 1996). The concept may be of particular significance to nurses working in community settings caring for terminally ill patients. Knowing about the patient and getting to know what the patient thinks about their situation helps the nurse to interpret concerns or anticipate needs (Luker et al 2000). Luker et al (2000) suggest that Community Nurses equate high-quality care with fundamental communication patterns which exist between nurses and patients, nurses and carers and/or carers and the patient. Furthermore, Luker et al (2000) go on to say that spending time in the home and ensuring continuity of care are seen as prerequisites to knowing the patient, and that nurses provided more than just physical care. By providing such care it is argued that nurses are able best to respond to individual needs (Luker et al 2000).

EVALUATING CARE: THE 'GOOD DEATH'

Roper et al (2000) suggest that like other Activities of Living, the activity of dying should be evaluated. Death should not be viewed as a failure by medical and nursing staff, indeed, a 'good death' can be achieved. It is suggested that there are 12 principles of a good death (Age Concern 1999) (see Box 14.9).

Exercise

Apply the principles of the good death to Bob's story.

1. Did he have 'a good death'?
2. Reflect on some of your other experiences. How do you feel about the notion of 'a good death'?
3. Can patients have a good death in different clinical settings?
4. Develop some strategies to ensure that patients in your care will have a good death.

Box 14.9	The good death

- To know when death is coming, and to understand what can be expected
- To be able to retain control of what happens
- To be afforded dignity and privacy
- To have control over pain relief and other symptom control
- To have choice and control over where death occurs (at home or elsewhere)
- To have access to information and expertise of whatever kind is necessary
- To have access to any spiritual or emotional support required
- To have access to hospice care in any location, not only in hospital
- To have control over who is present and who shares the end
- To be able to issue advance directives which ensure wishes are respected
- To have time to say goodbye, and control over other aspects of timing
- To be able to leave when it is time to go, and not to have life prolonged pointlessly.

From Age Concern (1999).

More recently Costello (2006) investigated hospital nurses' experiences of death and dying in two hospitals within the UK. Indeed Costello suggests that as nurses form the largest professional group to provide care for patients who are dying, it is vital that all nurses, not just those working in a palliative care environment, have an awareness of what constitutes a good death. Interestingly, Costello contends that the nurse's perceptions of the way a patient dies is influenced by the degree of disruption to ward routine and he goes on to say that good death has positive benefits for nurses, patients and relatives. In the study good deaths have a limited impact on the day-to-day activity or sentimental order of the ward, are socially constructed and are perceived by nurses to involve elements of control and implied passivity by patients. Similarly, bad death for the nurses in the study is characterised by limited control over the events leading up to and including the death event. In particular, nurses felt that a lack of preparation time to get to know the family and make an accurate assessment of patients' needs constituted a risk to the smooth running of the ward. Dying patients with unresolved physical and psychological problems, such as pain, nausea, vomiting or spiritual distress and who were unresponsive to treatment or nursing care were invariably regarded as experiencing a bad death (Costello 2006).

Roper et al (1996) suggest that the phases of the nursing process can be worked through rapidly, in an emergency, or quickly changing situation, such as cardiac arrest, or more time can be devoted to assessing and planning, as in Bob's story. However, all of the Activities of Living must be considered collectively (i.e. because of their interrelationships) although there may be some nursing goals that are specific to the AL of dying (Roper et al 1996).

SUMMARY POINTS

1. The therapeutic relationship is crucial in communicating with someone who is dying. Developing such relationships requires practice and expertise.
2. The model can be applied to the activity of dying and provides a clear framework to help the nurse through assessment, planning, implementation and evaluation.
3. The activity of dying exists alongside all the other Activities of Living as defined by Roper et al (2000).

References

Age Concern 1999 Debate of the Age Health and Care Study Group. The future of health and care of older people: the best is yet to come. Age Concern, London

Aldred H, Gott M, Gariballa S 2005 Advanced heart failure: impact on older patients and informal carers. Journal of Advanced Nursing 49(2):116–124

Benner P, Tanner C, Chesla C 1996 Expertise in nursing practice, caring, clinical judgement and ethics, 2nd edn. Springer, New York

BODY (British Organ Donation Society) 2001 (www.organet. co.uk/body/DoH.html)

Bond J, Bond S 1997 Sociology and health care. Churchill Livingstone, Edinburgh

Brysiewicz P 2002 Violent death and the South African emergency nurse. International Journal of Nursing Studies 39: 253–258

Buckman R 1988 'I don't know what to say': How to help and support someone who is dying. Macmillan, London

Carter H, MacLeod R, Brander P et al 2004 Living with a terminal illness: patients' priorities. Journal of Advanced Nursing 45(6):611–620

Costello J 1995 Helping relatives cope with the grieving process. Professional Nurse 11(2):89–92

Costello J 2001 Nursing older dying patients: findings from an ethnographic study of death and dying in elderly care wards. Journal of Advanced Nursing 35(1):59–68

Costello J 2006 Dying well: nurses' experiences of 'good and bad' deaths in hospital. Journal of Advanced Nursing 54(5): 594–601

Costello J, Trinder-Brook A 2000 Children's nurses' experiences of caring for dying children in hospital. Paediatric Nursing 12(6):28–31

Cowles KV 1996 Cultural perspectives of grief: an expanded concept analysis. Journal of Advanced Nursing 23:287–294

deAraujo MMT, daSilva MJP, Francisco MCPB 2004 Nursing the dying: essential elements in the care of terminally ill patients. International Nursing Review 51:149–158

Department of Health 1999 Saving lives: our healthier nation. HMSO, London

Dougherty L, Lister S 2004 The Royal Marsden manual of clinical nursing procedures, 6th edn. Blackwell Science, London

Dougan HAS, Colquhoun MM 2006 The patient receiving palliative care. In: Alexander MF, Fawcett JN, Runciman PJ (eds) Nursing practice: hospital and home (the adult). Churchill Livingstone, Edinburgh

Farrell M 1990 What to do after bereavement. Professional Nurse 5(10):539–542

Friedrichsen M, Erichsen E 2004 The lived experience of constipation in cancer patients in palliative hospital-based home care. International Journal of Palliative Nursing 10(7):321–325

Gill P 2000 Brain stem death – an anthropological perspective. Care of the Critically Ill 16(6):217–220

Glaser BE, Strauss AL 1965 Awareness of dying. Aldine, New York

Health Education Authority 1998 Older people in the population, Fact sheet 1. HMSO, London

Helman C 1996 Culture health and illness, 3rd edn. Butterworth-Heinemann, Oxford

Hindmarch C 2000 On the death of a child, 2nd edn. Radcliffe Medical Press, Oxford

Holland K, Hogg C 2001 Cultural awareness in nursing and health care. An introductory text. Arnold, London

Hopkinson JB, Hallett CE, Luker KA 2003 Caring for dying people in hospital. Journal of Advanced Nursing 44(5):525–533

Huda Abu-Saad H, Courtens A 2001 Developments in palliative care. In: Huda Abu-Saad H (ed) Evidence-based palliative care across the life span, Chapter 2. Blackwell Science, Oxford

Hughes N, Neal RD 2000 Adults with terminal illness: a literature review of their needs and wishes for food. Journal of Advanced Nursing 32(5):1101–1107

Human Organ Transplants Act 1989 (www.hmso.gov.uk)

Human Tissue Act 1961 (www.hmso.gov.uk)

Jamieson EM, McCall JM, Whyte LA 2002 Clinical nursing practices, 4th edn. Churchill Livingstone, Edinburgh

Johnston B, Smith LN 2006 Nurses' and patients' perceptions of expert palliative nursing care. Journal of Advanced Nursing 54(6):700–709

Kennedy CM 2003 Death and dying. In: Kindlen S (ed) Physiology for health care and nursing, 2nd edn. Churchill Livingstone, Edinburgh

King RA 2001 Psychosocial and risk behavior correlates of youth suicide attempts and suicidal ideation. Journal of the American Academy of Child and Adolescent Psychiatry 40(7):837–846

Kubler-Ross E 1969 On death and dying. Macmillan, New York

Laungani P, Young B 1997 Conclusion I: Implications for practice and policy. In: Parkes CM, Laungani P, Young B 1997 Death and bereavement across cultures, pp 218–232. Routledge, London

Limandri BJ, Boyle DW 1978 Instilling hope. American Journal of Nursing 78(1):79–80

Llamas KJ, Pickhaver AM, Piller NB 2001 Palliative care needs assessment for cancer patients in acute hospitals: a review. Progress in Palliative Care 9(4):136–142

Luker KA, Austin L, Caress A et al 2000 The importance of 'knowing the patient': community nurses' constructions of quality in providing palliative care. Journal of Advanced Nursing 31(4):775–782

McMahon R, Pearson A 1998 Nursing as a therapy, 2nd edn. Stanley Thornes, Cheltenham

Mok E, Chiu PC 2004 Nurse-patient relationships in palliative care. Journal of Advanced Nursing 48(5):475–483

Neuberger J 1994 Caring for dying people of different faiths, 2nd edn. Mosby, London

Nordgren L, Olsson H 2004 Palliative care in a coronary care unit: a qualitative study of physicians' and nurses' perceptions. Journal of Clinical Nursing 13:185–193

Office for National Statistics 2000 (www.statistics.gov.uk/ default.asp)

Peplau HE 1992 Interpersonal relations: a theoretical framework for application in nursing practice. Nursing Science Quarterly 5(1):13–18

Radwin LE 1996 'Knowing the patient': a review of research on an emergency concept. Journal of Advanced Nursing 23:1142–1146

Roper N, Logan WW, Tierney AJ 1996 The elements of nursing. A model for nursing based on a model of living, 4th edn. Churchill Livingstone. Edinburgh

Roper N, Logan WW, Tierney AJ 2000 The Roper, Logan, Tierney model of nursing. Churchill Livingstone, Edinburgh

Ross L 1994 Spiritual aspects of nursing. Journal of Advanced Nursing 19:439–447

Rutishauser S 1994 Physiology and anatomy: A basis for nursing and health care, Churchill Livingstone, Edinburgh

Smith P 1992 The emotional labour of nursing. How nurses care. Macmillan Press, London

Street AF, Love A, Blackford J 2005 Managing family centered palliative care in aged and acute settings. Nursing and Health Sciences 7:45–55

Sundeen SJ, Stuart GW, Rankin EAO et al 1998 Nurse–client interaction. Implementing the nursing process, 6th edn. Mosby, London

Waugh A, Grant A 2006 Anatomy and physiology in health and illness, 4th edn. Churchill Livingstone, Edinburgh

Webster J 1998 The effect of care planning on quality of patient care. Professional Nurse 14(2):85–87

Wilkinson R 2000 Organ donation: the debate. Nursing Standard 141(28):41–42

World Health Organization 1990 Cancer pain relief and palliative care. Report of a WHO expert committee. Technical report series No. 804. WHO, Geneva

World Health Organization 1998 Working party on clinical guidelines for managing cancer pain in adults. National Council for Hospice and Specialist Palliative Services, London

World Health Organization 2002 Brief on the consultation on child and adolescent health and development. WHO, Geneva Press release (www.who.int)

Wright B 1996 Sudden death. A research base for practice, 2nd edn. Churchill Livingstone, Edinburgh

Further reading

Henley A, Schott J 1999 Culture, religion and patient care in a multi-ethnic society. Age Concern, London

Parkes CM, Laungani P, Young B (eds) 1997 Death and bereavement across cultures. Routledge, London

Sahberg-Blom E, Ternestedt B-M, Johansson J-E 2001 Is good 'quality of life' possible at the end of life? An explorative study of the experiences of a group of cancer patients in two care cultures. Journal of Clinical Nursing 10: 550–562

Smith-Brew S, Yanai L 1996a The organ donation process through a review of the literature. Part 1. Accident and Emergency Nursing 4:5–11

Smith-Brew S, Yanai L 1996b The organ donation process through a review of the literature. Part 2. Accident and Emergency Nursing 4:95–102

Wright B 1996 Sudden death. A research base for practice, 2nd edn. Churchill Livingstone, London

Useful websites

www.argonet.co.uk/body/doh.html (British Organ Donor Society)

www.avert.org (an AIDS education and medical research UK based charity)

www.hospice-spc-council.org.uk (National Council for Hospice and Specialists Palliative Care Services)

www.who.int (World Health Organization)

www.worldaidsday.org (World AIDS Day website)

Appendices

Appendix 1

EXAMPLE OF A CARE PLAN DOCUMENTATION AUDIT TOOL

Area of Concern	Yes	Proof	No	Action
(Approach to care) Is there a ward philosophy which reflects/recognises individualised patient care? Is the philosophy displayed:				
a) for patients?				
b) for relatives/visitors?				
c) for other health carers?				
Are the nurses working on the ward familiar with the philosophy?				
Do the care plans reflect the use of a nursing model? Are named nurses easily identifiable:				
a) in the care plan?				
b) by the patient/family?				
Are the records kept securely and is confidentiality assured?				
Is there a list of signatories available?				
(Assessing) Does the care plan begin with assessment of the patient:				
a) biographically?				
b) needs/problems?				
Does the assessment contain information to reflect the individual needs of patients in an holistic way (bio-psycho-socio-cultural, spiritual & economic)? Are the problems/needs patient centred?				
Are the goals patient centred and achievable for the patient? Does the care plan demonstrate a systematic/problem solving and progressive approach to care? Does the care plan show that planning for discharge commenced during the assessment (and continuously throughout the need for care)? Is the time that it takes to admit a patient explicitly acknowledged?				
(Planning) Does the care plan accurately and clearly identify the care required by the nurse and other health care professionals? Are medical instructions explicitly documented and regularly reviewed? Does the care plan provide an accurate baseline upon which improvement or deterioration in patient progress can be measured? Can the patient(s) understand the information contained within the plan? Does the patient have easy access to his/her own care plans?				

(continued)

EXAMPLE OF A CARE PLAN DOCUMENTATION AUDIT TOOL *(continued)*

Area of Concern	Yes	Proof	No	Action
Does the nurse discuss the plan of care with the patient/family on a regular basis?				

(Planning/Implementing)

Area of Concern	Yes	Proof	No	Action
Do the records clearly demonstrate the chronology and accurate description of events throughout the patient's stay?				
Do the records accurately demonstrate that individualised care was delivered throughout the patient's episode of care?				
Are the care plans legible and easy to read?				
Is there evidence of continuous nursing input throughout the patient's episode of care?				
Are the care plans clearly signed for each entry?				
Is care delivered recorded for each shift on the progress sheet?				

(Implementing)

Area of Concern	Yes	Proof	No	Action
Are additional entries clearly signed and dated?				
Are signatures written in full?				
Are entries written in black/red ink only and no evidence of 'Tippex' being used?				
Do nurses who have not had contact with the patient make entries into the care plan?				
Does the care plan contain excessive abbreviation, meaningless phrases or offensive subjective statements?				
Does the care plan show evidence of the patient/family involvement in care planning/evaluation (i.e teaching/solving/alleviating/coping)?				

(Implementing/Evaluating)

Area of Concern	Yes	Proof	No	Action
Does the care plan show evidence of a collaborative approach to care by other health care professionals?				
Does the care plan contain evidence that care would continue after discharge and that appropriate referrals have been made?				
Are the problems identified fully evaluated in writing:				
a) per shift?				
b) upon achieving the goal?				
Do nurses make written entries as soon as care is given/completed?				
Does the nurse discuss progress/care with the patient per shift?				
Does the nurse make entries in the care plan in the presence of the patient (e.g. at the bedside)?				
Do the records reflect that the practitioner's 'duty to care' has been fulfilled at all times?				

(Developments)

Area of Concern	Yes	Proof	No	Action
Are regular ward meetings/discussions held to discuss the standard and progress of care delivery?				
Is commitment shown towards the monitoring and development of the standard of record keeping?				

Appendix 2

REFERENCE VALUES FOR THE MORE COMMON ANALYTES IN URINE

Analysis	Reference range	Units
Albumin	[See note 1]	
Calcium	1.2–3.7 (low-calcium diet)	mmol/24 h
	Up to 12 (normal diet)	
Copper	Up to 0.6	μmol/24 h
Cortisol	9–50	μmol/mol
Creatinine	10–20	mmol/24 h
Hydroxyindole-3-acetic acid (5-HIAA)	<60	μmol/24 h
Normetadrenaline	0.4–3.4	μmol/24 h
Metadrenaline	0.3–1.7	μmol/24 h
Oxalate	80–490 (M)	mmol/24 h
	40–320 (F)	mmol/24 h
Phosphate	15–50	mmol/24 h
Potassium[2]	25–100	mmol/24 h
Protein	Up to 0.3	g/l
Sodium	100–200	mmol/24 h
Urate	1.2–3.0	mmol/24 h
Urea	170–600	mmol/24 h

Notes

1. Albumin/creatinine ratio (ACR) and urinary albumin excretion rate (AER) are used to detect microalbuminuria, i.e. excessive albumin excretion in patients with diabetes mellitus, which is of predictive value in identifying patients at risk of progression to diabetic nephropathy. The test should only be carried out in the absence of overt proteinuria (Dipstix negative).

ACR

Reference range: <3.5 mg albumin/mmol creatinine

Borderline: 3.5–10 mg albumin/mmol creatinine

Sensitive test: >10 mg albumin/mmol creatinine

AER

Reference range: <20 μg albumin/min

Microalbuminuria: 20–200 μg albumin/min

2. The urinary output of electrolytes such as sodium and potassium is normally a reflection of intake. This can vary widely, especially on a cultural, worldwide basis. The values quoted are more appropriate to a 'Western' diet (Alexander M, Fawcett JN, Runciman PJ 2000 Nursing practice hospital and home. The adult, 2nd edn. Churchill Livingstone, Edinburgh, p. 1071).

Appendix 3

COMMONLY USED FORMS

| (Section 1) | Patient's nursing records | Biographical Data |

PATIENT'S NAME: **A**

WISHES TO BE KNOWN AS:

ADDRESS:

POST CODE:
TEL NO:
AGE: D.O.B:
MARITAL STATUS:
LANGUAGE(S) SPOKEN:
OCCUPATION:

PRACTISING FAITH: **B**
CONTACT No:

NEXT OF KIN: **C**
RELATIONSHIP:
ADDRESS:

CONTACT Nos:
(DAY)
(NIGHT)
(EMERGENCY)
SIGNIFICANT OTHER:

AWARE OF ADMISSION? Yes/No

G.P. NAME + ADDRESS: **D**

TEL No:

COMMUNITY NURSE:
TEL No:

SOCIAL WORKER:
TEL No:

HEALTH VISITOR:
TEL No:

MEALS ON WHEELS:

HOME CARE TEAM:

DAY CARE:

OTHER AGENCIES:

HOSPITAL: **E**
WARD:
ADMISSION STATUS:
ADMITTED FROM:

DATE: TIME:
CONSULTANT:

REASON FOR ADMISSION: **F**

PREVIOUS MEDICAL HISTORY:

CURRENT MEDICATIONS:

ALLERGIES:

TYPE OF HOUSING/ACCOMMODATION: **G**

LIVES WITH:

DEPENDENTS:

PRIMARY/NAMED NURSE: **H**

ADMITTING NURSE:

INFORMATION OBTAINED FROM:

PATIENT'S VIEWS/FEELINGS ON ADMISSION: **I**

ADMISSION DEPENDENCY SCORE: **J**
PRESSURE ULCER RISK SCORE:
MOVING & HANDLING RISK SCORE:

VALUABLES: Retained/Sent home   **K**

(Section 2)	Patient assessment	

ACTIVITIES OF LIVING	NORMAL HABITS & ROUTINES (Physical, Psychological, Sociocultural, Environmental & Economic)	ACTUAL & POTENTIAL PROBLEMS
Maintaining a safe environment		
Communicating		
Breathing		
Eating & Drinking		
Eliminating		
Personal cleansing & dressing		
Controlling body temperature		
Mobilising		
Working & playing		
Expressing sexuality		
Sleeping		
Dying		

Date: .... Time: .... Signature:.........................

(Section 3a)   **Patient care plan**

PATIENT'S NAME .... **WARD** ....

ACTIVITY CONCERNED.. **DATE ASSESSED** ....

PROBLEM
The patient

GOAL
The patient

To be achieved by ……...   ....……

NURSING INTERVENTION	

SIGNATURE ....……….

EVALUATION
The patient

DATE……….....................................…   SIGNATURE………...…

(Section 3b)   **Daily evaluation/communication/progress**   page ☐

PATIENT'S NAME ....   WARD ....

AL ....

Date/Time	Remarks	Designation & Signature

(Section 4)	Medically derived & collaborative care communication	page

PATIENT'S NAME .... WARD ....

Date/Time	Remarks	Designation & signature

(Section 5a)   Discharge planning

RECORD THE PROBLEMS IDENTIFIED & THE ACTION & REFERRAL AGENCY REQUIRED

Date ↓   FACTORS AFFECTING HEALTH RECOVERY   ACTION   Signature ↓

Physical

Psychological

Sociocultural

Environmental

Economic

(Section 5b)   **Discharge summary**

PATIENT'S NAME ....   DISCHARGE DATE ....

DISCHARGE ADDRESS ....

....

....

COMMUNITY CARE ASSESSMENT   NO ☐   YES ☐   DATE ....

INFORMATION	✓	DATE	SIGNATURE
Patient aware			
Relative/carer aware			
Mode of transport			
Social worker/services			
Community nurse			
Physiotherapy			
Other			
Specific care instructions			
Aids/prosthesis			
Follow-up appointment			
Medication & education			
Equipment to take home			
Valuables/property			
Medical certificate			
GP letter/informed			

COMMUNITY CARE OUTCOME

(Section 6)   Patient dependency/independency progress

DATE																
SCORE																
0																
1																
2																
3																
4																
5																

Moving and handling risk score

DATE	
SCORE	

Pressure ulcer risk score

DATE	
SCORE	

Dependency scoring criteria

1. Completely self caring within the environment.

2. Is vulnerable to difficulties with the AL, due to altered state or medical intervention.

   Problems are potential.

   Minimal or occasional assistance is required.

3. Is unsafe in the AL.

   Lacks the necessary ability to carry out the AL without assistance/supervision.

   Other ALs affected.

4. Acute/chronic disturbance resulting in an increasing number of actual and potential problems.

   Disturbances in most ALs.

   Requires trained nurse assistance/observation.

5. Unable to manage the AL independently.

   Needs assistance from one or more trained nurses (total nursing/medical support).

   Example states: Unconscious/semiconscious

   Very young/old

   Suicidal

Appendix 4

ASSESSMENT SCHEDULE USING THE ROPER–LOGAN–TIERNEY MODEL FOR NURSING
Possible questions to consider during the assessment stage of care planning

Activity of Living	Physical	Psychological	Sociocultural	Environmental	Politicoeconomic
Maintaining a safe environment	• Is the person able to prevent accidents or at risk from injury (day & night)? • Is the person at risk from infection, shock, haemorrhage, or unconsciousness? • Is the person aware or safe taking or receiving medications? • What are the vital sign baseline observations? e.g. pulse, blood pressure	• Does the person lack knowledge or ability to identify hazards or promote healthy living? • Does the person's mood, personality, behaviour or false perception put safety at risk? • Is the person under stress or anxious about safety/lifestyle?	• What are the person's beliefs and values concerning safety and healthy living? • Does the person require information or education regarding safety/ healthy living?	• Can the person recognise hazards within the environment hazardous to safety? • Are there any hazardous situations within the environment? • If in hospital – is the person aware of fire hazards and procedures, would they be able to leave the ward without assistance?	• Are there any lack of resources/ facilities compromising safety? • Are there any economic factors inhibiting the person's health/lifestyle?
Communicating	• Is the person able to fully communicate – speech, hearing, vision, non-verbal, read & write? • Is the person in pain – location, intensity, type, and pattern? • What is the person's current conscious level recording?	• Does the person's mood, perception, personality or behaviour affect communication? • Does the person feel anxious or threatened about being in hospital or other care setting? • Does the person lack knowledge, information or intelligence? • What are the person's experiences of pain?	• What is the person's native language? • Are there any social or cultural norms affecting communication, i.e. touch, clothing, relationships? • What are the person's beliefs about pain? • How does the person normally cope with pain episodes?	• Is the environment conducive to encourage good communications, i.e. privacy, layout, lighting etc. • Are there any factors precipitating pain?	• Can the person use or access telephones, newspapers and other media resources? • Are there any economic difficulties affecting communication?

ASSESSMENT SCHEDULE *(continued)*
Possible questions to consider during the assessment stage of care planning

Activity of Living	Physical	Psychological	Sociocultural	Environmental	Politicoeconomic
Breathing	• Does the person have difficulty in breathing and what are the causes? • Are there any abnormalities in the person's breathing pattern or habit? • Are there any activities which affect breathing? • Are there any physical risks related to breathing? • What is the person's respiratory rate?	• Are there any emotional responses which might affect breathing? • Does the person require any information or advice to aid breathing or promote healthy lifestyle?	• What are the person's beliefs related to coughing, spitting and smoking?	• Are there any factors which might alter/affect the person's breathing, i.e. O_2, temperature, ventilation position in bed, irritants, medications?	• Does the person have sufficient knowledge, information and resources to adopt a healthy lifestyle or overcome difficulties with breathing, i.e. medication, housing, emotional support?
Eating and drinking	• Does the person have difficulty in shopping and preparing a nutritious diet? • Is the person having difficulty in taking in, chewing, swallowing or digesting food or drink? If so due to what cause? • How does the person describe their diet? • What is the person's current weight?	• Does the person understand what a healthy balanced diet is? • Does the person express any views on body image? • Does the person have knowledge about food handling and hygiene? • What is the person's attitude towards eating and drinking, likes and dislikes of certain foods and drinks? • Is the person stressed or anxious about eating and drinking?	• Does the person have any cultural influences regarding eating and drinking? • Does the person have any traditional or restrictive dietary habits pre/post meals? • Could the person make any necessary adjustments to the diet if required?	• What kind of environment does the person normally take meals in? • What factors are likely to affect the person's ability to eat or drink? • Does the person have facilities at home to shop, store, cook and eat food/drink?	• Are there any factors affecting the person's choice and availability of diet, malnutrition? Safe handling? • Does the person have sufficient knowledge and assistance to provide a healthy diet?

ASSESSMENT SCHEDULE *(continued)*
Possible questions to consider during the assessment stage of care planning

Activity of Living	Physical	Psychological	Sociocultural	Environmental	Politicoeconomic
Eliminating	• Does the person have difficulty in passing urine or having bowels opened – what is the cause? • Does the person have difficulty in using or reaching toilets, bedpans or commodes etc? • Does the person have any other devices in situ which alters normal urinary or defaecatory function? • What is the person's normal habit and routine?	• Does the person have any psychological or emotional problems altering normal function? • What is the person's concept of privacy and modesty? • Is the person anxious or concerned about eliminating? • Does the person express the need for self care/privacy?	• What is the person's normal language for eliminating? • What are the person's normal pre/posteliminatory routines? • Does the person understand the need for hygiene? • Are there any cultural/religious or social traditions to be followed?	• Does the person know where the toilet and hand washing facilities are situated and how to use them? • Are the facilities within reach, safe and sufficient for the person to use? • Are the facilities conducive to privacy?	• Does the person have facilities appropriate to their needs? • Does the person have sufficient knowledge to prevent the spread of infection and to use appropriate hygiene?
Personal cleansing and dressing	• What are the person's normal habits and routines related to masculinity/femininity? • What difficulties are the person currently or likely to experience – cause? • What changes can be detected in relation to hair, mouth, teeth, hands, nails, feet, skin and overall dress and appearance? • Is the person at risk of any complications if unable to carry out this activity?	• What standards does the person normally achieve? • What knowledge does the person have – washing, bathing, dental care etc? • Does the person's anxiety, mood, perception or behaviour influence this AL? • Is the person likely to be embarrassed? • Is the person likely to be fearful, shocked or repulsed at the sight of skin trauma?	• What are the person's beliefs related to cleansing and dressing (day & night)?	• Are there sufficient facilities and resources to enable needs to be met? • Is the person worried about the facilities, privacy and dignity?	• Does the person have sufficient knowledge, finances and resources to meet their needs? • Does the person have essential items, i.e. clothing, footwear etc?

ASSESSMENT SCHEDULE *(continued)*
Possible questions to consider during the assessment stage of care planning

Activity of Living	Physical	Psychological	Sociocultural	Environmental	Politicoeconomic
Controlling body temperature	• Does the person have any difficulties with controlling body temperature, i.e. exercise, hormones, food and fluid intake or time of day? • Are there any difficulties/disorders affecting normal body temperature – cause? • What is the person's body temperature on admission?	• Does the person's personality, perception, temperament or behaviour alter body temperature? • Does the person's mood alter body temperature?	• Are there any social or cultural influences affecting appropriate wearing of clothing etc?	• Is the person able to detect or control temperature changes and make appropriate choices/actions?	• Is the person vulnerable to changes in temperature?
Mobilising	• Does the person normally manage to mobilise unaided, i.e. without a stick, chair, frame or another person? • What physical or medical factors are inhibiting mobilisation? • How are other ALs affected by mobility difficulties? • Is the problem temporary or permanent? • Are there any risks/complications which might occur as a result of limited/reduced mobility?	• How does the person feel about problems or limitations, in mobility? • Is the person normally active/adventurous? • Does the person understand the reasons for rest or exercise? • Is the person motivated towards appropriate recovery programme? • Does the person have sufficient information regarding mobility?	• How is the person likely to be affected socially as a result of temporary or permanent alteration in mobility, i.e. social – family, friends, holidays, leisure activities, shopping, domestic activities? • Are there any social or cultural restrictions upon the person's mobility?	• What is the person's moving/lifting risk factor score? • Are there any factors inhibiting the person's optimum mobility, i.e. walking and lifting aids, type of residence, visual/auditory impairment, temperature climate?	• Are there any factors affecting the person's ability to move around freely within the home environment? • Does the person have access to facilities/resources/adaptations to allow for optimum achievement of this AL?

ASSESSMENT SCHEDULE *(continued)*
Possible questions to consider during the assessment stage of care planning

Activity of Living	Physical	Psychological	Sociocultural	Environmental	Politicoeconomic
Working and playing	• What are the person's normal occupational and leisure activities and how physically demanding are they? • How does the person's current health status/ situation affect this activity?	• What are the emotional effects upon this activity caused by current health status? • Does the person have sufficient information to maintain safety and reduce harmful effects related to this activity, i.e. stress, overwork? • Does the person have sufficient intellect to receive and be motivated by appropriate information? • What are the person's reactions to hospitalisation, i.e. boredom, motivation, self-fulfilment? • What are the person's reactions to other life events, i.e. unemployment, redundancy, retirement, unpaid work?	• Has the person's social role been altered/ compromised as a result of current health status? • What moral and social obligations might be affected by a temporary or permanent change in this activity? • What support can the person expect from identified carers?	• Does the person have knowledge regarding Health and Safety at Work Act (1974) if appropriate? • Is the person aware of any environmental risks or hazards? • Can any environmental risks or hazards be identified?	• Does the person have any economic worries, i.e. safety worries, employment worries? • Does the person have sufficient information and access to statutory and voluntary advice and support?
Expressing sexuality	• What is the person's gender? • Are there any physical changes in gender structure and function affecting the person's health status? • Is the person comfortable with interaction/ communication contact – touch, opposite sex, undressing, etc? • Does the presence of disease, illness or handicap, disabilities have any effect on this activity?	• What are the person's attitudes, normal habits, and routines in relation to expressing sexuality, i.e. dress, appearance, intercourse? • Does the person have any unusual or inappropriate sexual behaviour to be considered? • Does the person have any fears, anxieties or lack of information regarding maintaining this activity?	• Does the person have any cultural or religious influences which are to be considered?	• Are there any factors inhibiting the maintenance of this activity, i.e. hospital, home, lack of information?	• Does the person have sufficient information regarding safe and healthy sexual lifestyles? • Are there any ethical, legal or economic factors influencing this activity?

ASSESSMENT SCHEDULE *(continued)*
Possible questions to consider during the assessment stage of care planning

Activity of Living	Physical	Psychological	Sociocultural	Environmental	Politicoeconomic
Sleeping	• What is the person's normal sleep, awakening routine? • What are the person's normal presleep routines? • Does the person snore, sleepwalk, fall out of bed, have nightmares? • What is the person's normal sleeping position? • Does the person take medication to aid sleep? • Are there any sleep deficits present? • What are the causes of any sleep deficits, problems?	• Does the person have any fears or anxieties which may inhibit or reduce sleep? • What are the person's attitudes, beliefs about sleep and rest, i.e. quality and quantity?	• Does the person normally share a bed or sleep alone? • What type of clothing does the person normally wear? • How many pillows, sheets, blankets does the person normally use? • Does the person's work or lifestyle influence sleep in any way, e.g. shift work?	• How might the current environment alter or inhibit the person's sleep pattern? • Is the person used to noise, light or other? • Are there any safety aspects to consider?	• Are there any difficulties which are having long term or harmful effects on sleep deprivation? • Does the person have appropriate and sufficient knowledge related to sleep, rest and healthy living?
Dying	• Are there any confirmed or diagnostic factors threatening the person's life? • What are the physical effects upon the person, family and friends? • Is the person aware of the diagnosis, stage and progress of the life threatening disorder? • Is the possibility actual or potential?	• Is the person expressing a 'desire to know', anxiety or fear of dying? • Does the person desire that significant others 'know'? • What is the person's behaviour, mood, personality? • What is the person's understanding of their own dying/death?	• What are the person's attitudes, beliefs and life experiences about death? • Does the person have any specific cultural, religious, social or personal requests? • Who needs to be contacted on behalf of the person – family, partners, friends?	• Choice of environment to facilitate a peaceful death, i.e. hospice, home, hospital? • What resources will be required to meet the needs of the person, family and carers?	• Are there any economic, legal, ethical, resource, social or domestic factors inhibiting a peaceful death? • What is the effect of the death and reduced life expectancy of the person upon others? • Are there any sufficient and appropriate support services within the hospital and the home for the dying and bereaved? • Does the person wish to donate any organs; do the family know?

Index